Oral Implant

Basics, ITI Hollow Cylinde

André Schroeder, Franz Sutter, Daniel Buser, and
Gisbert Krekeler

In collaboration with
U. Belser, J. P. Bernard, C. M. ten Bruggencate,
D. Hess, B. Maeglin, J. P. Martinet, R. Mericske-Stern,
S. Steinemann, H. Stich, E. van der Zypen

Foreword by Ray C. Williams
Translated by R. Jacobi

490 illustrations

Second, revised edition

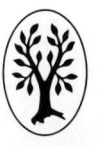

1996
Georg Thieme Verlag Stuttgart · New York
Thieme Medical Publishers, Inc. New York

Die Deutsche Bibliothek – CIP-Einheitsaufnahme

Oral implantology : basics – ITI hollow cylinder system /
André Schroeder ... In collab. with U. Belser ... Foreword by
Ray C. Williams. Transl. by R. Jacobi. – 2., rev. ed. – Stuttgart ;
New York : Thieme ; New York : Thieme Med. Publ., 1995
NE: Schroeder, André; Jacobi, R. [Übers.]

1st German edition 1988	1st Greek edition 1994
1st Italian edition 1993	1st Japanese edition 1995
1st Spanish edition 1993	1st Portugese edition 1995
2nd German edition 1994	

Important Note: Medicine is an ever-changing science. Research and clinical experience are continually broadening our knowledge, in particular our knowledge of proper treatment and drug therapy. Insofar as this book mentions any dosage or application, readers may rest assured that the authors, editors and publishers have made every effort to ensure that such references are strictly in accordance with the **state of knowledge at the time of production of the book. Nevertheless, every user is requested** to examine carefully the manufacturer's leaflets accompanying each drug to check on his own responsibility whether the dosage schedules recommended therein or the contraindications stated by the manufacturers differ from the statements made in the present book. Such examination is particularly important with drugs that are either rarely used or have been newly released on the market.

This book is an authorized and revised translation from the 2nd German edition, published and copyrighted 1994 by Georg Thieme Verlag, Stuttgart, Germany. Title of the German edition: Orale Implantologie. Allgemeine Grundlagen und ITI-Hohlzylindersystem.

Some of the product names, patents and registered designs referred to in this book are in fact registered trademarks or proprietary names even though specific reference to this fact is not always made in the text. Therefore, the appearance of a name without designation as proprietary is not to be construed as a representation by the publisher that it is in the public domain.
    This book, including all parts thereof, is legally protected by copyright. Any use, exploitation or commercialization outside the narrow limits set by copyright legislation, without the publisher's consent, is illegal and liable to prosecution. This applies in particular to photostat reproduction, copying, mimeographing or duplication of any kind, translating, preparation of microfilms, and electronic data processing and storage.

© 1996 Georg Thieme Verlag, Rüdigerstraße 14, 70469 Stuttgart, Germany
Thieme Medical Publishers Inc., 381 Park Avenue South, New York, N. Y. 10016

Typesetting by Müller, Heilbronn
Printed in Germany by Appl, Wemding

ISBN 3-13-744302-4 (GTV, Stuttgart)
ISBN 0-86577-545-1 (TMP, New York)   1 2 3 4 5 6

We would like to thank Dr. Hans Peter Weber,
Harvard School of Dental Medicine, Boston,
for his thorough and expert review of the English translation.

Addresses

Belser, U., Prof. Dr. med. dent.,
Abteilung für festsitzende Prothetik und Okklusion,
Zahnärztl. Institut der Universität Genf
19, rue Barthélemy-Menn, CH-1211 Geneva 4

Bernard, J. P., Dr. med.,
Abteilung für Oralchirurgie und Stomatologie,
Zahnärztl. Institut der Universität Genf
19, rue Barthélemy-Menn, CH-1211 Geneva 4

Buser, D., PD Dr. med. dent.,
Leiter der Station für zahnärztliche Radiologie und diagnostische Stomatologie, Klinik für Oralchirurgie, Zahnmedizinische Kliniken der Universität Bern
Freiburgstraße 7, CH-3010 Bern

Hess, D., Dr. med. dent.,
Externer Oberassistent, Abteilung für festsitzende Prothetik und Okklusion,
Zahnärztl. Institut der Universität Genf
19, rue Barthélemy-Menn, CH-1211 Geneva 4

Jacobi, R. D. D. S.
Professor, Dept. of Fixed Prosthodontics
University of Oklahoma College of Dentistry
P. O. Box 26901, Oklahoma City OK, 73190, United States

Krekeler, G., Prof. Dr. med. dent.,
Klinik für Zahn-, Mund- und Kieferkrankheiten der Universität Freiburg i. Br.
Hugstetter Straße 55, D-79106 Freiburg im Breisgau

Maeglin, B. †, Prof. Dr. med., Dr. med. dent.,
em. Vorsteher der Abteilung für Stomatologie und zahnärztliche Chirurgie,
Zahnärztliches Institut der Universität Basel
Spalenring 91, CH-4055 Basel

Martinet, J. P., Dr. med. dent.,
Calle Tristan Narvaja 1513
Apto 1307, Montevideo, Uruguay

Mericske-Stern, R., Dr. med. dent., lic. phil. hist.,
Oberassistentin der Klinik für zahnärztliche Prothetik der Universität Bern
Freiburgstraße 7, CH-3010 Bern

Schroeder, A., Prof. Dr. med. dent., Dr. h. c.,
em. Professor der Universität Bern und Direktor der Klinik für Zahnerhaltung
Brunnadernrain 3 a, CH-3006 Bern

Steinemann, S., Prof. Dr. phil.,
Institut de Physique expérimentale, Université de Lausanne
CH-1015 Lausanne-Dorigny

Stich, H., Dr. med. dent. h. c.,
Klinik für Zahnerhaltung der Universität Bern
Freiburgstraße 7, CH-3010 Bern

Sutter, F., Dr. h. c., Dr. h. c.,
Konstrukteur, Institut Straumann
CH-4437 Waldenburg

ten Bruggenkate, C. M., Dr. med., Dr. med. dent.,
St. Elisabeth Ziekenhuis
Simon Smitweg 1, NL-2353 GA Leiderdorp

Van der Zypen, E., Prof. Dr. med.,
Anatomisches Institut der Universität Bern
Bühlstraße 26, CH-3012 Bern

Foreword

I am delighted to be asked to write the foreword to this revised edition of *Oral Implantology*. Over the last eight years I have been privileged to have a warm friendship with André Schroeder and a wonderful association with the gifted people he surrounds himself with, collectively known as the International Team for Oral Implantology. I first met Andre through my colleagues H. P. Weber, Dany Buser and Klaus Lang. Shortly after these friends introduced me to Professor Schroeder, I of course was introduced to the ITI dental implant system. At that time the ITI dental implant system was just beginning to be known in the U.S. In working with Professor Schroeder and the Straumann Institute, I had the opportunity to introduce the ITI system to the department heads of the periodontal departments of U.S. dental schools. That seems like a long time ago now. In record time the ITI system has become known worldwide, and is enjoying immense success as the leader in non-submerged dental implant systems.

This book beautifully details the development and use of the ITI dental implant system. It was a fortunate day for dentistry indeed when André Schroeder of the University of Berne and Fritz Straumann of Straumann Institute began to collaborate. This innovative team subsequently introduced to the profession the unique non-submerged ITI dental implant. There have been, logically, a number of changes and improvements over time with the ITI system, but the concept of a non-submerged implant system which preserves and fosters the interaction of the soft-tissue with implant has not changed. The concept of a one-stage implant, so seemingly at odds with convention in the 1970's, is now becoming the standard for new implant designs. The profession is no longer focused primarily on osseointegration in the success of dental implants. Thanks to the ITI implant system, the profession also appreciates the importance of the soft tissue/implant interface in determining the long-term success of dental implants.

This book, full of updated and new information, will provide the reader with a rich appreciation of the field of implant dentistry in general, and the non-submerged ITI dental implant system in particular. This new addition also presents the exciting concepts of guided bone regeneration as a treatment method in implant dentistry. Guided bone regeneration offers dentistry the ability to restore the dentition in patients who until now were not candidates for dental implants. That alone is a wonderful advance in the field.

All told, given the track record of Professor Schroeder and his team over the past quarter of a century, I take this opportunity to say "kudos". I look forward to the exciting next quarter of a century in implant dentistry knowing that individuals such as André Schroeder and his team are pushing the frontiers forward in this dynamic branch of dentistry.

November 1995
Ray C. Williams, D.M.D.
Chairman, Department of Periodontics
University of North Carolina

Preface to the Second Edition

The first edition of this book in German was quickly sold out, making it apparent that we would soon have to consider a new printing. Naturally, this project required considerably more time than the authors first assumed.

This was not so much because conceptual changes regarding things such as anatomy, the material (titanium), histological findings, and the surgical procedures affected the fundamentals, but rather because there was a rapid succession of improvements in the already sound designs of rotationally symmetric implants and the superstructures that are attached to them.

These types of innovations had to be tested technically and clinically over several years before they could be included in a second edition.

In addition to the immense work of the constructor and of the manufacturer, it was, above all, PD Dr. Daniel Buser (now one of the principal authors), as well as Dr. med. dent. Regina Mericske-Stern, Lic. phil. hist., and last but not least, the Geneva group with Prof. Urs Belser and his co-workers Dr. med. Jean-Pierre Bernard, Dr. med. dent. Daniel Hess, and Dr. Jean-Paul Martinet, who brought the system to completion in an extremely impressive way, especially in regard to its aesthetic aspects.

To our deep regret, one of the authors of the first edition, Prof. Dr. med. Dr. med. dent. Benedikt Maeglin of Basel, died unexpectedly in September of 1992. Our entire team remembers him with love and respect.

Those whose names appear below are grateful to all the associate authors for their contributions to this book. We also thank all the other helpful individuals, beginning with the dental laboratory technicians, including the photography laboratory personnel, and extending to Mrs. Veronika Thalmann, who transcribed the final manuscript with her usual precision and efficiency, for their valuable and greatly appreciated work.

We owe a special debt of gratitude to the publisher, Georg Thieme Verlag and its associates, Dr. Christian Urbanowicz, Mrs. Roswitha Röhling, Mr. K. H. Fleischmann, Dr. C. Bergman, and Mrs. Allyson Famous-Thierauf, without whose cooperation this (second) edition could not have been realized.

Bern, Waldenburg, Freiburg i. Br. André Schroeder, Franz Sutter,
1994 Daniel Buser, and Gisbert Krekeler

Preface to the First Edition

Oral implantology has recently become the object of growing attention. Now that its scientific foundations have been laid, this branch of reconstructive dentistry has passed out of the phase of mere empiricism and sheer wishful thinking, and, as a result, is now taken much more seriously than was the case ten or twenty years ago. It has therefore been the authors' prime aim here to devote their attention to its theoretical basis, with reference to anatomy, materials, metallurgy, biomechanics, histology, surgical principles, periimplantal problems, and other subjects. At the same time, the authors wanted to give a comprehensive account of the ITI system and all its various aspects, such as construction, surgical techniques, indications, preparatory and followup treatment, and superconstructions, including findings since 1974.

In this translation, so-called extension implants, which seem to have receded into the background at present, have also been taken into consideration, as their inclusion renders the development of the Bonefit concept more intelligible.

The ITI (International Team for Oral Implantology) is a group which aims to promote study, experimental research, and practical and scientific exchange of experience in the field of oral implantology. The group conducts its work in close cooperation with a private venture, the Straumann Institute at Waldenburg (near Basel, Switzerland). The team consists not only of dentists, oral and maxillofacial surgeons, prosthodontists, periodontists, anatomists and histologists, but also of constructors, physicists, metallurgists, dental technicians, and other experts. The ITI organizes courses on a regular basis at which these experts have an opportunity to read papers and carry out demonstrations. In every theoretical and practical sense, it is these expert's findings and experience which are recorded in the present book. The keen reader will also find that the book may serve as a handy, extremely well illustrated manual for the ITI courses mentioned, as well as for his own practical work.

It seemed unnecessary to weigh down a book meant mainly to be used by practitioners with too many bibliographic references. A steadily increasing number of works on the subject of implantology is being published, and it would have been hard to make a satisfactory selection. The references at the end of each chapter are intended to serve merely as a guide to further reading.

The authors' special thanks go to Prof. van der Zypen for his valuable contribution on the anatomic foundations, as well as to Prof. Steinemann for his comprehensive study of titanium as a material, and to Prof. Maeglin, who took care of the chapters on the general principles of surgery and on difficulties and complications.

The authors are particularly obliged to Dr. D. Buser and Dr. H. Stich who, as coauthors, rendered outstanding services, and were a tremendous help when photographic material had to be obtained and made available. We should also like to thank the staff of the photographic laboratory at the dental clinics of Berne University, P. Wegmüller and his colleagues. The laboratory was put at the authors' constant disposal.

The first drafts of the German version were typed by Mrs. U. Keller and Mrs. H. Sutter. The fair copy of the final version, after many additions, was produced by Mrs. V. Thalmann with tireless energy and accuracy. We are most grateful to all three of them.

Dr. J. Simpson and D. J. Williams, B. Sc., translated the book into English. This was certainly no easy task, and they carried it out very conscientiously and efficiently.

Finally, the authors are greatly indebted to many other friends and colleagues who gave their assistance, and whose names are mentioned in the text. Last, but not least, we are indebted to Dr. F. Straumann, who over many years, up to his death in September 1988, always showed kindness and generosity towards ITI.

In conclusion, we should like to record our thanks to the editorial and production staff at Georg Thieme Verlag, particularly Margaret Hadler.

January 1990

A. Schroeder
F. Sutter
G. Krekeler

Table of Contents

General Basis

1 Preconditions for Long-Term Implantological Success 2
A. Schroeder

Introduction 2
The Materials Problem 3
    Mechanical Properties 3
    Biocompatibility 3

2 Anatomic Basis of Implantology 11
E. van der Zypen

Bone Structure of the Maxilla and Age-Related Changes 11
    Configuration of the Maxillary Alveolar Process 11
    Tooth Axes 12
    Structure of the Alveolar Wall 12
    Relationship of the Maxillary Teeth to Maxillary Sinus and
    Nasal Cavity 15
Bone Structure of the Mandible and Age-Related Changes 16
    Configuration of the Mandible 16
    Tooth Axes 17
    Structure of the Alveolar Wall 18
    Course of the Mandibular Canal 18
    Changes in Mandibular Form during Life 19
Remarks Concerning the Periodontal Ligament 21
Innervation of Teeth and Gingiva 24
    Innervation of Maxillary Teeth 24
    Innervation of Mandibular Teeth 26
    Innervation of the Maxillary and Mandibular Gingiva 28
Arterial Blood Supply to the Maxillary and Mandibular Teeth 29
    Arteries of the Maxillary Teeth 29
    Arteries of the Mandibular Teeth 31
Venous Drainage from Maxillary and Mandibular Teeth 33
Lymphatic Drainage from Maxillary and Mandibular Teeth and
    Gingiva 34
    Lymphatic Drainage from the Teeth 34
    Lymphatic Drainage from the Gingiva 34
Comments 34

3	**The Properties of Titanium**	37
	S. Steinemann	

Introduction	37
Material Properties	38
Corrosion – Chemical Compatibility	39
Behavior of Titanium in an Electrolyte	43
Biologic Compatibility	45
Titanium as an Implant Material	47
Plasma Coating	48
Osteointegration	51
Effectiveness	51
A Model of the Bond	55

The ITI System

4	**A Brief History of Implantology**	60
	A. Schroeder	

Introduction	60
Transfixation	60
Submucosal Implants	60
Subperiosteal Implants	60
Endosteal Implants	62
The Development of the ITI-System	63

5	**Stages in the Development of the ITI Implant**	66
	A. Schroeder and F. Sutter	

Implant Design	66

6	**Tissue Response**	80
	A. Schroeder and D. Buser with a contribution by H. Stich	

Response of Bone	80
Soft Tissue ("Gingival" Cuff)	92
Discussion of the Histological Findings and Conclusions	102
Producing of the Histologic Specimens	104
H. Stich	
Light Microscopy	104
Embedding in Acrylic	104

Final Embedding Mixture	104
Hardening of the Text Specimens (Polymerization)	105
Cutting with the Saw	105
Thin Grinding	107
Counter Staining	108
Preparation for Scanning Electron Microscopy	109
Chemicals, supplies, and apparatuses	110

Design of ITI Implants

7 The Concept of the ITI Implants 114
F. Sutter

Introduction	114
The Different ITI Implant Types	114
The Hollow Cylinder Implants (HC Type)	114
The Hollow Screw Implant (HS Type)	120
The Screw Implants (S Type)	124
Basic Design of the ITI System	129
The One-Part-Implant Design	129
The Two-Part-Implant Design	129
Characteristics of Perforated ITI Hollow Body Implants (HC, HS)	132
Characteristics of the ITI Solid Screw Implants (S)	137
Thread: Profile and Loading Characteristics	137
Overall ITI Concept as an Integrated System	140
Instruments	145
HC Implants	145
HS Implants	146
S Implants	151
Preparation of the Implant Bed	153
Biomechanics of the Implant-Bone Structural Unit	169
Implant Materials Considered in Terms of Their Design and the Technique of Implant Manufacture	174
Titanium as Implant Material	174
Surface Morphology of the Anchorage Element	175
Implant Production Technique	177
ITI Implants in Combination with Bone Grafts	178
Material and Methods	179
Design and Mechanical Testing	183
Discussion	187
Diameter-Reduced Screw Implants (ITI 3.3)	187
Special Implants, 6 mm Anchorage	192
Method of Operation	192

Reconstruction on Two-Part ITI Implants 195
    Conical Abutment System 195
    Octa System (Screw Retained Restorations) 205
    Step-by-Step Description of the Operation 207
    Base 211
    Precise Fit of the Prefabricated Gold and Plastic (Delrin) Copings
    and the Finished Restoration 212
    Outlook 218
Sterile Packaging 219

Clinic

8   **Questions Related to the Indications for ITI Implants** 226
    A. Schroeder

Contraindications 226
Age Limitations 227
Indications 227

9   **Preoperative Diagnosis and Treatment Planning** 231
    U. Belser, R. Mericske-Stern, D. Buser, J. P. Bernard,
    D. Hess, and J. P. Martinet

Initial Consultation and Ascertainment of the Patient's Desires 231
Principles of Treatment Planning 232
    Patient Evaluation 232
    Selection Criteria 232
Treatment Planning for Implant-Born Overdentures in Edentulous Jaws .. 233
    Planning Steps 233
    Number of Implants 240
    Evaluation Criteria 241
Implant-Specific Planning Principles for the Partially Edentulous Jaw ... 242
    Premolar Units 242
    Biomechanical Guidelines 244
    Connecting Implant Abutments to Natural Teeth 246
    Fixed-Detachable Implant-Borne Superstructures 246
Practical Planning Procedure 246
    Single Tooth Space in the Maxilla 247
    Shortened Mandibular Dental Arch 251
    Shortened Maxillary Dental Arch 253

10 Surgical Procedure with ITI Implants 256
D. Buser and B. Maeglin

Infrastructure and Preoperative Preparations 257
    Equipment 257
    Preparation of the Surgical Team 260
    Premedication and Disinfection 260
    Anesthesia 260
Surgical Procedure for Main Indications 261
    The Edentulous Mandible 261
The Single Tooth Gap in the Maxilla 297
Soft-Tissue Surgery for ITI Implants 310
Use of the GBR Technique with ITI Implants 318

11 Overdentures Supported by ITI Implants 330
R. Mericske-Stern

Patient Selection (Indications and Contraindications) 330
    Indications 331
Prosthetic Procedures 336
    Function of the Overdenture 336
    Design of the Overdenture with Implants 337
    Fabrication of the Implant-Borne Overdenture 337
    Insertion of the Overdenture 348
    Anchorage and Retention 349
Maintenance Care 364
    Hygiene and Peri-implant Marginal Tissues 364
    Follow-Up Care of the Prosthesis 367

12 Fixed Prosthetic Restorations 374
U. Belser, J. P. Bernard, J. P. Martinet, and D. Hess

Principles of Superstructure Design 374
Specific Indications 375
    Mandibular Distal Extension Cases 378
    Maxillary Distal Extension Cases 388
    The Edentulous Mandible 394
    Edentulous Spaces in the Posterior Region 394
    Edentulous Spaces in the Maxillary Anterior Region 399
    Single Tooth Spaces 401

13 Follow-Up-Care and Recall 420
G. Krekeler

14 Peri-implant Problems 428
G. Krekeler

Anchorage of the Implant Body 428
Thermal Trauma 428
Improper Loading 431
The Gingiva-Implant Seal 434
Microbial Plaque 434
Implant Surface 434
Marginal Infection 438
The Mucosa 441
Conclusions 441

15 Complications with ITI Implants 445
D. Buser and B. Maeglin

Intraoperative Complications 445
    Hemorrhage 445
    Intraoperative Nerve Damage 446
    Perforation of the Antrum or Nasal Cavity 446
    Damage to Adjacent Teeth 447
    Failure to Obtain Primary Stability 447
    Fracture of Implant or Instrument 447
    Foreign Bodies 449
    Emphysema in the Face and Neck Region 449
Postoperative Complications 449
    Early Complications 450
    Late Complications 452

16 Documentation and Statistics 477
A. Schroeder and G. Krekeler

Parameters of Documentation 477
Collection of Data 478
Statistics 479

17 Long-Term Results of ITI Implants 482
C. M. ten Bruggenkate

Participating Clinics 485
Discussion and Conclusions 487

18 Legal Considerations 489
A. Schroeder

Postgraduate Training.. 489
Undertaking of the Treatment 490
Establishing the Indication 490
Performance of the Therapy 491
Postoperative Follow-Up 491

19 Final Remarks 493
A. Schroeder

Index 495

General Basis

1 Preconditions for Long-Term Implantological Success

A. Schroeder

Introduction

A carefully planned full *rehabilitation of the mouth* using "state of the art" methods can free the patient of dental problems for decades. However, this can only be achieved with the complete cooperation of the patient, accompanied by regular supervision and care on the part of the dental surgeon and his assistants (e.g., the dental hygienist). If these conditions are met, we can seriously consider the treatment to have prospects of *long-term success.*

Endosteal implants should be so designed, tested and proven that they can be used routinely in such cases. Examining the situation today, this is still a very ambitious objective. Modern endosteal implantology has not been

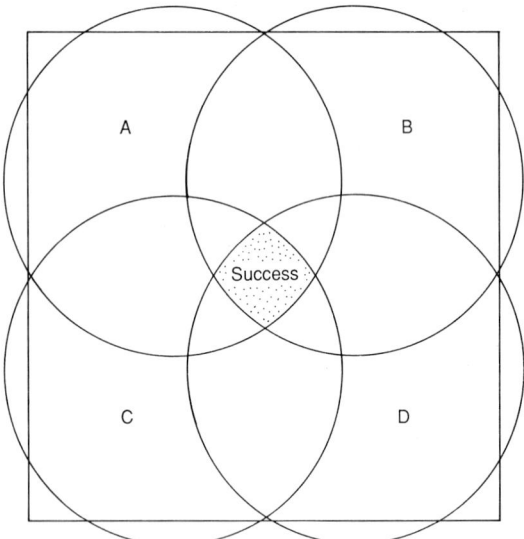

Fig. 1.1 □ = Suitable design (biomechanics), material and surface morphology.
A = Correct indication and favorable anatomic conditions (bone and mucosa), B = good operative technique, C = patient cooperation (oral hygiene), D = adequate superstructure

practiced long enough for "long-term success" to be defined on a timescale measured in decades. Nevertheless, we must not compromise our objective, since lower standards are not compatible with the painstakingly developed basic principles of modern dental medicine.

The minimum requirements and conditions that must be met to achieve long-term success as we have defined it are presented in Figure 1.**1**.

The Materials Problem

Practically all materials used clinically in dental medicine are evaluated by simultaneous consideration of two groups of parameters:
– the physical and mechanical properties;
– the biological properties.

This is most clearly the case for implant materials, wich must meet high standards, as they are subjected to high mechanical loads and are in direct contact with living tissue.

The success of an endosteal implant is totally dependent upon the material used being able to satisfy both sets of requirements fully.

Biocompatible metals or alloys and specially developed ceramic materials are the primary materials for endosteal implants.

Mechanical Properties

The mechanical properties of several implant materials are compared with those of bone by Newesely in Eichner's book on materials (1981). In his commentary he stated that "The aim of materials research is ... to develop a material with sufficiently good mechanical properties but with a stiffness which approaches that of bone. The relevant physical properties are tensile strength and Young's modulus." The values quoted in this reference indicate that certain *metals* and alloys exhibit favorable properties when judged by these criteria, whereas ceramic materials are at a disadvantage because of insufficient elongation to fracture. Figure 1.2 (Pohler) illustrates this point.

The characteristic brittle nature of ceramics can be countered in several ways, including an implant design which takes this property into account, or by restricting the use of ceramics to coatings.

Biocompatibility

Biocompatility can be defined as the compatibility of any (foreign) material with a living organism. It may be that absolute biocompatibility is plain utopia (Williams). It is also clear that there must be various degrees of biocompatibility. Defining the term more closely, biocompatible materials are those for which the interaction between the material and vital tissue is so minimal that the material is not detrimentally affected by the tissue nor the tissue by the material.

1 Preconditions for Long-Term Implantological Success

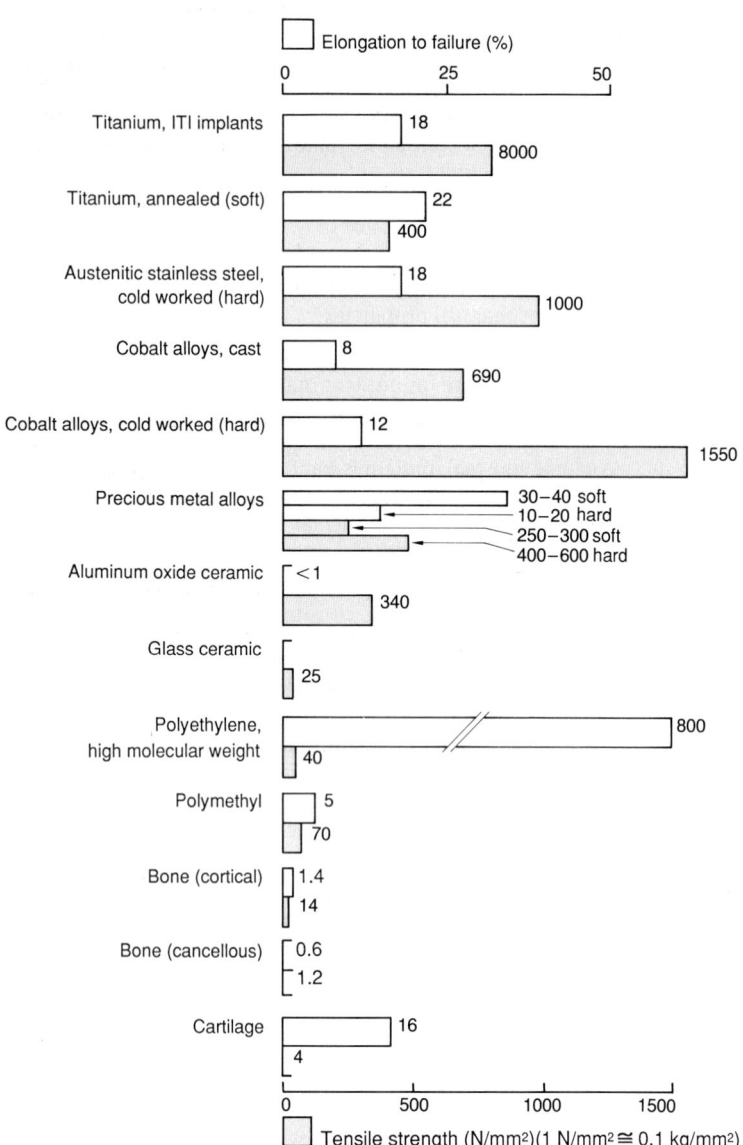

Fig. 1.2 Values for tensile strength and elongation of implant materials *(O. Pohler)*

Factors influencing biocompatibility include chemical, mechanical, electrical and surface-specific properties (Osborn, Kasemo). The biocompatibility of materials being considered for endosteal implants is evaluated primarily by the reaction of *bone* to the material, although the reaction with the mucosa at the implant neck is also significant. The reason for this is that the mainstream of work on biocompatibility of materials for use in and around bone is based on the requirements of skeletal surgery (endoprothesis and osteosynthesis development), i.e. "closed" implant systems in which the problem of mucosal penetration does not occur.

Various authors have attempted to classify materials with respect to their compatibility in bone. An example of such a classification, a simplified version based on that of Strunz, is presented in Figure 1.**3**.

Some Comments on the Material Groups

Metals, such as stainless steel, Co-Cr-Mo alloys, noble metal alloys, polymethylmethacrylate (PMMA), and other polymers are tolerated by bone to a certain extent, but cannot be said to integrate with it. Bone keeps its distance, so to speak; in this case the term "distant osteogenesis" is used to describe the

Material	Implant Tissue	Histological appearance "interface"	Type of osteogenesis
1 Stainless steel Co-Cr-Mo alloy Gold alloy, PMMA (biotolerated)		Connective tissue capsule (fibrous scar) possible osteoid or chondroid contact	Distant osteogenesis
2 Titanium, Tantalum Aluminum Oxide ceramic (bioinert)		Contact between bone and implant surface	Contact osteogenesis
3 Bioglasses Bioceramics Ca-phosphates Apatite (bioactive)		Chemical bond to bone	True bond osteogenesis
4 Titanium with rough surface e.g., flame-spray coatings (bioinert and "structure osteotropic")		Physical-chemical bond to bone	Bond osteogenesis

Fig. 1.**3** The possible histological reactions at the bone/implant interface for several implant materials [I = implant, K = bone (after *Strunz*)]

situation in which there is a more or less thick and fibrous layer of connective tissue between the implant and the bone (Fig. 1.**4**). This phenomenon is even observed when good congruity is achieved between implant and bone, and the implant is not loaded during the healing phase.

Titanium, tantalum and other metals (e.g., niobium) as well as aluminum oxide ceramics are described as being bioinert. When an optimal fit is achieved between the implant bed and the implant, new bone formation and bone remodelling occurs right up to the implant surface; this is termed "contact osteogenesis." However, a real bond between bone and implant does not normally form (Figs. 1.**5** and 1.**6**), except under circumstances that will be discussed later.

A full "bond osteogenesis," in which chemical reactions ply an important role, is characteristic of the so-called bioactive materials; these are described in the literature under the generic term "glass ceramics."

Hench and co-workers developed bioglasses in the early 1970s and histologically demonstrated direct bonding of foreign material to bone. These findings encouraged Broemer and his co-workers (cited in Strunz) to develop materials with a different chemical composition from those of Hench's group, and which are classified as ceramics because of the manufacturing process involved (Strunz).

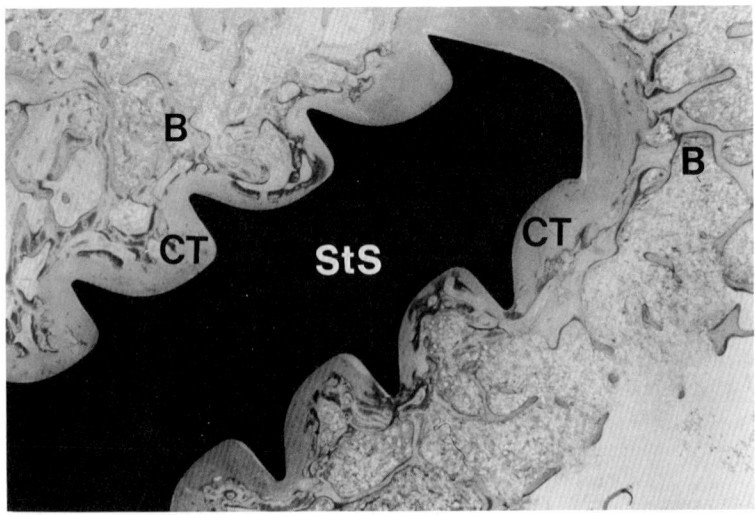

Fig. 1.**4** Stainless steel screw (AO/ASIF [Working Group on Osteosynthesis]) 3 months after implantation in a canine tibia. Typical example of distant osteogenesis (B = bone, CT = connective tissue, StS = steel screw)

The Materials Problem 7

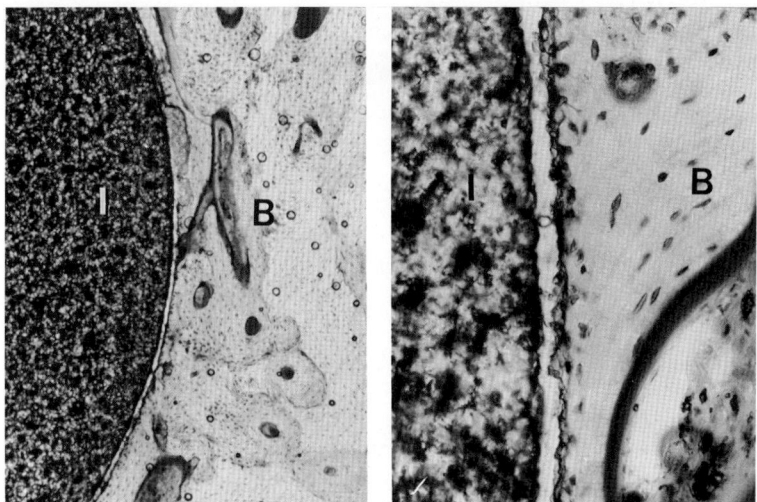

Fig. 1.**5a, b** Contact osteogenesis to an aluminum oxide implant (Sandhaus CBS implant): bone (B) has formed right up to the implant (I). Nevertheless – at least for a smooth surface – no true inseparable bond exists between the two materials (**b** at higher magnification)

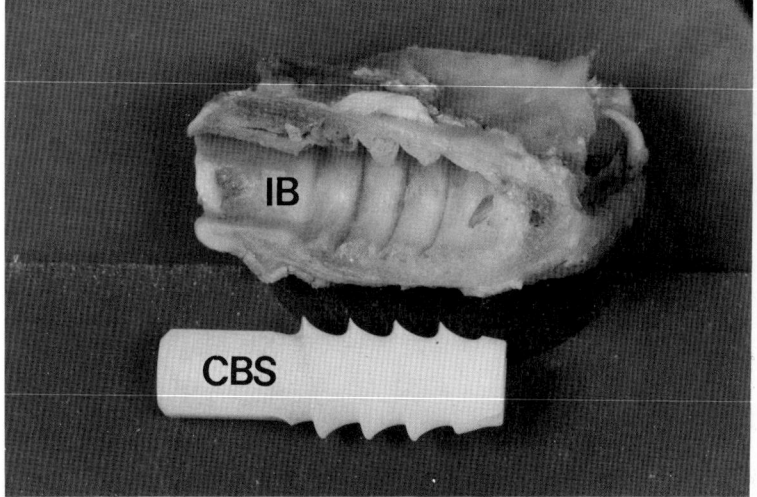

Fig. 1.**6** Al$_2$O$_3$ screw (CBS) can be screwed out of its implant bed (IB): no ankylotic bond formed (from *Sterchi*, A: Thesis, Berne 1968, published in Schweiz. Mschr. Zahnheilk. 82, 1972, 862)

8 1 Preconditions for Long-Term Implantological Success

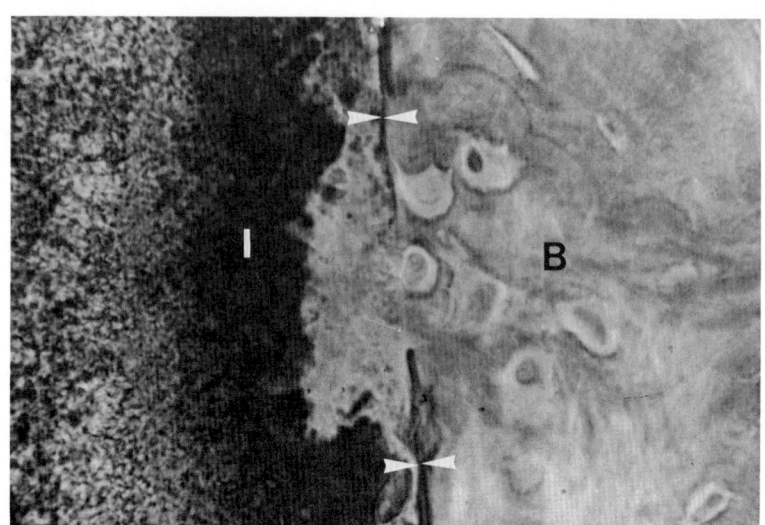

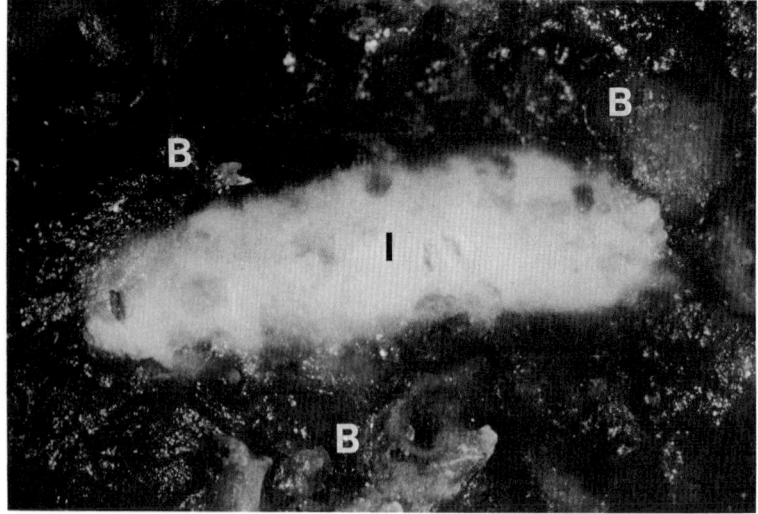

Fig. 1.7a Resorption of glass ceramic by tissue in an implant bed Arrows show original interface between implant material, I, (A2 glass ceramic, Leitz) and bone, B
b Bioceramic (A2 Leitz) implant after 6 weeks in the jaw of a monkey. The implant was originally cylindrical; a clear demonstration of macroscopic degradation

The most important constituents of this group of materials are SiO_2, $Ca_3(PO_4)_2$, CaO, MgO, Na_2O and K_2O. Other research teams are investigating bioactive materials that are made up entirely of *calcium phosphates* (Denissen, De Groot, Osborn, etc.), i.e., tri- and tetra-calcium phosphate and hydroxyapatite. The behavior and properties of this group of materials have provent to be extremely complex, and many problems remain to be solved.

These last groups of materials are similar in that they are not only tolerated as foreign materials but, in addition, bone growth originates at their surfaces, and a bond forms between implant and bone strong enough to withstand physiologic loading. The bond is formed at the molecular and crystalline level, and is thus clearly different from a simple mechanical interference anchoring.

Such bioactive materials would be of interest in oral implantology if they could provide implants with sufficient mechanical strength or be used as coatings for metallic implants.

In addition to these purely mechanical considerations, there is a further problem unique to bioactive materials: it is difficult to strike a balance between the activity of the material needed to trigger bond osteogenesis and the concurrent degradation of the material involved in the process (Fig. 1.**7**). These intimately linked phenomena are a function of the composition of the material.

Bond osteogenesis, as achieved by the use of a bioactive material, produces an implant/bone bond that cannot be separated mechanically. Failure on pullout or other mechanical tests occurs either in the implant material or in the bone but not at the (original) interface. An *"ankylotic"* bond is formed between the implant and bone.

It must, however, be pointed out that an ankylotic bond can also develop on bioinert (as opposed to bioactive) materials, but only under special circumstances. On the one hand, the implant must have a favorable micromorphologic surface structure (roughness, porosity), not only to ensure keying of bone into the implant surface, but also possibly to activate osteoinduction (see page 91); on the other hand, the implant and implant bed must be perfectly congruent.

References

Albrektsson, A., G. Zarb, P. Worthington, A. R. Eriksson: The long-term efficacy of currently used dental implants: a review and proposed criteria of success. Int. J. Oral Maxillofac Surg 1, 1986; 11–25

Brånemark P. I., G. A. Zarb, T. Albrektsson. Gewebeintegrierter Zahnersatz. Quintessenz, Berlin, 1985

Denissen, H., C. Mangano, G. Venini: Hydroxylapatite implants. Piccin Nuova, Padua, 1985

Deporter, D. A., B. Friedland, P. A. Watson et al: A clinical and radiographic assessment of a porous-surfaced, titanium alloy dental implant system in dogs. J. Dent. Res. 65 (1986), 1064–70

Deporter, D. A., P. A. Watson, R. M. Pillar et al. A histological assessment of the initial healing response adjacent to poroussurfaced titanium alloy dental implants in dogs. J. Dent. Res. 65 1986, 1071–7

Deporter, D. A., P. A. Watson, R. M. Pillar, T. P. Howley, J. Winslow. A histological evaluation of a functional endosseous poroussurfaced, titanium alloy dental implant system in the dog. J. Dent. Res. 67 (1988) 1190–5

Franke, J. Der heutige Stand der Implantologie. Hanser, Munich 1985

Hench, L. L., H. A. Paschall. Direct chemical bonding between bio-active glass-ceramic materials and bone. J. Biomed Mater. Res. 4 (1973) 25

Keller, J. C., F. A. Young, B. Hansel. Systematic effects of porous titanium dental implants. Dent. Mater. 1 (1985) 41–2

Klawitter, J. J., A. H. Weinstein, F. W. Cooke, L. J. Peterson, B. M. Pennel, R. V. McKinney. An evaluation of porous alumina ceramic dental implants. J. Dent. Res. 56 (1977) 768–76

McKinney, R. V. Jun., D. E. Steflick, D. L. Koth, B. B. Singh. The scientific basis for dental implant therapy. J. Dent. Educ. 52 (1988) 695–705

National Institutes of Health Consensus Development Conference Statement. Dental implants. J. Am. Dent. Assoc. 117 (1988) 509–13

Newesely, H. Implantatmaterialien. In: Eichner K. Zahnärztliche Werkstoffe und ihre Verarbeitung. Hüthig, Heidelberg 1981

J. F. Osborn, Implantatwerkstoff Hydroxylapatitkeramik. Quintessenz, Berlin 1985

Pohler, O. Personal communication. Waldenburg, Switzerland: Institut Straumann.

Sterchi, A. Histologische Untersuchung zweier enossaler Implantate (CBS-Schrauben nach Sandhaus) im Affenversuch. Schweiz Monatsschr. Zahnheilkunde 82 (1972) 862

Strub, J. R. Langzeitprognose von enossalen oralen Implantaten unter spezieller Berücksichtigung von periimplantären, materialkundlichen und okklusalen Gesichtspunkten. Quintessenz, Berlin: 1986

Strunz, V. Enossale Implantationsmaterialien in der Mund- und Kieferchirurgie. Hanser, Munich: 1985

Williams D. F. Biocompatibility of clinical implant materials. Vol. 1. Boca Raton, Florida: CRC Press, 1981

2 Anatomic Basis of Implantology

E. van der Zypen

Bone Structure of the Maxilla and Age-Related Changes

Configuration of the Maxillary Alveolar Process

The maxillary alveolar process provides minimal space for the roots of the teeth. For this reason, the roots of the incisors and particularly those of the canines protrude at the anterior maxillary aspect of the alveolar ridge (Fig. 2.1). These protrusions flatten out more occipitally, and are barely recognizable behind the infrazygomatic ridge.

The infrazygomatic ridge separates the anterior aspect of the maxillary body from the infratemporal fossa (Fig. 2.1). This ridge is distinctly palpable in the living state. It originates from the zygomatic process of the maxilla and approximates the region of the first molars in the buccal alveolar wall. The infrazygomatic ridge constitutes the most important supportive pillar

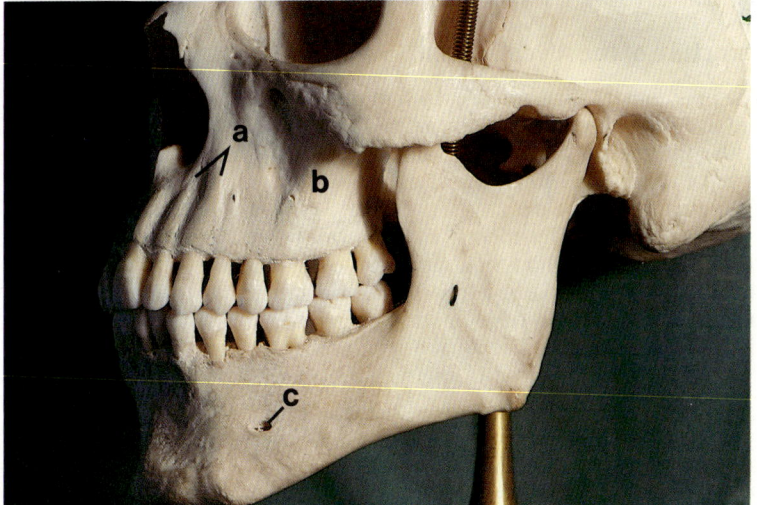

Fig. 2.1 Left side view of an adult skull.
a = alveolar process, **b** = infrazygomatic ridge, **c** = mental foramen

(zygomatic pillar) for dissipating the masticatory forces of the maxillary teeth (see below).

The alveolar process of the maxilla ends behind the last molar in the retromolar tuberculum, which delimits the pterygomaxillary fissure ventrally. It undergoes interesting changes during life, and may also vary considerably between individuals. Up to 7 years of age, the tuberculum exists only in rudimentary form (Fig. 2.**2a**); the alveolar canals into which the posterior superior alveolar nerves pass (see below) are present merely as alveolar sulci. Only after 20 years of age is the retromolar tuberculum fully differentiated; the alveolar foramina serve as the ports of entry into the alveolar canals (Fig. 2.**2b**). After 50 years of age, the retromolar tuberculum is increasingly subject to involution, and the alveolar canals are once again opened into alveolar sulci (Fig. 2.**2c**). It is thus evident that the retromolar tuberculum is an unsuitable site for insertion of an implant.

Tooth Axes

Maxillary teeth axes lie oblique to, and not aligned with, the vertical axis of the cranium (Fig. 2.**3**). Consequently, roots in the dental arch of the maxilla are more closely spaced than are the crowns of the teeth, which usually have the appearance of tilting slightly outwards. In relation to the vertical axis, the axes of incisor teeth deviate by 3°, and those of molar teeth by 1.5–2°. Accordingly, the vestibular alveolar wall is almost twice as thick as the palatal wall.

Structure of the Alveolar Wall

The interdental septae are 0.7–1.4 mm in thickness and, like other parts of the alveolar wall, consist of compact and cancellous bone. The compact bone, with a thickness of between 100 and 800 µm, is not comparable with that of the reamaining skeleton, because of its inwardly radiating cementoalveolar fiber bundles (see below).

The periodontal ligaments, which provide the resilient suspension of the teeth, load the cancellous bone adjacent to the roots in such a way that the osseous trabeculae take on a trajectional orientation. Due to the involvement of the infratemporal ridge in dissipating the masticatory pressure of maxillary teeth, this trajectional orientation of the cancellous bone trabeculae is most pronounced in the region of the first molar (Fig. 2.**4**). Ver-

---

Fig. 2.**2a** Cranium of a 5- to 6-year-old male child from the right side. A retromolar tuberculum has not yet developed. **a** = alveolar sulci.

b Cranium of an approximately 30-year-old man from the right side. Powerful development of the retromolar tuberculum. **a** = alveolar foramina.

c Cranium of a 62-year-old man from the right side. The retromolar tuberculum has largely regressed. **a** = alveolar sulci

Bone Structure of the Maxilla

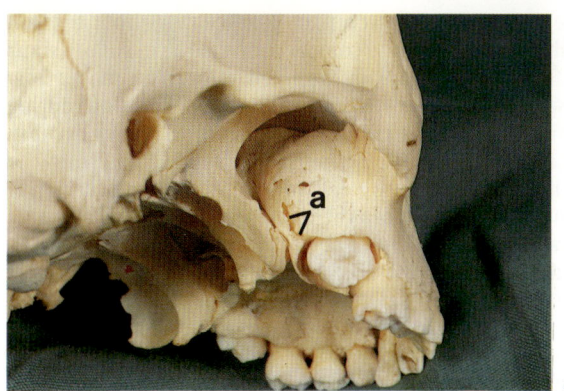

a

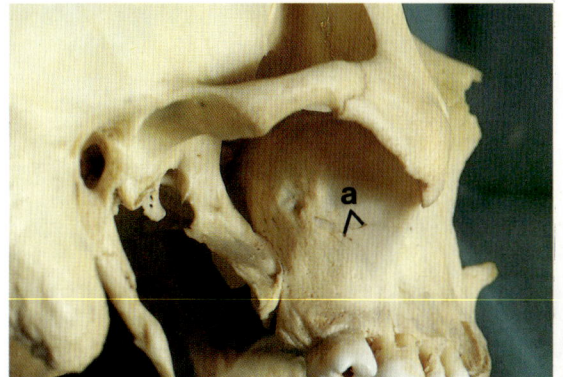

b

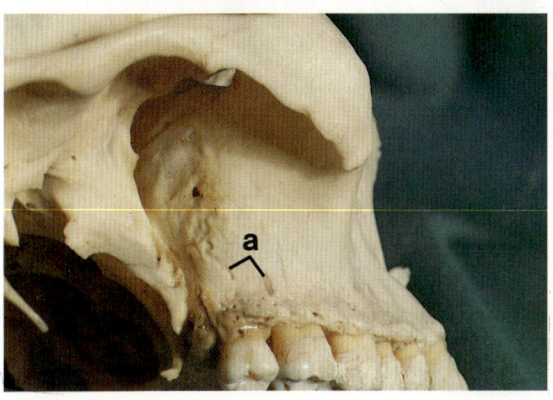

c

ticoradial trabeculae originate at the compact bone near the root tip, and diverge in fanlike fashion to insert in the compact bone of the maxillary sinus wall or nose floor. These verticoradially oriented trabeculae most likely reflect the response of the bone to a push-and-pull loading during mastication. The horizontoradially oriented bone trabeculae, which occur in the interdental and interradicular septae, must be distinguished from the verticoradial trabeculae. They are more clearly differentiated in the region of the premolars and molars than between the incisor teeth, and this probably reflects two functions. On the one hand, they counteract the traction forces exerted on the periodontium, and on the other, may be subject to differential loading produced by tilting of the teeth during chewing. Whether the theoretically conceivable rotational movement of a tooth around its longitudinal axis occurs in vivo is unclear; but if so, it would also influence the configuration of the interdental trabeculae, via traction on the cementoalveolar fibers.

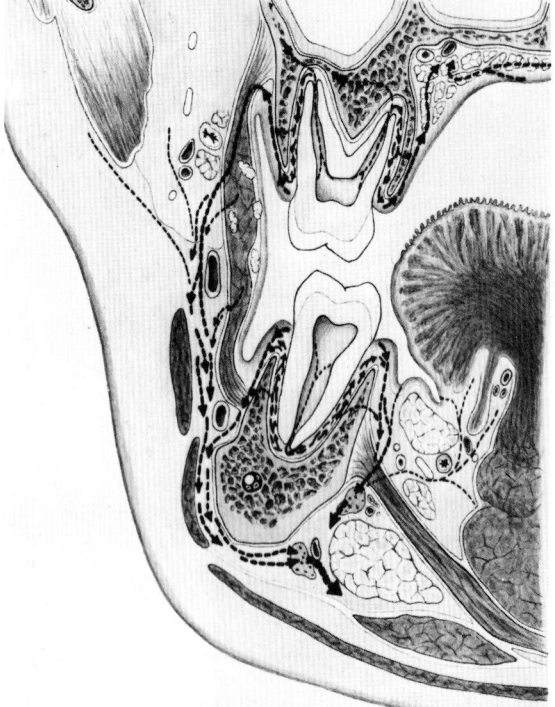

Fig. 2.**3** Tooth axes demonstrated in a frontal section at the level of the upper and lower second molars (after *Pernkopf* 1960)

Bone Structure of the Maxilla

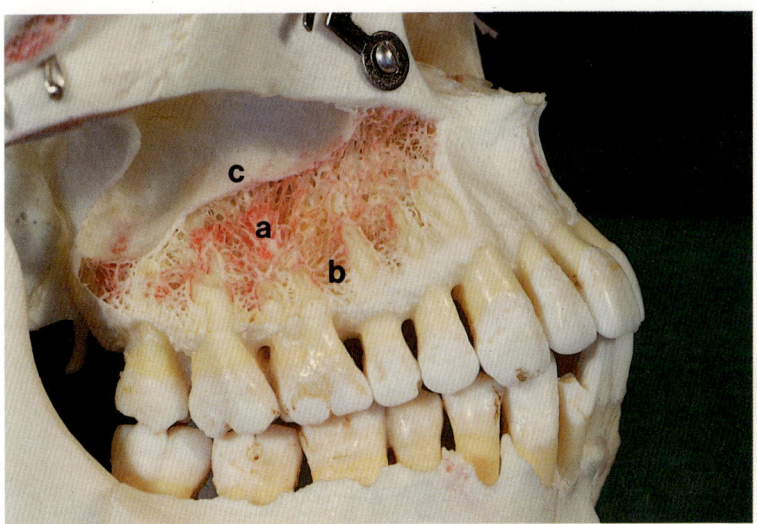

Fig. 2.4 Cancellous bone of the maxillary premolars and molars on the right side;
a = verticoradial trabeculae of the first molar (in the region of the infrazygomatic ridge),
b = horizontoradial (interdental) trabeculae,
c = compact bone of the maxillary sinus floor (partially sectioned)

Relationship of Maxillary Teeth to the Maxillary Sinus and Nasal Cavity

In the region of the incisors, the cancellous bone of the alveolar wall continues to the thin compact bone of the nasal floor. The long roots of the canine teeth often extend as far as the infraorbital foramen in the lateral nasal wall. The cancellous bone trabeculae radiating from the alveolar walls of premolars and molars borders on the thin compact bone of the maxillary sinus (Fig. 2.**4**).

In 70% of cases, the floor of the maxillary sinus lies below the level of the nasal floor, and is usually concave, having a smooth wall. The root tips of the second molar, and often also those of the first molar, are located at the smallest distance from the maxillary sinus. The alveolar wall of these two teeth can arch anteriorly over the floor of the maxillary sinus, such that the latter is more or less completely compartmentalized (Fig. 2.**5**).

After loss of teeth, not only does atrophy of the alveolar wall occur, but the sinus floor also sinks downwards, such that several years after tooth loss, only a thin bony lamella separates the floor of the empty alveolus from the maxillary sinus.

16 2 Anatomic Basis of Implantology

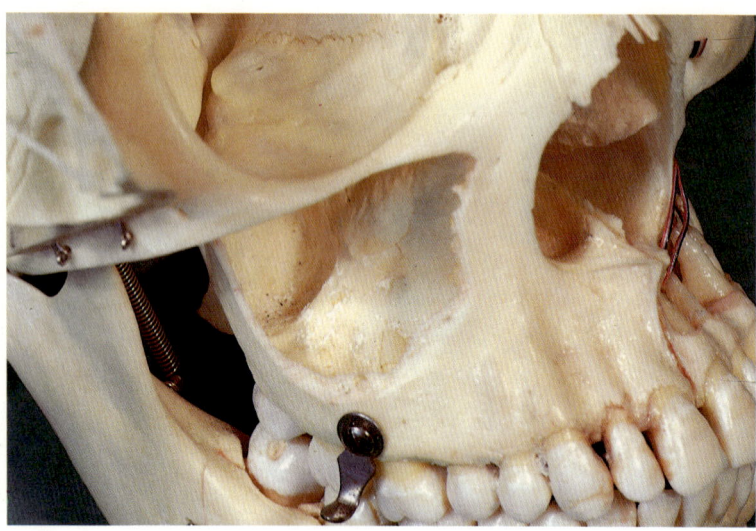

Fig. 2.5 Right maxillary sinus, opened. Septation of the maxillary sinus is incomplete owing to the presence of the roots of the second and third molars

Bone Structure of the Mandible and Age-Related Changes

Configuration of the Mandible

In the current context, only the body of the mandible is of interest, this consisting of a basal part on which the alveolar portion rests. The anatomic positioning of the prominences, lines and fossae will not be dealt with in more detail, since they are of only slight importance in this connection. Only the jugum mentale is of significance, and it should not be confused with the mental tubercle of the mental protuberance. Until 3 years of age, the jugum mentale is palpable in the region of the canine teeth, this being attributable to the root and definitive tooth anlage. It is thus situated in front of the mental foramen, which may be found dorsocaudal to the readily palpable jugum, at the level of the second premolars.

The retromolar trigonum, which is formed where the mandible body transforms into the ramus, corresponds to the retromolar tuberculum of the maxilla (Fig. 2.6). The trigonum is delimited lingually by the temporal crista, and buccally by the oblique line. In adolescents, it may be considered under certain circumstances as a site for inserting an implant, since the mandibular

Bone Structure of the Mandible

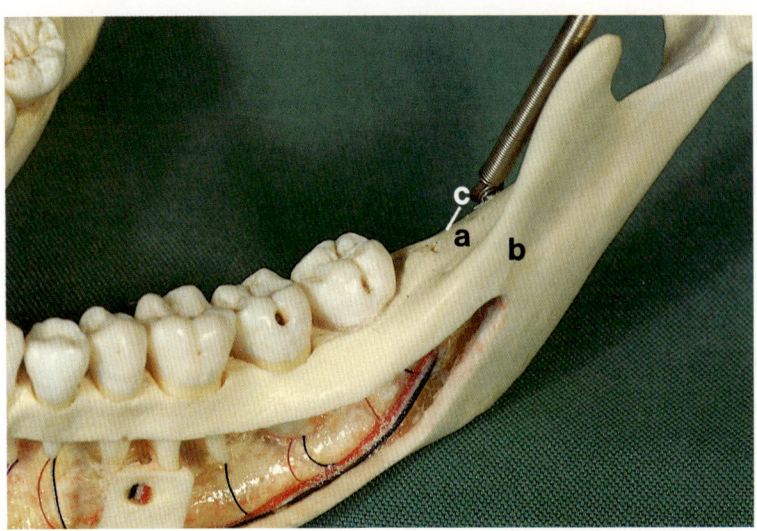

Fig. 2.**6** Mandible viewed from the left side with the mandibular canal opened; **a** = retromolar fossa, **b** = oblique lines, **c** = temporal crista

canal runs about 8 mm mediocaudally to the floor of the retromolar trigonum, with a normal mandibular angle of 120°.

The distance between the two retromolar trigona (trigonal distance) is 60–65 mm, which is somewhat greater than that between the maxillary retromolar tubercula (tubercular distance), which averages 50 mm. The maxillary arch is thus narrower than the mandibular arch. On the other hand, if the distance between the distobuccal protuberances of the second lower molars (molar distance) is compared with that between the midcrown surfaces of each mandibular molar, the dental arches are both about 55 mm across (Fig. 2.**3**). Owing to the oblique position of the teeth (see next section) and the different points of contact between them, the differences between bone arches are compensated for. If the retromolar trigonum is used as a site for implantation, these anatomical factors must be taken into consideration.

Tooth Axes

The axes of the mandibular teeth are inclined inwards relative to the vertical axis of the cranium, such that their crowns on opposite sides of the jaw lie closer together than the roots (Fig. 2.**3**). With regard to the alveolar wall, this means that the cortical bone is thicker lingually than buccally. However,

2 Anatomic Basis of Implantology

taken as a whole, the alveolar walls of the adult mandible are more completely differentiated, both lingually and buccally, than the corresponding structures of the maxilla.

Structure of the Alveolar Wall

The orientational relationships existing between cancellous bone trabeculae of the alveolar wall are principally the same as occur in the maxilla, except that the verticoradial pattern around individual teeth is more constant (Fig. 2.**7**). This may be explained by the absence of a buttress, which is developed in the infratemporal ridge of the maxilla to dissipate masticatory forces.

Course of the Mandibular Canal

The mandibular canal begins at the mandibular foramen, which is centrally located between the anterior and posterior margins of the mandibular ramus, about 1 cm above and 2 cm behind the crown of the third molar. The mandibular canal passes obliquely downwards through the cancellous bone of the mandibular ramus and reaches the mandibular body, lying equidistant between he lingual and buccal compact bone (Fig. 2.**8**). The distance of the horizontal part from the floor of the dental alveoli is 3–4 mm in the region of

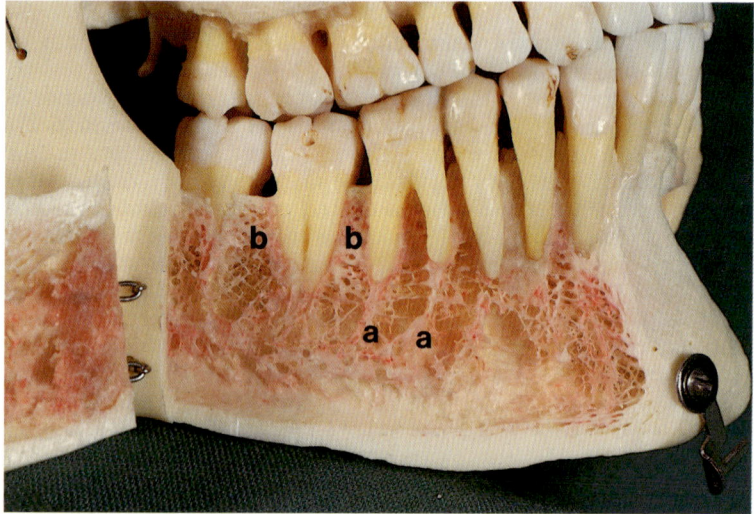

Fig. 2.7 Cancellous bone of the premolars and molars in the mandible, viewed from the rigth side; **a** = verticoradial trabeculae, **b** = horizontoradial trabeculae

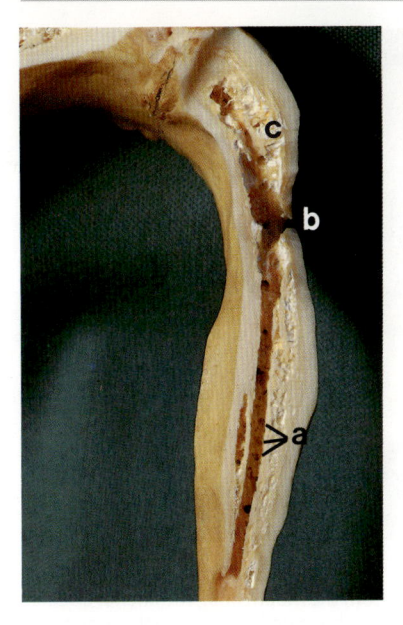

Fig. 2.8 Mandibular canal of the right half of the mandible opened caudally;
a = alveolar canaliculi,
b = mental foramen,
c = incisive (anterior inferior alveolar) canal

the third molar, and about 8 mm in the region of the first molar. At regular intervals, alveolar canaliculi of the mandible pass perpendicularly from the canal into the dental alveoli (Fig. 2.**8**). Between the first and second premolars, the canal deviates sharply towards the buccal side (mental canal), and opens to the outside as the mental foramen. Close to this opening, a small, curved canal located in the center of the cancellous bone deviates in the frontocaudal plane. This is the incisive canal (Fig. 2.**8**), within which nerves and vessels for the canine and incisor teeth course.

Changes in Mandibular Form during Life

In the neonate, the alveolar part of the mandibular body is twice as high as the basal part. However, from this time up to adolescence, the basal part increases in height by a factor of 4, and the alveolar part by a factor of approximately 2 only. After loss of teeth, it is principally the alveolar part that atrophies, although severe degenerative processes also occur in the basal part during aging; these involve the lingual aspect to a greater extent than the buccal or vestibular ones.

The pressure caused by a poorly fitting prosthesis may contribute to, or even trigger, the disappearance of compact bone on the lingual aspect of the mandible. For example, in the case of a 65-year-old wearer of a full pros-

20 2 Anatomic Basis of Implantology

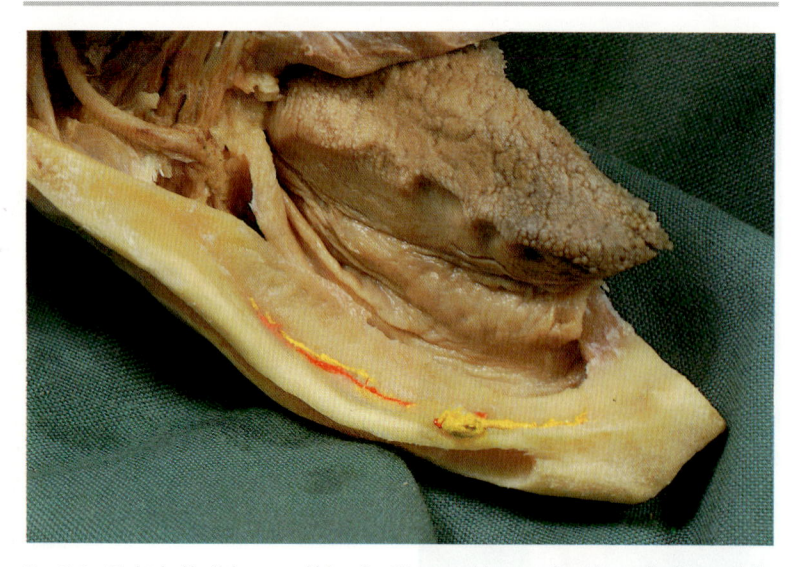

Fig. 2.**9** Right half of the mandible of a 65-year-old man tilted buccally. View of the lingual surface. After removal of the mucosa from the mouth floor, the inferior alveolar nerve and artery are exposed, owing to atrophic bone degeneration with consequent opening of the mandibular canal medially

thesis, the mandibular canal was found to be open lingually over a long stretch, such that the inferior alveolar nerve with its accompanying vessels coursed immediately subjacent to the lingual mucosa (Fig. 2.**9**).

In a different case involving a 62-year-old man, the incisor (anterior inferior alveolar) nerve was situated immediately below the mucosa of the mouth floor (Fig. 2.**10**). The topographic positions shown for this sensory nerve suggests that considerable prosthetic pain must have been suffered by both patients; indeed, this was confirmed by the medical history of the first case.

The atrophy of the mandibular alveolar process, which sets in with age or on loss of teeth, leads to an alteration of the mandibular angle. In neonates, this is 150°, and in adults, 120°. In old age, the mandibular angle once again approaches that of childhood, and may, indeed, increase to over 160°. This alteration of the angle, which accompanies atrophy, also affects the retromolar trigonum, which becomes depressed in bone, and thus comes into close topographic proximity with the oblique part of the mandibular canal. Hence, the retromolar trigonum can no longer be used as a site for implantation in age-atrophied bone.

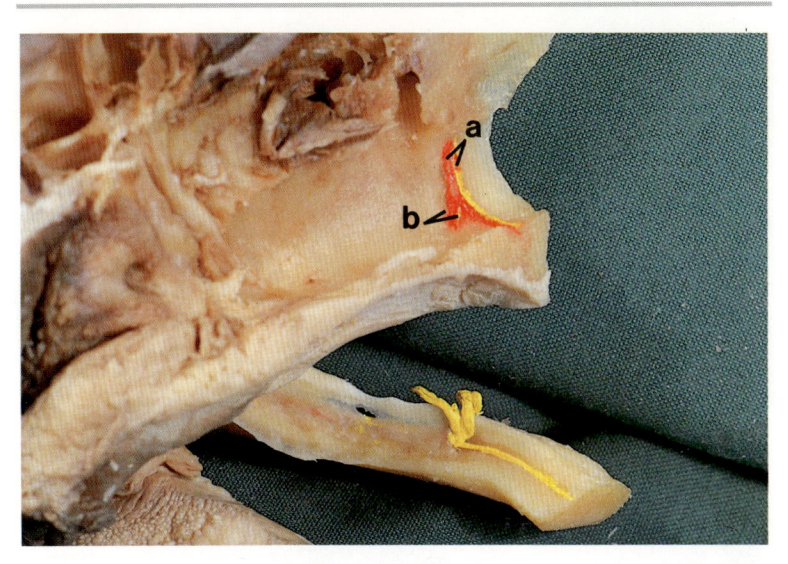

Fig. 2.**10** Mandible of a 62-year-old man. View of the lingual surface on the left side. Atrophy of the basal region with consequent opening of the incisor canal. The incisor (anterior inferior alveolar) nerve is situated immediately below the mouth floor mucosa. **a** = lateral nasal nerve and artery, **b** = perforating branch to the canine plexus

Remarks Concerning the Periodontal Ligament

The inside of the bony alveolar wall is lined by periosteal connective tissue. This consists of flat bundles of interwoven collagen fibers (Fig. 2.**11**). Between the meshes of this network, the cementoalveolar fiber bundles pass into the compact bone of the alveolar wall.

It has been shown by scanning electron microscopy of human teeth that, at least along the middle two-thirds of the septal sides, Sharpey's fibers are not so strongly interwoven as is often assumed. Collagen fiber bundles penetrate the surface of the cementum in parallel (Fig. 2.**12**), and are associated into functional, morphologic units over long stretches. We have been able to demonstrate a periodontal venous plexus only in the basal root region of the human periodontal ligament. Indeed, in increasingly complex animals, there is a trend towards vestigiality of such systems: in monkeys they are markedly less well developed than in rabbits (Rohen et al. 1984).

Sharpey's fibers, designated in general as the alveolar-dental ligaments, become anchored in the compact bone after penetration of the periosteal alveolar wall (Fig. 2.**11**). The width of anchorage holes within the compact

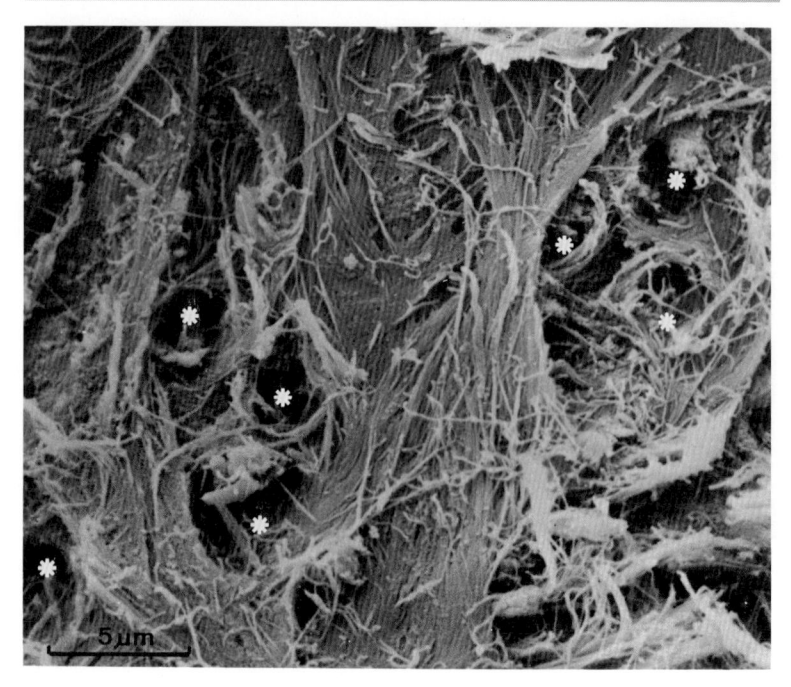

Fig. 2.**11** Periosteum of the alveolar wall. Between the collagen fiber bundle sheets, arranged in scissorlike fashion, groups of three discontinuities (asterisks) are found, through which bundles of cementoalveolar fibers pass into the bony alveolar wall. Scanning electron micrograph; negative magnification: 1600 times

Fig. 2.**12** Cementoalveolar fiber bundles of a premolar tooth; middle third. The fiber bundles leave the cementum at right angles (W.) In each case, three fiber bundles form a functional, morphologic unit (**a, b, c**). **F** = fibroblast process. Scanning electron micrograph; negative magnification: 780 times

bone increases from about 100 µm in adolescence to up to 10 times their original size with increasing age (Fig. 2.**13**). The alveolar wall then resembles cancellous, more closely than it does compact, bone. It is more than likely that the described alterations occurring in the compact bone of the alveolar wall contribute to the loosening of teeth in patients with marginal periodontitis.

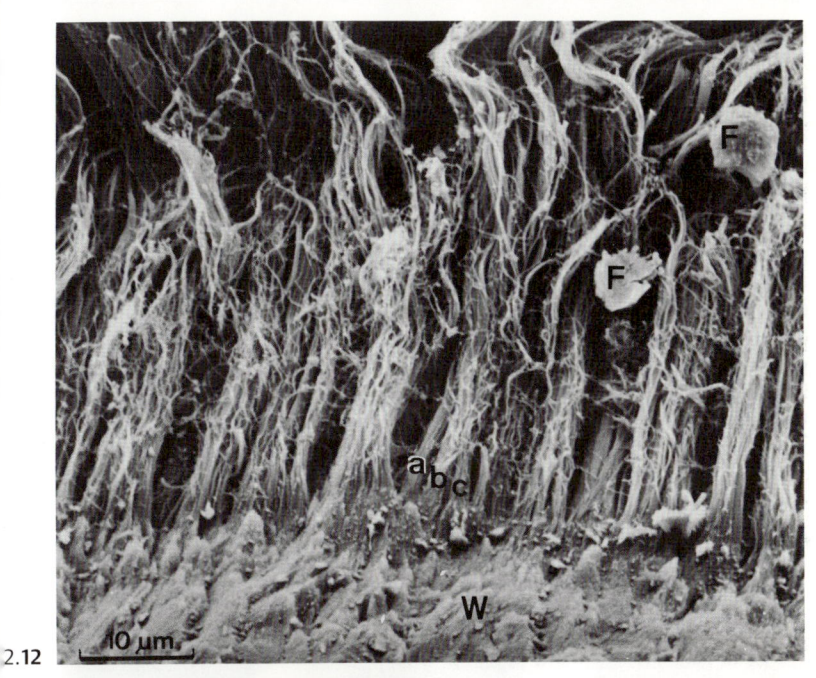

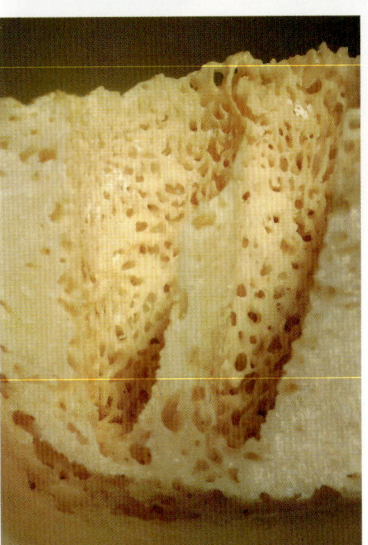

Remarks Concerning the Periodontal Ligament 23

Fig. 2.13 Bony lingual alveolar wall of the first molar, mandible of a 55-year-old man. The cementoalveolar anchorage zone extends up to the point of transition from compact to cancellous bone. Negative magnification: 8 times

Innervation of Teeth and Gingiva

Innervation of Maxillary Teeth

Sensory afferent nerve fibers from the maxillary teeth pass centrally, mostly via branches of the maxillary nerve. However, fairly recent dissection findings have demonstrated that afferent nerves from the incisor and canine teeth are also conducted via the ophthalmic nerve (Van der Zypen 1985). The perikarya of all sensory nerves are located in the trigeminal ganglion.

In the following account, the anatomic course of the nerves will be described in the opposite direction to their impulse conduction, namely, from the thicker to the thinner branches. The posterior superior alveolar nerves leave the infraorbital nerve, before it enters the orbit, through the inferior orbital fissure. The nerves pass through the pterygomaxillary fissure from the pterygopalatine fossa and run obliquely downwards across the maxillary tuberculum. They pass through the alveolar foramina into the alveolar canals, from which dental and interdental (interalveolar) branches descend to the roots of the molars and the interdental and interradicular septae (Fig. 2.**14**). The cranial branch of the posterior superior alveolar nerves runs further forward after giving off smaller branches to the mucosa of the

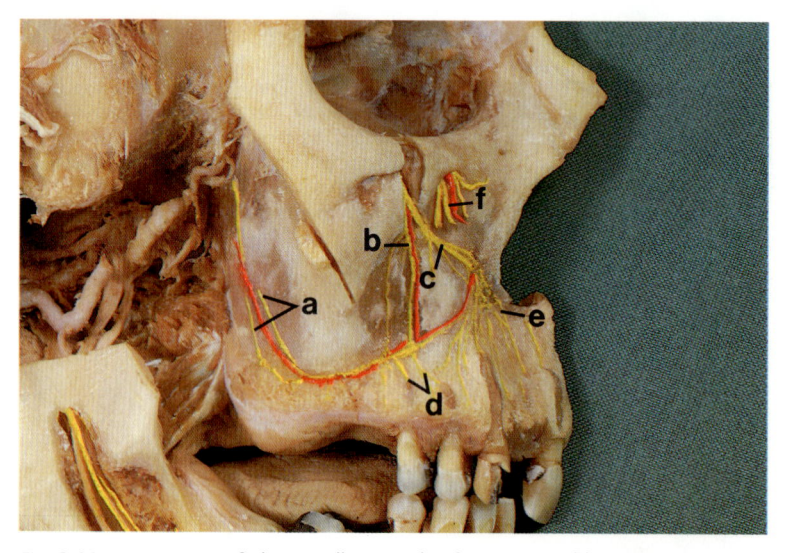

Fig. 2.**14** Innervation of the maxillary teeth of a 79-year-old man. **a** = posterior superior alveolar nerves, **b** = middle superior alveolar nerve, **c** = anterior superior alveolar nerve, **d** = dental plexus, **e** canine plexus, **f** = infraorbital nerve

maxillary sinus, and fans out in the cancellous bone of the anterior maxilla in the dental plexus (Fig. 2.**14**). The middle and anterior superior alveolar nerves also enter this plexus. They branch from the infraorbital nerve during its course through the similarly named canal, and penetrate the compact bone of the maxillary body lateral to the canine fossa, either together or separately. Via the dental plexus, the afferent fibers are directed centrally from the premolars and associated gingiva.

The dental plexus is particularly dense in the region of the canine fossa, which lies in the maxillary body below the infraorbital foramen. This anterior part of the plexus would appear to qualify for a separate designation, the canine plexus (Fig. 2.**15**), since it also incorporates the lateral nasal nerve. This is a terminal branch of the anterior ethmoid nerve, which, in turn, is a branch of the nasociliary nerve, and, accordingly, it is part of the ophthalmic nerve. It is particularly interesting that sensory afferent fibers from the canine and incisor teeth are conducted away via the ophthalmic nerve; this explains why patients with toothache in the region of these teeth complain of pain radiating into the frontotemporal plane. It is possible that the popular designation of "eye tooth" for the canine also derives from these pains, conducted via the ophthalmic nerve and radiating into the region of the eye. Accompanied by the similarly named artery, the lateral nasal nerve

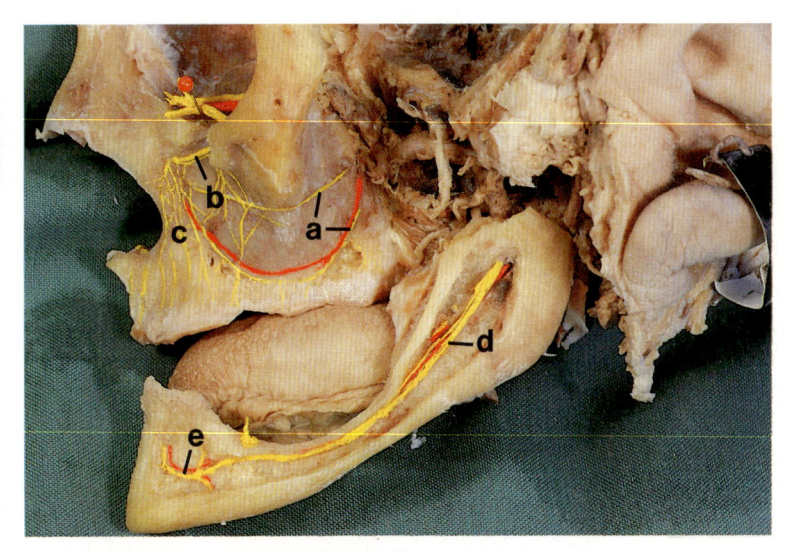

Fig. 2.**15** Innervation of the maxillar teeth of a 72-year-old woman. **a** = posterior superior alveolar nerves, **b** = anterior superior alveolar nerve, **c** = canine plexus, **d** = inferior alveolar nerve, **e** = incisor (anterior inferior alveolar) nerve

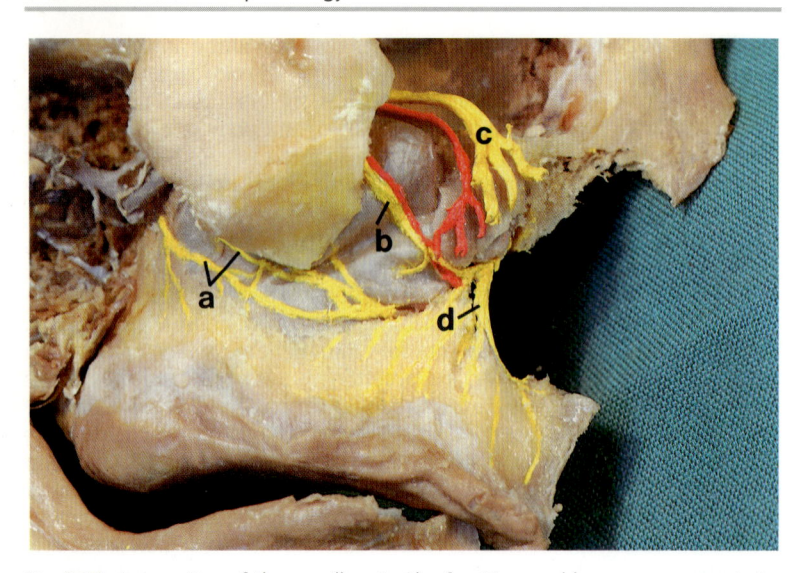

Fig. 2.16 Innervation of the maxillary teeth of a 65-year-old woman. **a** = posterior superior alveolar nerves, **b** = anterior superior alveolar nerve, **c** = infraorbital nerve, **d** = lateral nasal nerve, after dissecting away part of the lateral bony wall of the nose. Note branching of the lateral nasal nerve into the canine plexus

passes downwards under the mucosa of the lateral nasal wall (Fig. 2.**10**). A thick branch penetrates this wall and disperses in the canine plexus (Fig. 2.**16**).

After leaving the infraorbital foramen, the infraorbital nerve and its branches, the minor pes anserinus, are no longer involved in the innervation of the teeth or gingiva.

Innervation of Mandibular Teeth

The sensory afferent fibers of the mandibular teeth pass via the inferior alveolar nerve into the third branch of the trigeminal, namely, the mandibular nerve. As in the case of maxillary teeth, the perikarya of the pain tract fibers are situated in the trigeminal ganglion.

Within the mandibular canal, the inferior alveolar nerve runs in a tough periosteal sheath (Fig. 2.**17**), which extends from the mandibular to the mental foramen. This periosteal coat also envelops the inferior alveolar artery and vein, as well as the central lymphatic vessel of the mandibular teeth. Hence, it cannot be referred to as a perineural sheath, but may be most

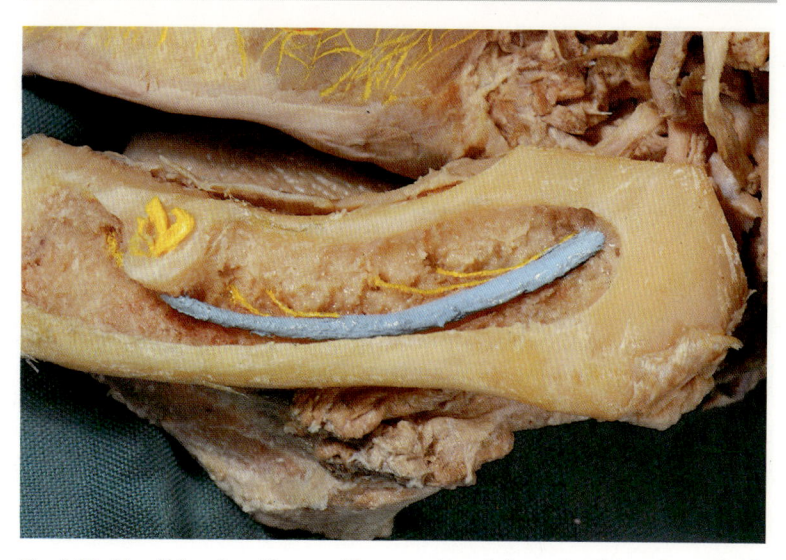

Fig. 2.17 Mandible of a 68-year-old man, viewed from the left side, with the mandibular canal opened. The tough periosteal sheath, which extends from the mandibular foramen to the mental foramen, is stained blue

readily compared with the carotid vagina of the throat. At irregular intervals, this sheath is penetrated by nerve branches which run freely through the cancellous bone and give rise to the dental and interdental rami, which pass almost perpendicularly upwards. An inferior dental plexus is formed either not at all, or only in the form of occasional nerve bridges (Figs. 2.**17**, 2.**18**). Just distal to the mental foramen, the incisor nerve for the canine and incisor teeth branches off from the inferior alveolar nerve. It crosses medial to the mental nerve and passes forward in its own bony canal within the cancellous bone, and is not enveloped by a periosteal sheath. It appears appropriate to designate this nerve as the anterior inferior alveolar nerve, and to name its canal similarly, since otherwise it may, and indeed usually is, confused with the incisor canal of the maxilla in the anatomic nomenclature. As mentioned above, the anterior inferior alveolar nerve, as a rule, crosses medial to the mental nerve; a crossing above this nerve, as is usually described in textbooks, has never been observed.

On opening up the periosteal sheath, the dentogingival rami and their accompanying vessels may be seen to branch off at an early stage, but they run for some distance further within the periosteal sheath before penetrat-

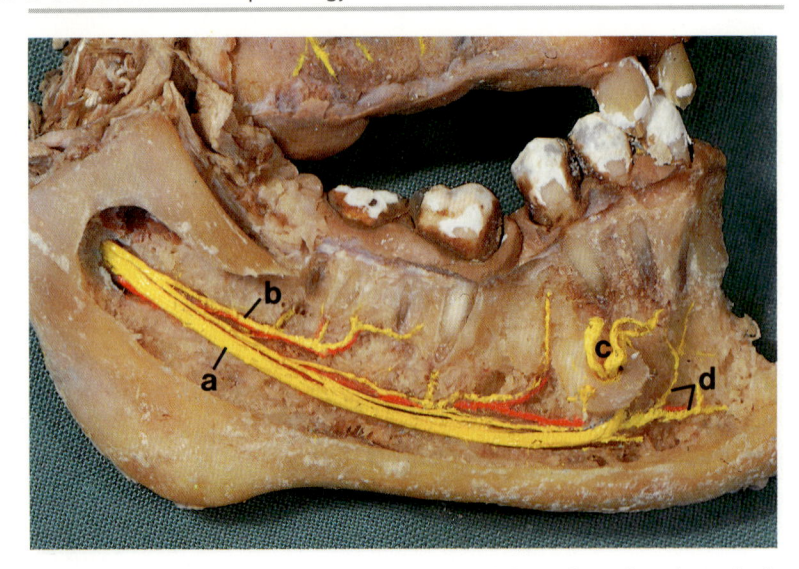

Fig. 2.**18** Mandible of a 57-year-old man, viewed from the right side, with the mandibular canal opened and periosteal sheath removed. **a** = inferior alveolar nerve, **b** = dentogingival nerve, **c** = mental nerve, **d** = incisor (anterior inferior alveolar) nerves

ing it (Fig. 2.**18**). In one-third of the cases investigated, the inferior alveolar nerve divides, before entering the mandibular canal, into its terminal branches: 1. the mylohyoid nerve, which passes as a motor branch in the mylohyoid sulcus, on the inner side of the mandible, into the area it innervates; 2. as a rule, two dentogingival nerves; 3. the anterior inferior alveolar (incisor) nerve, the longest branch; and 4. the mental nerve, the thickest branch (Fig. 2.**19**).

Innervation of the Maxillary and Mandibular Gingiva

The palatal gingiva receives its sensory innervation from the palatine and nasopalatine nerves. The sensory innervation of the vestibular gingiva is via the dental plexus, and that of the labial gingiva via the canine plexus. The infraorbital and buccal nerves do not participate in the sensory innervation of the gingiva (Fig. 2.**20a**).

In the mandible, the buccal nerve possesses a small innervation field situated buccally, in the region of the first molar. The rest of the gingiva is innervated, buccally, from the dentogingival nerves of the inferior alveolar nerve, labially, from the anterior inferior alveolar (incisor) nerve and lingually, from the lingual nerve (Fig. 2.**20b**).

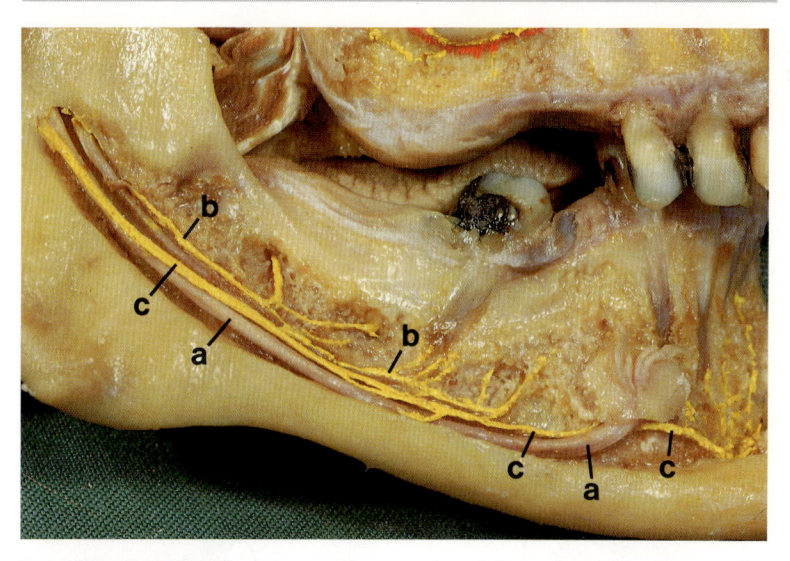

Fig. 2.**19** Mandible of a 79-year-old man, viewed from the right side, revealing pronounced division of the inferior alveolar nerve. The following nerves run in the mandibular canal: **a** = mental nerve (not colored), **b** = dentogingival nerve, **c** = incisor (anterior inferior alveolar) nerve

Arterial Blood Supply to the Maxillary and Mandibular Teeth

Arteries of the Maxillary Teeth

The maxillary teeth are supplied with blood via an outer and an inner vascular circuit. From the dorsal side, the posterior superior alveolar arteries participate in the development of the outer vascular circuit; they arise directly from the maxillary artery before it enters the pterygopalatine fossa via the pterygomaxillary fissure (Figs. 2.**14** and 2.**21**). These dorsal branches combine with the middle and anterior superior alveolar arteries, which both arise from the infraorbital artery, one of the terminal branches of the maxillary artery. Finally, the lateral nasal artery also participates in the formation of the outer vascular circuit; it is accompanied by the similarly named nerve, and arises from the ophthalmic artery via the nasociliary artery. Hence, there are five arteries which form a superior external dental arch (Fig. 2.**21**).

30 2 Anatomic Basis of Implantology

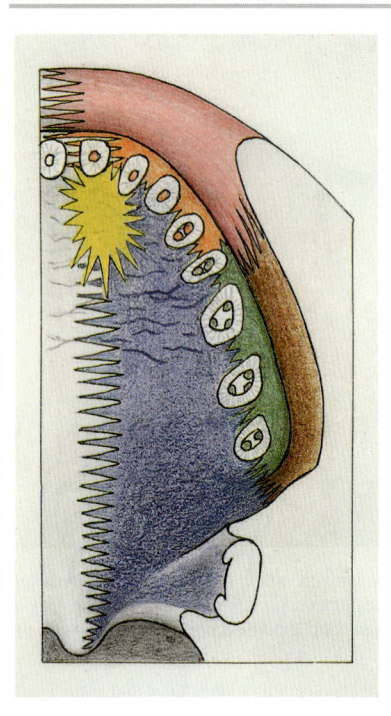

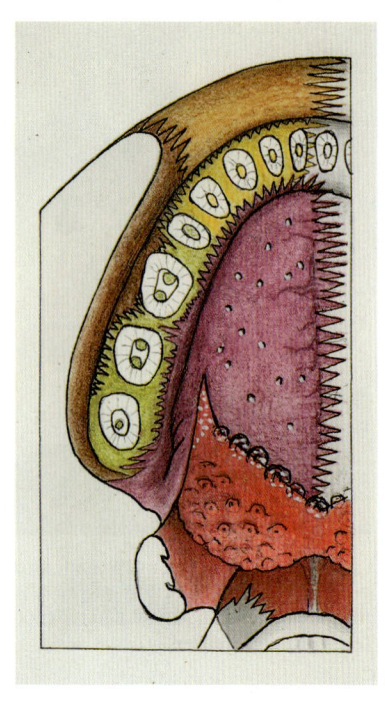

Fig. 2.**20a** Sensory innervation of the maxillary gingiva (after *Pernkopf* 1960). Labiovestibular: orange = canine plexus, green = dental plexus (posterior superior and middle alveolar nerves); palatal: blue = greater palatine nerve, yellow = nasopalatine nerve. The infraorbital (violet) and buccal (brown) nerves do not participate in the sensory innervation of the maxillary gingiva.
b Sensory innervation of the mandibular gingiva (after *Pernkopf* 1960). Labiobuccal: yellow = incisor (anterior inferior alveolar) nerve, brown = buccal nerve, green = dentogingival nerve; lingual: violet = lingual nerve. The mental nerve (light brown) does not participate in the sensory innervation of the mandibular gingiva

The inner vascular circuit which supplies the maxillary teeth and adjacent gingiva is formed exclusively from the terminal branches of the maxillary artery. The descending palatine artery, which forms the posterior tributary of the medial arch under the mucosa of the hard palate (Fig. 2**22**), also participates. From the front, the anastomotic ramus passes through the incisive foramen into this vascular circuit. This branch arises from the posterior nasal septal artery of the sphenopalatine artery.

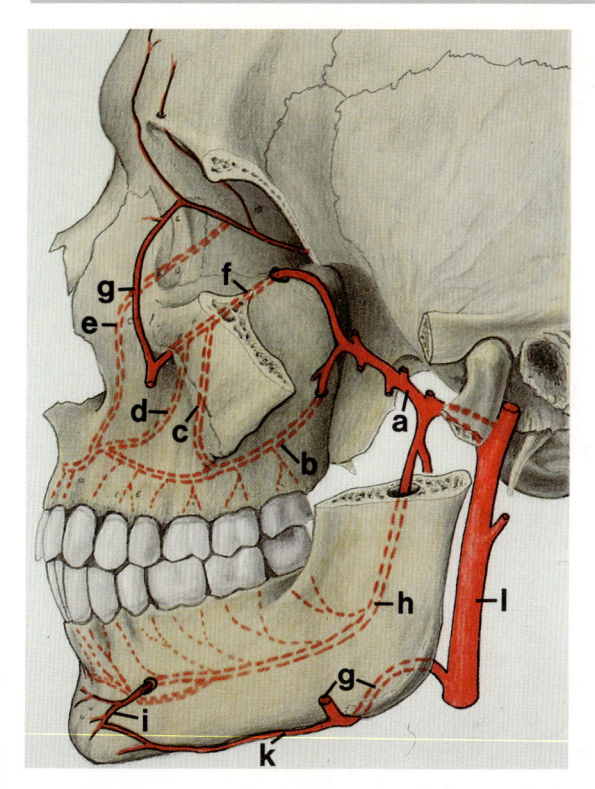

Fig. 2.21 Outer arterial vascular circuit of the maxillary and mandibular teeth. **a** = maxillary artery, **b** = posterior superior alveolar artery, **c** = middle superior alveolar artery, **d** = anterior superior alveolar artery, **e** = lateral nasal artery, **f** = infraorbital artery, **g** = facial artery, **h** = inferior alveolar artery, **i** = mental artery, **k** = submental artery, **l** = external carotid artery

Arteries of the Mandibular Teeth

The mandibular teeth are also supplied via a vascular circuit. The main vessel is the inferior alveolar artery, which runs in the alveolar canal and reaches the mandibular teeth via the dental rami. The inferior alveolar artery forms an outer vascular arch to the facial artery via the mental and submental arteries (Fig. 2.**21**). An inner vascular arch connects the inferior alveolar artery to the deep lingual artery via the supragenoid ramus, and to the sublingual artery via the interincisor rami (Fig. 2.**23**).

32 2 Anatomic Basis of Implantology

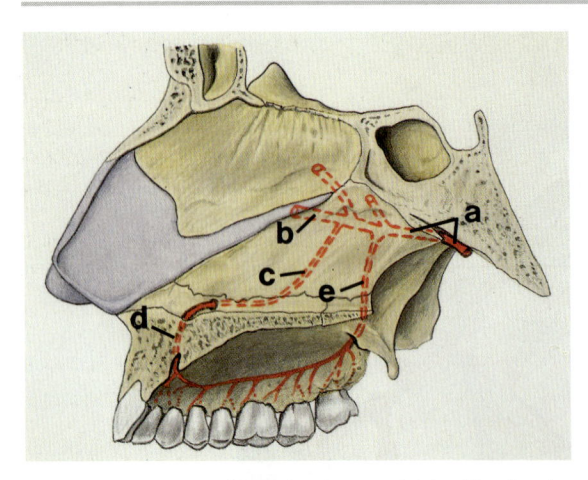

Fig. 2.22 Inner arterial vascular circuit supplying blood to the gingiva of the maxillary teeth. **a** = maxillary artery, **b** = sphenopalatine artery, **c** = posterior nasal septal artery, **d** = anastomotic ramus, **e** = descending (greater) palatine artery

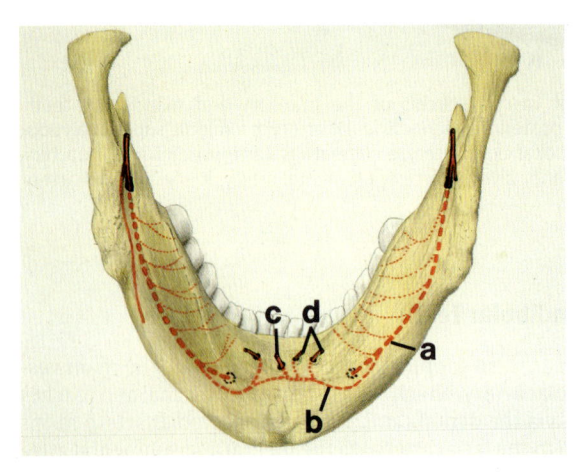

Fig. 2.23 Inner anastomoses of the inferior alveolar artery. **a** = inferior alveolar artery, **b** = incisor (anterior inferior alveolar) artery, **c** = supragenoid ramus of the deep lingual artery, **d** = interincisor rami of the sublingual artery

Venous Drainage from Maxillary and Mandiubular Teeth

Venous blood from the dental pulp flows via the superior and inferior alveolar veins into the pterygoid plexus, which expands on the lateral surface of the medial pterygoid muscle. This venous plexus conducts the blood into the retromandibular vein via the maxillary veins (Fig. 2.**24**). It is of particular significance that the pterygoid plexus possesses four outlets that finally run into the cavernous sinus: 1. the plexus of the oval foramen; 2. the medial meningeal vein; 3. an anastomosis between the inferior and superior

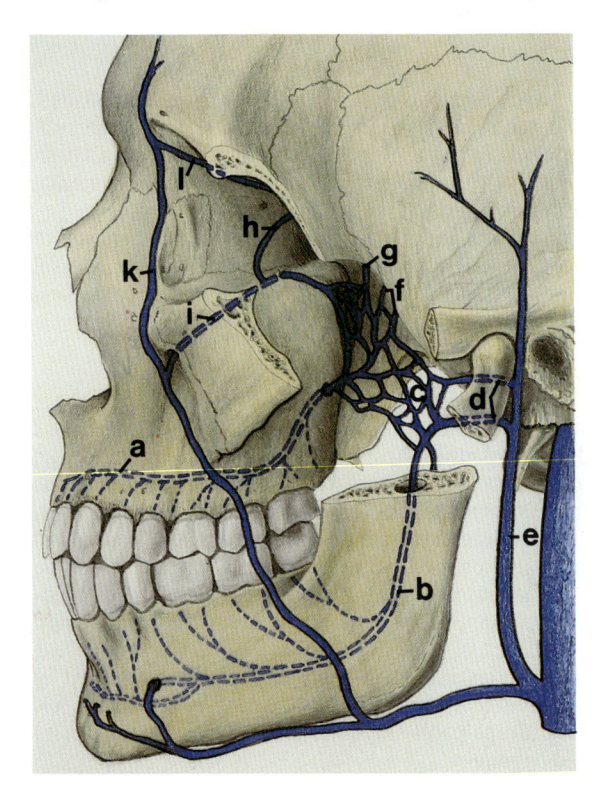

Fig. 2.**24** Venous drainage from the maxillary and mandibular teeth. The venous blood flows from the teeth via the superior (**a**) and inferior (**b**) alveolar veins into the pterygoid plexus (**c**), and from there via the maxillary veins (**d**) into the retromandibular vein (**e**). Various connections to the cavernous sinus are present: via the oval foraminal plexus (**f**), the middle meningeal vein (**g**), the inferior opthhalmic vein (**h**) and the infraorbital vein (**i**). The latter forms an anastomosis to the facial vein (**k**), which joins the dorsal vein of the nose (**l**), arising from the superior opthalmic vein

ophthalmic veins; and 4. the infraorbital (or deep facial) vein to the facial vein, and from there, via the angular and dorsal nasal veins, into the superior ophthalmic vein. These connections to the cavernous sinus are of clinical importance because infections carried here from the maxillary and mandibular teeth via the specified routes may lead to a sinus cavernosus thrombosis or meningitis.

Lymphatic Drainage from Maxillary and Mandibular Teeth and Gingiva

Lymphatic Drainage from the Teeth

The existence of lymphatic vessels in the pulp has now been established. Lymph from the molars and premolars of the maxilla flows to the submandibular lymph nodes via lymphatics in the alveolar canals; lymph from the incisors and canine teeth is conveyed to the parotid and submental lymph nodes via the infraorbital canal.

Lymph from the premolars and molars of the mandible is believed to drain directly to the deep cervical lymph nodes via a central lymphatic vessel in the mandibular canal. Incisor and canine teeth of the mandible possess their own regional submandibular lymph nodes (Fig. 2.**25**).

Lymphatic Drainage from the Gingiva

The gingiva is also traversed by fine lymphatic vessels, and both vestibular and oral lymphatic drainage pathways can be distinguished (Fig. 2.**25**). The vestibular drainage route of the gingiva from the maxilla and mandible leads to the submandibular and submental lymph nodes. In the oral drainage tract, lymphatics from the maxilla and mandible take separate routes. The palatal lymphatic tracts join the lymphatics of the nasal mucosa via the incisive canal, and pass into the lateral pharyngeal lymph nodes via the pterygopalatine canal. The lingual lymphatics flow to the submandibular lymph nodes.

Supraregional lymph nodes of the teeth and gingiva are represented by the deep cervical lymph nodes, which are mostly covered by the sternocleidomastoid muscle, and are palpable, in some cases, solely at the dorsal boundary of the carotid trigonum.

Comments

From the detailed description of anatomic structures and topographic relationships given above, one recognizes at this stage that physiological restrictions are imposed upon implantology within bone. In particular, one must consider:

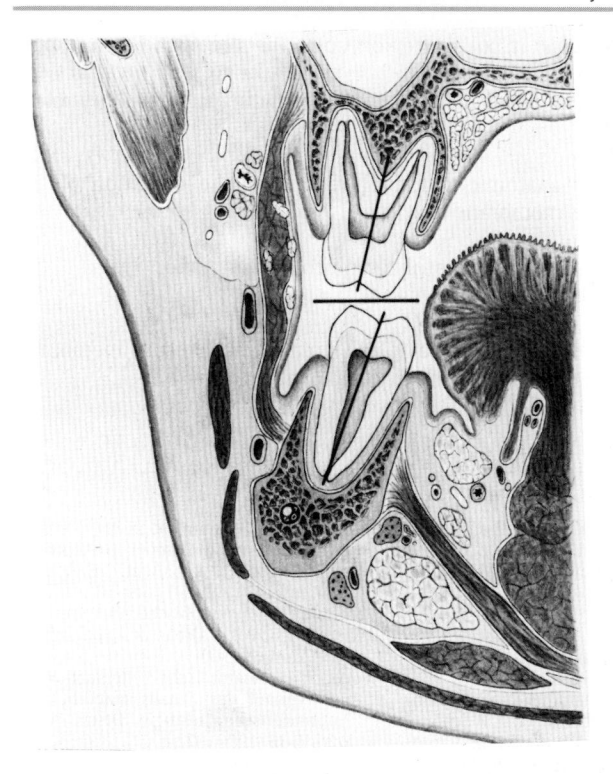

Fig. 2.**25** Lymphatic drainage from the teeth and gingiva (after *Pernkopf* 1960). See text for details

- bone layout;
- bone structure;
- vascular and nerve supply to the various regions of the jaw;
- the topographic relationship of the maxillary teeth to the nasal cavity and maxillary sinus.

It is then possible to classify the potential implantation sites as follows:
Favorable:
- anterior mandible (between the two mental foramina)
- mandibular region near posterior teeth, and as far forward as natural dentition exists. (If implants are being considered only after several years of total tooth loss, then the posterior mandibular region is usually no longer a suitable site.)

Conditionally favorable: maxillary region up to the site of the second premolars
Unfavorable: posterior region of the maxilla, including the maxillary retromolar tubercle

From a purely anatomic-structural viewpoint, the condition of the suprajacent mucous membrane covering also plays an essential role.

Favorable: taut, attached and keratinized mucous membrane
Unfavorable: mobile mucous membrane

In contrast to skeletal considerations, unfavorable mucous membrane conditions may be improved operatively at no great expense.

References

Bastide, G., J. Bécue, R. Combelles. La vascularisation artérielle du maxillaire inférieur chez l'homme. C. R. Assoc. Anat. 1971; 56 (1971) 951–5

Benninghoff, A. Über die Anpassung der Knochenkompakta an geänderte Beanspruchungen. Anat. Anz. 63 (1927) 289–99

Gysi, B. E., S. Kubik. Anatomie-Orale Implantologie. In J. R. Strub, B. E. Gysi, P. Schärer. Schwerpunkte in der oralen Implantologie und Rekonstruktion. Quintessenz, Berlin 1983

Härle, F. Die Lage des Mandibularkanals im zahnlosen Kiefer. Dtsch. Zahnärztl. Z. 32 (1977) 275–6

Jacques, P., M. Bleicher. La vascularisation artérielle du sinus maxillaire chez l'adulte: étude anatomique avec considérations médico-chirurgicales. Ann. Otolaryngol. Chir. Cervicofac. 4 (1932) 353–66

Jensen, O. Site classification for the osseointegrated implant. J. Prosthet. Dent. 61 (1989) 228–34

Kubik, S. Anatomische Grundlagen der Implantologie. Dent. Rev. 1–2:11–19, 3:13–23 (1984)

Kubik, S. Die Anatomie der Kieferknochen in bezug die enossale Blatt-Implantation, 1. Mandibula. Zahnärztl. Welt 85 (1986) 264–71

Motsch, A. Spannungsoptische Untersuchungen zur funktionellen Anatomie des Unterkiefers. Verh. Anat. Ges. Erg. Bd. Anat. Anz. 120 (1966–7) 419–30

Pernkopf, E. Topographische Anatomie des Menschen. Vol 4. Urban and Schwarzenberg, Munich 1960

Reich, R. H. Anatomische Untersuchungen zum Verlauf des Canalis mandibularis: Präprothetische Chirurgie. Dtsch. Zahnärztl. Z. 35 (1980) 972–5

Rohen, J. W., W. H. Arnold, M. Wachter. Rasterelektronenmikroskopische Untersuchungen über die Architektur der Wurzelhautgefäße. Dtsch. Zahnärztl. Z. 39 (1984) 958–64

Schroeder, H. E.: Orale Strukturbiologie. 2 nd ed. Thieme, Stuttgart 1982

Testut, L. A. Laterjet. Traité d'anatomie humaine. Doin, Paris 1948

Van der Zypen, E. Anatomische Grundlagen zur Implantation. Schweiz. Monatsschr. Zahnmed. 95 (1985) 827–37

Van der Zypen, E. Zur Anatomie des Splanchnocranium. Grundlagen für eine Implantologie. Phillip. J. 5 (1988) 235–40

Wetzel, G. Lehrbuch der Anatomie für Zahnärzte. Fischer, Jena 1951

3 The Properties of Titanium

S. Steinemann

Introduction

Titanium has been used for fracture treatment and in orthopedics for more than 20 years without one case of incompatibility having been documented.

There are also good reasons to consider this material to be ideal for dental (endosteal) implants:
- Titanium is a reactive metal. This means that in air, water or any other electrolyte an oxide is spontaneously formed on the surface of the metal. This oxide is one of the most resistant minerals known, building a dense film which protects the metal from chemical attack, including that of aggressive body fluids.
- Titanium is "inert" in tissue. The oxide film in contact with the tissue is practically insoluble; in particular, no ions are released that could go on to react with organic molecules.
- Titanium possesses good mechanical properties. Its tensile strength is very close to that of the stainless steel used for load-bearing surgical implants. Titanium is also many times stronger than either cortical bone or dentin, allowing dental implants of slender form, which are nevertheless capable of supporting large loads. Equally important is the fact that the metal is tough and malleable, which makes it insensitive to shock loading and ensures that a heavily loaded implant will yield but not fail.
- Titanium does not simply behave passively in tissue and bone; bone grows into the rough surface and bonds to the metal, a reaction which is normally only attributed to the so-called bioactive materials. This ankylotic anchoring, often termed osseointegration, forms the best possible basis for a functional dental implant, as it can withstand all possible load types, e.g., tensile, compressive and shear forces.

These few statements summarize the results of many years of multidisciplinary study of titanium as a biomaterial. Interested users and critics alike would expect these facts to be more fully explained and documented; the aim of the remainder of this chapter is to fulfill this need, in spite of the largely technical and theoretical nature of the subject.

Material Properties

Unalloyed titanium grade 4 is used in ITI implants; the chemical composition and mechanical properties of this grade are given in Table 3.**1**. This material is also used for orthopedic implants and is standardized in ISO 5832/II. Grade 4 indicates a material with a raised oxygen and iron content; these elements are in solution in the titanium metal, and their main effect is to improve the mechanical properties. The strength of the plain wrought material is, however, still insufficient for highly loaded dental implants, and greater strength is produced by cold work and suitable heat treatment.

With data on the material's mechanical strength, the question of the magnitude of lateral forces which can be supported by a 3-mm diameter titanium implant pillar or the endangered cross section at the upper end of the hollow cylinder, without the implant deforming or even breaking, can be addressed (Fig. 3.**1**). Calculation and experiment both show that lateral forces up to about 20 kg can be tolerated. Much greater axial loads can be supported. This strength level is more than adequate to satisfy the requirements placed upon a dental implant.

Table 3.1 Properties of unalloyed titanium for implants

a) *Chemical composition of grade 4 titanium*

% O	Fe	C	N	H	Ti
0.4 max.	0.5 max.*	0.1 max.	0.05 max.	0.015 max.	Trace

* typically under 0.1%

b) *Mechanical properties*

	Tensile Strength	Elongation	Young's modulus
Wrought/annealed	550 MPa min.	20% min.	110 GPa
Cold worked	800 MPa typical	15% min.	110 GPa

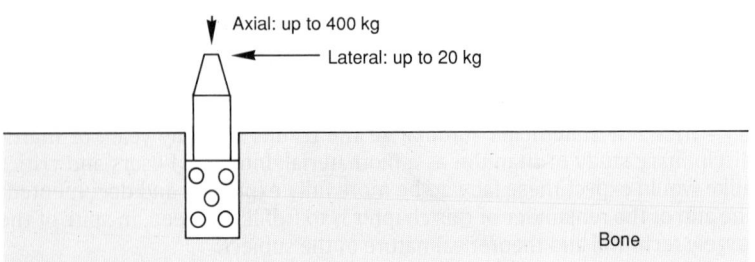

Fig. 3.**1** Maximum loads an implant can support; limit determined by design and material strength

Corrosion – Chemical Compatibility

Standard electrode potential electrochemical series are often used as a basis for the discussion and explanation of corrosion reactions (Fig. 3.2). The standard electrode potential is defined as the potential at which the oxidation rate – metal atoms are oxidized to metal ions setting free electrons – is equal to the reduction rate – the metal ion loses its charge consuming electrons – in a 1 molar solution of ions in the electrolyte. This reaction scheme is depicted in Figure 3.3.

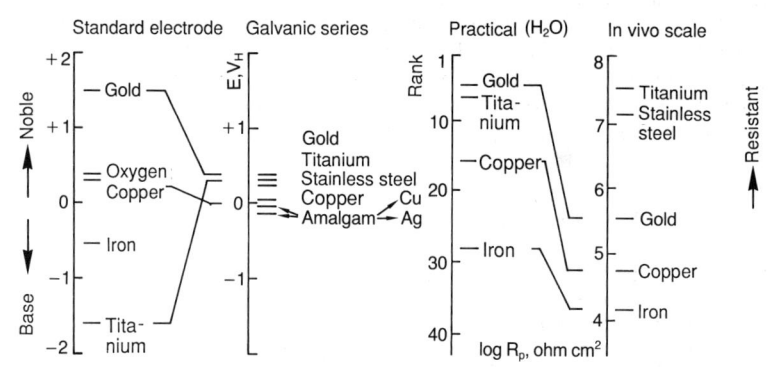

Fig. 3.2 Four series and practical scales for corrosion resistance of selected metals: standard electrode potential series (left), galvanic series in synthetic saliva after *Stegemann* (mid-left), scale of practical nobility after *Pourbaix* (mid-right), and the in vivo scale after *Steinemann* (right). Instead of the classification "noble – base," the use of "resistant – not resistant" would be better, as the corrosion rates vary by a factor of 10 000 and more

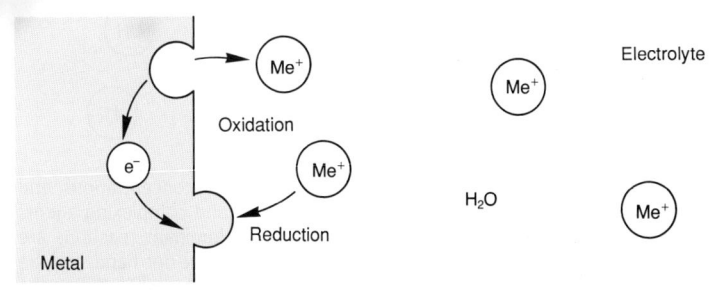

Fig. 3.3 The potential series only considers the reactions involving oxidation of metal and reduction of metal ions, which is unrealistic

As one can imagine, the electrochemical series is nothing more than a theoretical concept used by chemists. The high concentration of ions referred to in the definition may be likened to a concentrated acid and it is certainly not correct to neglect the other electrolyte constituents. Titanium is a classic example of how thoughtless use of the electrochemical series can be misleading. Titanium is classified in the series as a reactive metal, but in reality it is one of the most resistant materials available for surgical implants and chemical apparatus.

Galvanic series such as that for sea water (Fontana and Greene) or synthetic saliva (Stegemann) are more realistic (Fig. 3.**2**). As the name suggests, these series are useful in predicting which pairs of metals should not be (galvanically) coupled. The nearer a material is to the top of the series, the more corrosion resistant or "chemically compatible" it is.

Metals are in a different order in the electrochemical series than in the galvanic series, and the values of the potentials are much closer together in the latter. The electrochemical explanation for this is that in reality, the influence of the partial reaction involving metal ions is negligible because of the low concentration of these ions. The corrosion reaction is dominated by a "reaction with water," i.e., the reduction of dissolved oxygen to hydroxyl ions (Fig. 3.**4**). This reaction is the driving force which "polarizes" the metal and thus governs all reactions on a corroding metal. The standard electrode potential for oxygen reduction (+ 0.40 V_H) is included in the electrochemical series in Figure 3.**2**. A glance at the two galvanic series then shows that the potentials for many metals are indeed grouped around this value. Aqueous electrolytes, which include sea water, tissue fluid and saliva, show this effect.

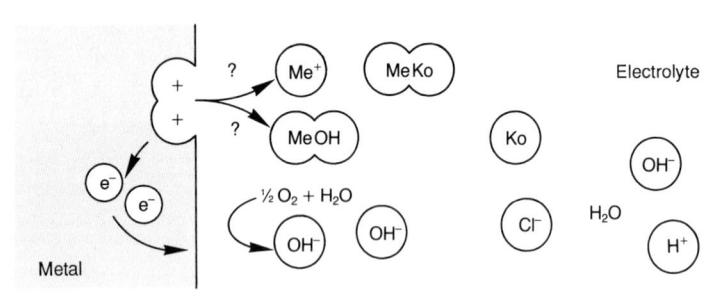

Fig. 3.**4** In reality, the metal ions (Me⁺) are only present in low concentrations, and other reactants, e.g., oxygen (O_2), chlorine (as the ion Cl⁻), and complexing agents (Ko, typically organic molecules) become important. The dominant reactions are normally the reduction of oxygen to form hydroxyl ions (OH⁻) on the one hand, and the formation of metal ions, metal hydroxides (MeOH) or metal complexes (MeKo) on the other. One or another of these "unwanted corrosion products" will form, depending upon its chemical affinity

The concept of "oxidizing strength" of a solution is used; it is expressed as the redox potential and can be measured with a platinum electrode (ca. 0.3 V_H in tissue).

In the 1960s, Pourbaix developed a new concept to describe corrosion processes. He made a distinction between "thermodynamically noble" and "practically noble:" The corrosion mechanism can only be predicted if one knows which reactions occur spontaneously and which corrosion products (of all those possible) are stable (see Fig. 3.**4**). Metal ions are not the only reaction products; metal oxides, halogen compounds (Cl, F, etc.) and others may form.

For a metal to be corrosion resistant, it must either be immune or passive. Noble metals and mercury are immune in water. A metal is said to exhibit passive behavior when the metal spontaneously oxidizes to produce an insoluble oxide in a compact layer, which acts as an extremely effective protective coating against corrosion. Whether a metal is immune or passive depends naturally upon whether the medium is acid or alkaline, and whether it contains oxidizing or reducing substances (e.g., chlorate or hydrochloric acid). The fewer such factors a metal is sensitive to, the more corrosion resistant it is. The practical scale (Pourbaix's "noblesse pratique") presented in Figure 3.**2** is derived in this way.

When the theoretical and the two practical scales in Figure 3.**2** are compared, it becomes clear that the theoretical classification of metals as noble or active is no longer valid in the practical series. Titanium is directly below gold in the practical series, which means that hese two materials exhibit very similar corrosion resistance. A thin, electrically insulating oxide film protects the reactive titanium from the corrosive medium.

The three series are useful as they identify resistant metals; however, they say nothing about the corrosion rate or intensity, i.e., about the amount of corrosion products produced. But precisely this value is required for a discussion of "chemical compatibility" because in the end, all tissue responses depend on the amounts of "unwanted" reaction products produced.

Corrosion of metallic biomaterials can only be studied by electrochemical methods, as corrosion is neither visible nor detectable by weight loss. Hoar and Mears used a hybrid method to measure corrosion rates; they measured the corrosion potential in vivo and then determined the anodic partial current (corrosion current) in oxygen-free physiologic solutions at this potential. There are many possible processes that can promote or inhibit corrosion in living tissue; thus direct measurement in vivo (Steinemann) must be preferred. This involves the measurement of the polarization resistance, using small implanted plates of metal as electrodes (Fig. 3.**5**). The polarization resistance is inversely proportional to the corrosion current which, in turn, is directly proportional to the amount of oxidized or corroded metal.

Such experiments were performed for several pure metals and most of the alloys in practical surgical use; a selection of results is presented in Table 3.2. One can see that the corrosion rate of resistant metals such as stainless steel or titanium is very low indeed; corrosion removes less than one layer of metal atoms per day, which means that it would take more than a million years to fully oxidize a titanium dental implant. The corrosion rate of gold is also quoted in the table; it is about 100 times greater than that for titanium

Table 3.2 Corrosion data for four metals as current and amount

	Current density, in vitro	$\mu A/cm^2$ in vivo	Oxidized or dissolved $\mu g/d$ for implant 2 cm^2
Stainless steel, Cobalt alloys	0.0004–0.3	0.002–0.003	0.1
Titanium	0.0002–0.03	0.0003–0.005	0.03
Gold	--	0.06	7

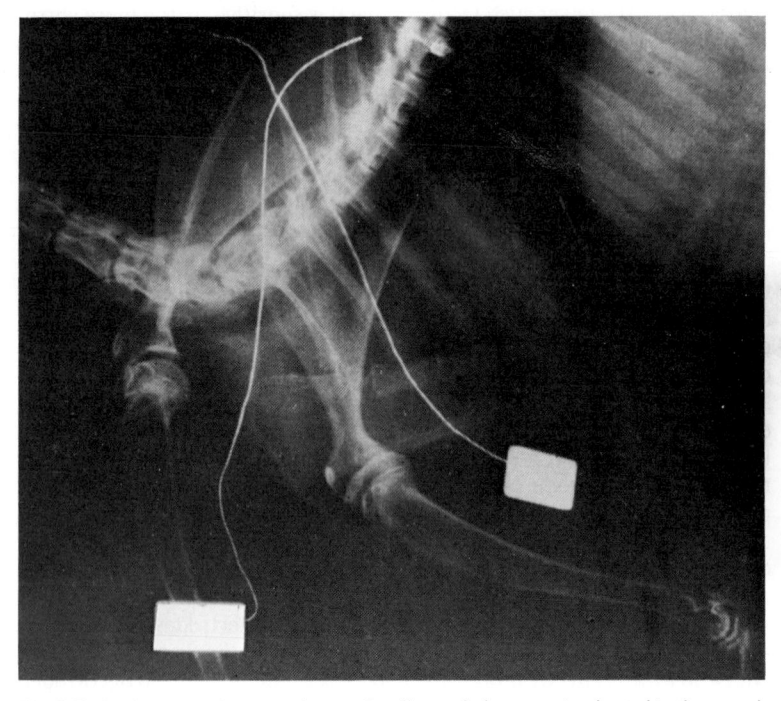

Fig. 3.5 In vivo corrosion experiment. Small metal plates are implanted in the muscle with measuring leads to the back of the animal (radiograph)

or stainless steel! This may come as a surprise, but it is due to the presence of complexing agents (chloride, sulfur compounds, etc.) in tissue.

A high polarization resistance indicates good corrosion resistance; therefore the results of the in vivo corrosion experiments can be presented as a corrosion-resistance scale and compared with the potential series in Figure 3.**2**. This scale is logarithmic; a change of one unit on the scale means a change in corrosion speed by a factor of 10 (e.g., iron at 4 corrodes 1000 times faster than stainless steel at 7). Examination of this last scale reveals that the descriptions noble or active cover an enormous range of corrosion rates, which could never have been predicted from the differences of the potentials alone.

The term "chemical compatibility" has been used, implying intentionally or unintentionally that corrosion is a normal process (there is no such thing as "zero corrosion"). But is a minimal corrosion rate sufficient to guarantee "(bio)chemical compatibility"?

Behavior of Titanium in an Electrolyte

First an explanation of the term "reactive metal" is necessary. Titanium oxide is a much more stable substance than either titanium metal or its ions in solution. The reaction energy set free when titanium oxidizes is even greater than that necessary to decompose water, which is why the oxide-forming reaction is always spontaneous. The reaction mechanism is illustrated in Figure 3.**6**. The spontaneously produced oxide always forms a thin film on the metal about 3 nm or 20 atomic layers thick.

The solubility of metal oxides in electrolytes varies. The solubility of active (freshly precipitated) titanium oxides in given in Figure 3.**7**. This shows that the oxide is only soluble in acids below pH 2 and in strongly alkaline solutions; in neutral solutions the solubility is only about 3 micromolar

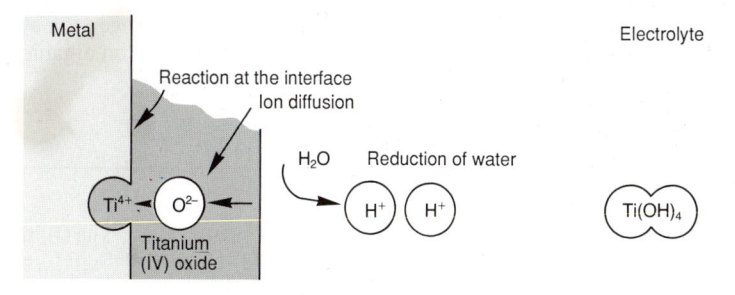

Fig. 3.**6** Schematic representation of the processes that occur at the surface of reactive titanium. The oxidation is spontaneous and rapid; water is broken down and oxygen combines with titanium ions. At neutral pH values (pH ≈ 7), no titanium ions are present; only electrically neutral titanium hydroxide is dissolved in the electrolyte

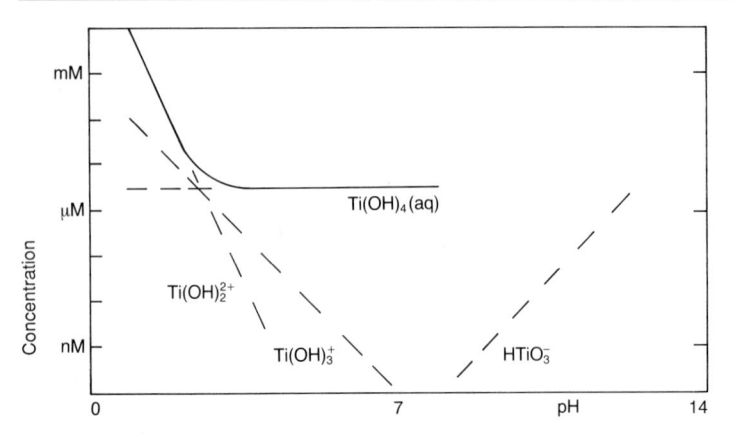

Fig. 3.7 Solubility of titanium oxide in chloride and chlorate solutions as a function of pH (after *Baes and Mesmer*). The solid line gives the total dissolved titanium as titanium hydroxide in moles (1 mole = 1 gm molecular weight per liter)

(equivalent to 1 titanium hydroxide molecule in 19 million water molecules). Chemistry further teaches that the dissolved species is the electrically uncharged hydroxide.

Similar concentrations of titanium have been found in in vitro experiments (Table 3.3). These have been interpreted as loss of metal in the form of ions; this is not correct, as standad analytical chemistry cannot distinguish the chemical state (species) of a dissolved element! It is important to differentiate between ions and neutral species in solution, as only the former can react, e.g., with proteins. The dissolved ion concentration for titanium is only about 0.1 nanomolar, 10 000 times lower than that of the neutral species. This concentration is also 100 times lower than that of the hydrogen ion at pH 7, which means that the probability of titanium binding with an organic molecule is always very small.

Table 3.3 Chemical data for titanium in an electrolyte

a) *Solubility of titanium oxide* in chloride and chlorate solutions at pH ≈ 7 (*Baes* und *Mesmer*)	
as uncharged Ti(OH)$_4$(aq)	$3 \cdot 10^{-6}$ M = 0.15 µg (Ti)/g
as ion (cation) Ti(OH)$_3^+$	ca. 10^{-10} M = 0.000005 µg (Ti)/g
b) *Amount of metal* found in an in vitro experiment (*Dörre; Ducheyne et al.; Steinemann* and *Perren*)	
in synthetic saliva at 37 °C	0.075–0.35 µg (Ti)/g
in Hanks solution + EDTA at 37 °C	0.01 µg (Ti)/g

Biologic Compatibility

An in vivo corrosion experiment can always be followed up by a tissue examination. The observed tissue reaction can then be compared with the amount of "unwanted" corrosion product that was measured in the electrochemical experiment. Correlations are to be expected.

Certain characteristic types of tissue reaction have been repeatedly observed; it is sufficient to discriminate between toxicity (pyknosis, sterile abscess), sequestration (thick, nonvascular connective tissue in contact with the implant, absence of pathologic cells) and inertness (loose, vascularized connective tissue). This scale is the abscissa in Figure 3.**8**. The ordinate is the polarization resistance; the values are those from the corrosion experiments described earlier in the chapter. The figure shows that the toxic reaction to Co, Cu, Ni, and V correlates with a high corrosion rate; also, the inert metals that do not trigger a tissue response, namely, Pt, Ta, Nb, Zr, and Ti, are all highly corrosion resitant. A certain pattern can thus be identified; there appears to be a rough correlation between chemical and biologic compatibility.

A sequestration reaction is obseved between the two extremes of toxicity and tolerance. The foreign body is encapsulated, a harmless form of

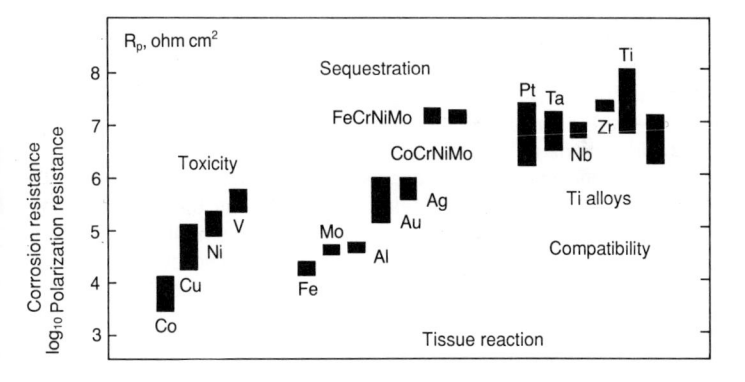

Fig. 3.**8** Corrosion resistance and tissue reaction for pure metals and alloys (FeNiCrMo is stainless steel, CoCrNiMo is the cobalt base alloy used for endoprostheses in orthopedics, Ti alloys include Ti-6Al-4V, Ti-15Mo, etc.). The diagram shows the relationship between "chemical compatibility" and "biologic compatibility." The toxic metals corrode at a much higher rate (about 10 000 times faster) than the inert metals. However, the toxic reaction is specific, and many metals – despite corrosion rates – only trigger the less harmful sequestration-rejection reaction. In contrast, a high corrosion resistance does not guarantee compatibility; stainless steel and cobalt alloys, despite a minimal release of toxic corrosion products, nevertheless provoke an encapsulation reaction

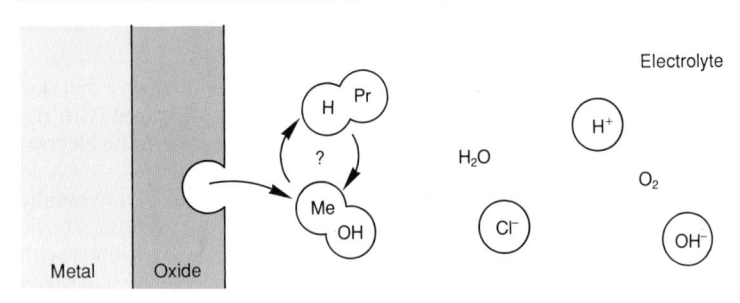

Fig. 3.9 The primary corrosion product, either a metal ion or a hydroxide (MeOH) can react with protein (HPr), forming metalloprotein complexes that are potentially toxic

rejection. This type of tissue reaction is observed for both corrosion resistant materials – stainless steel (FeCrNiMo) and cobalt-chromium-molybdenum alloys – and for the strongly corroding metals Fe, Mo, and Al. It must be assumed that the unwanted corrosion product itself is the determinig factor. Iron, molybdenum and aluminum as nontoxic metals do not trigger an extreme tissue reaction, despite high corrosion rates (about 300 times that of stainless steel). On the other hand, the very small corrosion of stainless steel and cobaltchromium alloys, comparable to that of Ti, Nb, and Zr, releases sufficient quantities of the highly toxic elements nickel and cobalt to trigger a noticeable tissue reaction. It should be mentioned at this point that no limiting concentration is commonly admitted for an allergic reaction. Gold and silver are also to be found in this middle group, as these noble metals can also corrode in living tissue.

As demonstrated above, a low corrosion rate alone is not sufficient to guarantee compatibility, nor is the elemental dose the only determining factor. It would appear that the intrinsic toxicity of the element and its ability to bind to macromolecules is equally important (Zitter; Luckey and Venugopal; Steinemann and Perren). The mechanisms of reactions of this type are well known; the basic reaction paths are shown in Figure 3.9. Is the conversion of a metal hydroxide to a potentially toxic metal-protein possible or not? Chemical data for titanium, zirconium, niobium and tantalum show that organic complexes of this type are unlikely and it is also known that organometallic compounds of these elements, as far as they exist, are unstable.

Titanium as an Implant Material

Attempts have been made to compare titanium with aluminum oxide ceramics and the so-called bioactive materials such as Bioglass and sintered hydroxyapatite. However, this is not entirely correct, as neither the metal itself nor its ions in solution are present. The chemical behavior of titanium is determined solely by its surface oxide. The mass of available physiologic data must be interpreted in the light of this fact.

Human beings ingest a considerable amount of titanium in many chemical forms per day in their diets (see Table 3.**4**). About 40% of the total amount ingested or about 300 µg per day are metabolized. Even though this figure may not be very accurate, it is clearly very much higher (about 10 000 times) than the amount the oxidation of a titanium implant can "deliver" (see Table 3.**2**). Therefore, the presence of a titanium implant is irrelevant to the total titanium "load" in the body, and systematic reactions (allergy) or deposition in the organs do not occur. Furthermore, the biologic half-life (320 days) is far too short for titanium to accumulate in the body.

Table 3.**4** contains the results from a collection of tissue analyses. If the titanium analysis for the whole body or for muscle tissue is compared with the data in Figure 3.**3** or Table 3.**3**, some correspondence is obvious. Is this purely coincidental? Surely not; rather, the titanium concentration found in the tissue is identical to the saturation solubility of the oxide, i.e., the maximum possible level. More of the oxide simply cannot go into solution, which means that if a foreign body in the form of a titanium implant is added to the system, then its surface oxide will not dissolve. The metal, described in terms used in radiation protection, is neither "available" nor "transportable." This explains, on the basis of chemical principles, why titanium is inert in body tissue.

Further analyses describing the amount of titanium found in tissues adjacent to titanium implants are presented in Table 3.**4**. The concentrations reported are often very much higher than the normal levels for titanium in

Table 3.**4** Chemical data for titanium in the body

a) *Metabolic data* (*Bowen*; *Steinemann* und *Perren*)	
Titanium compounds in diet	ca. 800 µg (Ti)/g
Metabolized (excreted in urine)	ca. 300 µg (Ti)/g
b) *Typical analyses of tissue,* based on fresh tissue (FT) (ICRP, *Ferguson* et al.; *Bowen*; *Willems* et al.; *Ducheyne* et al.; *Meachem* and *Williams*; *Simpson* et al.; *Moosmann*; *Steinemann* and *Perren*)	
Average for whole body (15 mg out of 70 kg)	0.21 µg (Ti)/gFT
Normal amount in muscle	0.13/0.19–0.47 µg (Ti)/gFT
Around an implant in muscle or spongiosa	2.6/30/3.9 µg (Ti)/gFT
Around a fracture-fixation implant	109/280/27 µg (Ti)/gFT

3 The Properties of Titanium

tissue around single implants and, in particular, in connection with fracture plates. Inter- and intracellular impregnation of the tissue is observed; the source is either residues from implant surface treatment or products of mechanical wear because implants are in contact. Despite this impregnation, cell function was not impaired (Riede et al., Simpson et al.). Even the fine wear particles are inert.

Plasma Coating

The reason for coating is to produce a rough implant surface that greatly improves implant anchorage power in bone. The industrial process is not new, and is used for both metals and ceramics. The process functions as follows: an inert gas is blown through an intense electric arc and the coating material, in this case titanium hydride, is introduced into the extremely hot gas immediately downstream of the arc (Fig. 3.**10**) (see also pages 72–3). The inert gas is broken down into ions and electrons in the arc; physicists describe this state as a plasma. The titanium hydride decomposes in the gas stream and forms droplets of molten metal that are projected onto the

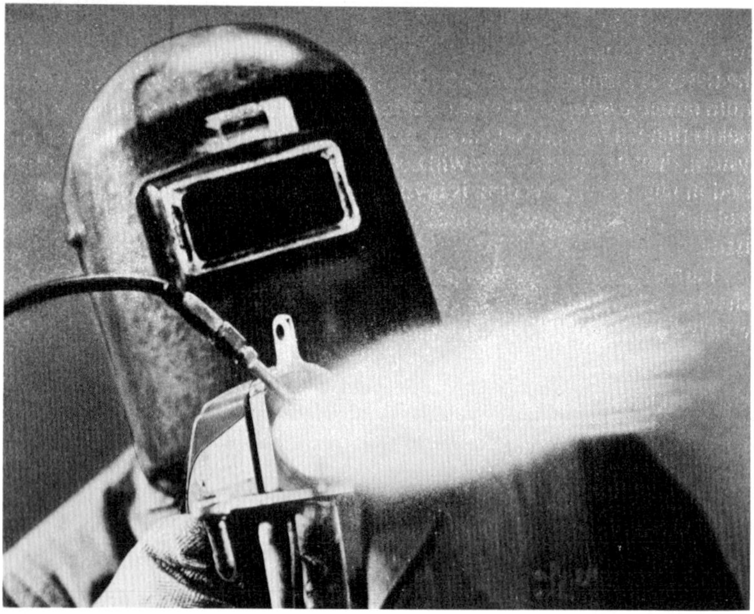

Fig. 3.**10** The plasma spraying process. The plasma gun is a high-intensity electric arc burning in a gas stream; titanium is introduced as a powder into this gas stream, where it melts

implant suface to build up a coating. The layer is typically 20–30 μm thick with a roughness of about 15 μm. The surface of the coating is rough with round forms, although highly porous but continuous. Figure 3.**11** shows that the coating is also partially "welded" to the substrate.

The molten metal droplets come into contact with air between the plasma gun and the implant, and absorb some oxygen and nitrogen. Chemical analyses of the plasma-deposited coating show that it contains about 9% oxygen, 3% nitrogen and 0.1% carbon; X-ray diffraction analysis reveals about 15% ∂-titanium oxynitride along with some rutile (titanium dioxide) in an α-titanium matrix. The gases dissolve in the molten metal, where they partially react to form oxide phases. The gas uptake also increases the solidification temperature, and this helps to produce a rougher surface.

The electrochemical behavior of plasma-coated titanium in physiologic saline at 40 °C is very similar to that of normal titanium with respect to its oxidation and corrosion properties. The potentials in the galvanic series are almost identical (see Fig. 3.**2**), namely, +0.34 V_H for the plasma coating, +0.18 V_H for a freshly pickled coating (dilute HF and HNO_3), and +0.32 V_H for pickled unalloyed titanium. The currents measured on these materials at the above potentials are, however, different: 3.5, 11 and 0.9 mA per cm^2 geometric surface, respectively. This variation is entirely due to the porosity of the layer; the plasma coating has an effectives surface areal 12 times that of a piece of solid titanium of identical shape. The chemical nature of the surface itself has been investigated by X-ray excited photoelectron spectroscopy (ESCA). This technique gives information on the state of the material to a depth of about 5 nm (i.e., about 20 atomic layers). The spectra from plasma-sprayed and massive titanium surfaces are virtually identical and are characteristic of a an oxide film containing IV-valent titanium. The spectral lines from titanium are weak; the thickness of the oxide film is about 3 nm. All these observations lead to the conclusion that the plasma coating is chemically compatible, and, more important, that its biological compatibility is at least as good as that of normal titanium.

Gases in titanium harden the metal, an enhancement that is advantageous for the surface of an implant. Gases also render titanium brittle, but this is inconsequential, as dental implants are not loaded outside the elastic range. The bond strength between the porous plasma layer and the substrate is limited, but brutal treatment is required to cause this bond to fail, e.g., bending the implant or exposure to an intense ultrasound source, e.g., the tip of an ultrasonic scaler. In practice, the bond between the coating and the bulk metal must only withstand the modest shear and tensile forces generated between implant and bone; experiments have shown that either the bone fractures or the implant head is broken off before the plasma coating separates from its substrate.

3 The Properties of Titanium

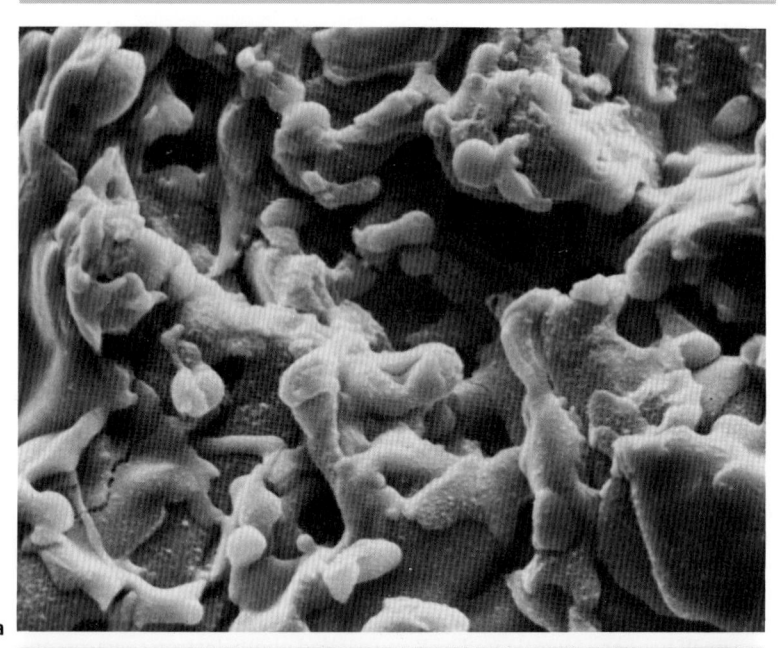

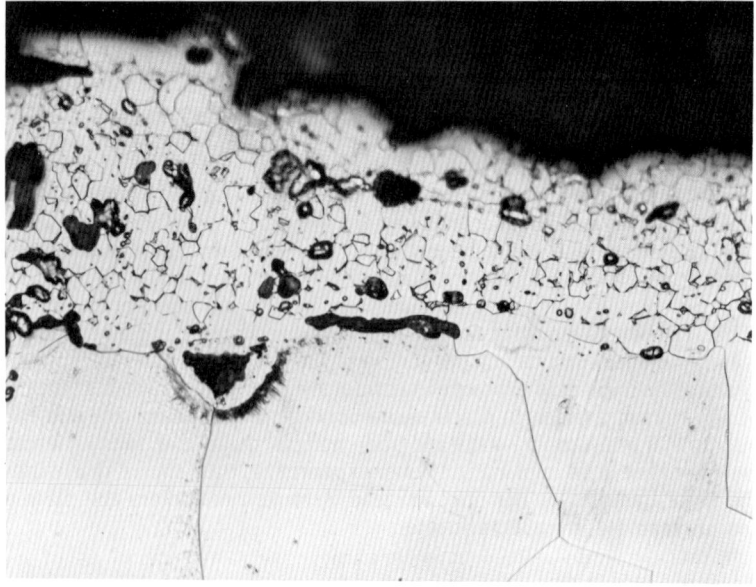

Osteointegration

Effectiveness

A solid bond is observed in vivo between a titanium implant and bone. This ankylotic anchorage, also termed osteointegration, is accepted today as the most promising method of stabilizing endosteal implants and endoprostheses (see pages 100–7).

Histologically, osteointegration is recognizable by the presence of regenerated bone right up to the metal surface (see pages 91–100). The structure in the contact region can be studied in detail using X-ray microanalysis. Histologic preparations are perfectly adequate for this purpose. Figure 3.**12** shows a highly magnified contact region of functionally loaded hollow cylinder implant after more than a year in situ. The plasma titanium particles are clearly recognizable in the scanning micrograph using secondary electrons; lamellar bone with its characteristic lacunae seems to have penetrated

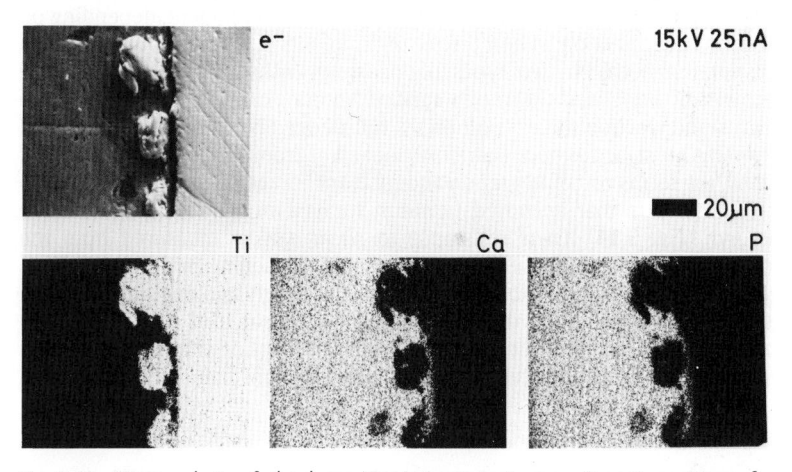

Fig. 3.**12** Microanalysis of the bone-titanium contact zone. Scanning picture for secondary electrons (e) and characteristic X-ray emissions of titanium (Ti), calcium (Ca) and phosphorus (P). The distribution of elements shows perfect integration, since the calcium and phosphorus images exactly replicate the titanium

◀ Fig. 3.**11** Scanning electron micrograph of the plasma coating (**a**), and metallography of a plasma-coated implant surface (**b**). The rough surface structure is clearly visible in the scanning micrograph; the porosity of the coating and grain structure of the wrought implant material are shown in the section (Magnifications: **a** 2450 x, **b** 350 x)

into the porous surface. Scanning pictures using the characteristic elemental X-ray emissions for titanium, calcium and phosphorus show how complete the anchorage is; the Ca and P regions are exact replicas of the titanium picture. It is noteworthy that the relative intensities of Ca and P are constant throughout, which is a good indication that the osseous tissue is fully mineralized. Quantitative analyses along single-line scans through the contact zone further show that bone has approached to within less than 0.5 µm of the metal surface, leaving a gap which is so small that the presence of any organized tissue between bone and metal can be ruled out. Osteointegration must therefore be a process that functions at the molecular level.

The interaction between tissue or bone and a biomaterial is always a complex physicochemical and ultrastructural process. The question that has to be answered in the case of functional dental implants is: "Can an effective and lasting bond be formed that can also transmit loads?"

The implant and hence the implant/bone interface is loaded in all possible directions (Fig. 3.**13**). The load can be directed along the interface as shear force or as tension or compression. Most loads are complex in that they are made up of a shear and a tensile or compressive component, depending on the loading direction. When discussing implants it is important to make a distinction between two types of loads; to withstand shear forces, the growth of bone into the rough surface (interlocking) is sufficient, but to withstand traction forces (pull-off), a full-fledged bond between bone and implant must be formed. Therefore, looked at from the functional point of view, the terms osteointegration and total anchorage must be synonymous.

The loads that anchored titanium-sprayed implants can sustain are known (Fig. 3.**14**). Their resistance to *shear* can be measured from the moment required to loosen bone screws. This loosening moment increases greatly with time as the bone grows into the rough implant surface, and a simple conversion gives the shear strength as shear load per unit contact area. The *pull-off* resistance is measured by implanting titanium discs with specially prepared surfaces in a milled bone implant bed and pulling them

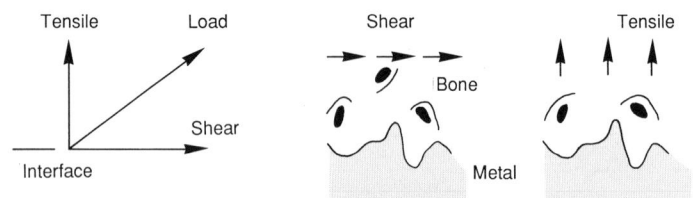

Fig. 3.**13** The loads acting on the metal surface can come from any direction. Growth of bone into the rough surface interlocks the two materials and effectively transmits shear loads acting parallel to the interface. Resistance to tensile (pull-off) loads requires more than this, namely: a bond between metal and bone

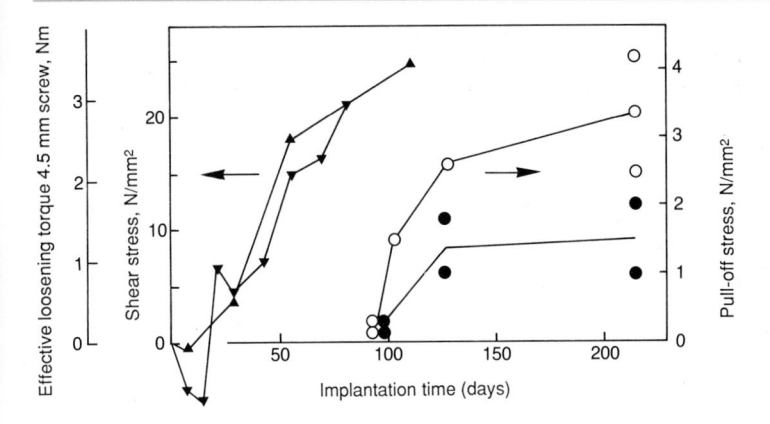

Fig. 3.14 Anchoring ability of implants in cortical bone. The graph shows the results of experiments to determine the turn-out torques for bone screws (▲▼), and pull-off loads for titanium discs (● ○). Clinically, the incubation period is important; the anchorage can resist shear forces after about 3 weeks, but a bond to resist pull-off requires 3 months to form

out (vertically) after various implantation times. Nothing happens for quite a long period until, after about 100 days, it becomes evident that a bone/implant bond has formed.

The strength of a titanium implant anchorage can never reach that of bone itself. The comparison in Table 3.5 shows that the maximum shear strength of the interface is about $1/3$ that of cortical bone and that the pull-off strength is about equal to the tensile strength of low-density cancellous bone. Nevertheless, these are good results. How high are the functional forces that can be supported by a typical implant (Figure 3.15)? Axial forces

Table 3.5 Mechanical data for bone and anchored implants

a) Anchorage of titanium implants with rough surfaces		
	Strength	Latency for anchorage
Shear strength at the interface	up to 25 MPa	20–30 days
Pull-off strength	ca. 3 MPa	ca. 100 days

b) Strength of human bone	
Tensile strength of cortical bone	ca. 150 MPa
Shear (tortional) strength of cortical bone	ca. 70 MPa
Compressive strength of cancellous bone	1–10 MPa

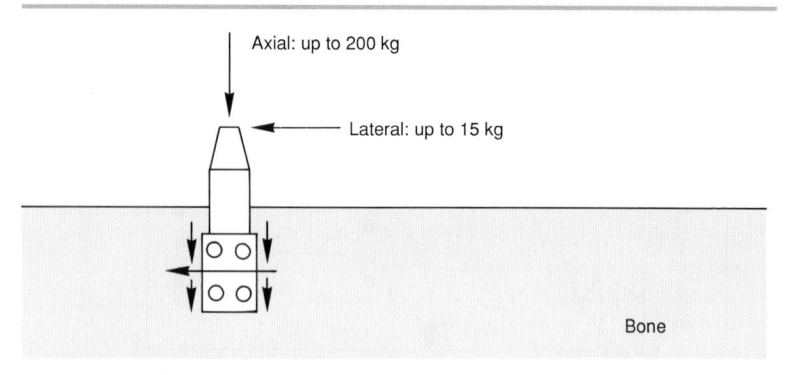

Fig. 3.**15** Maximum loads an implant can support; limit given by the anchorage of a rough implant in bone

of over 100 kg and shear forces of about 15 kg are necessary to break off a 4-mm diameter, 10-mm long hollow cylinder from bone. Such an anchorage can rightly be described as ankylotic.

The importance of osteointegration goes beyond simple load-bearing considerations. In Figure 3.**15** an arrow is drawn right through the implant; it symbolizes that the forces are transmitted through the implant into the bone when total anchorage is present; this is not the case without bonding, i.e., for press-fit or congruent anchorage, as tensile forces are not transmitted. This can be demonstrated using photoelastic stress-analysis techniques (see pages 80–5). The uninterrupted flow of stresses is the favorable precondition for functional adaptation of bone, and these mechanisms – a central aspect of Wolff's law – are carefully considered in bone surgery.

Clinical experience has shown that implants should first be loaded only about 3 to 4 months post implantation (except when primarily stabilized). Micromovements seem to disturb the osteogenesis process; this applies to both titanium and bioactive materials such as bioglasses and phosphates. The results given in Figure 3.**14** are for unloaded implants. They show a latency period of about 20 days for the bone to begin to grow into the rough implant surface and about 100 days, or $3^{1}/_{2}$ months, for bone to grow onto the implant surface. This timetable for incorporation in two stages is paralleled in the healing of bone fractures (Schenk), whereby the gap is quickly bridged by less organized bone, followed by stabilization through generalized bone remodelling. These processes can be followed by sequential labeling. Using this technique in the late healing-in phase of a dental implant, it was demonstrated that bone remodelling occurs *from the metal surface outwards,* a clear indication of total integration.

A Model of the Bond

The rather surprising fact that a bond is formed between bone and titanium begs the question as to whether there is any stimulus for bone attachment or bioactivity present. According to Hench, a bioactive material induces a specific biologic reaction at its surface, which results in a bond being formed between the implant and tissue or bone. Titanium does not fit into this classification because, as has been discussed earlier in this chaper, the metal with its protective oxide is inert in tissue and is neither mobile nor available. The vehicle for the attachment of bone lies elsewhere, probably in specific surface chemical processes.

A layer of organic matter 5 nm thick is found on fracture treatment plates when routinely removed after about 2 years. This layer can only be broken down by the strongest oxidizing agent (chlorax, chloric acid) or the strongest complexing agent (EDTA). This intensive interaction between metal and living tissue clearly indicates the presence of a genuine physicochemical bond.

Albrektsson used high-resolution electron microscopy to study the bonetitanium interface. He found a layer or matrix material about 20 nm

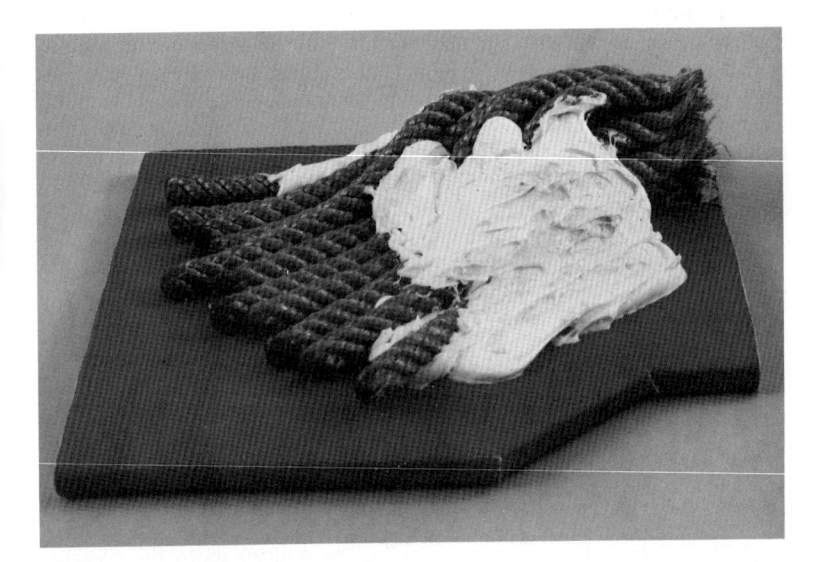

Fig. 3.**16** Model of the submicroscopic structures and bodies involved in osteointegration. The organic structural elements of bone, the collagen fiber bundles, are "glued" to the oxide surface of reactive titanium. The molecules of the "glue material" are of roughly the same size as the thickness of the "glue layer"

thick and then, at a distance of about 100 nm, massively mineralized collagen fibers; in between, the fibrils and mineral deposits were not organized. The main components of the bone ground substance were proteoglycans, giant molecules about the same size as the contact region. Biochemists have identified these substances as the "glue" between cells and between cells and other surfaces, including those of foreign bodies. These findings lead to a model for bonding on an atomic and molecular scale (Fig. 3.**16**).

The "gluing" of tissue or biomolecules to titanium or, more correctly, to its surface, is distinctive. It is otherwise only observed on so-called bioactive substances (bioglasses, hydroxyapatite), but not in conjunction with plastics, aluminum oxide or other metals used in bone surgery.

The surface of a metal oxide is normally hydroxylated, i.e., the free metal ligands in the surface of the crystal break up water molecules and saturate or screen their strong positive charge with negatively-charged hydroxyl ions (Boehm). In the case of titanium oxide (Fig. 3.**17**), for every water molecule split, two hydroxyl groups are produced, which are differently positioned on the surface and produce an acid or base property in their vicinity. These bipolar or amphoteric forms can function like tongs or a claw (Greek χηλη), hence the term chelate. An important characteristic of amphoteric materials is their point-of-zero charge. This is measured as the pH value at which the positive and negative charges at the surface are exactly balanced. The point for titanium oxide is at pH ≈ 6.2. Amino acids, the elementary building blocks of all biologic molecules, are also bipolar; they are ampholytes that can react as an acid (because of the carboxyl groups) or as bases (because of the amino groups). These hybrid ions are naturally ideal partners for chemisorption,

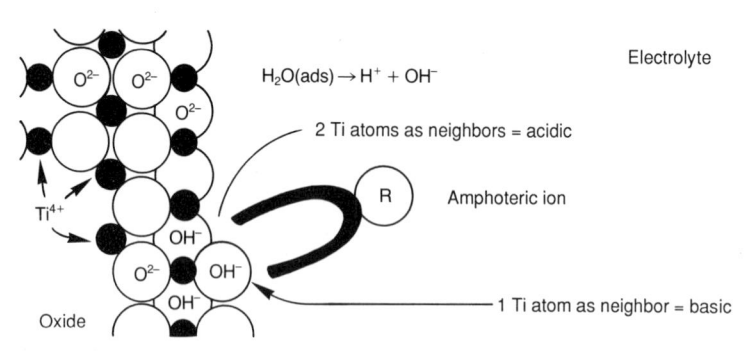

Fig. 3.**17** Surface reaction of titanium oxide. The diagram shows the crystalline (layered) structure of small Ti ions and large O ions. At the interface, hydroxyl ions are formed from the splitting of water molecules; positive and negative charges are produced, which locally give the surface an acidic or basic character – conditions favorable for a strong, permanent bond to organic molecules

forming a strong double bond with amphoteric hydroxylated titanium oxide. This reaction has been confirmed by photoelectron spectroscopy.

It is also interesting to note that hydroxyapatite has a point-of-zero charge (pH ≈ 7) similar to that of hydroxylated titanium oxide. This relation between electrical properties and absorption is very important in relation to the observed attachment of bone and tissue to titanium; it seems, to put it simply, that "living tissue mistakes reactive titanium for bone mineral."

References

Titanium in Surgery

Perren, S. M., M. Russenberger, S. Steinemann, et al. A dynamic compression plate and clinical experience with a new compression plate "DCP". Acta. Orthop. Scand. Suppl. 125 (1969) 31–61

Riede, U. N., T. Rüedi, Y. L. E. Rohner, S. Perren, R. Guggenheim, F. Limacher. Quantitative und morphologische Erfassung der Gewebeaktion auf Metallimplantate (Osteosynthesematerial), 1: Eine morphometrische, histologische, mikroanalytische und rasterelektronenmikroskopische Studie am Schafsknochen; 2: Untersuchungen am Menschen. Arch. Orthop. Unfallchir. 78 (1974) 199–215; 79:215–25

Simpson, J. P., V. Geret, S. A. Brown, K. Merritt. Retrieved fracture plates: implant and tissue analysis. In A. Weinstein, D. Gibbons, S. Brown, W. Ruff. Implant retrieval: material and biological analysis. NBS Spec. Publ. 601 (1981) 395–422

Corrosion

Fontana, M. G., N. D. Greene. Corrosion engineering. McGraw-Hill, New York 1967

Hoar, T. P., D. C. Mears. Corrosion-resistant alloys in chloride solutions: materials for surgical implants. Proc. R. Soc. London 294 A (1966) 486–510

Pourbaix, M., et al.: Atlas d'équilibres électrochimiques. Gauthier-Villars, Paris 1963

Stegemann, K. Korrosionserscheinungen an Dentallegierung, Part 1 and 2. Dtsch. Zahnärztl. Z. 11 (1956) 391–401, 13 (1958) 104–13

Steinemann, S. G. Corrosion of Titanium and -Ti-Alloys for Surgical Implants. In G. Lütjering, U. Zwicker, W. Bunk. Titanium, science and technology. Proc. 5th Int. Conf. Dtsch. Ges. Metallkd, Oberursel 1985 (p. 1373–1379)

Tissue Tolerance

Luckey, T. D., B. Venugopal. Metal toxicity in mammals. Vol 1. Physiologic and chemical basis for metal toxicity. Vol 2: Chemical toxicity of metals and metalloids. Plenun, New York 1977–8

Steinemann, S. G. Korrosion, Verträglichkeit und mechanische Eigenschaften von metallischen Allenthesen. In K. Schuchardt, B. Spiessl. Fortschritte der Kiefer- und Gesichts-Chirurgie. Vol 19. Thieme, Stuttgart: 1975 (p. 50–56)

Steinemann, S. G., S. M. Perren. Titanlegierungen für Implantate: physiko-chemische Prinzipien. In 5. Vortragsreihe des DVM-Arbeitskreises Implantate. Deutscher Verband für Materialprüfung, Berlin 1985 (p. 63–73)

Zitter, H. Schädigung des Gewebes durch metallische Implantate. Unfallheilkd. 79 (1976) 91–100

Properties of Titanium Oxide

Baes, C. F., R. E. Mesmer. The hydrolysis of cations. Wiley, New York 1976

Boehm, H. P. Funktionelle Gruppen an Festkörper-Oberflächen. Angew. Chem. 78 (1966) 617–28

Osseointegration

Albrektsson, T., P. I. Brånemark, H. A. Hansson, et al. The interface zone of inorganic implants in vivo: titanium implants in bone. Ann. Biomed. Eng. 11 (1983) 1–27

Carlsson, L., T. Rostlund, B. Albrektsson, T. Albrektsson. Removal torques for polished and rough titanium implants. Int J. Oral. Maxillofac. Surg. 3 (1988) 21–4

Eulenberger, J., F. Keller, A. Schroeder, S. G. Steinemann. Haftung zwischen Knochen und Titan. In 4. Vortragsreihe des DVM-Arbeitskreises Implantate. Deutscher Verband für Materialprüfung, Berlin 1984 (p. 131–134)

Hench, L. L. The interfacial behavoir of biomaterials. J. Biomed. Mater. Res. 1980; 14 (1980) 803–11

Lausmaa, J., L. Linder. Surface spectroscopic characterization of titanium implants after separation from plastic-embedded tissue. Biomaterials 9 (1988) 277–80

Mäusli, P. A., P. R. Bloch, V. Geret, S. G. Steinemann. Surface characterization of titanium and Ti-alloys. In P. Christel, A. Meunier, A. J. C. Lee. Biological and biomechanical performance of biomaterials. Elsevier, Amsterdam 1986 (p. 57–62)

Schenk, R. K. Die Histologie der primären Knochenheilung im Lichte neuer Konzeptionen über den Knochenumbau. Unfallheilkd. 81 (1978) 219–27

Skalak, R. Biomechanical considerations in osseointegrated prostheses. J Prosthet. Dent. 49 (1983) 843–8

Steinemann, S. G., J. Eulenberger, P. A. Mäusli, A. Schroeder. Adhesion of bone to titanium. In P. Christel, A. Meunier, A. J. C. Lee. Biological and biomechanical performance of biomaterials. Elsevier, Amsterdam 1986 (p. 409–414)

Sundgren, J. E., P. Bodö, I. Lundström. Auger electron spectroscopics studies of the inerface between human tissue and implants of titanium and stainless steel. Academic Press, San Diego 1986

The ITI System

4 A Brief History of Implantology

A. Schroeder

Introduction

The wish to replace lost teeth in one way or another with implants has occupied man's spirit for centuries or even milennia. A Honduran skull dating from pre-Columbian times is often mentioned in the literature; one of the lower lateral incisors was a black stone. It can be assumend that the stone was in place for a considerable time, as it was covered with the same amount of calculus as its natural neighbors.

A good summary of historical data from the 16th to 20th centuries can be found in Sandhaus' (1975) book on implantology and in Wahl's (1985) inaugural paper. In the course of the last 50 years, four different implantation methods have been developed and put into practice, albeit with varying success:
- transdental fixation (transfixation);
- submucosal implants;
- subperiostal implants;
- endosteal implants.

Transfixation

This method is advantageous because it does not have to deal with the problems of a pillar penetrating the mucosa. The natural tooth root and epithelial attachment are retained; in this sense it is, in principle, a *closed* implant system, in contrast to the other methods.

Submucosal Implants

This method involves implanting small button-like retention elements under the mucous membrane, with the purpose of providing retention for a total prosthesis, particularly in the maxilla. Submucosal implants can claim some success, but the method has not gained wide acceptance.

Subperiosteal Implants

The basic idea was conceived half a century ago (Müller 1937) and followed up by many practitioners and clinical researchers (Dahl, Gershkoff, Goldberg, Ogus, Hammer, Reichenbach, Marziani, Schwindling, Obwegeser, Kallenberger and Maeglin, Koele, Wunderer and Spiessl, just to mention a few). The first author of the present book implanted a few vitallium subperiosteal

Introduction

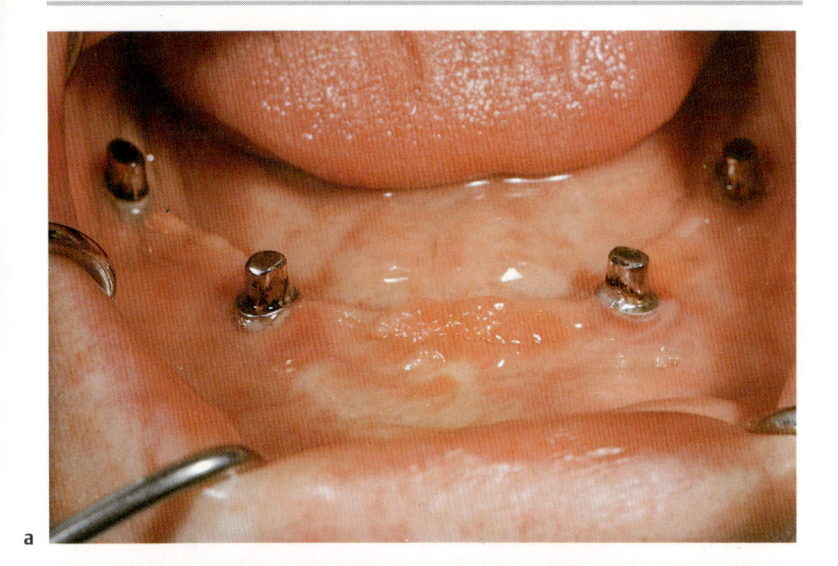

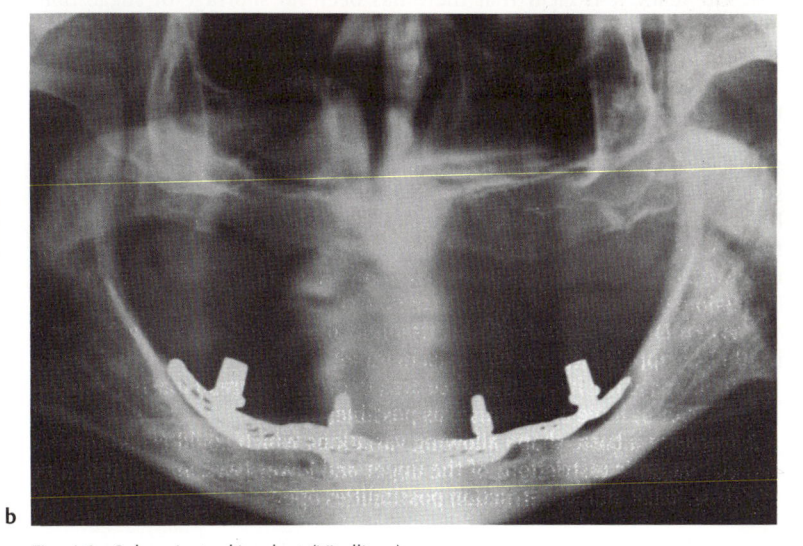

Fig. 4.1 Subperiosteal implant (Vitallium)
a Clinical condition 20 years after implantation
b radiograph 28 years after implantation, shortly before removal

supports in the mandible in a two-stage procedure 40 years ago. One of these remained functional for 29 years before its removal because of sporadic recurrent infections (Fig. 4.**1**). This isolated case is only mentioned here in order to give those people who remain sceptical towards, or completely reject, oral implantology cause to reconsider their position. Even if, as in this case, the subperiosteal support was clinically only tolerated rather than accepted, when looked at from the patient's point of view, it provided invaluable service for over a quarter of a century.

In other words: to show an interest in the problems of oral implantology is not a priori equal to showing a complete lack of common sense!

To return to subperiosteal implants, the high failure rates have led to a loss of interest in this type of implant since the 1960s. However, it would not be proper to ignore the potential of subperiosteal implants, as there will always be cases in which, because of insufficient bone mass, the problem cannot be solved by either an endosteal implant or preprosthetic surgery.

Endosteal Implants

Looking at the history of endosteal implants and their development over the last 100 years, it is clear that there has been no shortage of suggestions involving all imaginable *designs.* It was, however, exceptional for these to be supported by any form of basic research and development.

As early as 1913, Greenfield presented a paper on a cagelike implant made of platinum-iridium to the Academy of Stomatology in Philadelphia. 25 years later, the Strock brothers experimented with vitallium screws, using a passive (inert) material for the first time. Various screw designs were subsequently developed by Formiggini, Zepponi, Cherchève, Tramonte, Heinrich, Sandhaus, Brånemark, and others, whereby alongside stainless steel and chrome-cobalt-molybdenum alloys, titanium, tantalum and aluminum oxide were often recommended. Nail-like implants were propagated by Scialom ("tripod") and Pruin ("nail road").

When Linkow introduced his titanium-blade implants ("blade-vents") in 1967, he apparently had two aims in mind:
1. To increase the implant surface area in order to spread masticatory forces over as large a bone mass as possible;
2. To create a basic shape allowing variations which could accommodate all anatomic restrictions of the upper and lower jaws, and, at the same time, leave all reconstruction possibilities open.

Linkow's blade implants and many similar designs (Cranin, Muratori, Pasqualini, Heinrich, and others) have achieved worldwide acceptance.

Yet other designs have emerged in the last 20 years: Koch and Kirsch (IMZ-implants), Schulte (Tübingen immediate implant), Mutschelknauss, Brinkmann, Doerre (anchor and arrowhead pin). The system developed by the Göteborg group of Brånemark has attained a special status, as their basic experimental work dates back as far as the mid 1960s. In the meantime, an impressive amount of data has been collected, which is continuously being evaluated and updated. The basic element is a titanium screw (Fig. 4.2).

The Development of the ITI-System

The ITI hollow cylinder implants were developed in the course of close cooperation between the Department of Operative Dentistry, University of Berne, Switzerland, and the Straumann Institute, Waldenburg, Switzerland (a private research company), after both institutions had originally started on the clinical evaluation and possible improvement of Herkovits' tantalum implants.

The double-blade implant suggested by Herkovits and first described by Schroeder was not followed up, because both sides soon became aware of the lack of biomechanical and histological supporting data. It was then decided (1973) that before progress could be made, some basic research was necessary, independent of any preconceived implant design.

The clinic in Berne was willing and able to perform animal experiments and histologic evaluation, and the biomechanical and materials-science aspects could be handled by the Straumann Institute with their long experience in osteosynthesis. Of primary interest were the following material/surface combinations:

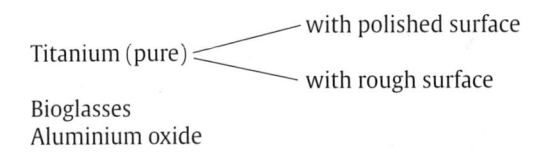

Titanium (pure)
- with polished surface
- with rough surface

Bioglasses
Aluminium oxide

The latter material was included despite the fact that several years before, the clinic in Berne had studied the tissue reaction to Sandhaus's (CBS) aluminum oxide implant (thesis, Sterchi 1972) (see page 7). The results of

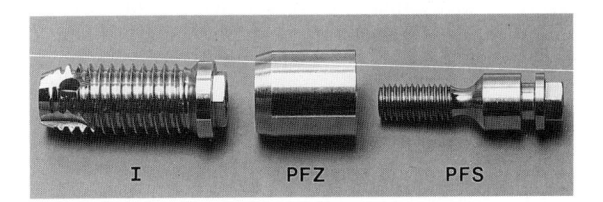

Fig. 4.2 Screw implant ("fixture") after Brånemark
(**I** = implant, **PFZ** = post cylinder, **PfS** = abutment screw)

64 4 A Brief History of Implantology

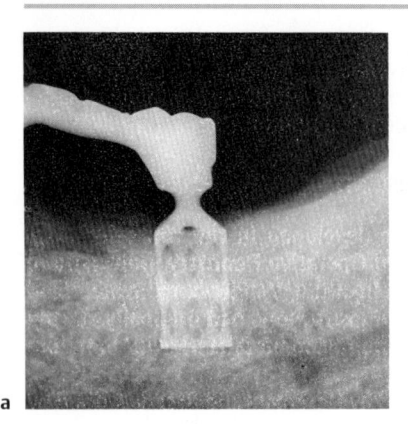

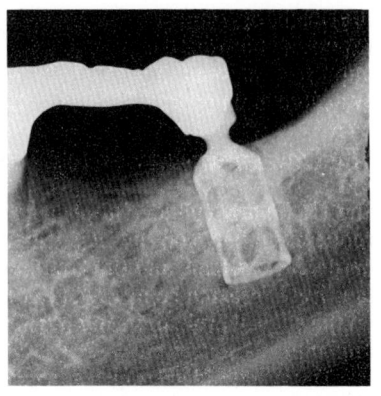

Fig. 4.**3a, b** X-rays of the first hollow cylinder implant, introduced into a patient in 1974. **a** One year after implantation, **b** Twenty years after implantation

this work will not be discussed here, with the important exception of the data on titanium (see Chap. 6).

The work on pure titanium has shown that this is the material of choice with respect to its biologic-histologic behavior. It must be said at this point that much of the material-technological background and testing methods which are necessary for oral implantology have antecedents and equivalents in the field of orthopedic surgery.

A simple hollow cylinder, which was primarily thought to be suitable for animal experiments in *Macaca speciosa* monkeys, was designed by Sutter. This implant was used in a patient as early as 1974, more by accident than intent, only because implantation of a Heskovits implant had failed. Despite the fact that the use of the hollow cylinder was premature, if for no other reason than a lack of adequate instruments, this implant is still in place today – 1995 (Fig. 4.**3**). It has never been cause for any complaint; bone and mucosal margin are healthy. Apart from this unplanned use of a "pioneer hollow cylinder," clinical tests were only started after satisfactory results in animals were achieved and the instrumentation was sufficiently advanced to justify implantation in humans. This procedure is one of the fundamental guidelines of the research program.

References

Adell, R., U. Lekholm, P. Rockler, P. I. Brånemark. A 15-year study of osseointegrated implants in the treatment of the edentulous jaw. Int. J. Oral. Maxillofac. Surg. 10 (1981) 387

Babbush, C. A. Implantationen im Kieferbereich – Indikationen und Techniken. Zahnärztlich-medizinisches Schrifttum, Munich 1984

Brånemark, P. I., U. Breine, R. Adell, B. O. Hansson, J. Lindström, A. Ohlsson. Intraosseous anchorage of dental prostheses. Scand. J. Plast. Reconstr. Surg. 3 (1969) 81

Dahl, G. S. A. Om möjligheten för Implantation i käken av metallskelett sombas eller retention för fasta eller avtagbare proteser. T. Odont. 51 (1943) 440

Franke, J. Der heutige Stand der Implantologie. Hanser, Munich 1980

Frenkel, G. Erfahrungen mit der subperiostalen Gerüstplantation im Unterkiefer. Dtsch. Zahnärztebl. 7 (1957) 227

Goldberg, N. I., A. Gershkoff. The implant lower denture. Dent. Dig. 55 (1949) 490

Hammer, H. Indikation und Kontraindikation zur subperiostalen Gerüsteinpflanzung. Dtsch. Zahnärztl. Z. 10 (1955) 1101

Herschfeld, J. J. Classics in dental history: E. J. Greenfield and artificial implants. Bull. Hist. Dent. 1 (1984) 33–41

Kallenberger, K., B. Maeglin. Zur Frage der Einheilungsvorgänge bei Gerüstimplantaten. Schweiz. Monatsschr. Zahnheilkd. 67 (1967) 300

Kirsch, A. Fünf Jahre IMZ-Implantat-System – Grundalgen, Methodik, Erfahrungen. In Franke J. Der heutige Stand der Implantologie. Hanser Munich, 1980

Koch, W. L. Die zweiphasige enossale Implantation von intramobilen Zylinderimplantaten IMZ (2). Quintessenz 27 (1976)

Lindquist, L. W., G. E. Carlsson, P. O. Glantz. Rehabilitation of the edentulous mandible with a tissue-integrated fixed prothesis: a six-year longitudinal study. Quintessence Int. 18 (1987) 89–96

Maeglin, B. Über langjährige Erfahrungen mit subperiostalen Gerüstimplantaten in der Mundhöhle. Schweiz. Monatsschr. Zahnheilkd. 77 (1967) 232

Marziani, L. Subperiostale Gerüstimplantate zu prothetischen Zwecken. Dtsch. Zahnärztl. Z. 10 (1955) 1115

Obwegeser, H. Implantate zur Verankerung von partiellem und totalem Zahnersatz. In K. Schuchardt. Die Zahn-, Mund- und Kieferheilkunde, vol 3:2. Urban and Schwarzenberg, Munich 1959

Sandhaus, S. Neue Aspekte der Implantologie. Medica, Stuttgart 1975

Schroeder, A. Histologische und klinische Beobachtungen bei der Erprobung von Hohlzylinder-Implantaten unter besonderer Berücksichtigung der Titanspritzschicht-Oberfläche. In J. Franke. Der heutige Stand der Implantologie. Hanser, Munich 1980

Schulte, W. Das enossale Tübinger Implantat aus Al_2O_3 (Frialit®): der Entwicklungsstand nach 6 Jahren; 1, 2. Zahnärztl. Mitt. 71 (1981) 1114, 1181

Sutter, F., A. Schroeder, F. Straumann. ITI-Hohlzylindersysteme – Prinzipien, Methodik. Swiss. Dent. 4 (1983) 21

Tetsch, P. Systeme der Implantologie. In W. Ketterl. Deutscher Zahnärztekalender 1982. Hanser, Munich 1982

Wahl, G. Neuere Möglichkeiten zur Kontrolle enossaler Einheilungsvorgänge in der zahnärztlichen Implantologie mit Hilfe der Szintigraphie. [Postdoctoral thesis]. Bonn, 1985

Zarb, G. A., F. L. Zarb. Tissue-integrated dental prosthesis. Quintessence Int. 16 (1985) 39–42

5 Stages in the Development of the ITI Implant

A. Schroeder and F. Sutter

Following the emergence of technically pure titanium as the preferred material for implants, the authors, as previously mentioned, succeeded in making implants that were ideally suited for animal experiments on macaque monkeys (*Macaca speciosa*).

The mechanical design criteria placed upon an implant led to the choice of a hollow implant as a basic design concept. (F. Sutter). This concept is used in both the hollow cylinder and the hollow screw. In the case of the hollow cylinder, it has evolved into several different forms.

In all of its variations, the implant is shaped so that even under heavy loading, it produces no points of excessive stress concentration in the bone.

All other critical factors, such as strength and biocompatibility of the materials, microstructure of the implant's surface, and a high degree of primary stability were also taken into account.

Implant Design

Transverse openings in the side walls and oblique holes at the shoulder were characteristic of the early hollow cylinders (and hollow screw implants with outside diameters of 5.5 mm) (Fig. 5.**1**). In the expectation that bone would grow over the shoulder, provided it was sunk deeply enough, the neck of the implant was made as narrow as strength requirements would permit at the point where it emerges from the tissue.

The considerations of bone healing and overgrowth were explored by Schroeder and co-workers through clinical observations, experiments on animals, and above all, histological studies (1976 and 1978, p. 83 f.).

Minor modifications of these first trial implants led to the standard implant, designated as Type C, which was subsequently inserted and tested in patients (Fig. 5.**2**).

To accommodate the less-than-ideal jaw conditions that are frequently encountered, especially in the lateral and posterior regions of the mandible, various other types of implants were developed (Fig. 5.**3**).

These so-called extension implants are no longer in use and have been completely replaced by the rotationally symmetrical, one-and two-part implants of today's ITI concept (chapter 7). While the extension implants (Types E, K, and H) had certain advantages over the C type, especially in ridges distal to shortened dental arches ("free-end" situations), there were

Implant Design

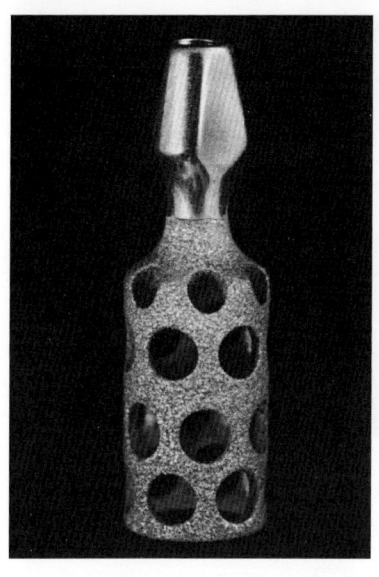

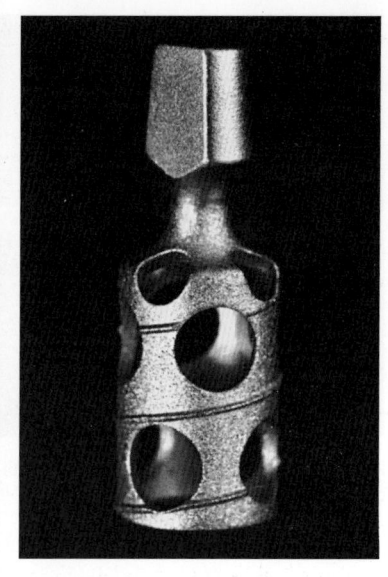

Fig. 5.1 Implants developed in 1974: **a** = hollow cylinder; **b** = hollow screw
These have both transverse holes and holes through their shoulders

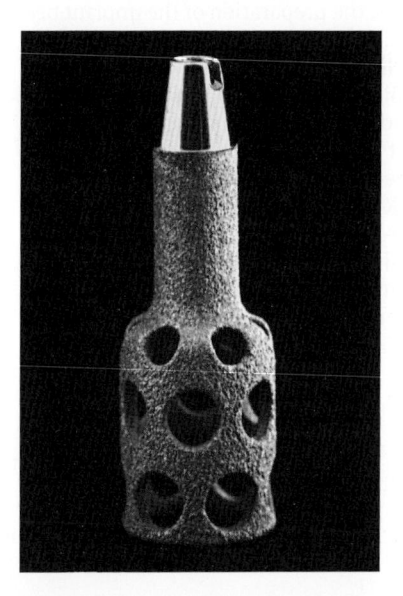

Fig. 5.2 The standard Type-C hollow cylinder implant

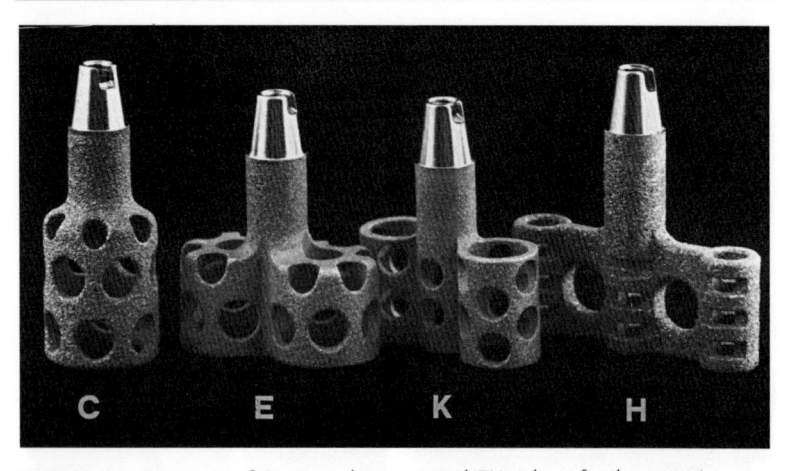

68 5 Stages in the Development of the ITI Implant

Fig. 5.3 An assortment of titanium plasma-coated ITI implants for the posterior dental region

also some disadvantages, most importantly the less routine and familiar technique.

For example, in some circumstances, the preparation of the implant bed posed certain difficulties because a drill guide had to be used and precisely placed-something not everyone is inclined to do. Furthermore, removal of the implant (if necessary) could be problematic, especially if the base of the implant has remained firmly ankylosed to the bone. In such cases, removal of the implant results in a bony defect that is considerably larger than one left by removal of a rotationally symmetrical implant.

Figure 5.**4a** and **b** shows a Type K extension implant that was placed distal to a shortened dental arch (free-end extension) in 1982. The patient was an unusually young female (born in 1960) with a surprisingly reduced bone height remaining between the mandibular canal and surface of the alveolar ridge. The implant has now been in place for 13 years with no pathologic changes in bone or soft tissue.

Implant Design **69**

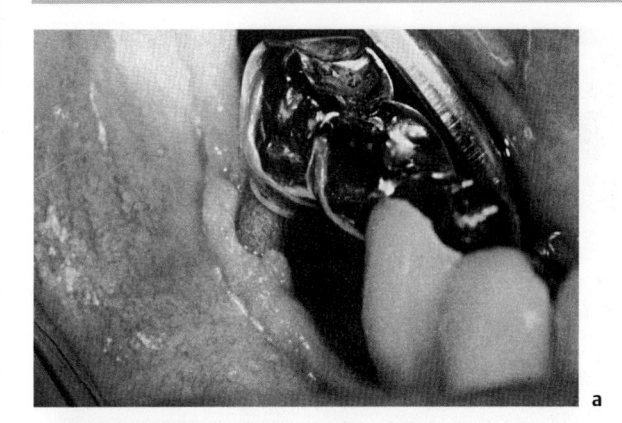

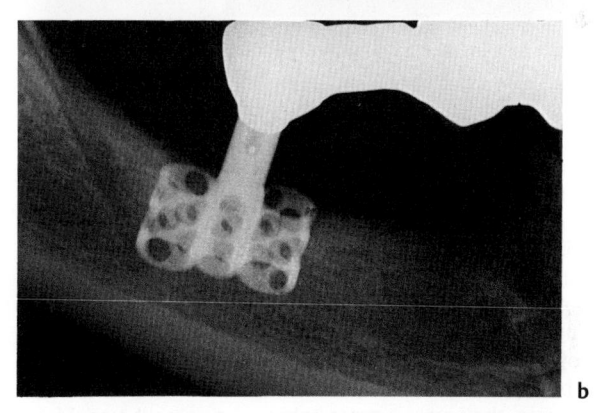

Fig. 5.**4a** and **b** A terminal implant in the lower first molar region (bridge from first premolar) with very little available bone that has been in place for 10 years

Between May of 1980 and April of 1987, Dr. G. Krekeler (Freiburg im Breisgau) placed 153 Type H extension implants in 126 patients. In accordance with the basic concept, most of these were in thin mandibular ridges distal to shortened dental arches. A typical case is seen in figure 5.**5**.

Approximately one hundred of these extension implants were placed over a period of about 10 years in patients in Bern, Freiburg, and other cities. The indications varied, but most were in ridges distal to shortened dental arches. The indications varied, but most were in ridges distal to shortened dental arches. The average failure rate of between 12% and 15% apparently depended less on the type of implant than on the care of the surgeon, the knowledge and skill of the prosthodontist and technician, and the general

70 5 Stages in the Development of the ITI Implant

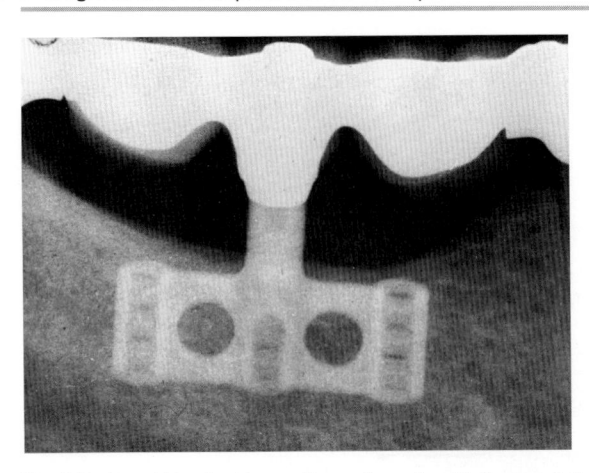

Fig. 5.**5** Type H implant in a radiograph made with the parallel technique

ability of the operator to correctly evaluate the case as a whole, which means taking *all* determining factors into account.

The most important step in the development of the ITI concept, which will be described in detail in chapter 7, was the development of the Type F hollow cylinder implant. The basic shape of the Type F implant was the same as that of the first simple Type C hollow cylinder, but the outer diameter was reduced to 3.5 mm and it was made in an assortment of five different lengths for bone-embedment depths of 8, 10, 12, and 14 millimeters.

Combinations of one-piece F implants between the two mental foramina were found to be especially suited for retaining dentures in edentulous mandibles. In these cases, they were a great help to patients who could not adapt to conventional complete dentures. In this region, the implants impinge on neither the mandibular canal nor the mental nerve if proper technical procedures are followed. Even in severely resorbed mandibles, enough bone height is usually available to allow the use of this type of implant.

Histological findings and more than ten years of clinical experience have shown that following *splinting* of the implants with a bar, *loading* is possible after only a short time (Fig. 5.**6**).

Implant Design

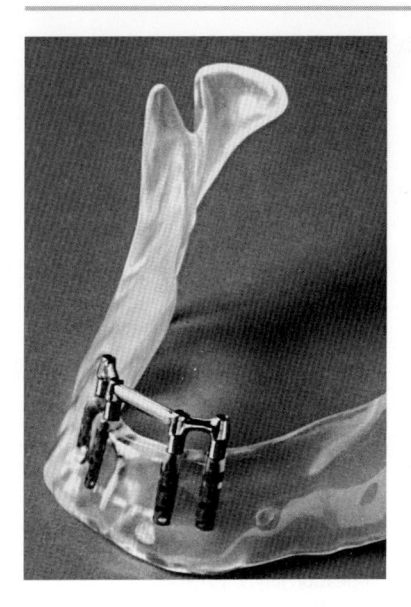

Fig. 5.**6** A model with four one-piece Type F implants splinted together by a bar

The following figures 5.**7**–5.**12** show a few examples of cases from the period between the years 1979 and 1984.

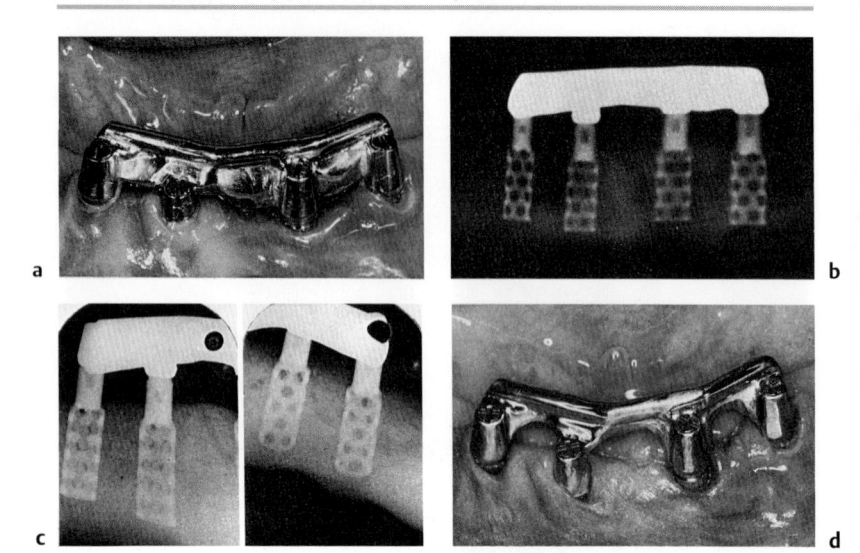

72 5 Stages in the Development of the ITI Implant

Fig. 5.7 Patient F., female, born 1930; date of opeation July 5, 1979
Commentary and prognosis 1986: three abutments in mucosa that, although movable, is for the most part free of inflammation. The superstructure as seen in **a** is not conducive to good oral hygiene. For this reason it was reshaped by grinding at a later recall appointment to facilitate cleaning under the bar (**d**). **b** and **c**: Follow-up radiographs made in 1979 and 1986. Prognosis: favorable. Overall evaluation: success

Implant Design **73**

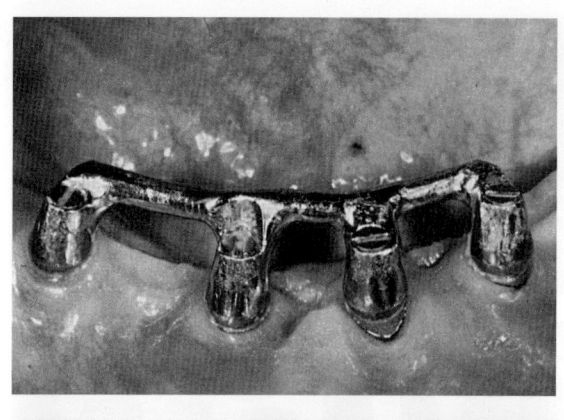

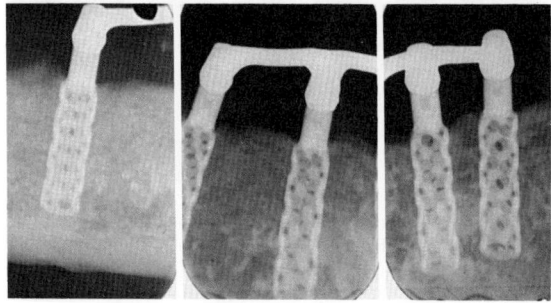

Fig. 5.**8** Patient B., male born 1908; Date of operation July 3, 1979
Commentary and prognosis 1986: Abutments partially in mucosa that is movable but not inflamed (**a**); satisfactory superstructure and hygiene. **b** Follow-up radiographs 1985. Prognosis: favorable, except for the implant in the lower-left lateral incisor position. Overall evalutaion: success

5 Stages in the Development of the ITI Implant

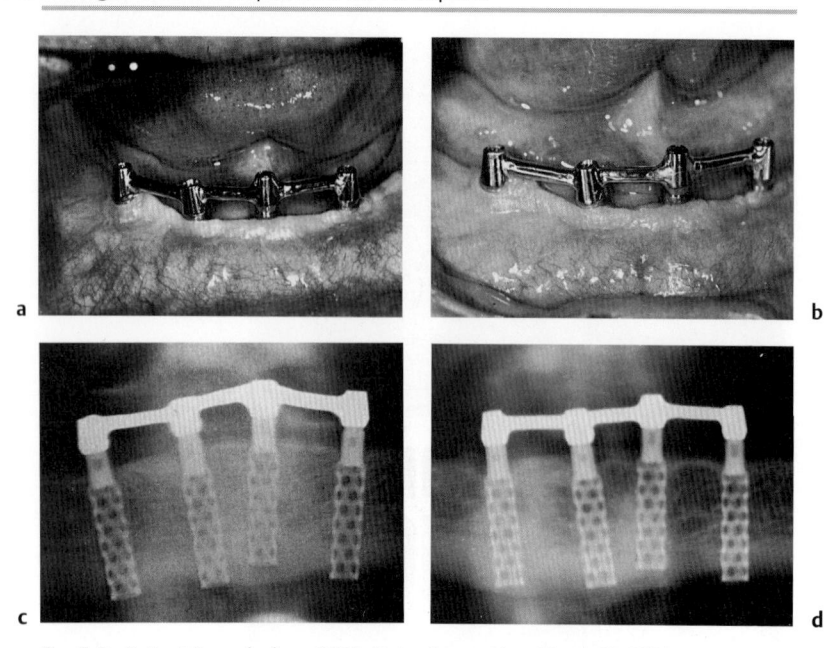

Fig. 5.**9** Patient R., male, born 1935; Date of operation, March 13, 1981
Commentary and prognosis 1986: Abutments in noninflammed, keratinized mucosa (**a** 1981, **b** 1986)
Follow-up radiographs show nothing abnormal (**c** 1981, **d** 1986). Prognosis: good. Overall evaluation: success. Follow-up 1992: no changes

Implant Design **75**

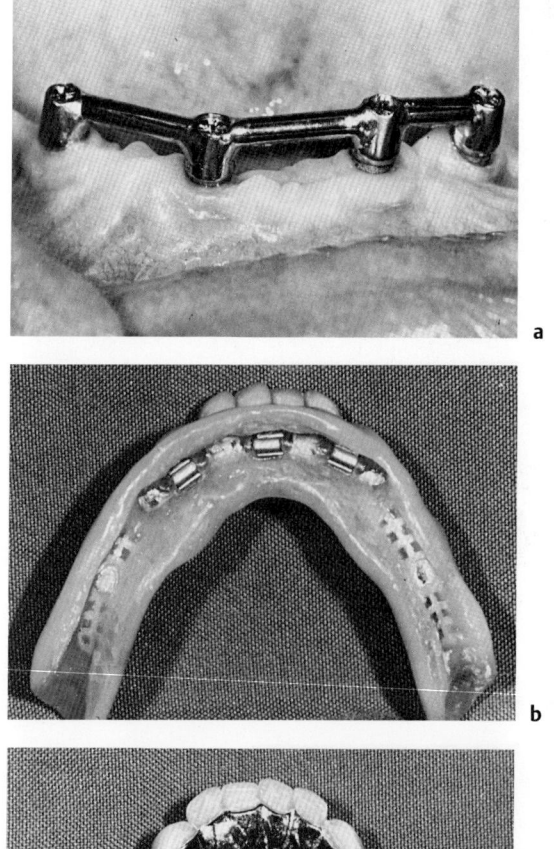

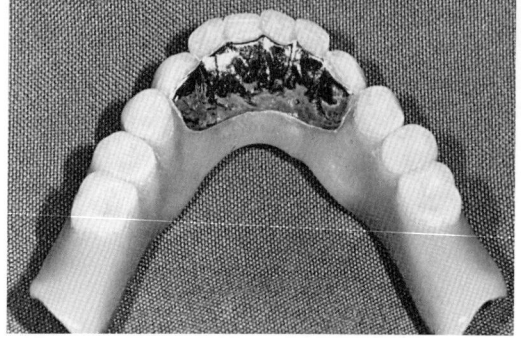

Fig. 5.**10** Patient G., female, born 1927; date of operation Nov. 2, 1982
Commentary and prognosis 1986: all abutments in inflammation-free, keratinized mucosa (**a** 1982, **d** 1985)

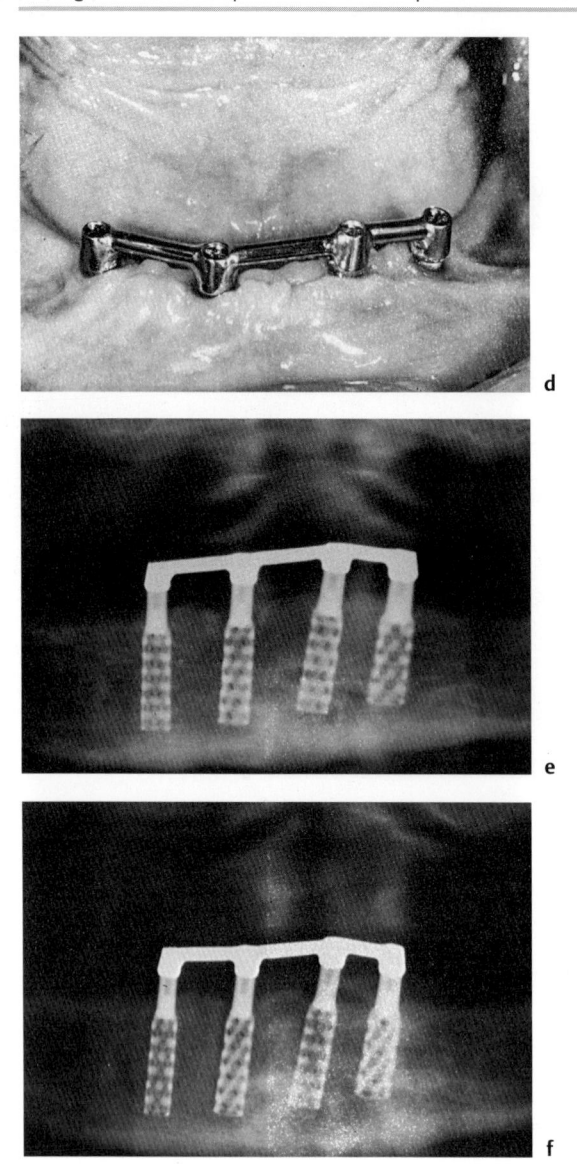

76 5 Stages in the Development of the ITI Implant

Fig. 5.**10** Follow-up radiographs show nothing abnormal (**e** 1983, **f** 1986). Prognosis: favorable. Overall evaluation: success. Figures **b** and **c** illustrate the recommended reinforcement of the denture base with a vitallium framework including a lingual plate "backing"

Implant Design **77**

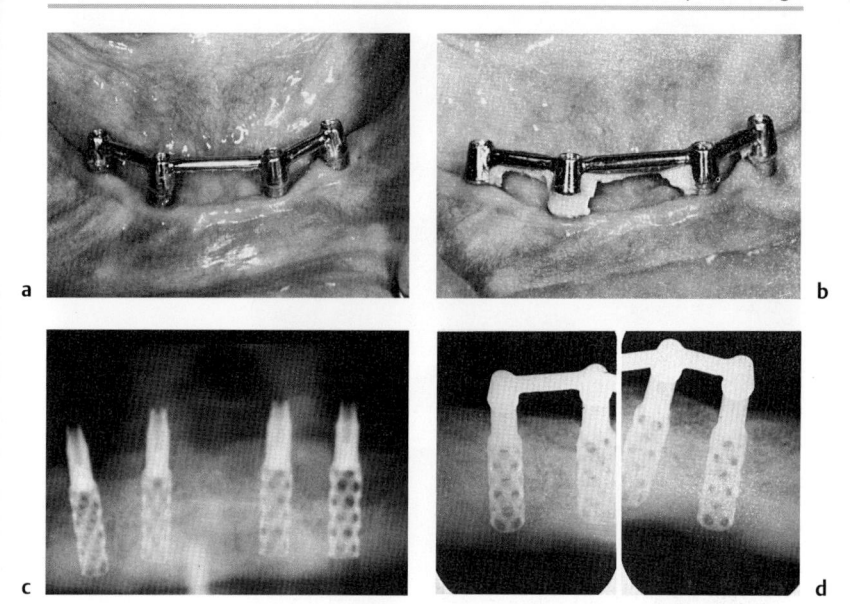

Fig. 5.**11** Patient K., female, born 1929; date of operation Jan. 11, 1983
Commentary and prognosis 1986: Abutments in mucosa that is immovable and macroscopically free of inflammation (**a**) in spite of the massive accumulation of calculus (**b**). Follow-up radiographs show nothing abnormal (**c** 1983, **d** 1986). Prognosis: favorable because the abutments lie within attached, keratinized mucosa.
Overall evalutaion: success in spite of poor oral hygiene

5 Stages in the Development of the ITI Implant

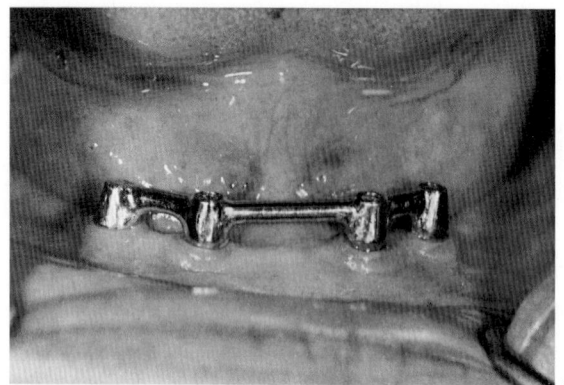

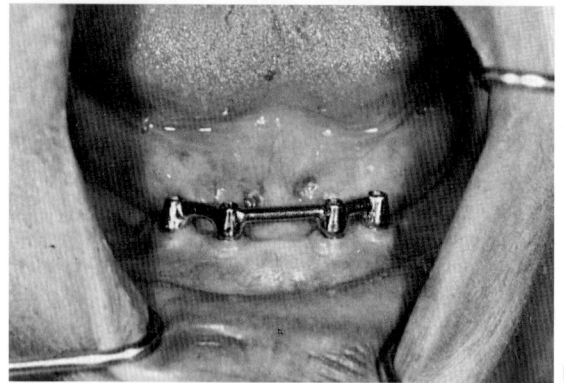

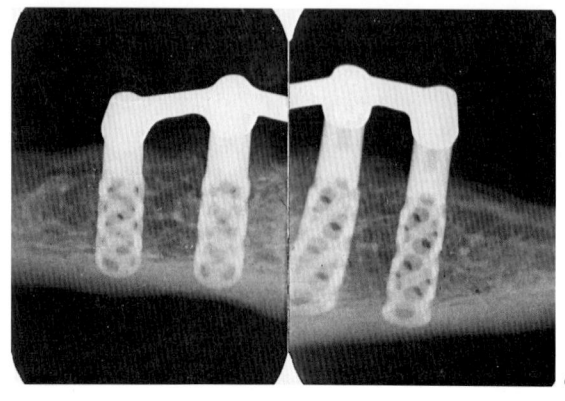

Implant Design

During the years in which the various types of ITI implant were developed and tested, the cardinal questions of implantology–namely the healing of the bone on one hand, and the reaction of the soft tissue on the other–manifested themselves in an obvious manner. Experience was gained that further helped to reduce the incidence of failures. Obtaining a gingival seal proved to be more of a problem than achieving bony anchorage.

Even if it cannot be claimed that placement of the abutments in immobile keratinized mucosa is the condito sine qua non for long-term success, it nevertheless greatly improves the prognosis. Where there is doubt as to whether there will be a wide enough band of attached mucosa around the abutment, placement of the implant should be preceded by a free-mucosal graft.

Just as there must be a wide band of attached mucosa, it is absolutely essential for an adequate labiolingual width of bone to be available. The implants must be embedded up to the abutments in the greatest mass of bone possible. If a sharp alveolar ridge prevents this requirement from being met, then the crest of the ridge must be broadened to the desired width either by removing the sharp edge until there is at least a 1.5 mm thickness of bone, both labial and lingual to each implant, or by some other method.

Our observations during the first 10 years have made us aware of other criteria necessary for success, pricipal among which are correct superstructure design and optimal oral hygiene. These will discussed later in detail.

Fig. 5.**12**   Patient D., female, born 1918; date of operation May 1, 1984
Commentary and prognosis 1986: abutments in completely inflammation-free, attached mucosa (**a** 1984, **b** 1986). Good oral hygiene. Follow-up radiograph 1987 with no abnormalities (**c**). Prognosis: favorable. Overall evaluation: success

6 Tissue Response

A. Schroeder and D. Buser
with a contribution by H. Stich

As has been emphasized many times previously (p.37 f.), *pure titanium* is one of the *bioinert* implant materials. Its biocompatibility has been known for a long time and has been repeatedly confirmed in the literature. This biocompatibility due to a surface oxide layer (p. 43 f.), which prevents direct contact of the metal with the surrounding tissue.

The histological findings described on the following pages document the results of numerous studies of titanium-plasma-coated ITI implants and other experimental titanium implants conducted over a time span of more than 20 years, beginning in 1974. More detailed accounts can be found in the publications cited.

Response of Bone

The bone reaction around the implant can be classified as a functional ankylosis or osseointegration (better grammatically, osteointegration). The total integration of an implant in bone that is regenerating after the trauma of implant bed preparation was postulated by Brånemark and co-workers in 1969, and was demonstrated histologically for the first time in 1976 in decalcified sections with pure titanium (Schroeder and co-workers 1976). One could say that the bone regeneration progressed as if the foreign body were not there at all. According to Albrektsson (1985), a border zone of necrosis at the defect site is unavoidable even when implant bed preparation is carried out as atraumatically as possible. The author begins: "Following severe trauma of a physical, chemical, or other nature, the osseous tissue heals through the formation of an irreversible layer of fibrous tissue. Healing is completely impeded if revascularization of the necrotic area does not occur."

It has been demonstrated that with a porous titanium implant, there is a rapid ingrowth of blood vessels, accompanied by both osteoclastic resorption and new bone formation, through osteoblastic activity. The cancellous bone that is laid down first is replaced within a few weeks by mature lamellar bone. This regenerated tissue is both qualitatively and quantitatively indistinguishable from bone that would have been formed if *no* implant had been placed.

Experimental findings, which have been repeatedly reproduced over many years, have led to the conclusion that new bone is laid down *directly upon the implant surface,* provided that the rules for atraumatic implant

Response of Bone **81**

placement are followed (rotation of the cutting instrument at less than 800 rpm, cooling with sterile physiologic saline solution) and the implant exhibits primary stability.

The *shape* of the implant is of secondary importance (Fig. 6.**1**–6.**4**). Higher magnifications have shown that bone follows all irregularities and surface invaginations such as those found on a porous titanium plasma layer, and that vital osteoblasts and osteocytes lie directly against the surface of the implant (Figs. 6.**5a** and **b**, Fig. 6.**6**). In areas that were apparently subjected to

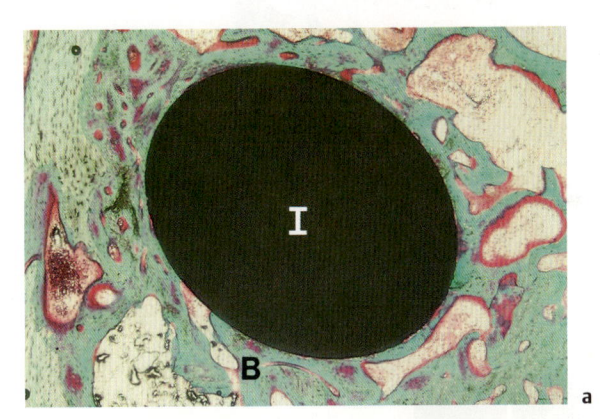

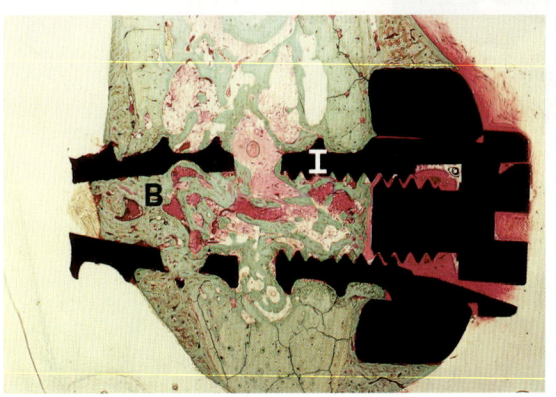

Fig. 6.**1** In achieving an ankylotic, direct union of bone to rough titanium, the shape of the implant is not decisive, provided there is a close fit between implant and bone
a Cylindrical implant
b Hollow screw (used here for osteosynthesis)
B = bone
I = implant

82 6 Tissue Response

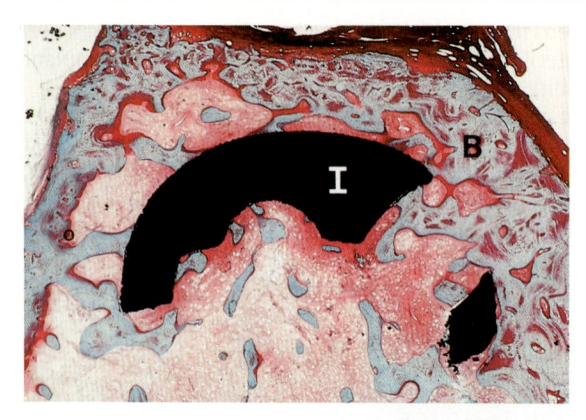

Fig. 6.2 The shoulder portion of an unloaded ITI implant, Type C (1974) anchored to bone in monkey through ankylosis ("osteointegrated")

B = bone
I = implant

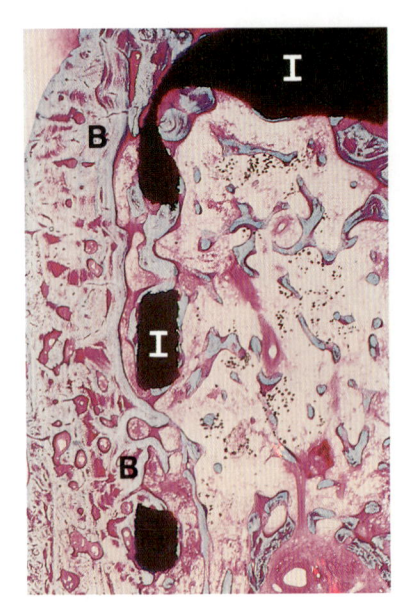

Fig. 6.3 Central portion of a hollow cylinder after 2 years of loading (monkey)

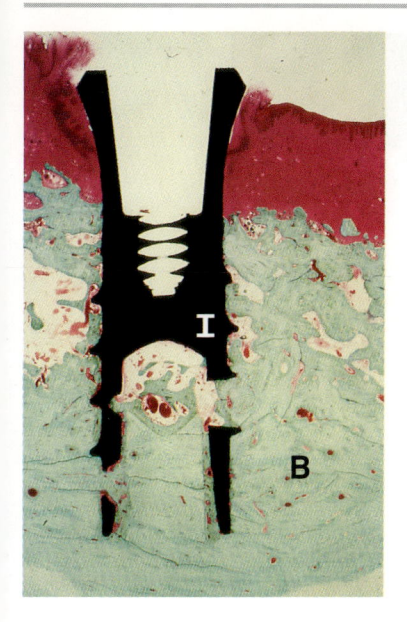

Fig. 6.4 Osteointegrated ITI hollow cylinder implant (beagle, 3-month healing period without loading)

B = bone
I = implant

high levels of tensile stress during embedding of the histological preparation, part of the plasma layer was separated from the body of the implant, but bone was still attached to the plasma layer (Fig. 6.**7**). These pictures illustrate the phenomenon of ankylotic bonding (or osteointegration) in a striking way, considering the fact that in vitro, a tensile force of 90 N/mm² is required to separate the plasma-sprayed layer from the implant.

Pictures obtained with the scanning electron microscope (SEM) confirm the light microscopic findings, as they also show the bone permeating the rough implant surface (Fig. 6.**8a**). When tension-induced tears occur, the separation occurs within the bone (Fig. 6.**8b**). This again demonstrates the strong microbond between the bone and the titanium plasma layer.

Recently, the ultrastructure of the bone-implant interface has also been studied with the transmission electron microscope (TEM) by Listgarten and co-workers (1992). In this study, epoxy implants were coated with a titanium plasma layer that was only 1000 Å (100 nm) thick to make the ultra thin sections necessary for ultrastructural investigation (Fig. 6.**9a** and **b**). Ultrastructural study of the bone-implant interface was undertaken following a 3-month-long unloaded healing phase. Nondecalcified sections showed direct contact of apatite crystals with the titanium surface (Fig. 6.**9c**), which was confirmed in decalcified sections by the presence of collagen fibrils in direct contact with the titanium surface (Fig. 6.**9d**). These findings contradicted the

6 Tissue Response

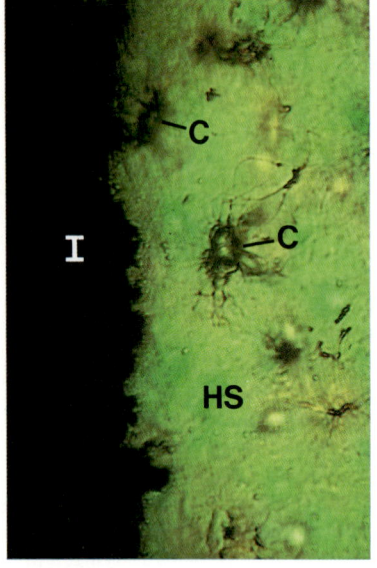

Fig. 6.5
a An ITI Implant healed through ankylosis ("osteointegration"): bony trabeculae with regularly formed osteons bonded directly to the rough surface
b Intimate bonding between the rough implant surface and bone

I = implant
B = bone
O = osteocytes

earlier findings of Albrektsson et al. (1985), who, in their studies, had described a layer of proteoglycans approximately 1000 Å (100 nm) wide between the mineralized bone tissue and the titanium oxide layer.

Response of Bone 85

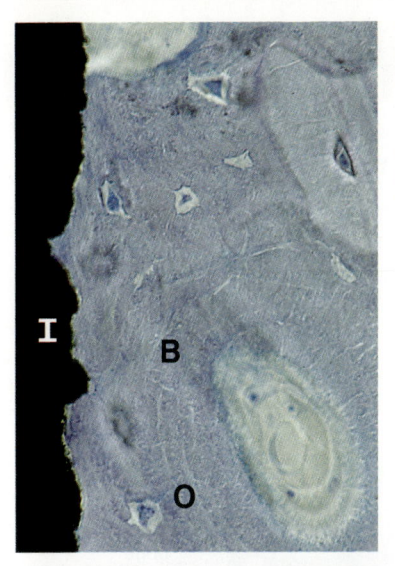

Fig. 6.**6** Direct contact of bone to extremely rough surface of a healed transgingival titanium implant (beagle, 3-month healing period)

I = implant
B = bone
O = osteocytes

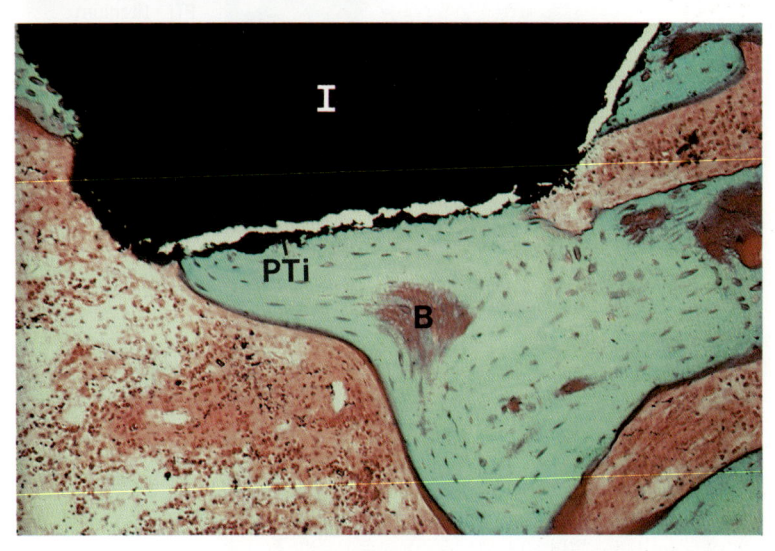

Fig. 6.**7** Tensile stresses, regardless of how they are produced, do not result in separation of bone from metal but, depending upon conditions, can cause the sprayed layer to separate from the body of the implant. This clearly illustrates the strong, resistant bond to bone. B = bone, I = implant, PTi = titanium plasma coating

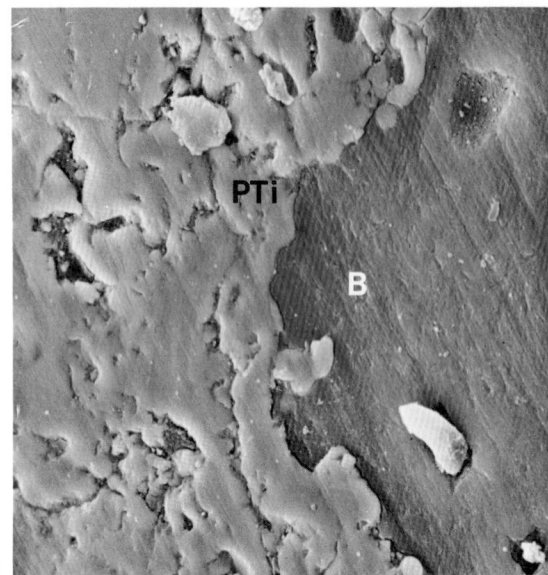

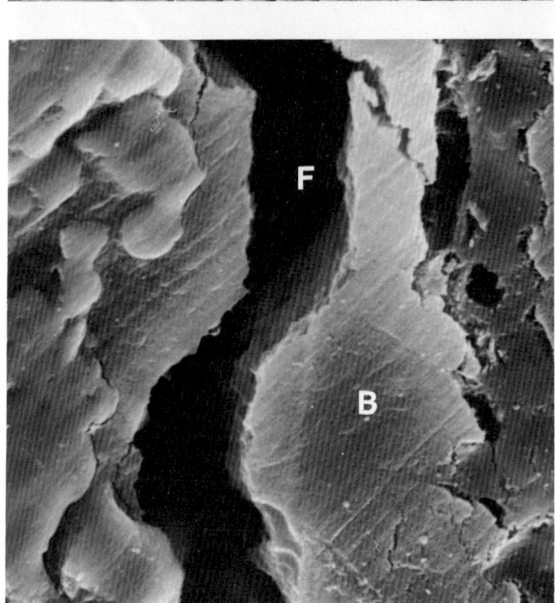

Fig. 6.**8a** and **b**
Confirmation of the light microscopic findings through SEM (scanning electron microscopy). Even the finest porosities and irregularities of the titanium plasma-sprayed coating (PTi) are filled with bone (B). The tension rupture occured within the bone itself and not between bone and the plasma-sprayed coating

B = bone
F = fracture within bone
PTi = titanium plasma-sprayed surface

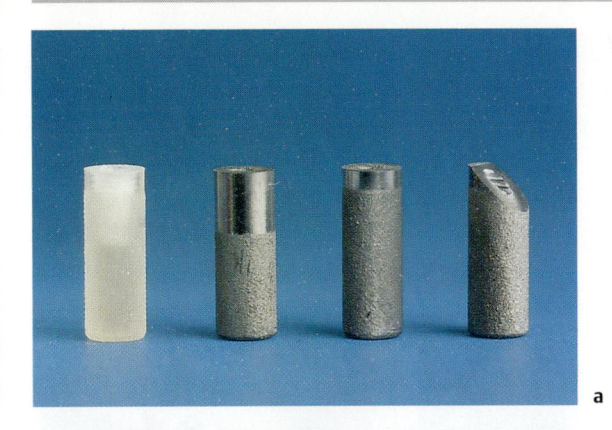

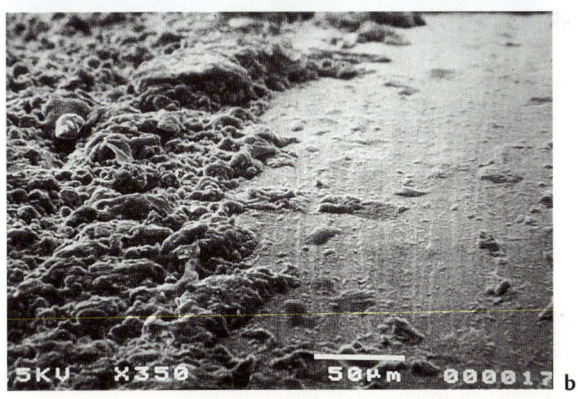

Fig. 6.9 Results of a TEM (transmission electron microscopy) study of the bone-implant interface (courtesy of Listgarten and co-workers 1992)
a Titanium implants with a TPS surface were duplicated with epoxy resin (left). This was then coated with an extremely thin (1000 Å or 100 nm) film of titanium vapor
b This SEM picture of the titanium-coated epoxy replica reveals the extremely rough surface of the endosseous portion of the implant

Fig. 6.9
c The direct deposition of apatite crystals onto the titanium film is seen in this non-decalcified histologic section (magnification approx. 16 000X)

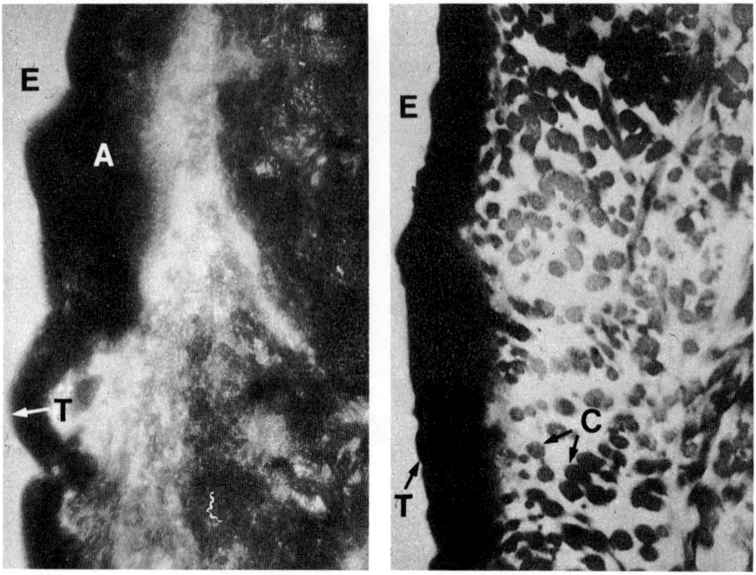

E = epoxy resin
T = titanium film
A = apatite crystal

d In this decalcified section, transversely cut collagen fibrils can also be seen in contact with the titanium film (magnification approx. 16 000X)

E = epoxy resin
T = titanium film
C = collagen fibrils

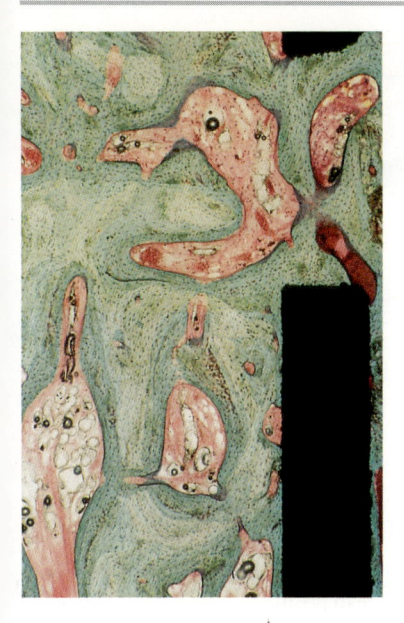

Fig. 6.**10** Human histological specimen of an implant that was removed 3 years after placement because of chronic inflammation in the alveolar ridge region. The implant exhibits the typical signs of osteointegration

Of course, it could not be assumed from these results alone that the ankylotic attachment of nonloaded implants would also be achieved with *loaded* implants. One could assume that under the influence of occlusal forces, there might be a rearrangement of tissue in the boundary region between implant and bone, resulting in the formation of a periodontium-like attachment apparatus. However, this was not observed in any of the specimens (Schroeder and co-workers 1978). Instead, there is the distinct impression that osteointegration is even enhanced under loading and at the same time, that the bone becomes more dense and compact over longer periods of implantation (Fig. 6.**10**).

In this way, it has been proven that the loaded implant experiences an anchorage in the bone without interpositioned connective tissue. An example from orthopedic surgery (Fig. 6.**11**) shows that this can also be achieved in other parts of the body. This case involves a titanium acetabulum (hip joint fossa) with a titanium plasma layer that was placed without cement in a dog (as therapy, not as animal experimentation). The resulting true union between implant and bone is unmistakable and impressive.

As previously mentioned, since 1974 the endoseous portion of the ITI implant has had a rough, porous surface produced by the plasma spray technique (p. 48). From a clinical standpoint, the titanium plasma spray coating (TPS) offers three advantages over a fine or smooth structured

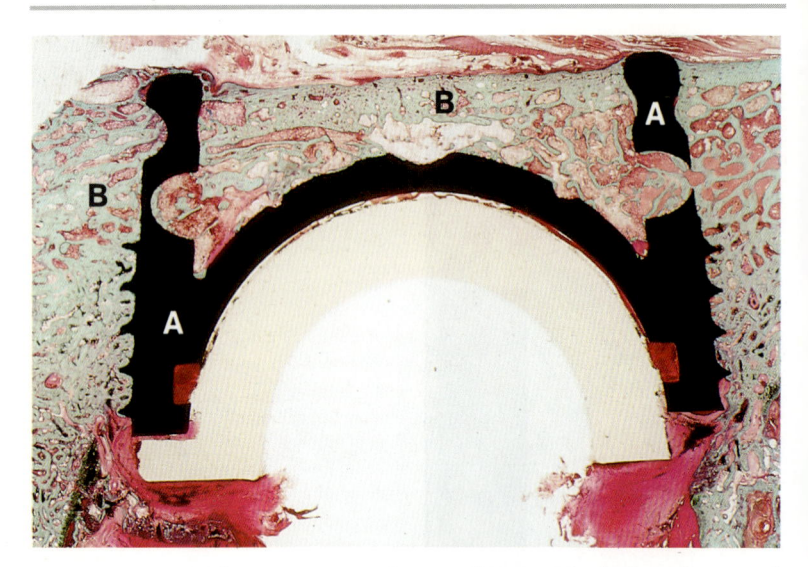

Fig. 6.**11** Example of osteointegration from another specialty (orthopedic surgery). A titanium acetabulum (hip socket) with titanium plasma-sprayed coating integrated into the bone with no intervening connective tissue (see text)

A = acetabulum
B = bone

titanium surface: (1) accelerated apposition of bone in the early healing phase, (2) increased area of contact surface between implant and bone, and (3) improved implant anchorage.

The acceleration of bone apposition can be demonstrated by comparing two histological sections taken from the same implant. One is from a highly polished area and the other from a titanium plasma-coated area. The test specimen was implanted in the femur of a rat, with attention given to achieving good primary seating, and left for 10 days. It must be kept in mind that bone formation takes place much more rapidly in the rat than in man. After 10 days in place, the polished surface still shows no contact with bone, while on the opposite side, bony trabeculae can already be identified resting directly against the rough surface (Fig. 6.**12a** and **b**). These findings have been confirmed in an animal study by Kirsch and Donath (1984).

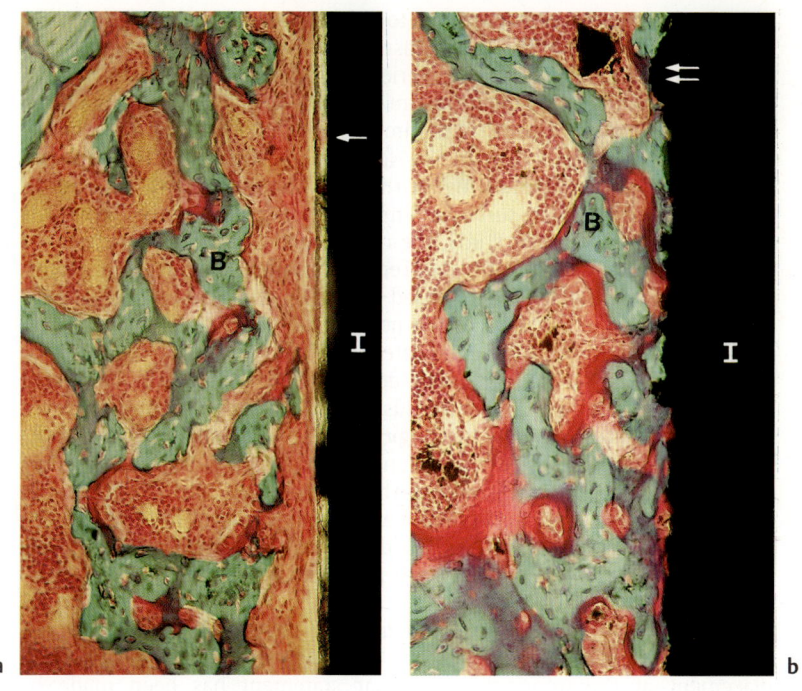

Fig. 6.**12** Osteogenesis near a small titanium implant (rat femur, implant duration: 10 days) with one side polished and the other side rough (titanium plasma coated)
a polished surface: still no bone contact
b rough surface: direct contact of bone trabeculae with the surface

B = bone
I = implant
⇐ rough surface
← smooth surface (the apparent unevenness is due to an optical effect)

The increase in the percentage of bone-implant contact surface was demonstrated in a histomorphometric study by Buser et al. (1991). Titanium implants with TPS coatings had an average bone-implant contact (BIC) in cancellous bone of nearly 40%, which was significantly higher than smoothly polished or finely structured titanium implants. These had average BIC values of slightly over 20%. Still higher values, reaching an average BIC of 52–58%, have been achieved with a new surface produced by sand blasting and acid etching.

The improvement in attachment to bone has been documented by Wilke and co-workers (1990) through measurements of the torque necessary to unscrew titanium implants with various surface structures from bone in sheep. The study showed that titanium implants with a TPS coating required significantly higher torque than did implants with polished or fine-grained surfaces. Measurements of up to 530 Ncm were obtained with TPS implants, which were at least 8 times higher than measurements with polished or fine-structured titanium surfaces. Similar to the results in the previously mentioned morphometric study, the coarse sand-blasted and acid-etched implants required somewhat higher removal torques than did TPS implants, with a maximum of 690 Ncm. Based upon the favorable results in these animal studies, clinical tests of the newer titanium surfaces on a limited number of patients seem to be indicated.

There is a lack of connective tissue membrane around osteointegrated implants. It remains unknown how this lack should be interpreted. Evidence has been presented (not only histologically, but also clinically), that in some ways implants do not differ in their function from natural teeth, in that they transmit chewing forces directly to the bone. This is related to both the magnitude of the force and the subjective perception of the patient. *The patient perceives the implant-supported tooth as no different from a natural tooth,* regardless of the absence of a periodontal membrane and its proprioceptors.

According to Skalak, "Osteointegration makes possible direct transmission of force from titanium implant to bone with no relative displacement at the interface." A similar statement has been made by Steinemann (1986): "...from a functional point of view osseointegration should be reserved to the case of a full force-transmitting attachment" (see also p. 51 f.).

Soft Tissue ("Gingival" Cuff)

In contrast to orthopedic implants, which are fully enclosed in the body, oral implants are "open" implants, in that they are permanently in contact with the germ-laden oral cavity. Even the lay person recognizes that this is a site of minimum resistance, and this has given rise to skepticism concerning implantology.

While the problem of achieving attachment of a foreign body in bone appears to have been largely solved, the second principal problem, the maintenance of the peri-implant soft tissue around the abutment, remains the object of further research and discussion. Different interpretations have arisen in this area. Here we shall attempt to narrow the field of speculation somewhat by considering a few facts.

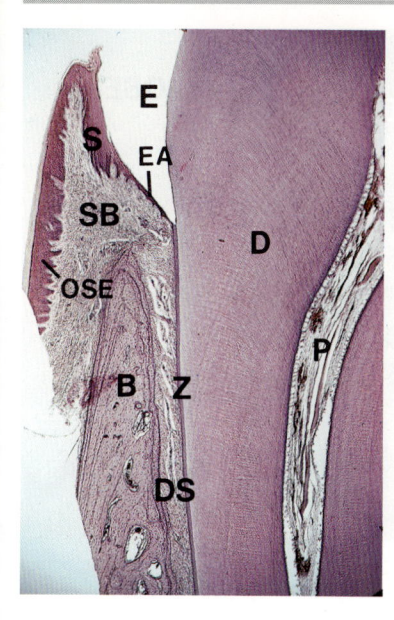

Fig. 6.**13** The marginal periodontium of a natural tooth

B	bone
D	dentin
DS	periodontal membrane
E	enamel
EA	epithelial attachment
OSE	outer junctional epithelium
P	pulp
S	junctional epithelium
SB	subepithelial connective tissue with collagen fiber bundles
Z	cementum

It is known that the integrity of the integumentum, where the soft tissue meets the hard tissue (enamel, cementum), is guaranteed through the dentogingival seal (Fig. 6.**13**). This is made up of the keratinized gingival epithelium, the nonkeratinized sulcular and junctional epithelium, and the subepithelial connective tissue with its complex system of fibers. The latter has several important functions. Above all, it gives the gingival "collar" its high resistance to mechanical shearing forces that it encounters during chewing. In a real sense, the epithelial attachment secures the attachment of the junctional epithelium to the hard substance by means of a basal lamina and hemidesmosomes. It extends from the apical part of the junctional epithelium to the botom of the gingival sulcus (Schroeder, H. E. 1987).

It is still unknown whether similar structures and mechanisms can be also assumed for the implant abutment and to what extent they can be demonstrated histologically. This can be resolved by referring to a low magnification view of the marginal "periodontium" of an implant abutment (Fig. 6.**14**).

Because bone, with its ground substance and fibrils, bonds tightly to the rough surface of a titanium implant, one might hope to also find a similar attachment in the case of the nonmineralized *supracrestal connective tissue*. This expectation was confirmed in two histological animal studies (Schroe-

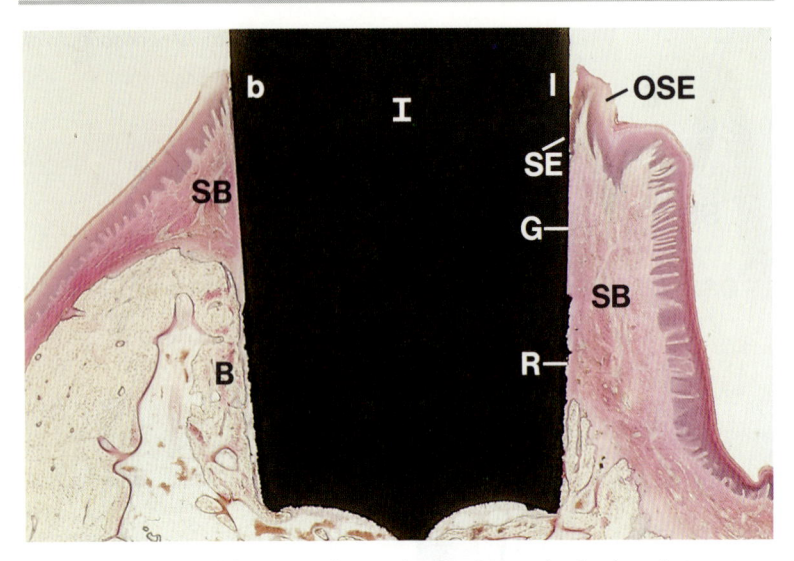

Fig. 6.**14** Overview of the marginal "periodontium" around an implant abutment

B	bone	R	rough surface
b	buccal	SB	subepithelial connective tissue
G	polished surface	SE	junctional epithelium
l	lingual	OSE	outer junctional epithelium

der et al., 1981; Buser et al., 1989), in which perpendicularly oriented connective tissue (CT) fibers were demonstrated. This arrangement of fibers could only be found at the porous surface of plasma-coated titanium implants with abutments located in keratinized mucosa (Fig. 6.**15a** and **b**). The light microscopic findings have also been confirmed by SEM (Fig. 6.**16**).

Since 1985, the supracrestal portions of ITI implants have been made smooth to reduce plaque accumulation and facilitate plaque removal by the patient. This made it imperative to perform one further animal experiment to investigate the soft-tissue reaction around nonporous titanium surfaces (Buser et al., 1992). This study showed that adjacent to smooth or sandblasted titanium implants, the connective tissue fibers ran predominantly parallel with the implant surface, while the perpendicular fibers stopped short of the implant surface (Fig. 6.**17a** and **b**). Adjacent to the implant, only circularly arranged CT fibers were found. These were especially evident in sections made at right angles to the long axis of the implant (Fig. 6.**18a** and **b**). The 50–100 μm-wide band of CT adjacent to the implant was also devoid

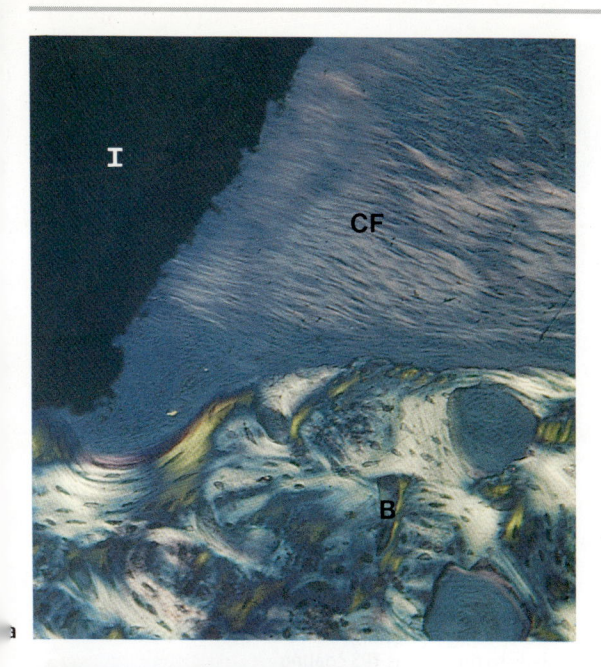

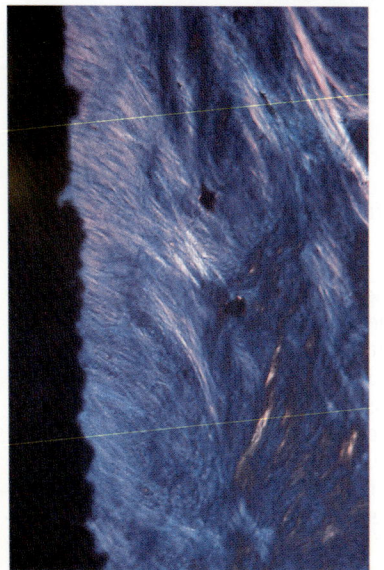

Soft Tissue **95**

Fig. 6.**15**
- **a** Subepithelial connective tissue in the abutment region. Connective tissue on the rough TPS implant surface (I). Collagen fiber bundels (CF) that are inserted more or less perpendicular between the junctional epithelium and the bone at the crest of the ridge (B)
- **b** Detailed view of a titanium implant (I) with a TPS surface. The collagen fibers are attached more or less perpendicular ($\rightarrow$) to the porous TPS coating (beagle, 3-month healing period)

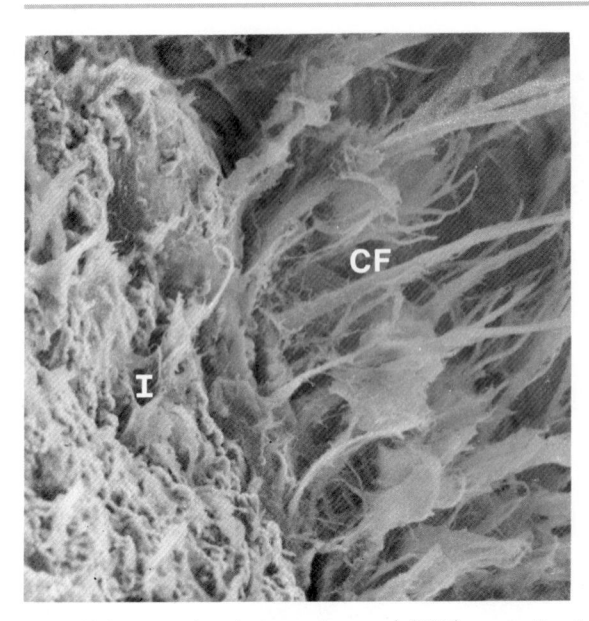

Fig. 6.**16** In a scanning electron micrograph (SEM), connective tissue fibers are likewise found attached perpendicularly to the porous TPS coating
I = implant
B = bone
CF = collagen fiber bundles

of blood vessels and bore a strong resemblance to an inflammation-free ring of scar tissue with closely packed, circularly arranged CT fibers. These findings were also confirmed in a TEM study by Listgarten et al. (1992). A well-structured, three-dimensional framework of collagen fibers with perpendicular, vertical, and circularly arranged CT fibers was found at a distance from the implant.

The next question that arises is whether the *epithelium* is in a position to attach to the titanium surface. This question can essentially be answered in the affirmative, and it has been proven many times that epithelial cells do indeed have the ability to accumulate on nonbiological materials to form an actual attachment. It has also been possible to demonstrate a basal lamina and hemidesmosomes through electron microscopy, despite the fact that technical difficulties in this type of investigation are considerable (Gould and co-workers, 1981). These difficulties are caused by the fact that it is extremely difficult to preserve the hemidesmosomes during preparation of the necessary ultrathin sections at the interface between epithelium and implant material without tearing or detaching them.

Soft Tissue **97**

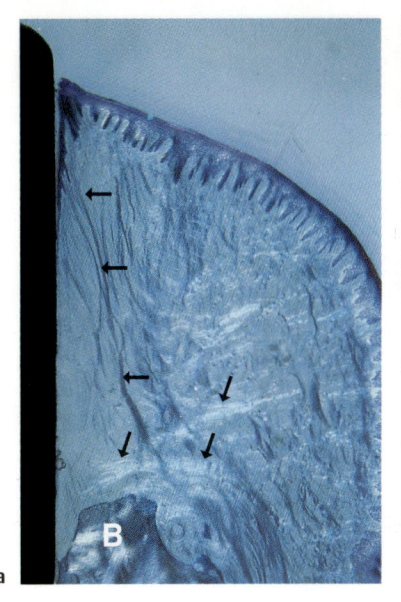

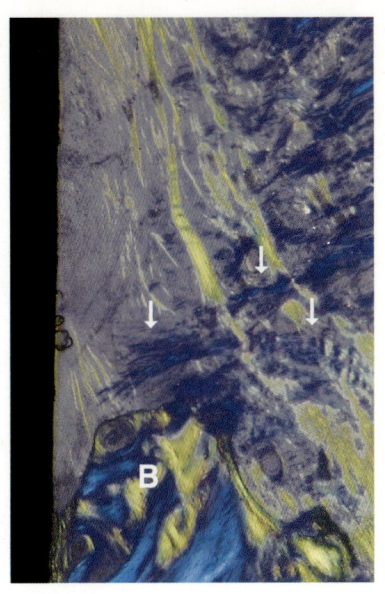

Fig. 6.**17** A buccolingual section through a finely structured titanium implant (polarized light, beagle, 3-month healing period)
a The overview shows a network of horizontal and vertidal connective tissue fibers (→) on the vestibular side of the supracrestal region (B = bone of the alveolar crest)
b The more detailed view just above the crest of the ridge (B) clearly shows that the perpendicular fibers (→) do not reach the surface of the implant

In an experimental study on beagles (Buser and co-workers 1992), epithelial structures, corresponding more or less to the epithelial structures surrounding teeth, were demonstrated around healing transgingival titanium implants that carried no functional load. During healing of the soft tissues, a peri-implant sulcus was formed (Fig. 6.**19a**) that was covered on the tissue side by a nonkeratinized sulcular epithelium (Fig. 6.**19b**). The sulcular epithelium was 8–15 cell layers thick and consisted of individual basal and suprabasal cells arranged more or less parallel with the surface of the implant. Occasionally, evidence of a mild inflammation in the form of leukocytes migrating through sulcular epithelium was found, which had no clinical manifestations (Fig. 6.**19b**). Farther apically, the epithelium lays directly against the implant surface, resembling a junctional epithelium.

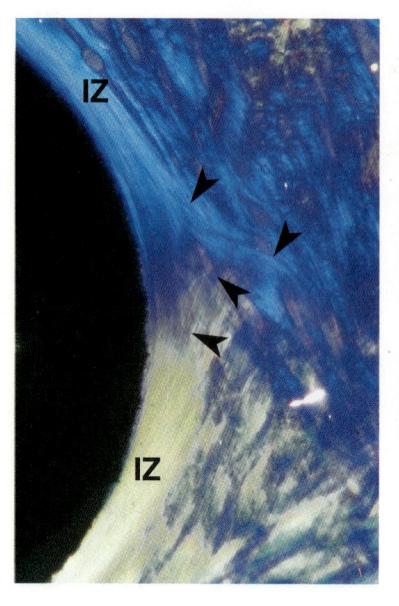

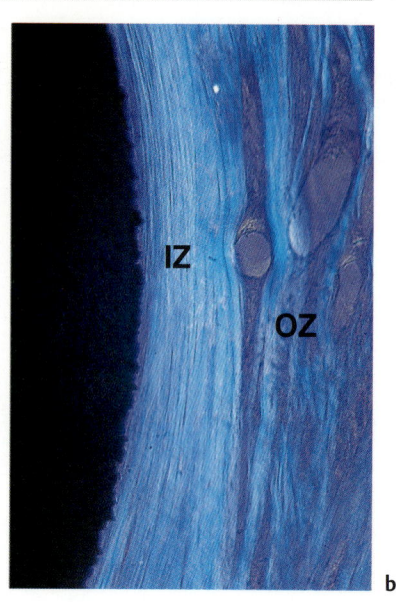

Fig. 6.**18** A transverse section through a coarsely structured, nonporous titanium implant in the supracrestal region (polarized light, beagle, 3-month healing period)
a The overview makes the circular course of the peri-implant CT fibers in the immediate vicinity of the implant (IZ = inner zone) apparent. Perpendicularly directed CT fibers enter this ring of fibers from more peripheral tissues (→)
b The close-up view shows the circular CT fibers. The absence of blood vessels within this inner CT zone (IZ) is very noticeable. They are found only at a certain distance from the implant surface in the outer CT zone (OZ)

Fig. 6.**19** Epithelial structures around a healed transgingival titanium implant (beagle, 3-month healing period. By courtesy of Buser and co-workers 1992)
a The overview shows the formation of a peri-implant sulcus
  I – Implant
  S – Sulcus
  SE – Sulcus epithelium

b Greater magnification allows identification of the sulcus epithelium(SE) and transmigrating leukocytes (→). The epithelial cells are arranged parallel with the implant's surface and are clearly separated from one another by intercellular spaces
c Farther apically, the junctional epithelium can be seen. It is 5–8 cells in width and comprised of basal cells (B) and suprabasal cells (S)
d Still farther apically, the junctional epithelium has become even narrower. The cellular structure is clearly visible with nuclei, nucleoli, and a mitotic figure (M)

Soft Tissue **99**

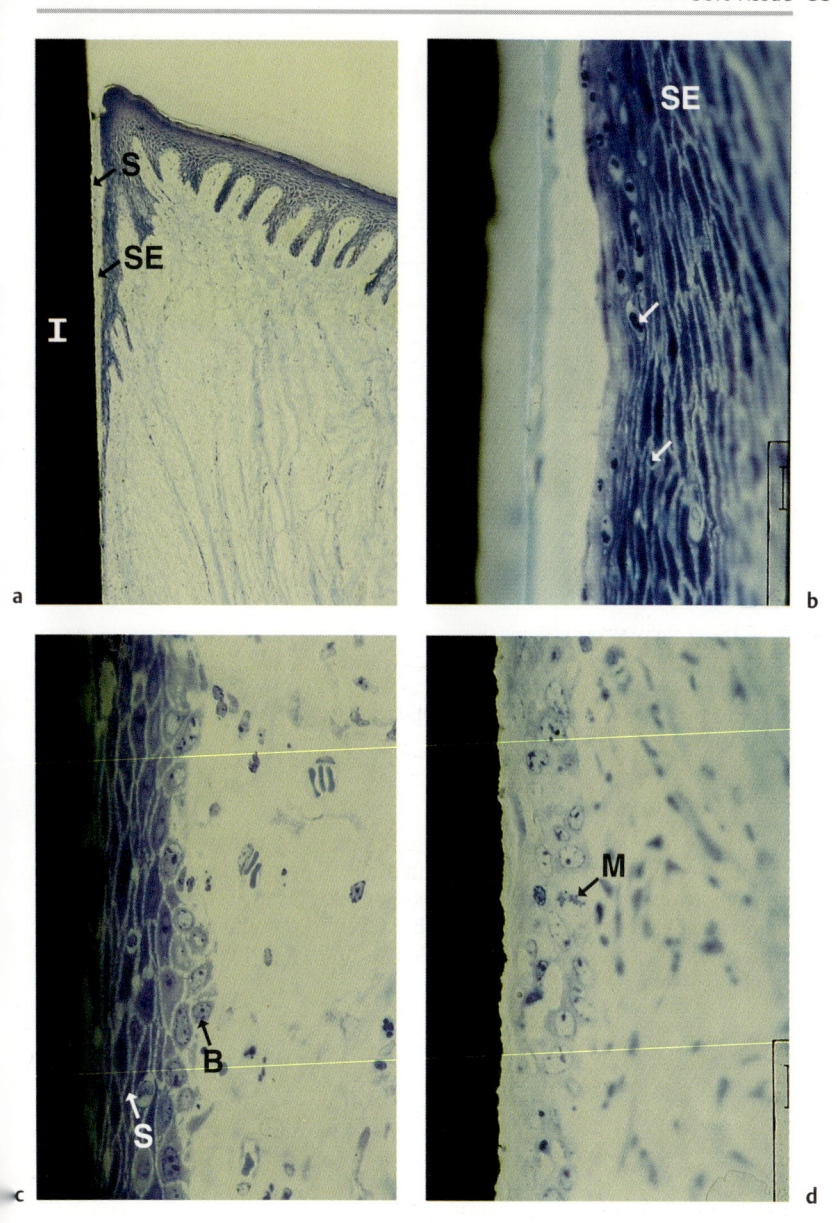

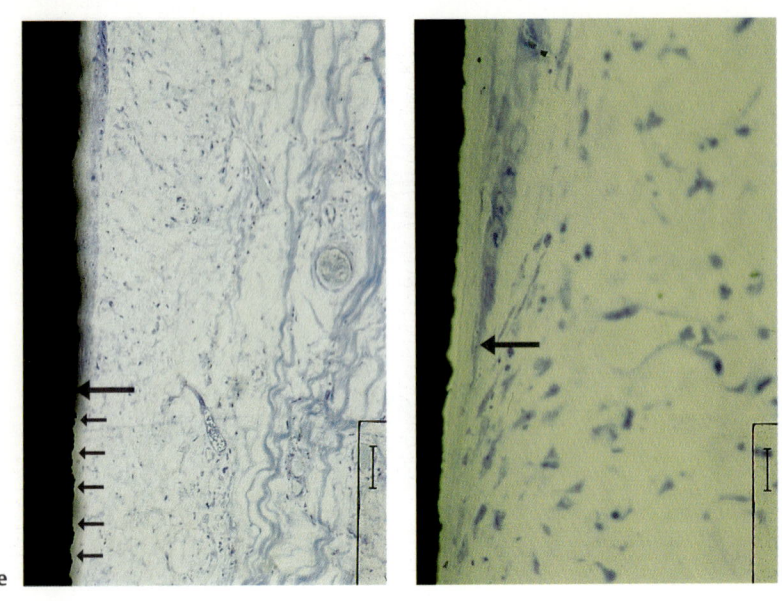

e The most apical epithelial cell is located approximately 1 mm above the bone (large arrow). Farther apical, the supracrestal CT is in direct contact with the surface of the implant (→)

f Higher magnification of the most apically located epithelial cell (→)

The width of the "junctional epithelium" decreased progressively toward its apical extent (Fig. 6.**19c** and **d**). In all prepared sections, the most apical portion of the "junctional epithelium" was clearly seen to lie above the bony ridge (Fig. 6.**19e** and **f**). The height of the direct contact of CT to titanium surface was barely 1 mm. These results confirm earlier findings with ITI implants in beagles (Fig. 6.**20a** and **b**).

Soft Tissue **101**

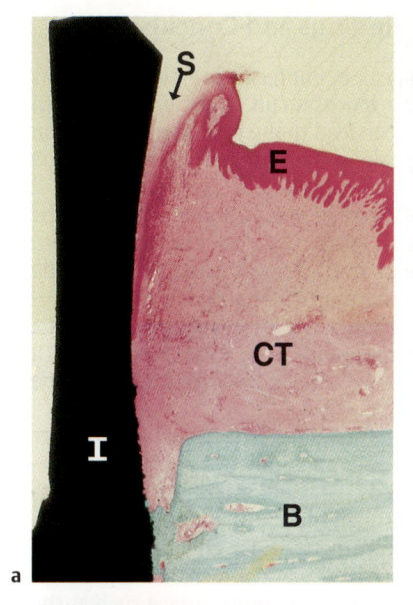

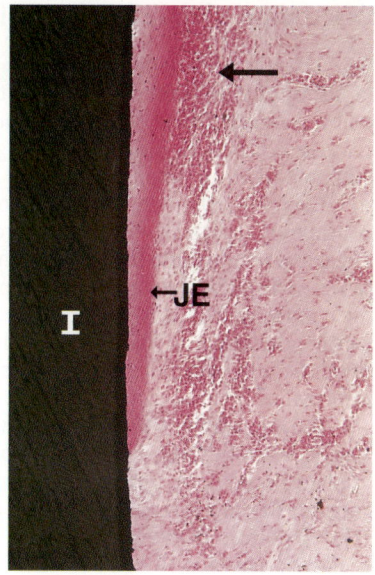

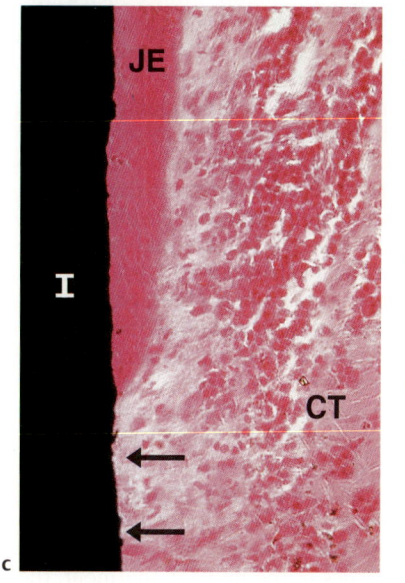

Fig. 6.20 Tissue integration of a ITI hollow screw implant (beagle, 3-month healing period)
- **a** This low-magnification view of the soft-tissue passage shows osteo-integration of the implant (I) in the crestal area (B), the supracrestal connective tissue (CT), the formation of a peri-implant sulcus (S), and the oral epithelium (E)
- **b** Moderate magnification of the junctional epithelium (JE). Notice the lymphocytic infiltration (→) in the subepithelial CT due to inefficient plaque control
- **c** High magnification of the most apical extent of the junctional epithelium (JE). Farther apical, the supracrestal connective tissue (CT) lies in direct contact with the titanium surface (→)

Discussion of the Histological Findings and Conclusions

Very often, publications and lectures speak in imprecise oversimplifications of an "epithelial seal," even though the mucosal cuff is comprised of both epithelium *and* connective tissue. This can lead to the incorrect assumption that the epithelium plays the leading role in the formation of a soft-tissue cuff around an abutment.

The optimum tissue integration of an endosseous implant should not be considered separately for each different type of tissue, but rather as a unit. Thus, it is not possible for an adherent and self-renewing attachment of the junctional epithelium to the surface of the abutment to occur if the underlying connective tissue is inadequately organized or if it is inflamed beyond a certain physiological limit. Instead, there is more likely to be deep ingrowth of epithelium, which begins a process that finally ends with the loss of the implant.

The organization of the connective tissue of the type necessary to create a tight, resistant "gingival" cuff is favored by rigid, ankylotic anchorage of the implant in the bone. Other factors, such as the condition of the surface that contacts the supracrestal connective tissue in the abutment area, also play a role. A porous titanium surface is recommended for the sake of tissue integration because it has been demonstrated that supracrestal connective tissue fibers attach perpendicularly to a porous titanium surface such as the TPS layer. For the sake of tissue *maintenance,* however, such a rough surface can be disadvantageous if it comes into direct contact with the oral cavity. A rough surface favors plaque accumulation and the development of soft-tissue inflammation around the implant. We made a fundamental decision in 1985 to make the ITI implants smooth in the supracrestal region, limiting the TPS layer to the endosseous portion. This can be viewed as a compromise, in that preference is given to considerations of prophylaxis and tissue maintenance. The decision has proven to be correct in retrospect. Results of more recent animal experiments have shown that the supracrestal connective tissue is able to establish a tough, functional soft-tissue cuff, even around titanium surfaces that are highly polished. As has already been pointed out, this cuff is characterized by a ring of circularly arranged fibers immediately adjacent to the implant. It resembles a ring of scar tissue with perpendicular connective tissue fibers streaming into it from the surrounding area. This "scar ring" is apparently able to prevent deep proliferation of epithelium to the bone level. Another possible interpretation of these repeatedly observed findings is that the epithelial cells, which are genetically programmed to cover over defects in connective tissue, consider the defects already healed. So far, these findings have been obtained exclusively in animal studies and remain to be confirmed in human histological preparations.

In additon to the surface characteristics of the implant abutment, the preliminary condition of the mucosa also plays a role. It appears that mature keratinized alveolar mucosa is superior to nonkeratinized alveolar mucosa. One reason for this could be the different manner in which the subepithelial connective tissue is built up. The alveolar mucosa contains mostly elastic fibers and practically no collagen fibers. There are also clinical reasons for recommending placement of the implant abutment in keratinized mucosa. The most important of these is the fact that the nonkeratinized alveolar mucosa is vulnerable to injury from the toothbrush, and this can lead patients to neglect their oral hygiene when there are painful lesions present from brushing.

The outcome of the preceding discussion is that as far as *tissue reactions* are concerned, an endosseous implant system can stand up under critical evaluation only if all of the separate relevant conditions are combined with one another in a logical manner.

To summarize the most important points: The formation of a rigid, ankylotic (connective tissue-free) attachment of the implant to bone (osteointegration) during healing requires:

1. a bionert implant material;
2. the least amount of trauma possible during preparation of the bony bed (low rotational speed, sharp burs and drills, a generous supply of cooling saline solution);
3. an optimal congruence between implant and implant bed that assures primary stability without wedging;
4. a healing period of *at least* 3 months, during which the implant is largely undisturbed in regard to occlusal loading.

The attachment to bone without intervening connective tissue is one of the most important prerequisites for the formation of a functional *supracrestal connective tissue,* which is the foundation for a resistant, gingiva-like soft-tissue cuff encircling the implant abutment. In this regard, the following points must be observed as secondary conditions:

1. gentle, atraumatic operative technique also in the soft tissue (sharp incisions and careful reflection of the mucoperiosteum);
2. placement of the implant abutment in an area of attached keratinized alveolar mucosa or, if that is not possible;
3. mucogingival surgery with free mucosal grafts from the palate;
4. close, clean suturing.

If these points have been observed, then the requirements for an epithelial attachment will also have been met, provided that:

1. immaculate oral hygiene is instituted from the very beginning, i.e. chemical plaque control with chlorhexidine 0.1–0.2% for the first 2–3 weeks after surgery followed by mechanical plaque control;
2. the supracrestal portion of the implant has a smooth surface.

Producing the Histologic Specimens

H. Stich

The majority of histological preparations shown in this section were prepared according to the following technique.

Light Microscopy

Dehydration and simultaneous block staining is carried out on the trimmed and well-fixed bone specimens (fixing solution: neutral buffered 10 % formalin solution).

The specimens are dehydrated and simultaneously stained with a succession of increasing concentrations of 60, 80, 90, and 100% alcohol mixed with 5% basic fuchsin. They remain in each of the colored alcohol solutions for 24 hours each.

In the rare cases where a block staining in blue is desired, aniline blue is added to the alcohol baths instead of the red dye.

Alcohol and remaining water are removed from the bone preparations with acetone.

The alcohol and excess dye material must be flushed out with at least 5–6 separate acetone baths that are separated by at least 4 weeks. After that, the preparations are ready for the embedding medium.

Embedding in Acrylic

A methyl methacrylic acid ester* is used as the embedding medium. To remove all traces of acetone from the bone specimen, the acrylic bath must be changed frequently. For a preparation of approximately 20 x 30 mm, the following steps are taken:

1. change of bath after 24 hours;
2. change of bath after about 72 hours;
3. change of bath after about 10 days, combined with a 5-minute vacuum treatment;
4. change of bath after 20 days; this bath contains a few milliliters of Plastoid-N* (one more brief vacuum treatment);
5. change of bath after approximately 4 weeks with 2% Plastoid-N*.

Final Embedding Mixture

In the fifth to sixth weeks, the preparations are placed in the final methacrylate bath, to which plasticizers and catalysts have been added.

Mixture:
120 ml	Methyl methacrylate
16 ml	Plastoid-N*
1.1 g	Parkadox*, dried powder; mix well until the powder is dissolved! Finally, 1 g of Celloidin* is stirred in (magnetic stirrer).

This mixture can be stored for up to 2 months in a refrigerator.

* see list at end of chapter

Hardening of the Test Specimens (Polymerization)

The specimens are placed together with the above mentioned mixture into suitable *glass* cylinders (e.g., pill bottles) with polyethylene stoppers. The stoppers are secured with tape (Scotch tape). To prevent premature hardening, the glass bottles are placed in a container of water (Fig. 6.**21**), allowing the acrylic to harden slowly at room temperature. The container should be kept out of bright sunlight. After 10–14 days, the specimens will be hard. They are then cured in an incubator at approximately 38 °C for 12 hours and undergo final curing in a 50 °C warming box for an additional 4 hours.

Cutting with the Saw

After the specimens have cooled, the glass bottles are broken. Finally, the specimens are mounted in a diamond saw* and sectioned with slow advancement of the saw. The specimens should be continuously cooled under a 85% glycerin solution. To avoid artifacts, the slice thickness is adjusted to just under 0.3 mm (Fig. 6.**22** and 6.**23**).

The side of the section that is to be made adhesive (the future microscope slide side) is planed smooth with the rotor and silicon carbide paper (1000 and 4000 grit). For this, a microscope slide covered with double-sided clear adhesive tape (Scotch tape) is used. If necessary, the surface of the preparatation is polished on the polishing rotor with 3 μm diamond abrasive.*

6 Tissue Response

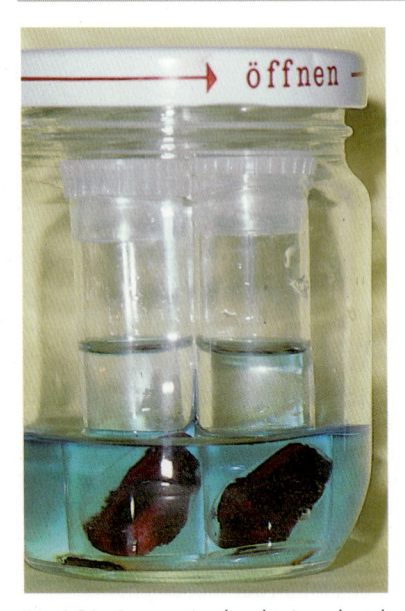

Fig. 6.**21** Preparation bottles in a closed water bath at room temperature

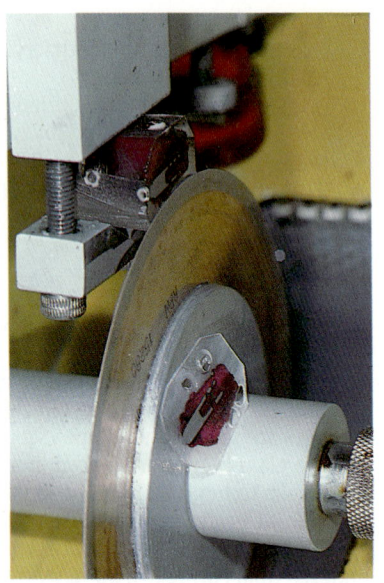

Fig. 6.**22** Bone specimen embedded in an acrylic block and mounted in the diamond saw

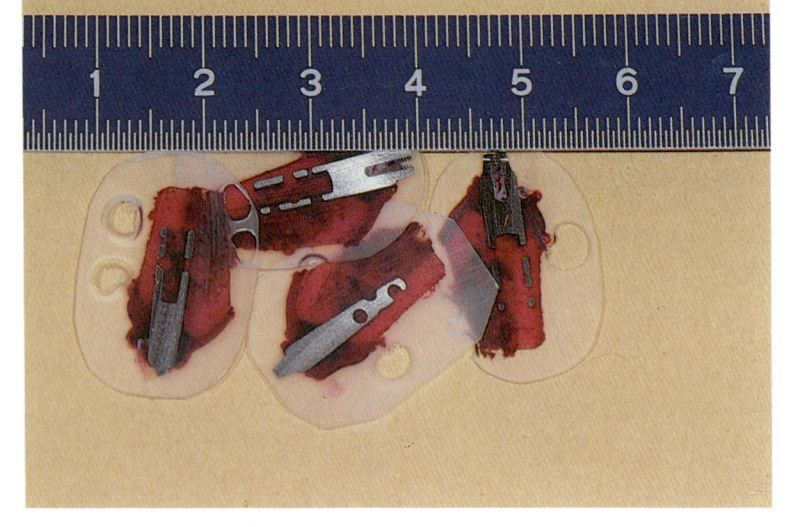

Fig. 6.**23** Coarse-cut sections

Thin Grinding

The specimens that have been cut and polished on one side are freed from the adhesive strip, washed thoroughly in clean benzene, and dried with cellulose. Using a clear epoxy resin, the preparation is bonded (polished side down) to a slide that has been freshly cleaned with benzene. Specimen and slide are pressed together with a clamp. Care must be taken to spread only a small amount of adhesive over the slide and eliminate all air bubbles (Fig. 6.**24**). The prepared specimens are then placed in the warming box for at least 3 hours at a temperature of 40 °C.

The next step is the actual thin-polishing procedure. For this, silicon carbide paper on a water-cooled rotor is utilized. Double-sided adhesive tape is placed on the underside of the slide for a finger hold. The first grinding stage is carried out with 500 grit paper. When the preparation becomes slightly transparent, the paper is changed to 1000 grit. Here it is important that the grinding is done in a parallel manner and under light pressure. Grinding is continued with this grit until the preparation is transparent or until the desired thickness has been reached. (a micrometer is used, compensating for the thickness of the adhesive.) Finally, the surface is polished with 4000 grit paper (Fig. 6.**25**). The specimen should be thoroughly rinsed before each change of grit!

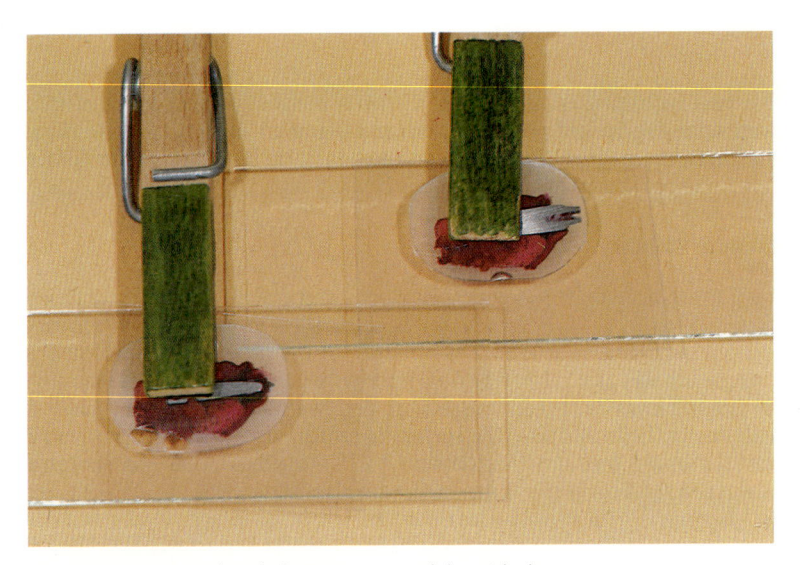

Fig. 6.**24** Specimens bonded to microscope slides with clamps

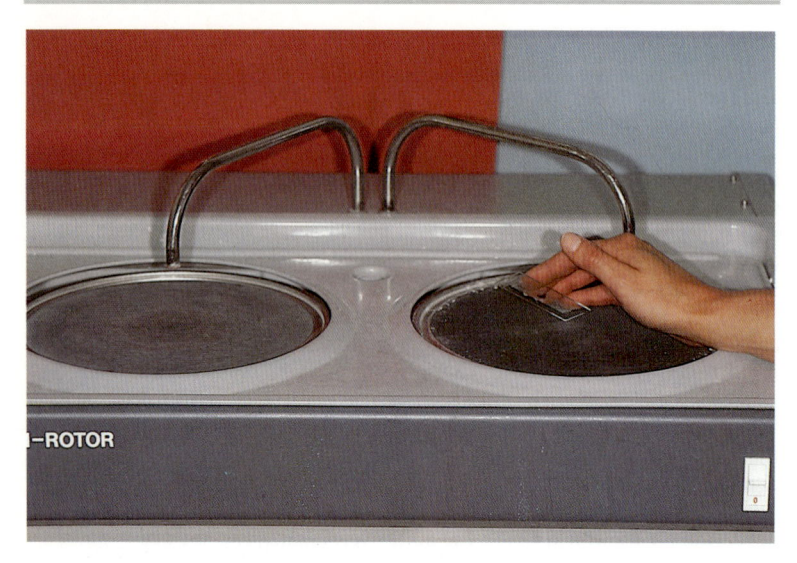

Fig. 6.25 Thinning a specimen on the rotary grinder

Final polishing is accomplished with a polishing wheel, fitted with a hard, adhesive-backed polishing cloth and Diamond Spray* (3 µm). To avoid forming a sharp relief between metal and bone, fine scratches on the surface remain unpolished. The preparation is cleaned with 90% alcohol (Fig. 6.26).

Counter Staining

Light green acetate (0.25% with 0.2% glacial acetic acid), is used for staining bone.

Staining time is at least 2–3 minutes. In the interim, the specimen is rinsed with 94% alcohol. After a final rinse with pure alcohol, the preparation is dried (blown with compressed air and warmed for approximately 8 minutes in the incubator). The surface is protected with a coating of liquid cover slipping medium (Merckospray*). If the preparation has become warped, a glass cover slip is used with the glass slide.

Fig. 6.**26** Rotary polisher

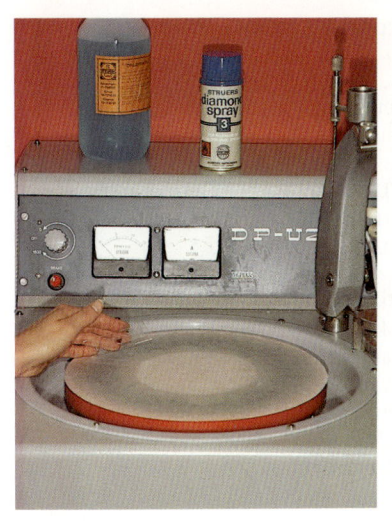

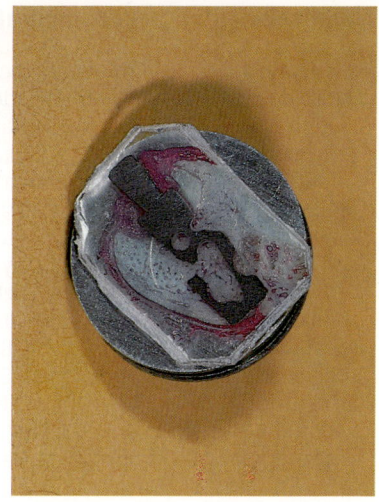

Fig. 6.**27** Prepared specimen bonded to glass and placed on SEM target

Preparation for Scanning Electron Microscopy

The dehydration, embedding, and sawing procedures are the same as for light microscopy. The preparations are also bonded to a microscope slide, ground, and well polished (Diamond Spray* 3 µm or, if necessary, 1 µm). The sections need not be as thin as is necessary for light microscopy.

The specimen is trimmed to fit on the SEM target by marking the size and cutting through both slide and specimen simultaneously with a dental diamond disk under water coolant. This procedure minimizes artifacts because the thin slice (metal with bone) remains bonded to the glass surface.

Finally, the preparation is cycled through multiple changes of pure acetone over a period of about 2 weeks to remove all traces of the methylmethacrylate embedding medium.

The Critical Point Dryer* drying apparatus is prepared with pure acetone, and the fluid exchange is accomplished with several CO_2 procedures. The preparations are immediately bonded to targets using Leit C*, and dried in a desiccator (Fig. 6.**27**). Sputter coating with gold (approx. 4000 nm) is the final step in this procedure.

Chemicals, supplies, and apparatuses

Araldite, slow curing – Ciba-Geigy Inc., Basel, Switzerland
Benzoyl peroxide, dry powder – Bender & Holbein, Basel, Switzerland
Celloidin – Fluka AG, Buchs, Switzerland
Methylmethacrylate monomer – Fluka Inc., Buchs, Switzerland
Plastoid-N. No. 5866 – Röhm-Pharma Ltd., Weiterstadt, Germany
Merckoglas. No. 3972 – Merck Inc., Darmstadt, Germany
Diamond spray, Struers – ABS Inc., Dietikon, Switzerland
Leit-C – Neubauer, Münster, Germany
Polishing cloth, Pan-W – ABS Inc., Dietikon, Switzerland
Silicon carbide papers – ABS Inc., Dietikon, Switzerland
Critical Point Dryer – Balzers Union, BaLzers, Liechtenstein
Diamond saw. Isomet – Buehler Ltd, Evanston, Illinois
Polisher DP-U2, Struers – ABS Inc., Dietikon, Switzerland
Grinder Knut-rotor, Struers – ABS Inc., Dietikon, Switzerland
Sputter apparatus – Balzers Union, Balzers, Liechtenstein

References

Albrektsson, T.: Knochengewebsreaktionen. In Brånemark, P. I., G. A. Zarb, T. Albrektsson (eds.): Gewebeintegrierter Zahnersatz. Quintessenz, Berlin 1985

Brånemark, P. I., U. Breine, R. Adell, B. O. Hansson, J. Lindström, A. Ohlsson: Intraosseous anchorage of dental prostheses. Scand. J. plast, reconstr. Surg. 3 (1969) 81

Buser, D., H. Stich, G. Krekeler, A. Schroeder: Faserstrukturen der periimplantären Mukosa bei Titanimplantaten – Eine tierexperimentelle Studie am Beagle-Hund. Z. zahnärztl. Implantol. 5 (1989) 15–23

Buser, D., R. K. Schenk, S. Steinemann, J. P. Fiorellini, C. Fox, H. Stich: Influence of surface characteristics on bone integration of titanium implants. A histomorphometric study in miniature pigs. J. biomed. Mater. Res. 25 (1991) 889–902

Buser, D., H. P. Weber, K. Donath, J. P. Fiorellini, D. W. Paquette, R. C. Williams: Soft tissue reactions to non-submerged unloaded titanium implant in beagle dogs. J. Periodontol. 63 (1992) 225–235

Gould, T. R. L., D. M. Brunette, L. Westbury: The attachment mechanism of epithelial cells to tianium in vitro. J. Periodont. Res. 16 (1981) 611

Grube, M., K. R. Paatz, H. Schmidt: Die Herstellung von Zahn- und Knochenschliffen. Zahn-, Mund- u. Kieferheilk. Zbl. 69 (1981) 200 u. 241

James, R. A., R. L. Schultz: Hemidesmosomes and the adhesion of junctional epithelial cells to metal implants, a preliminary report. Oral Implant. 4 (1974) 294

Jansen, J. A., R. de Wijn, J. M. L. Wolters-Lutgerhorst, P. J. van Mullem: Ultrastructural study of epithelial cel attachment to implant material. J. dent. Res. 64 (1985) 891

Kasemo, B., J. Lausmaa: Metallauswahl und Oberflächenbeschaffenheit. In Brånemark, P. I., G. A. Zarb, T. Albrektsson (ecs.): Gewebeintegrierter Zahnersatz. Quintessenz, Berlin 1985

Kirsch, A., K. Donath: Tierexperimentelle Untersuchungen zur Bedeutung der Mikromorphologie von Titanimplantatoberflächen. Fortschr. Zahnärztl. Implantol. 1 (1984) 35–40

References

Listgarten, M. A., D. Buser, S. Steinemann, K. Donath, N. P. Lang, H. P. Weber: Light and transmission electron microscopy of the intact interface between bone, gingiva and nonsubmerged titanium-coated epoxy resin implants. J. dent. Res. 71 (1992) 364–371

Mühlemann, H. R.: Zur Mikrostruktur der Implantatoberflächen. Schweiz. Mschr. Zahnheilk. 85 (1975) 97

Schenk, R.: Zur histologischen Verarbeitung von unentkalkten Knochen. Acta anat. 60 (1965) 3

Schroeder, A., O. Pohler, F. Sutter: Gewebsreaktion auf ein Titan-Hohlzylinderimplantat mit Titan-Spritzschicht-Oberfläche. Schweiz. Mschr. Zahnheilk. 86 (1976) 713–727

Schroeder, A., H. Stich, F. Straumann, F. Sutter: Über die Anlagerung von Osteozement an einen belasteten Implantatkörper. Schweiz. Mschr. Zahnheilk. 88 (1978) 1051

Schroeder, A., E. van der Zypen. H. Stich. F. Sutter: The reaction of bone, connective tissue and epithelium to endosteal implants with sprayed titanium implants. J. max.-fac. Surg. 9 (1981) 15–25

Schroeder, H. E.: Orale Strukturbiologie. 3. Aufl. Thieme, Stuttgart 1987

Skalak, R.: Biomechanische Betrachtungen. In: Brånemark, P. I., G. A. Zarb, T. Albrektsson (eds.): Gewebeintegrierter Zahnersatz. Quintessenz, Berlin 1985

Steinemann, S. G., J. Eulenberger, P. A. Mäusli, A. Schroeder: "Adhesion of bone to titanium." In Christel, P., A. Meunier, A. J. C. Lee (eds.): Advances of Biomaterials, Elsevier, Amsterdam 1986 (S. 409–414)

Strunz, V.: Enossale implantatmaterialien in der Mund- und Kieferchirurgie. Hanser, München 1985

Ten Cate, A. R.: Der gingivale Abschluß. In Brånemark, P. I., G. A. Zarb, T. Albrektsson (eds.): Gewebeintegrierter Zahnersatz. Quintessenz, Berlin 1985

Thomas, K. V., St. D. Cook: An evaluation of variables influencing implant fixation by direkt bone apposition. J. biomed. Mater. Res. 19 (1985) 875

Wenziker, K.: Methakrylate als Einbettmedien in der Zahnhistologie. Schweiz. Mschr. Zahnheilk. 75, 51 (1964)

Wilke, H. J., L. Claes, S. Steinemann: "The influence of various titanium surfaces on the interface shear strength between implants and bone". In: Heimke, G., U. Soltész, A. J. C. Lee (eds.): Advances in Biomaterials. Vol. 9. Clinical Implant Materials. Elsevier, Amsterdam (1990) 309–314

Design of ITI Implants

7 The Concept of the ITI Implants

F. Sutter

Introduction

The current ITI concept is based on the perforated hollow cylinder and hollow screw implants developed in 1974 and the TPS screw implants developed in 1977 (see pages 69 f.). The experience with the various ITI extension implant types, which were designed during the period between 1975 and 1979, affected the development of the new ITI system in a positive manner. Experimental biological tests of the tissue reaction to various implant materials and surfaces were carried out for many years with these pioneering implants.

The essential characteristics of these constructional designs were good physiological loadability, precise preparation of the implant site (characterized by minimal bone trauma), small volume of the implant anchoring element, and large bone surfaces. In all variations, the implant geometry was designed in such a way that excessively high specific pressure peaks do not act on the bone, even under severe functional stress. Furthermore, all other important factors, namely stability and biocompatibility of the material used, microstructure of the implant surface, and adequate primary stability, were also taken into consideration. Once again, technically pure titanium, which is characterized by its excellent biocompatibility and high mechanidal stability, was chosen for all implant types.

The anchoring part of the implant is coated with titanium plasma, which creates an optimal micromorphological surface, and thus favors direct growth of the bone to the implant surface. A transmucosal design was chosen for the two-part implants. The instruments are standardized.

The Different ITI Implant Types

The Hollow Cylinder Implants (HC Type)

The basic design of the new hollow cylinder (HC) implant corresponds to that of the classic ITI Type F implant, which has been used clinically since 1978. It was modified in certain respects on the basis of the clinical experience obtained and was integrated as the basic design geometry into the new ITI concept. The external diameter is still 3.5 mm. The anchoring surface is coated with titanium plasma. The cylinder has systematically arranged perforations up to about 4 mm below the bone crest. The HC implants are polished smooth in their neck regions to reduce the danger of plaque deposition and to engender good conditions for epithelial attachment. Depending on the indication, one-part or two-part HC implants can be used.

The One Part Hollow Cylinder Implants

The standardized range is produced in five lengths with 8, 10, 12, 14, and 16 mm anchorage depths (Fig. 7.**1a–d**). The anchorage depth corresponds to the plasma-coated part of the implant. The one-part HC implants were designed specifically for the edentulous atrophied mandible in combination with bar prosthetic superstructures. Generally, four implants are inserted between the mental foramina and are preferentially interconnected with a bar within 24 hours. Histological findings and 10 years of clinical experience have shown that early functional loading of the implants is possible because of the bar interconnection (22, 24). However, the phase of soft-tissue healing of 2 to 3 weeks should be allowed to pass first (Fig. 7.**2**).

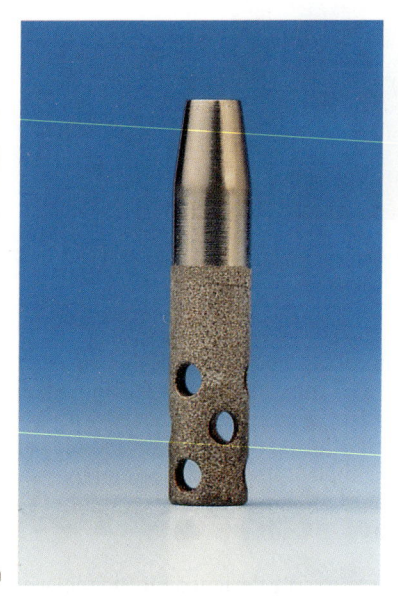

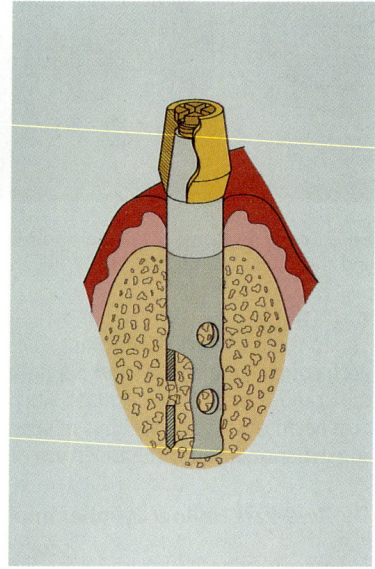

Fig. 7.**1a** and **b** Photographic and schematic representation of a one-part hollow cylinder implant (HC type)

116 7 The Concept of the ITI Implants

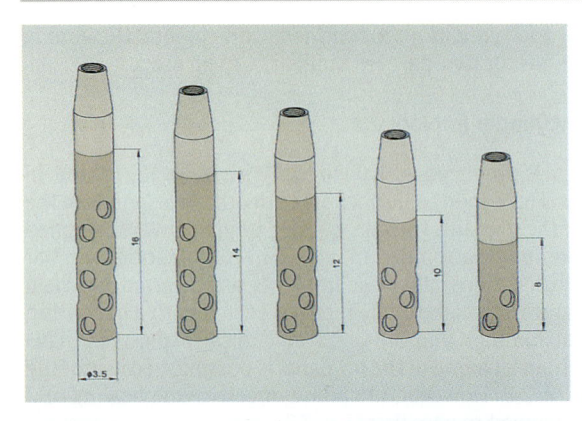

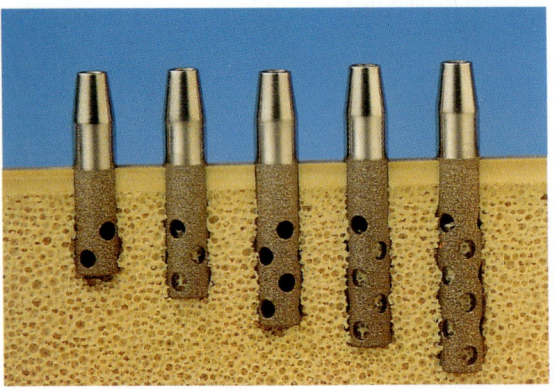

Fig. 7.**1c** and **d** Range of one-part hollow cylinder implants with a diameter of 3.5 mm and anchorage lengths of 8, 10, 12, 14, and 16 mm

In the one-part HC implant, the conical head part is precisely machined with concial angle of 8° and a height of 3.65 mm; it serves to accommodate the standardized gold copings. This implant head is also provided with a 2 mm occlusal thread, which is necessary for the fixation of the removable bar construction and for the insertion of the implant ifself (Fig. 7.**3a** and **b**).

The Two-Part Hollow Cylinder Implants

The two-part hollow cylinder implant was mainly designed for the replacement of single teeth in the maxilla. This indication entails high specifications, especially from an aesthetic point of view. In order to meet the latter

The Different ITI Implant Types 117

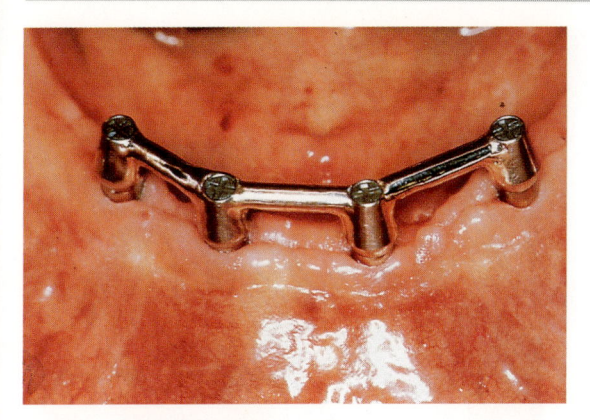

Fig. 7.2 Finished and screwed-in bar

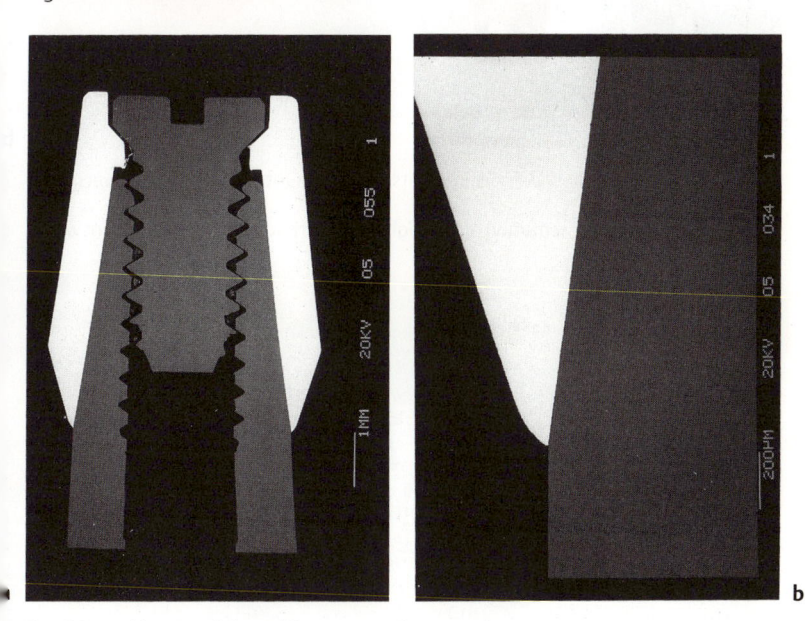

Fig. 7.3a and b Fit of the gold coping on the 8° implant conus

requirements, the body of the implant transforms above the bone level into a trumpet-like configuration with a diameter of 4.8 mm, which, roughly corresponds to the cervical diameter of a front tooth. The implant is available in two variants, a straight form and a form at an angle of 15° (Fig. 7.4a and b)

118   7   The Concept of the ITI Implants

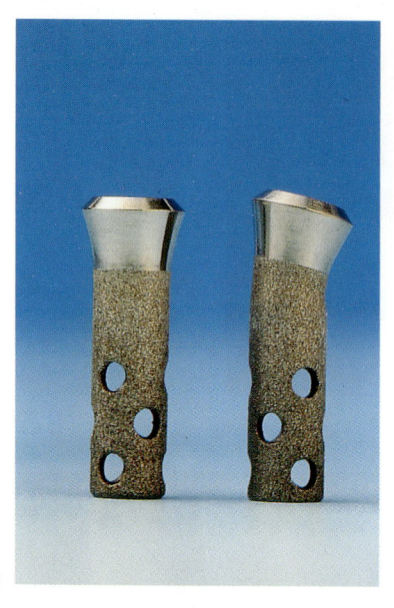

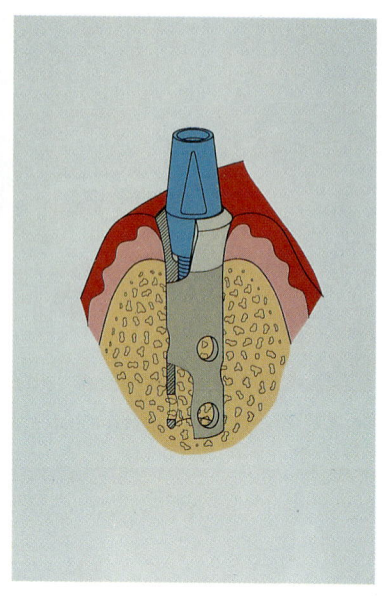

Fig. 7.**4a**   Two-part hollow cylinder implants in the straight and a 15° angled version

Fig. 7.**4b**   Graphic representation of a straight, two-part hollow cylinder implant with a conical secondary part

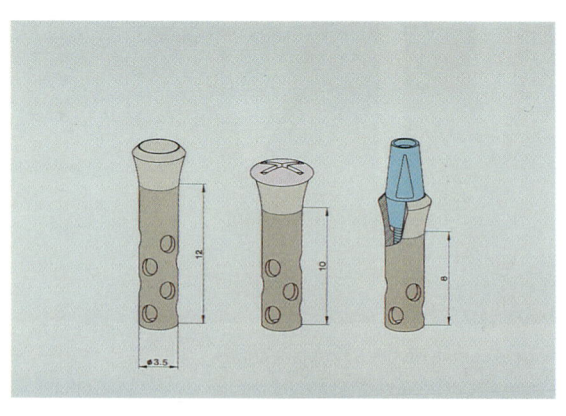

Fig. 7.**5a** and **b**   Range of straight and 15° angled two-part hollow cylinder implants in lengths of 8, 10, and 12 mm

Fig. 7.**5c** and **d**   Original size of the two-part hollow cylinder range

The Different ITI Implant Types

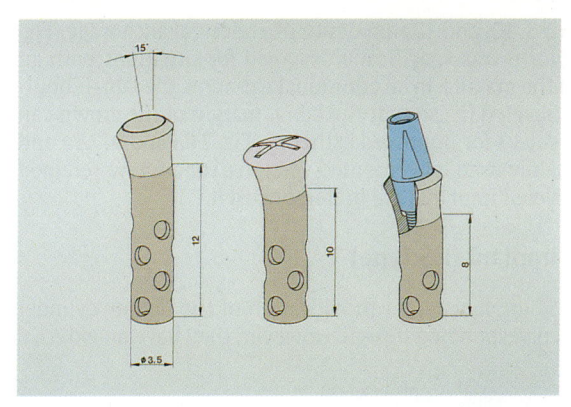

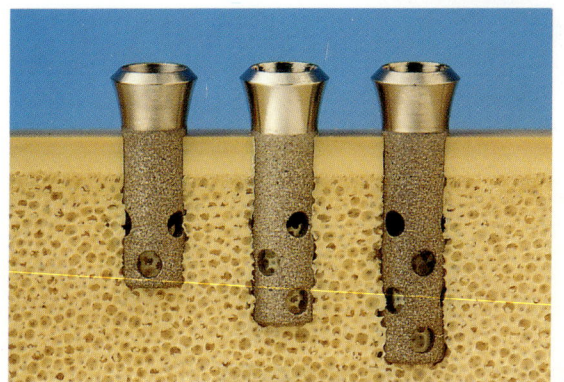

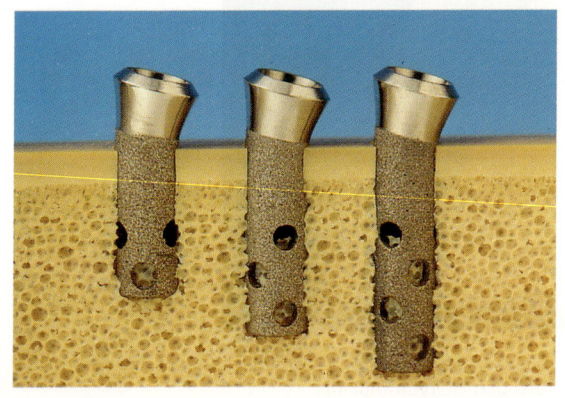

and in three lengths of 8, 10, and 12 mm depth of endosteal anchorage (Fig. 7.**5a–d**). The angular form was specifically designed for situations with an alveolar protrusion in the maxilla. In an additional variation, the labial shoulder of the implant is beveled (K) so that the labial margin of the crown can be placed within the sulcus for improved esthetics (Fig. 7.**6a** and **b**, 7.**7a** and **b**). This variation is mainly used for cemented versions. For a screw-retained procedure, the nonbeveled implants are preferably used.

The Hollow Screw Implant (HS Type)

The hollow screw (HS) implants are a modification of the hollow cylinder implants and have a corresponding design. However, they have an external

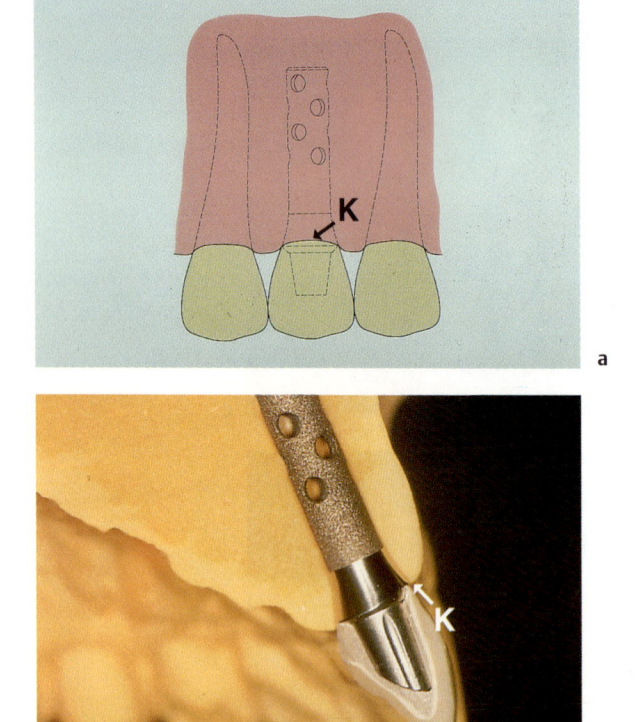

Fig. 7.**6a** and **b** Representation of the aesthetically advantageous bevelled buccal crown margin "K" in the two-part HC type implant

thread in addition, with an outer diameter of approx. 4.1 mm and a core diameter of 3.5 mm. The head and neck part, the arrangement and size of the perforations, and the titanium plasma coating of the implant anchoring element correspond exactly to the hollow cylinder implants. One-part and two-part variants of this implant are also available for different clinical indications. In addition to the properties of the hollow cylinder implants already described, the HS implants have the following further characteristics:
1. Optimal primary stability even in less dense cancellous bone
2. Slight and even primary compression by tapping the thread, since the tapped thread profile is about 0.05 mm smaller than the implant profile (see following section "Thread-profile and loading characteristics")

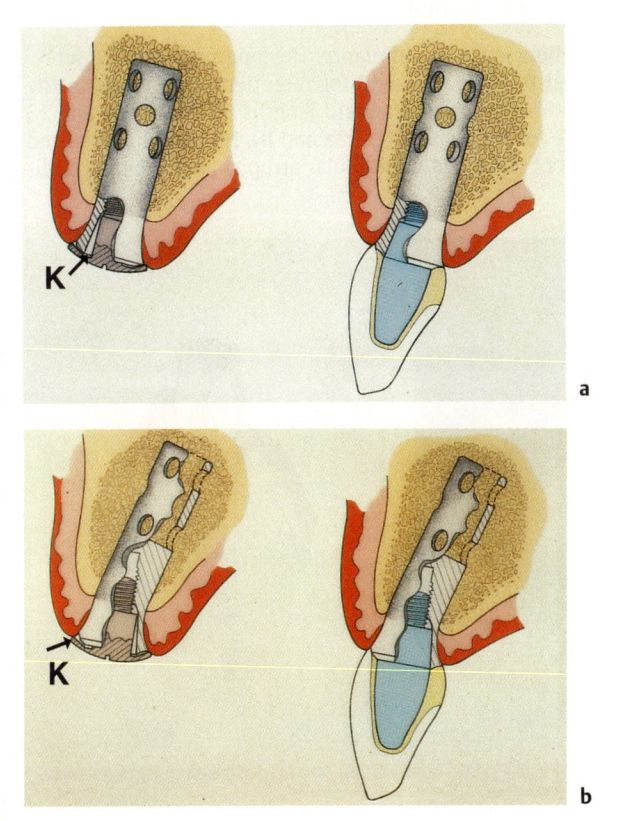

Fig. 7.7a and b Graphic representation of the two-part HC implants in the maxilla in the straight (**a**) and angulated (**b**) version

7 The Concept of the ITI Implants

In general terms, the HS implant combines the advantages of the hollow cylinder design with those of a screw implant. The hollow cylinder principle in additon to a suitable thread geometry will increase the stability of the inserted implant.

Axial pull out tests with various thread geometries were used to optimize the thread design. According to our testing results, the chosen profile gives the best overall results. Since 1980, such hollow screws have also been used in maxillofacial surgery for fixation of titanium reconstruction plates. The clinical results attained since then show that due to the characteristics described, and despite the large alternating stress, an increase in stability and anchorage can be attained, with time.

The One-Part Hollow Screw Implants

As with one-part hollow cylinder implants, the one-part hollow screw implants (Fig. 7.**8a** and **b**) were designed for retention of dentures in the edentulous mandible. Five different standard lengths (8, 10, 12, 14, and 16 mm) are also available for this type (Fig. 7.**9a** and **b**). HS implants are used preferentially in cases of advanced mandibular atrophy and in bone condi-

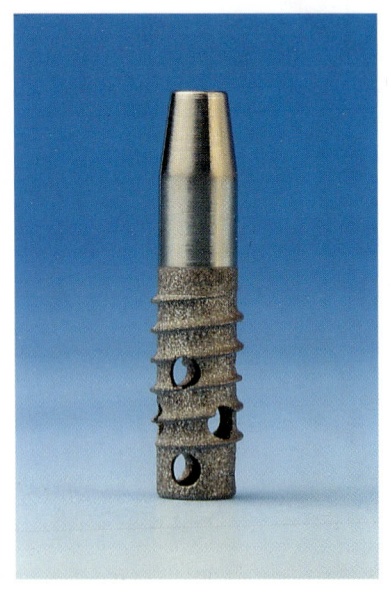

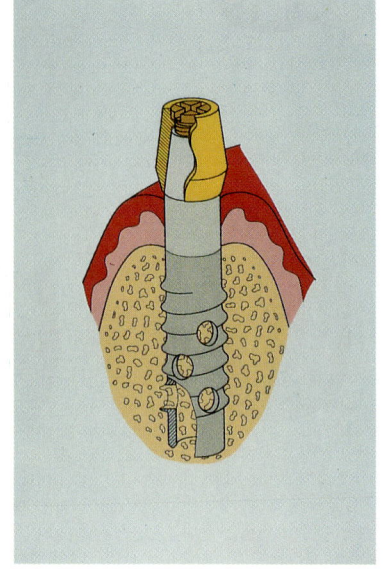

Fig. 7.**8a** and **b** Photographic and graphic representation of a one-part screw implant (HS type)

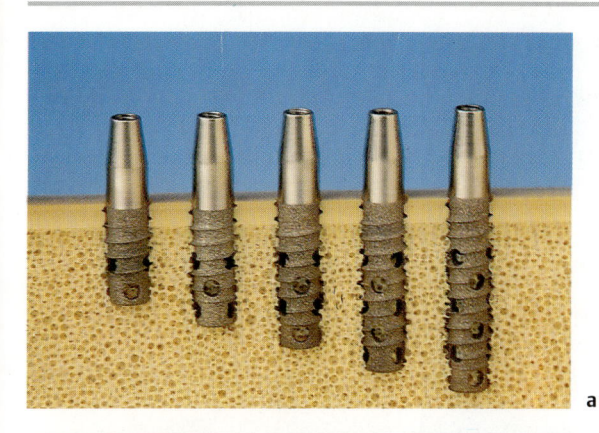

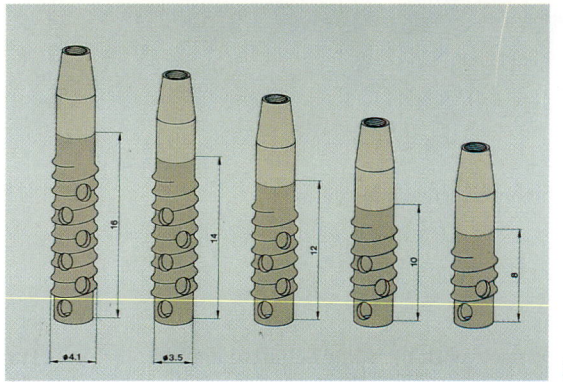

Fig. 7.**9a** and **b** Range of one-part hollow screw implants with an external diameter of 4.1 mm and anchorage lengths of 8, 10, 12, 14, and 16 mm

tions with low cancellous bone density, since the additional screw thread ensures adequate primary stability even under unfavorable conditions.

The Two-Part Hollow Screw Implants

Two-part HS implants (Fig. 7.**10a** and **b**) are mainly indicated in distal extension conditions in the mandible and maxilla, in which they serve as abutments for fixed prosthetic devices (bridges), and in single-tooth spaces in the region of the premolar and molar teeth. These two-part implants are highly suitable for retaining dentures in the edentulous mandible. Like the two-part hollow cylinder implants, these types are produced in three lengths of 8, 10,

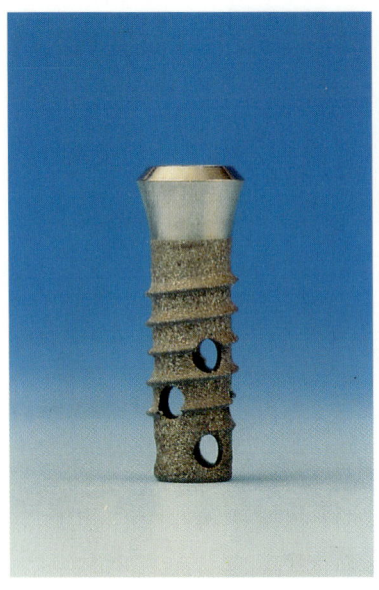

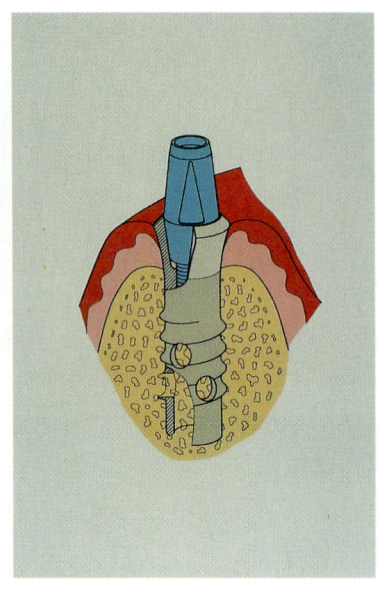

Fig. 7.**10a** and **b**   Two-part hollow screw implants

and 12 mm and can be used with the same standard abutments (Fig. 7.**11a** and **b**). For implantation in transplants, there are two additional lengths (14 and 16 mm) available. (Fig. 7.**16**).

The Screw Implants (S Type)

Another classic ITI implant, the TPS screw implant, has been used clinically in the edentulous mandible for more than 10 years. In the development of the new ITI concept, it was also logical to integrate this implant into the overall concept, since existing inadequacies of the implant could be eliminated at the same time. One major difference is that the screw implant is no longer self-tapping. Like the HS implants, it is only screwed in after pretapping the screw thread, at least in cortical bone.

The risk of thermal damage to the surrounding bone during the insertion in of the implant was thus substantially reduced. Moreover, the external profile of the one-part and two-part S implants exactly corresponds to that of the hollow-screw implant, allowing the same thread tap to be used.

The Different ITI Implant Types 125

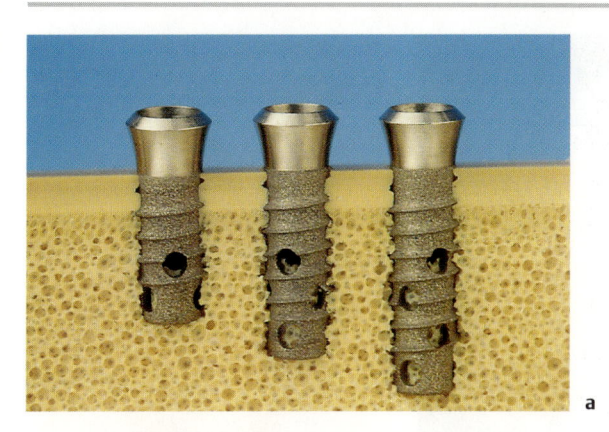

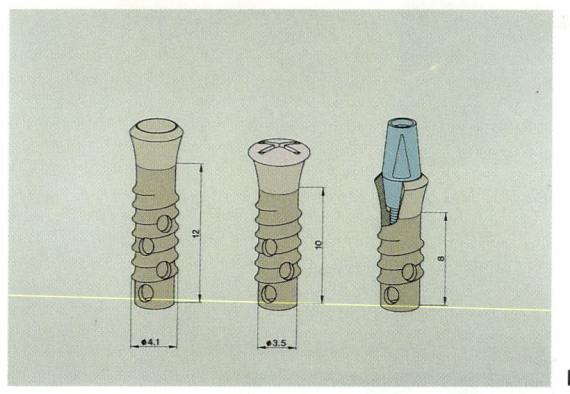

Fig. 7.**11a** and **b** Range of two-part hollow screw implants in standard lengths of 8, 10, and 12 mm

The One-Part Screw Implants

These implants are also produced in five standard lengths of 8, 10, 12, 14, and 16 mm endosteal anchorage depth. The length over which the plasma coating is applied also corresponds to the anchorage depth (Fig. 7.**12a** and **b**). Experience up to the present shows that these implants are mainly indicated in the edentulous mandible in combination with a bar prosthetic superstructure. The one-part S implant has the same head design as the one-part hollow cylinder and hollow screw implants (Fig. 7.**13a** and **b**).

126 7 The Concept of the ITI Implants

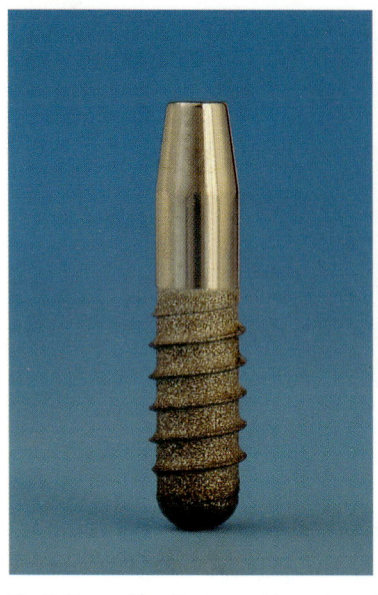

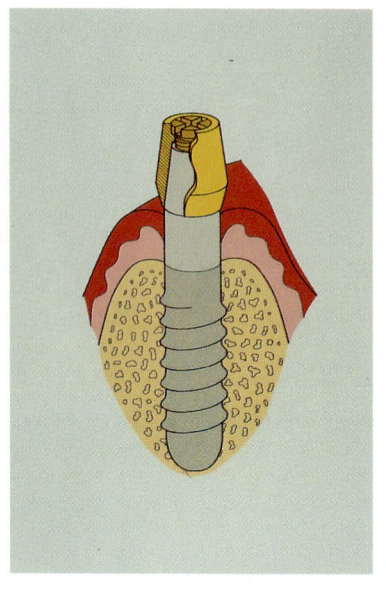

Fig. 7.**12a** and **b** Photographic and graphic representation of a one-part solid screw implant (S Type)

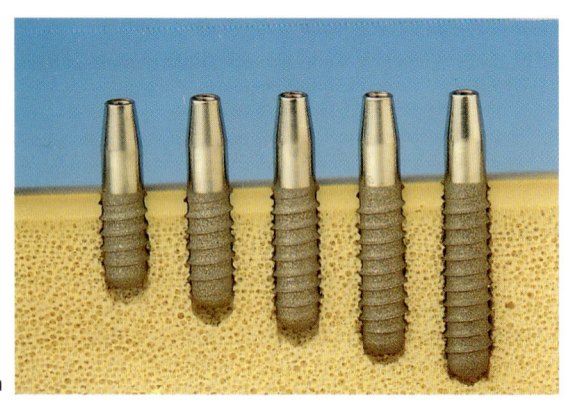

Fig. 7.**13a** and **b** Range of one-part screw implants with an external diameter of 4.1 mm and standard lengths of 8, 10, 12, 14, and 16 mm

The Different ITI Implant Types

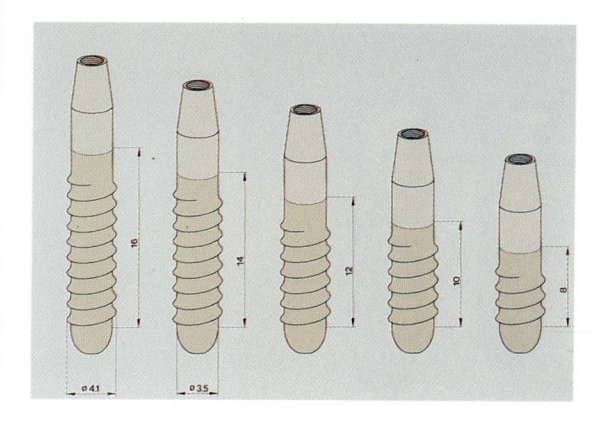

7.**13b**

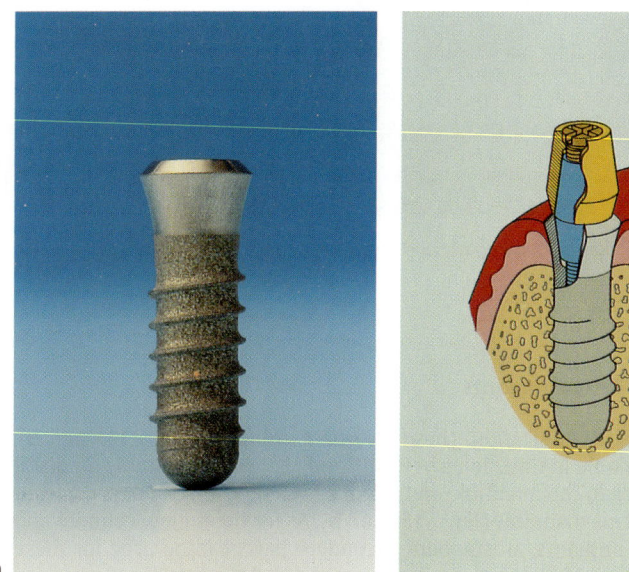

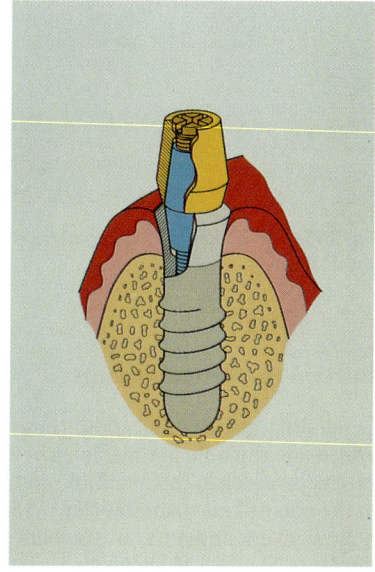

Fig. 7.**14a** and **b** Two-part solid screw implants that have the same thread profile as the hollow screw implants

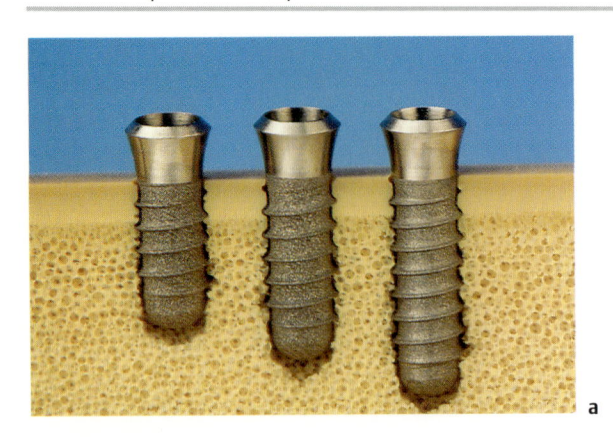

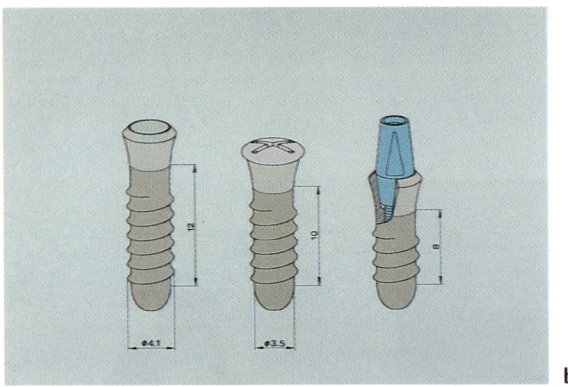

Fig. 7.**15a** and **b**   Range of two-part solid screw implants in standard lengths of 8, 10, and 12 mm

The Two-Part Screw Implants

Depending on the indication, these two-part implants (Fig. 7.**14a** and **b**), which are available in three lengths (8, 10, and 12 mm) are suitable for distal extension cases in the mandible and maxilla and for retention of prostheses in the edentulous mandible (Fig. 7.**15a** and **b**). As for the hollow cylinder and hollow screw implants, all standard secondary parts can be used for these implants. Figure 7.**16** shows two-part screw and hollow screw implants with anchorage lenghts of 14 and 16 mm. These implants are mainly used for implantation in transplants.

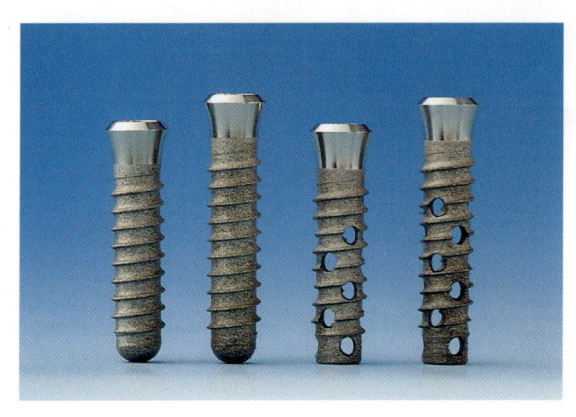

Fig. 7.**16** Additional hollow cylinder, hollow screw, and solid screw implants in lengths of 14 and 16 mm

Basic Design of the ITI System

The One-Part Implant Design

The investigations carried out during the last 20 years, and histological findings derived from ITI implants inserted in a single phase prove that an osteointegrated anchorage between the implant surface and the bone does not depend on a two-stage surgical procedure. This particularly applies to one-part implants, which are used for prosthesis retention in the edentulous mandible in multiple linkup, and which are interconnected postoperatively using a bar splint. With regard to plaque deposition and cleaning the part of the implant with mounted gold copings or bar interconnections projecting from the tissue, this method is preferable because of the simple and niche-free geometry.

The Two-Part Implant Design

Theoretically, there are two possibilities for the two-part implant design, which are used for the entire indication category:
1. the closed mucosal system, in which the primary part of the implant is sunk to the level of the bone crest, so that the mucoperiosteal flap can be sutured over the implant (Fig. 7.**17a**).
2. the open transmucosal system, in which the primary part is inserted such that the top remains about 3 mm above the bone crest. The wound margins are adapted around the neck of the implant, and primary soft-tissue sealing takes place involving the implant surface (Fig. 7.**17b**).

130 7 The Concept of the ITI Implants

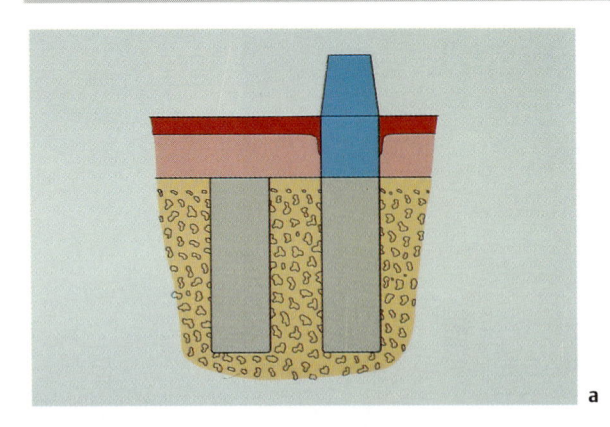

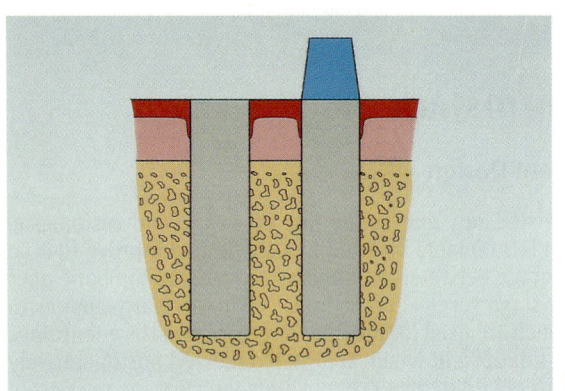

Fig. 7.**17a** The closed subgingival concept
Fig. 7.**17b** The open transgingival concept

For the following reasons, the ITI has decided in favor of the open or non submerged system:
1. in the transmucosal system, reoperation is not necessary to expose the implant and to insert a secondary part. (Fig. 7.**18a**);
2. the insertion of the secondary part can be carried out under clinical conditions that permit optimal vision. This is in contrast to the two-stage method, where as a result of the need for surgical exposure of the implant, the abutment insertion procedure is made more difficult by blood, saliva, and tissue residues (Fig. 7.**18b**);
3. the mucosal seal is formed during the healing phase in the transmucosal method and is not disturbed by insertion of the secondary part. In the

Basic Design of the ITI System **131**

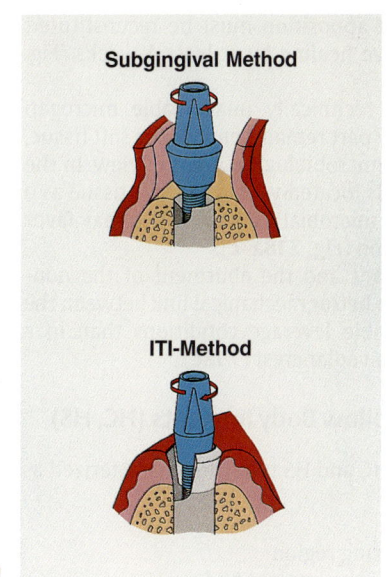

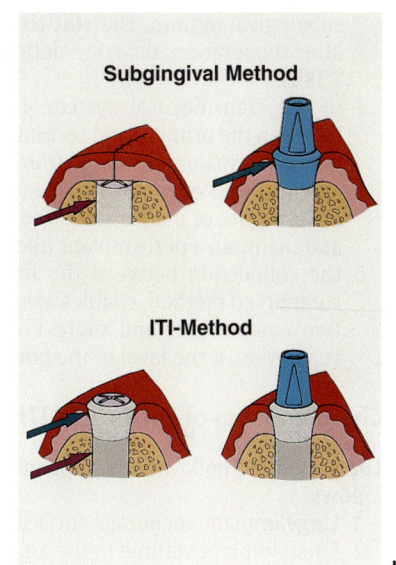

Fig. 7.18a Insertion of the secondary part under clinically clean conditions and optimal visual control in the ITI system

Fig. 7.18b The ITI method enables a single-phase operation. Reoperation is not necessary. The microgap between the primary and secondary part is outside the soft tissues

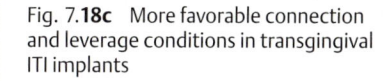

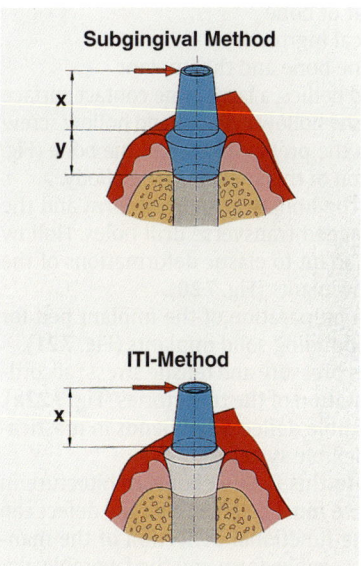

Fig. 7.18c More favorable connection and leverage conditions in transgingival ITI implants

subgingival system, the soft-tissue apposition must be reconstituted after reoperation, delaying definitive healing by at least 4 weeks (Fig. 7.**18b**);
4. in the transmucosal system, the technically unavoidable microgap between the primary and secondary part remains *outside* the soft tissue, which is a major advantage from a microbiological point of view. In the submucosal system, this microgap is located within the soft tissue as a possible site of plaque retention or microbial leakage, which may favor and maintain a peri-implant infection (Fig. 7.**18a–c**);
5. the connection between the implant and the abutment of the non-submerged method, enables a much better mechanical link between the two components and more favorable leverage conditions than in a separation at the level of the bony alveolar crest (7.**18c**).

Characteristics of Perforated ITI Hollow Body Implants (HC, HS)

The perforated hollow body implants (HC and HS type) are characterized as follows:
1. Large implant anchorage surface
2. Small implant volume in the anchoring region
3. Little bone loss in the preparation of the implant bed
4. Implant stiffness approximating that of bone
5. Promotion of the process of biological ingrowth
6. Reduction of the tension between the bone and the implant

1. Compared to the corresponding solid bodies, a large bone contact surface (anchorage surface) is attained with the hollow cylinder and hollow screw implants, which specifically reduces the pressure strain of the bone (Fig. 7.**19**) and enables favorable integration of the implant foreign body.
2. The implant volume is low, due to the hollow cylindrical form and the periodically and systematically arranged transverse drill holes. Hollow body implants can therefore better adapt to elastic deformations of the jaw than corresponding solid body implants (Fig. 7.**20**).
3. Far less bone removal occurs in the preparation of the implant bed for hollow implants than for the corresponding solid implants (Fig. 7.**21**).
4. The functional load in the jaw causes pressure and tensile stress; accordingly, there is a corresponding orientation of the trajectories (Fig. 7.**22a**). Moreover, it is known that the mandible deflects and bends in mastication and is therefore considered a flexible system.
   If a foreign body is incorporated into this flexible bone architecture in the form of an endosteal implant, care must be taken that the defect can be kept as small as possible and the functional deflection of the mandible is not impaired. The open and cagelike form and the favorable elastic properties of the ITI hollow body implants fulfill these requirements (Fig. 7.**22b**), due to the material and the design.

Basic Design of the ITI System

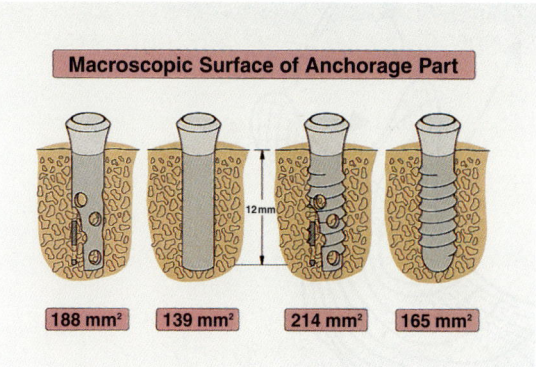

Macroscopic Surface of Anchorage Part

188 mm² | 139 mm² | 214 mm² | 165 mm²

Fig. 7.**19** Comparisons between hollow and corresponding solid implants with regard to the anchorage surface

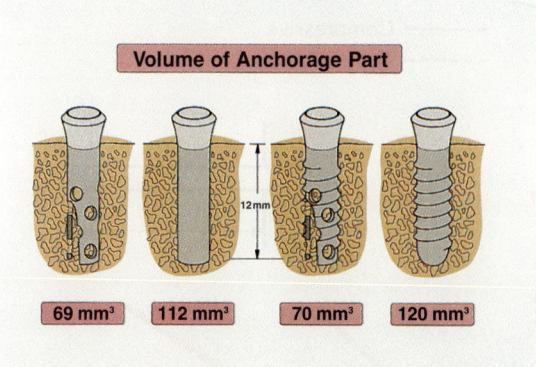

Volume of Anchorage Part

69 mm³ | 112 mm³ | 70 mm³ | 120 mm³

Fig. 7.**20** Comparisons of the hollow and solid implants with regard to the volume of the implant anchorage element

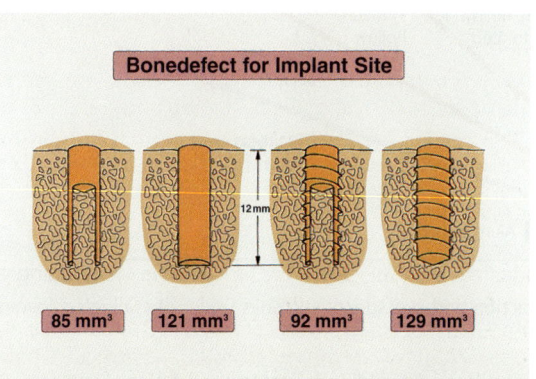

Bonedefect for Implant Site

85 mm³ | 121 mm³ | 92 mm³ | 129 mm³

Fig. 7.**21** Representation of the amount of bone removal required in implant bed preparation for hollow and corresponding solid implants

134 7 The Concept of the ITI Implants

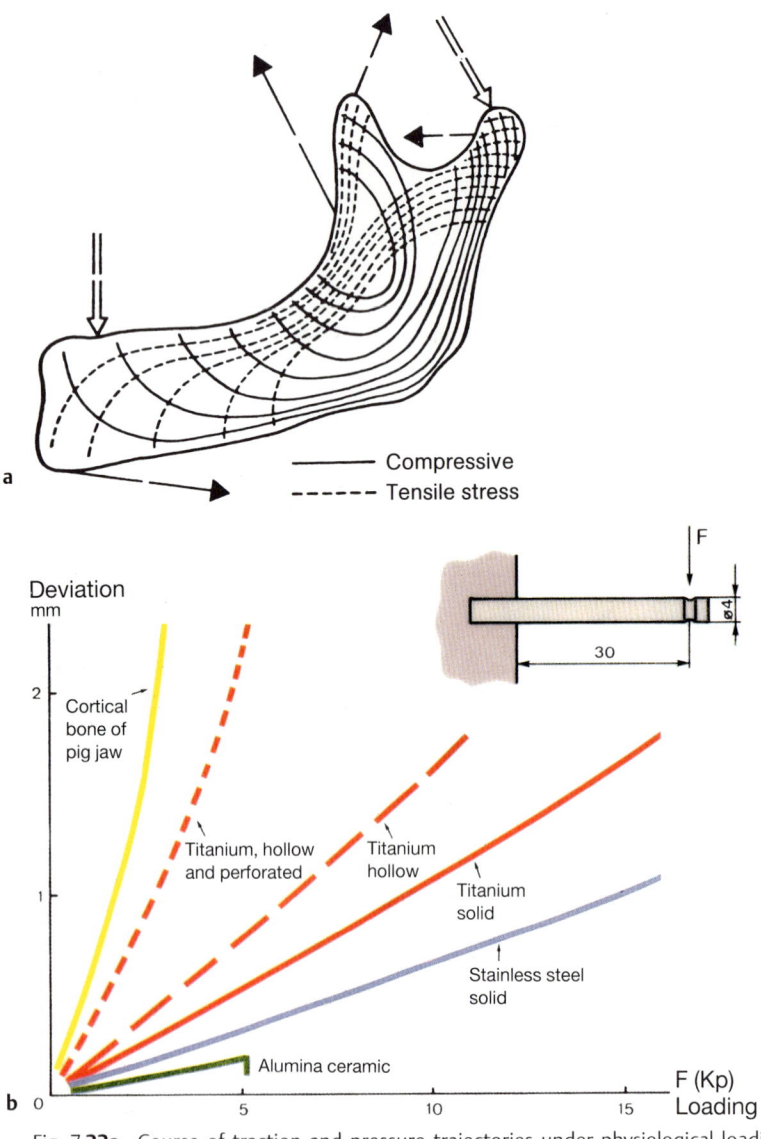

Fig. 7.**22a** Course of traction and pressure trajectories under physiological loading (according to Küppers)

Fig. 7.**22b** Comparison of stiffness depending on material and design of implants

Basic Design of the ITI System

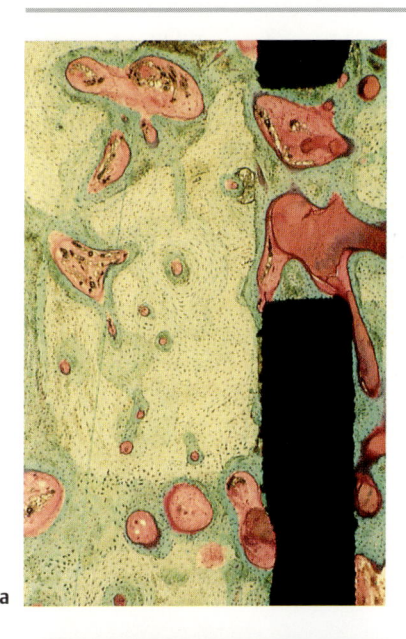

Fig. 7.**23a** Longitudinal histological section through a human implant removed after 3 years in function shows that bone has grown through the hollow cylinder perforations and that ankylotic anchorage has occurred (histology: Dr. H. Stich, Bern)

Fig. 7.**23b** Photographic representation of the perforations in hollow cylinder and hollow screw implants

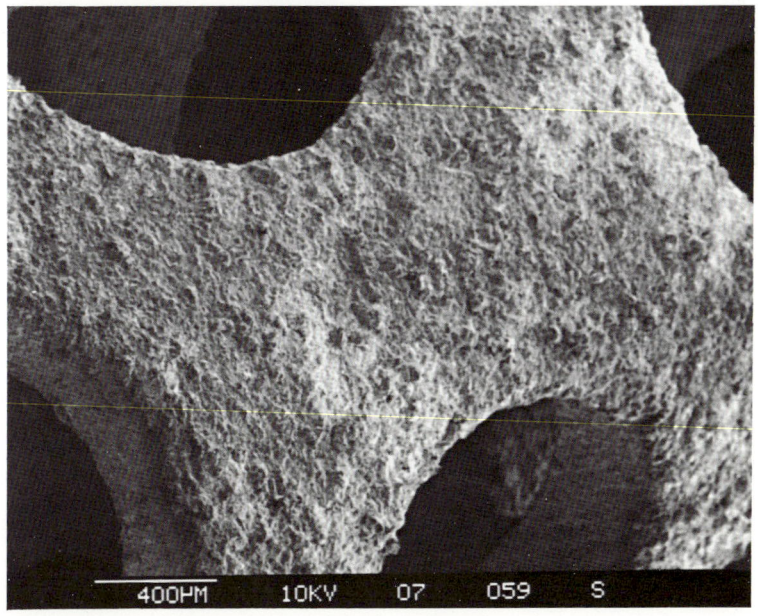

5. The open implant form permits favorable conditions for blood vascularization and regeneration of bone substance through the open implant aspects, which leads (in a relatively short period of time) to a bond between the central core of bone and the bone mass surrounding the implant (Fig. 7.**23a** and **b**).
6. The bone substance that has grown in and through the systematically and periodically arranged perforation has a dampening action on physiological implant loading and reduces the surface shear forces between the bone and the implant surface (Fig. 7.**24**).

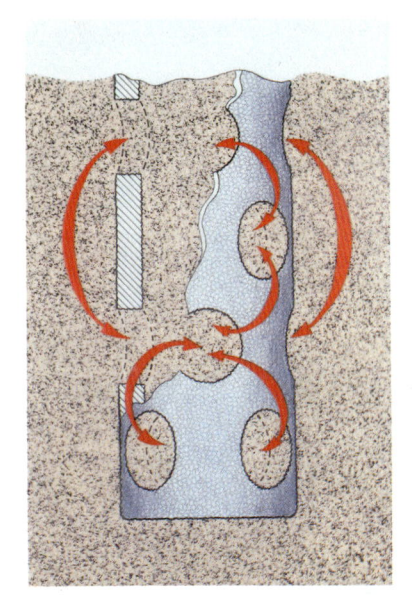

Fig. 7.**24** The most important constructional features of the hollow cylinder form in a schematic representation

Characteristics of the ITI Solid Screw Implants (S)

The solid screws have the following characteristics:
1. good mechanical stability, i.e., high maximum stress tolerance;
2. good primary stability;
3. simple method of implantation.

1: The high mechanical stability of the material (pure titanium) used for the ITI implants and the favorable maximum moment of fracture enables the greatest possible stress tolerance without danger of fracture.
2: By tapping the thread with a tap roughly 0.05 mm smaller, the risk of thermal damage during the insertion of the implant is largely eliminated, and good primary stability can be achieved.
3: For the implant site preparation, there are standardized instruments available; the round burrs and the 2.20/2.80 and 3.50 mm drills, as well as the depth gauge and the taps.

Thread: Profile and Loading Characteristics

To achieve optimum primary stability, even in low-density cancellous bone, the hollow and solid screw implants, in addition to the hollow cylinder implants, have been developed. The external profile of the solid screws (S Type) corresponds precisely to that of the perforated hollow screws (HS Type). Our objective of achieving optimal adherence of the bone to the implant surface and also of retaining it under physiological stress, was achieved by means of a special thread geometry and by the porous microstructure of the implant anchoring surface.

Due to the lower mechanical strength of the bone compared to titanium, the proportion of bone must predominate compared to the proportion of metal in the longitudinal section of the screw thread. To take this into account, a thread depth of 0.35 mm and a thread pitch of 1.25 mm were chosen. The load-bearing thread surfaces have an inclination of about 75° to the axis, which results in a more even spread of the compressive load over the complete screw thread surface, at the expense of a slight increase in the radial forces. Since the forces largely continue at right angles to the thread flank, the pressure forces "F" are directed into the bone mass outside the external diameter of the screw because of the flank inclination, which further improves the holding strength of the implants (Fig. 7.**25a** and **c**). However, the force is only transmitted inadequately to the bone mass when the holding flank of the thread is at a right angle to the axis (Fig. 7.**25b**). Experience has shown that slight precompression between implant and bone promotes the ankylotic bonding between bone and the titanium plasma-sprayed implant. To achieve this, the thread tap must be slightly smaller in diameter than the corresponding hollow and solid-core screw

138 7 The Concept of the ITI Implants

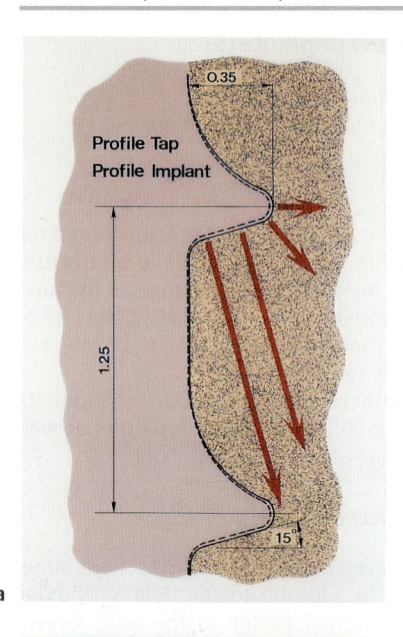

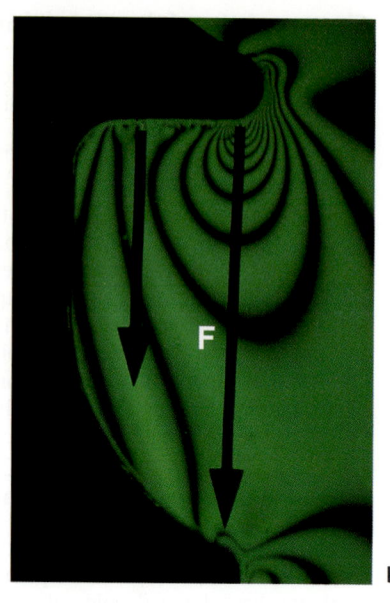

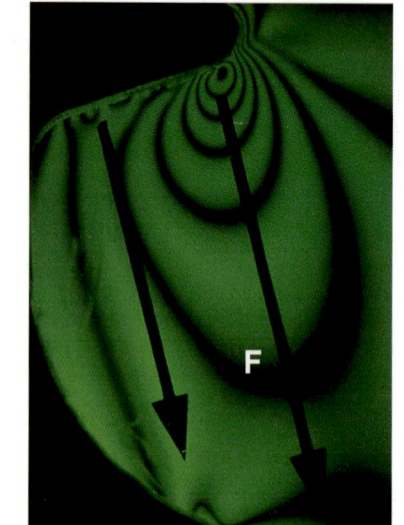

Fig. 7.**25a** An even, primary distribution of pressure over the entire thread profiles made possible by the smaller dimensions of the precut thread and the 15° inclination of the pressure surface to the plane of the transverse section. In axial loading, the force flow continues approximately at right angles to the pressure surface into the bone mass outside the implant

Fig. 7.**25b** and **c** Photoelastic experiments show the force flow F acting at right angles to the pressure surface

Basic Design of the ITI System

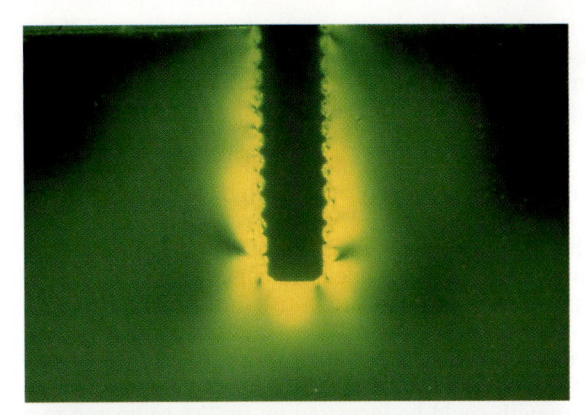

Fig. 7.**26a** This tension optical photograph shows the even primary pressure distribution of a hollow screw implant to the inside bone bed. The tensions decrease after removing a 1000 N axial load as shown in this figure

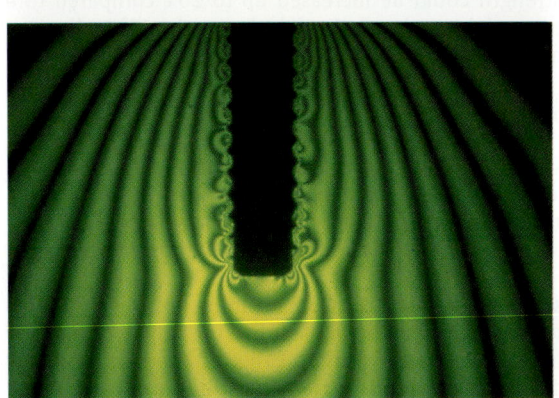

Fig. 7.**26b** The same situation as in **a**, with 1000 N axial loading. The tensions remain evenly distributed. No residual tensions after unloading (see **a** above)

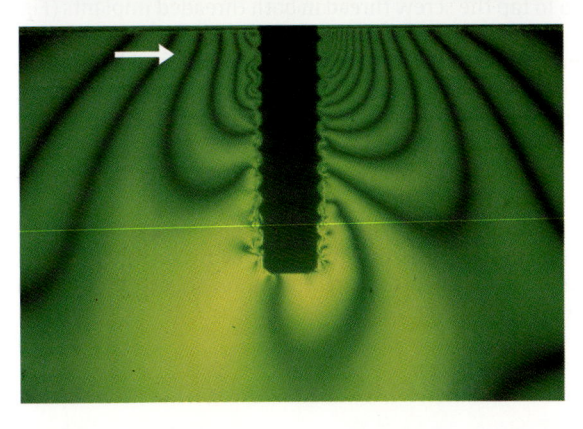

Fig. 7.**26c** Constellation with 500 N lateral loading of an ITI hollow screw implant

profiles (Fig. 7.**25a**). The photoelastic stress analysis shown in Figure 7.**26a–c** illustrates that these considerations do indeed lead to an extremely favorable stress distribution in these screw implants. Figure 7.**26b** shows the situation with an axial loading of 1000 N. The stresses are evenly distributed despite the high load.

As illustrated in Figure 7.**26a**, there is no residual stress at unloading. A similar constellation results from lateral loading with these screw implants (Fig. 7.**26c**).

In contrast to this, the photoelastic diagrams in Figure 7.**27a–c** clearly show that these characteristics of favorable force application could not be attained in implants with metric or standard British threads with rounded-off thread tips.

The new ITI thread configuration was determined by detailed experiments and comparative measurements. It was established inter alia that the maximum holding strength could be increased up to 20% compared to a thread flank geometry at right angles to the axis due to the 15° inclination angle thread flank shown in Figure 7.**25a**.

Overall ITI Concept as an Integrated System

An overall concept is available that has the following advantages:
1. individual choice of implants. Depending on bone quantity and quality, as well as personal preference, hollow cylinder, hollow screws, or screw implants can be chosen and used according to the indications described (Fig. 7.**30a**);
2. standardized instrument set (predrill, trephine mills, and depth gauges) which can be used for preparing the implant bed for hollow cylinder or hollow screw implants. Standardized twist drills are used for the screw implants instead of the predrill and the trephine mill. Moreover, a thread tap is required to to tap the screw thread in both threaded implants (Fig. 7.**28**);
3. standardized and uniform design of the implant head for all ITI implant types. In this way, the same standardized accessories (impression caps, transfer pin, gold copings, and occlusal screws) are used to manufacture the bar construction in all one-part implants (Fig. 7.**29**);
4. standardized and interchangeable range of secondary elements for all two-part implant types (Fig. 7.**29** and 7.**30b**);
5. wide range of indications. With the various implant types shown in Figure 7.**30** and the implant head design optimized for prosthetic work, the entire range of requirements in oral implantology can be covered with the system presented (Fig. 7.**31**).

Basic Design of the ITI System **141**

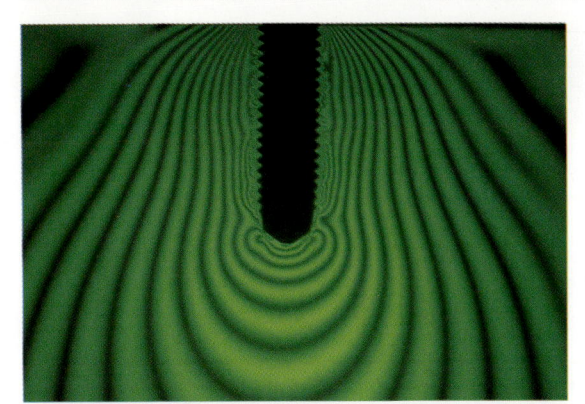

Fig. 7.**27a** This implant with a rounded-off metric profile at 1000 N axial loading

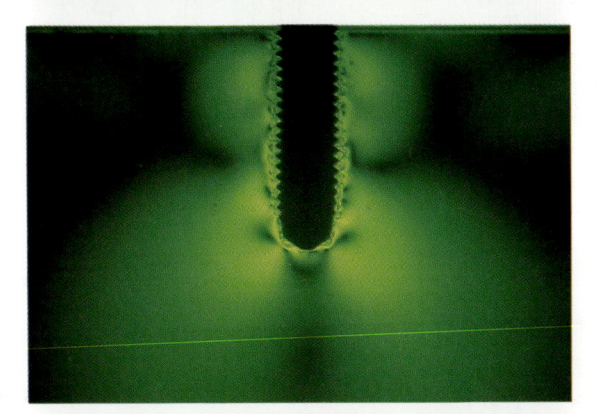

Fig. 7.**27b** In contrast to the ITI thread profile, this screw implant shows residual tension after unloading

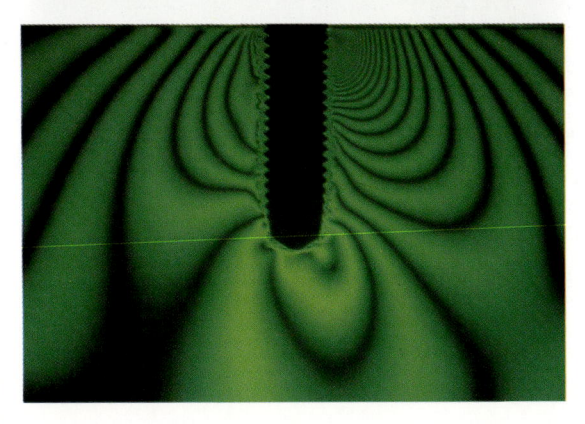

Fig. 7.**27c** Situation in 350 N lateral loading

142 7 The Concept of the ITI Implants

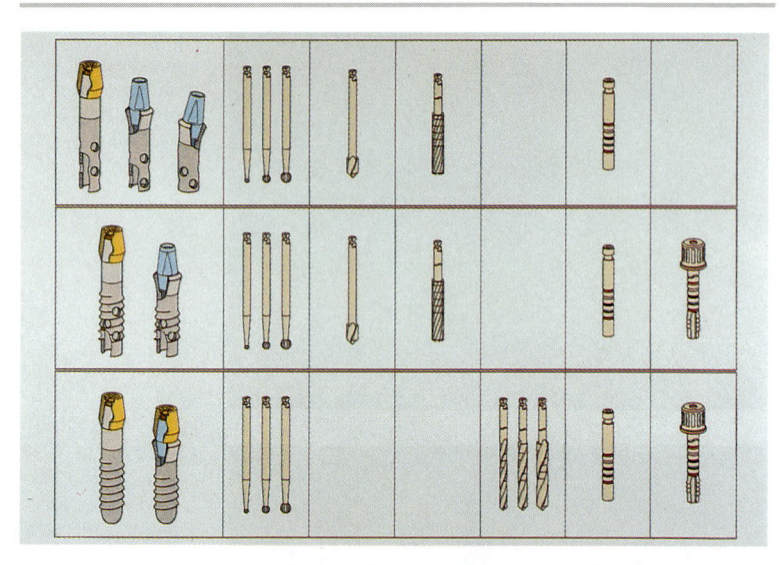

Fig. 7.**28** Representation of the overall concept. Fundamental features and instruments for preparation of the implant bed

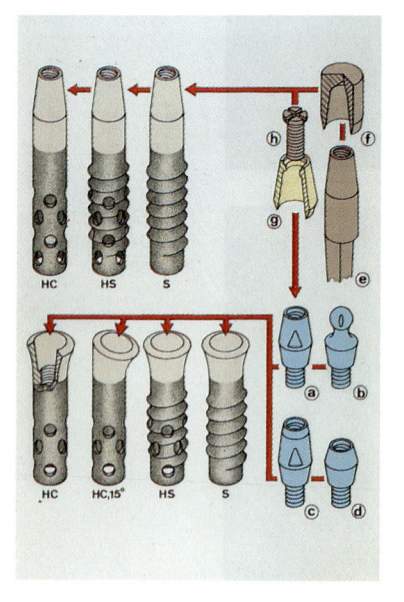

Fig. 7.**29** Graphic representation of the implant system with the seven implant types and the standardized secondary parts (abutments) and prosthetic accessories available

Basic Design of the ITI System **143**

a

b

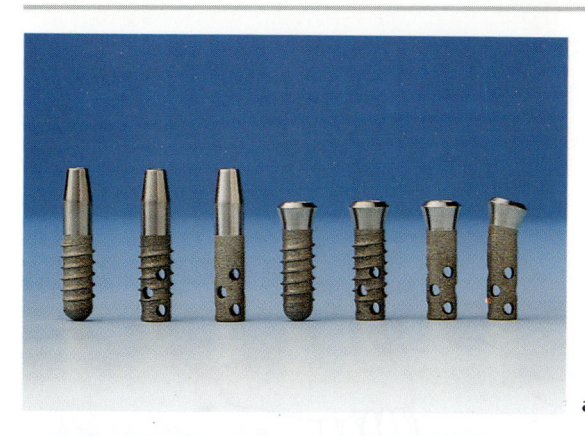

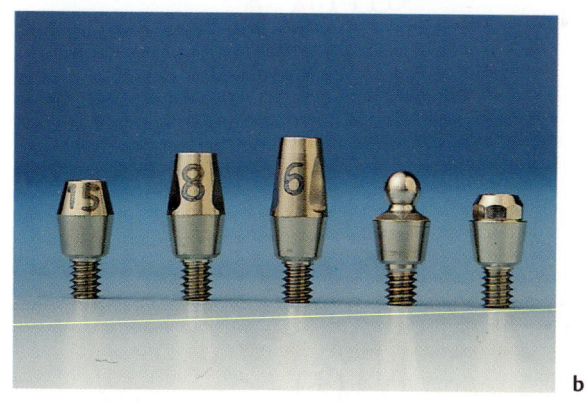

Fig. 7.**30a** and **b** Photographic representation of the ITI implant types and the standard secondary parts (abutments)

144 7 The Concept of the ITI Implants

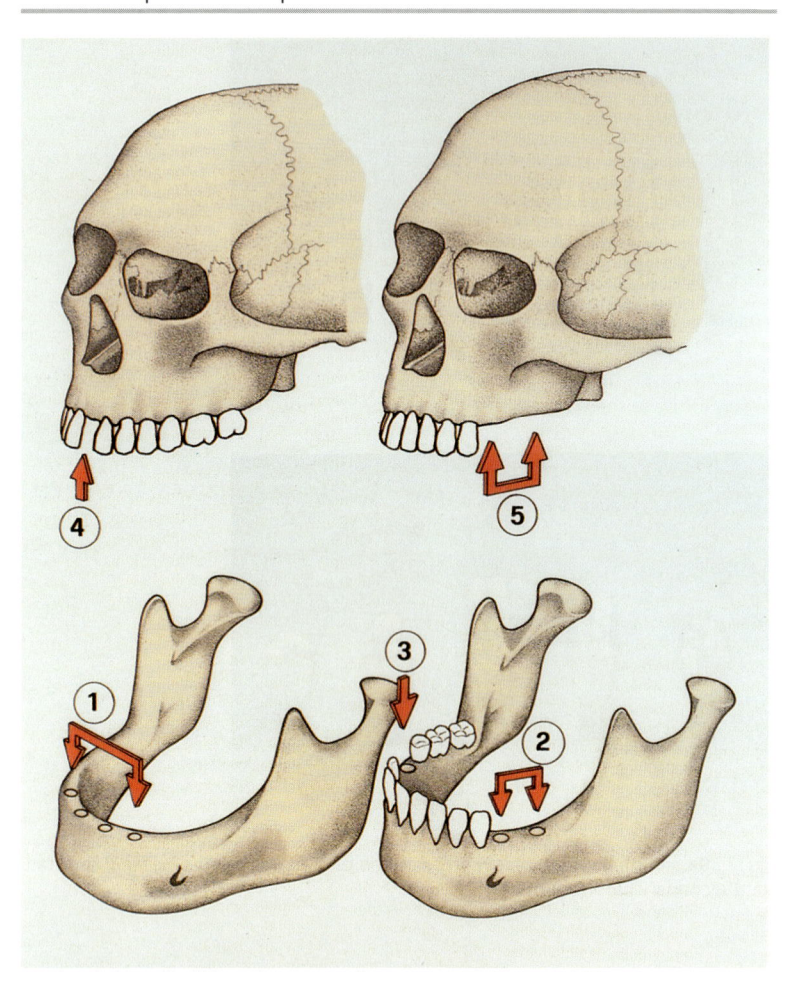

Fig. 7.**31** The main indications (1–5) for the ITI implants

Instruments

HC Implants

To prepare the implant bed for the three variants of ITI implants, the following instruments are available:
- Round burs; Clinical experience has shown that a range of three different diameters is useful (Fig. 7.**32**);
- predrill; this triple-fluted predrill, which is sunk up to the shoulder (i.e., about 4 mm deep into the bone) is available in two shaft lengths (Fig. 7.**33**);
- trephine mills; the trephine mills have three or five radial markings that correspond to the various anchorage depths (Fig. 7.**34** and 7.**36**). In this way, the anchorage depth determined preoperatively can be exactly prepared and checked with the color-coded depth gauge. Since the implants are also color-coded, it is simple to make the right choice; if, for example, the depth gauge is sunk to the groove marked red, a red-marked implant is chosen and inserted. The limited bone depth for

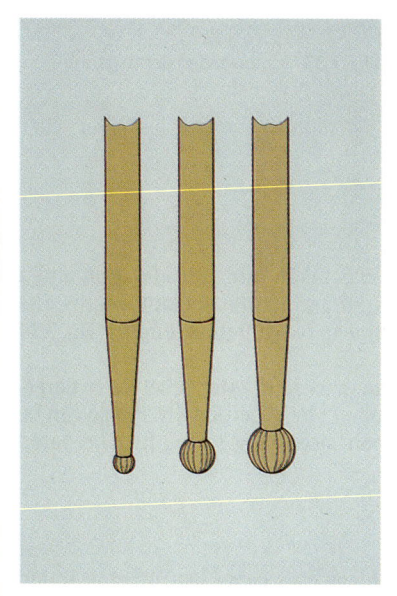

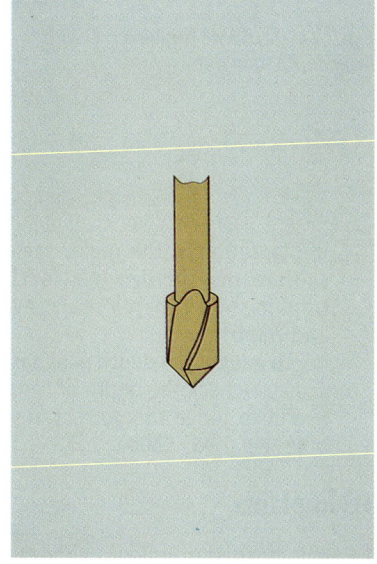

Fig. 7.**32** The spherical-headed drills are available in three diameters of 1.4, 2.3, and 3.1 mm

Fig. 7.**33** Representation of the pre-drilling device, which is sunk up to its shoulder level (about 4 mm)

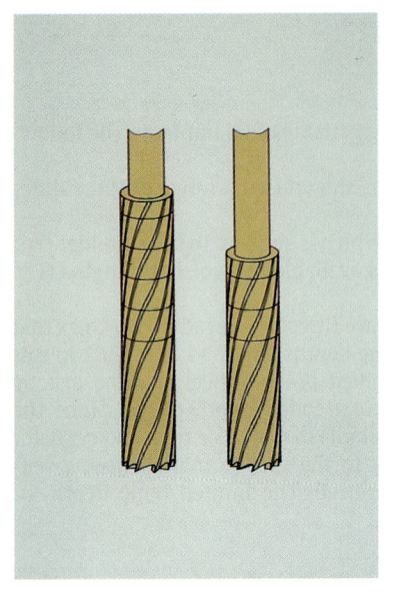

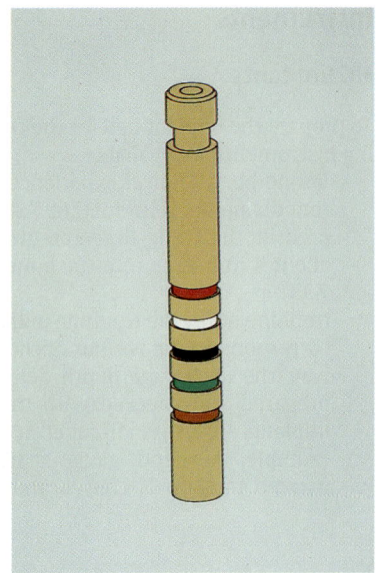

Fig. 7.**34** Standard trephine mill with laser depth markings

Fig. 7.**35** Color-coded depth gauge

implantation in the molar region was taken into consideration and a short reamer was designed for the 8, 10, and 12 mm implant lengths. The trephine mill is therefore also available in two different lengths (Fig. 7.**34** and 7.**39b**);
– depth gauge; the depth gauge is also marked in color. It serves to determine or check the depth of the implant site. Additionally, it also can be useful to judge the correct alignment according to the first prepared hole (Fig. 7.**35**, 7.**36b**).

HS Implants

In analogy to the hollow cylinder implant, the same instruments round burrs, predrill, trephine mill, and depth gauge) can be used with the HS implant (Fig. 7.**39a** and **b**). In addition, the following instruments are required:

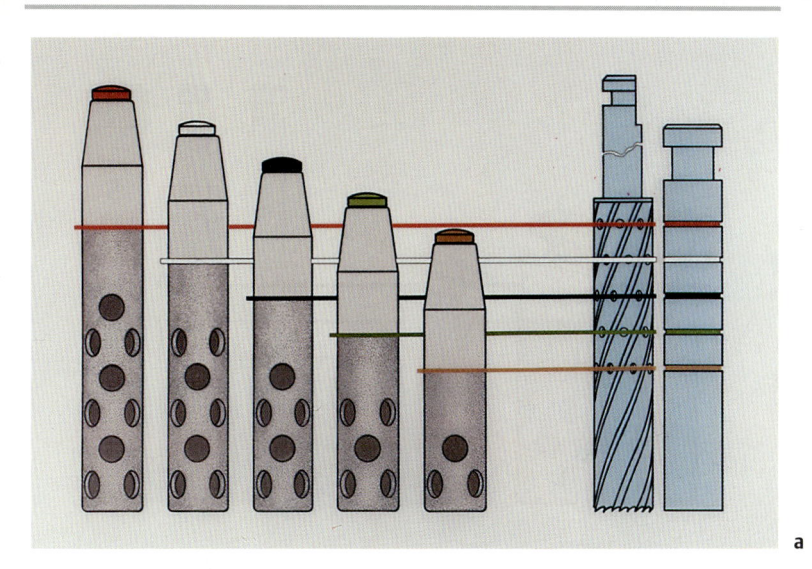

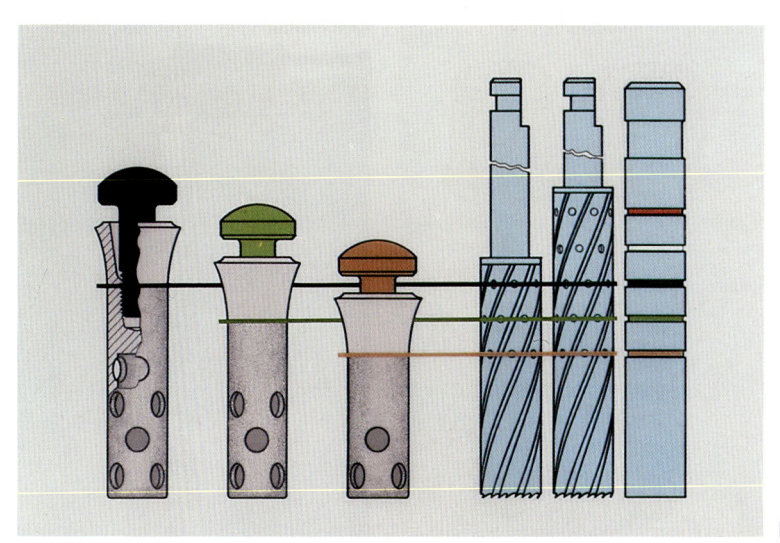

Fig. 7.**36a–c** Implant sinkage depth in relation to the corresponding markings on the trephine mill and the depth gauge. An appropriately shorter hollow trephine is available for implant procedures in the posterior regions of the oral cavity

148 7 The Concept of the ITI Implants

c

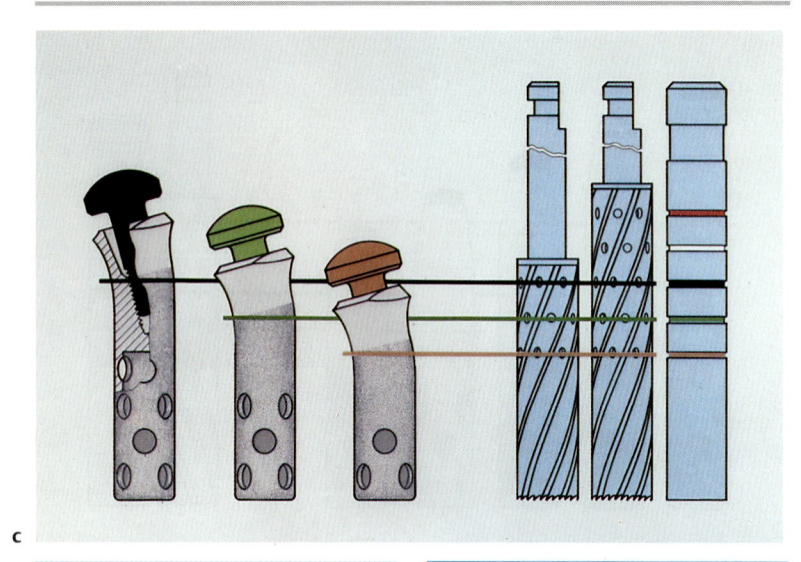

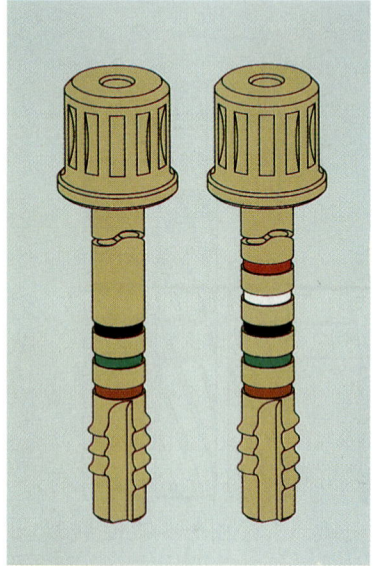

Fig. 7.**37** Color-coded thread cutter (tap) available in two lengths

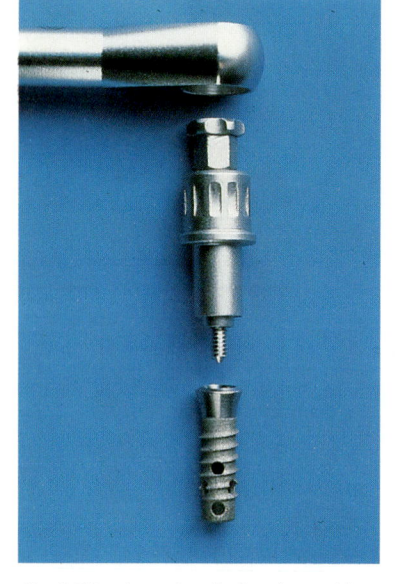

Fig. 7.**38a** Inserting devices in combination with a ratchet for one-part and two-part hollow screw and solid screw implants, as well as for the various abutments

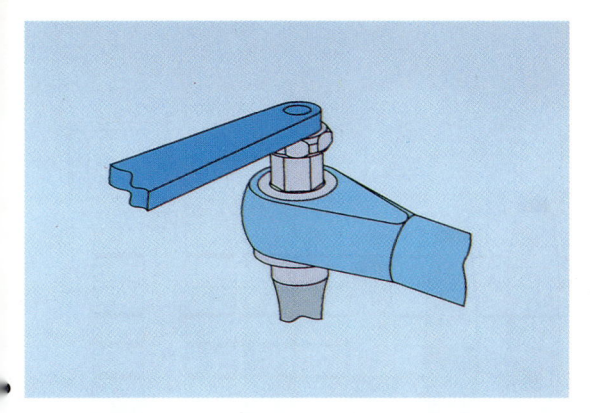

Fig. 7.**38b** and **c**
The guide key serves on the one hand to tighten or fix the inserting device to the implants or secondary parts (abutments), on the other hand to maintain the axial orientation while placing a screw-type implant

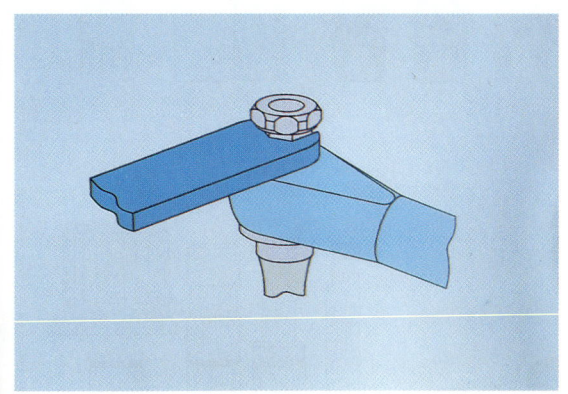

- thread tap; the thread taps are produced in two different lengths for the same reasons as for the trephine mill and are color-coded identically (Fig. 7.**37**);
- ratchet; the ratchet is used for tapping and for inserting the solid-screw or hollow-screw implants. In case of malfunction, the mechanism can be activated without having to take the ratchet apart or removing it from the instrument (thread tap or implant inserting device).

Even if the direction of rotatory movement is changed, the ratchet can stay fixed in position. Only a rotation of the pin "a" with two surfaces and directional markings by 180° is necessary (Fig. 7.**38a**, 7.**115**, and 7.**116**). For the future, it is planned that a mechanism for limiting the moment of rotation for abutments (about 0.35 Nm) and for occlusal screws (about 0.15 Nm) will be integrated into the ratchet.

150 7 The Concept of the ITI Implants

a

b

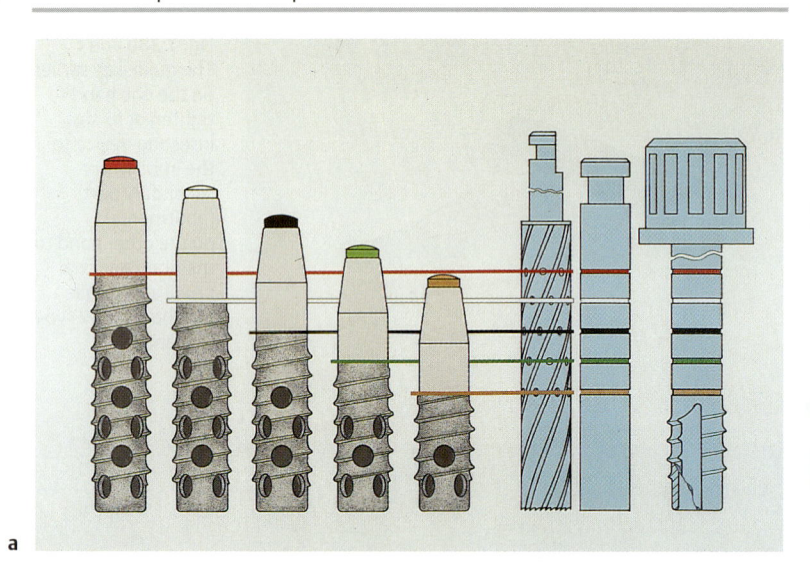

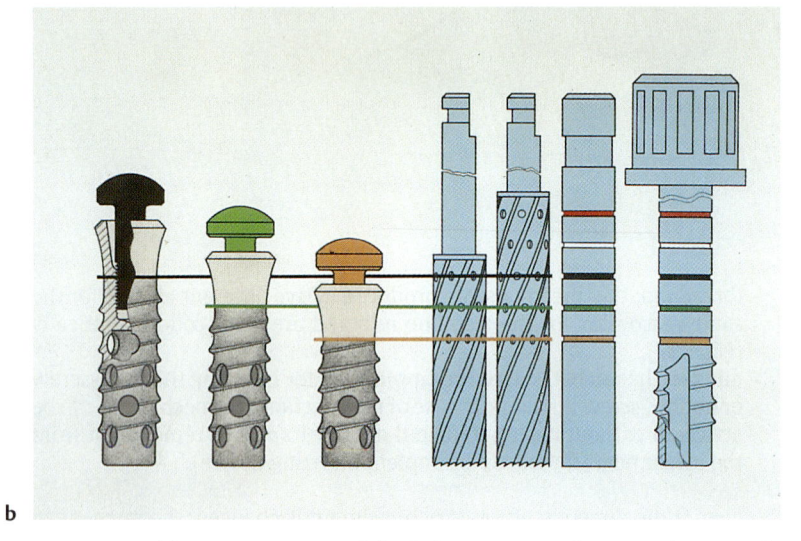

Fig. 7.**39a** and **b** Representation of the hollow screw implants in relation to the corresponding instruments with depth markings

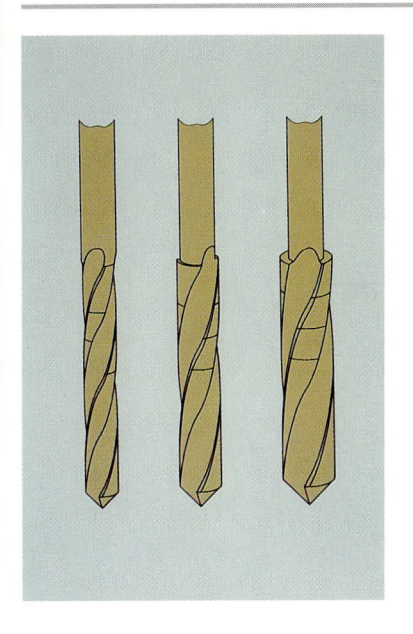

Fig. 7.**40** Three standard fluted drills of 2.2 mm, 2.8 mm, and 3.5 mm diameter

- guide key; the guide key serves to maintain the axial direction while tapping the threads with tap and ratchet, as well as for inserting in the implant. The open end of the key is used to rigidly attach the parts to be screwed into implants or abutments with the inserting device (Fig. 7.**38b** and **c**).

S Implants

With regard to the instruments for working the S implant bed, the round burs, the thread tap, and the depth gauge from the HC and the HS instruments are used. For the S implants, the following drilling instruments are used instead of the predrill and the trephine mills:
- twist drill (pilot drill) diameter 2.2; it is used for the first stage of drilling. Analogous to trephine mills, it has markings enabling determination of the depth (Fig. 7.**40**, left);
- twist drill (pilot drill) diameter 2.8; it is used for the second drilling stage and also has depth markings (Fig. 7.**40**, middle);
- twist drill (twist drill) diameter 3.5; this drill, with which the preparation of the implant site is completed, has three spiral longitudinal grooves. This enables dimensionally precise clatter-free cutting with the drill. The drill lengths and the depth markings have also been adopted from the trephine mills (Fig. 7.**40** on the right, 7.**41a** and **b**).

152 7 The Concept of the ITI Implants

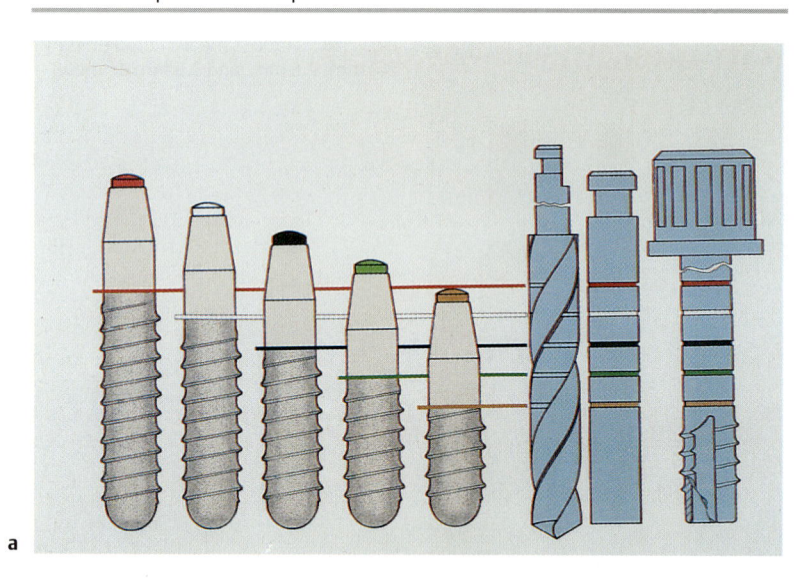

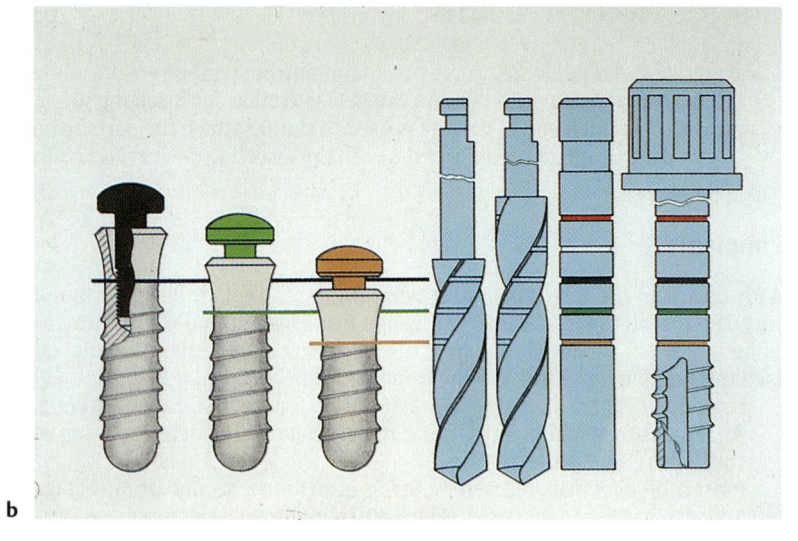

Fig. 7.**41a** and **b** Anchorage depth of the one-part and two-part solid screw implants in relation to the corresponding depth-marked instruments

Preparation of the Implant Bed

The success of an endosteal implant largely depends on its definitive healing. This is substantially affected by preparing the implant bed congruent to the implant base with preservation of bone vitality. This in turn is only ensured when the bone structure is damaged neither thermally nor mechanically in preparation. Rotation-symmetrical implants enable preparation of a congruent implant bed in a relatively simple way. A standardized range of drills, which is restricted to a minimum, is available for preparing the bed for the various implant types (Fig. 7.**42a–c**).

With hollow cylinder and hollow screw implants, preparation of the implant bed (with minimal traumatization of the jawbone) is possible due to the thin-walled trephine mill with outer grooves. The form of the cutting teeth at the end of the mill enables vibration-free and clean cutting of the bone. Microscopic investigations on traumatized bone confirm the high cutting quality of this instrument.

Even if the form of the jawbone is not ideal, the milled circular hole can always be cut on the desired axis. In addition to the cutting quality, the rate of cutting by the trephine is also crucial for preparation of the implant bed. When using of a double-reduction green-angle handpiece (two green rings, reduction ratio to the speed of the motor.), the speed of rotation is reduced to about 800 rpm. For preparation of the screw implant site (S-Type), three twist-drills are available (diam. 2.30, 2.80 and 3.50 mm). Due to the three spirally arranged grooves, clatter is avoided, the precision of the drillhole diameter is increased, and an ideal cutting process is ensured. A speed of rotation of maximum 800 rpm is also recommended for these drilling instruments. Besides the reduced rate of cutting, cooling with sterile physiological saline is absolutely necessary. In principle, this can be carried out by external or by internal irrigation.

Measurements of temperature with internally and externally cooled ITI drilling instruments were carried out on freshly removed calf humeri. Care was taken that the bone samples (cut in dices) were as homogeneous as possible and that the cortical bone layer had approximately the same thickness (Fig. 7.**48**). The following ITI drilling instruments were included in this experiment: a round bur, a predrill and trephine mill for the hollow bodies (hollow cylinder and hollow screw types), a round bur and 3.5 mm twist drill for the screw implants (S Type) Fig. 7.**42d**).

The speed of rotation of 800 and 3500 rpm chosen for the drilling experiment was reliably ensured by means of an electric motor. The milling and drilling process typical for an implantation was simulated well with the device shown in figure 7.**48**. The bone dices were fixed in a water container with a special device; the top side of the dice was not covered with water.

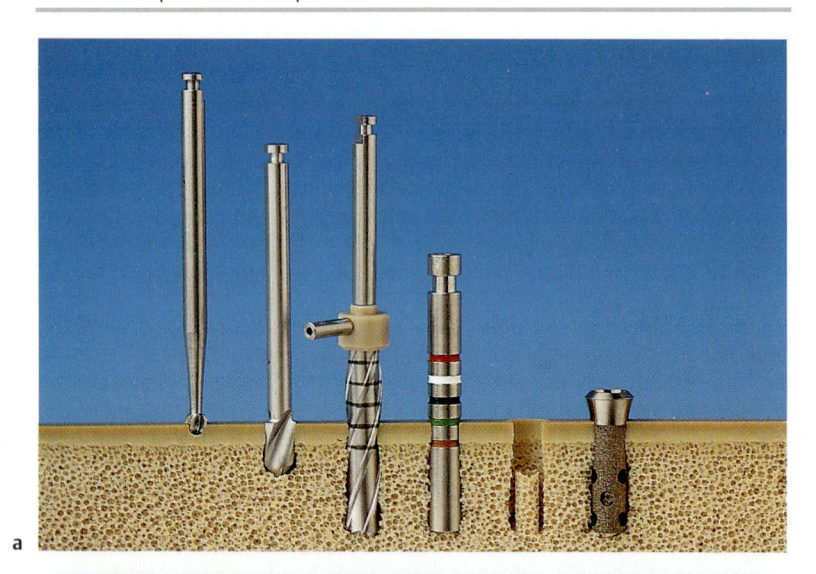

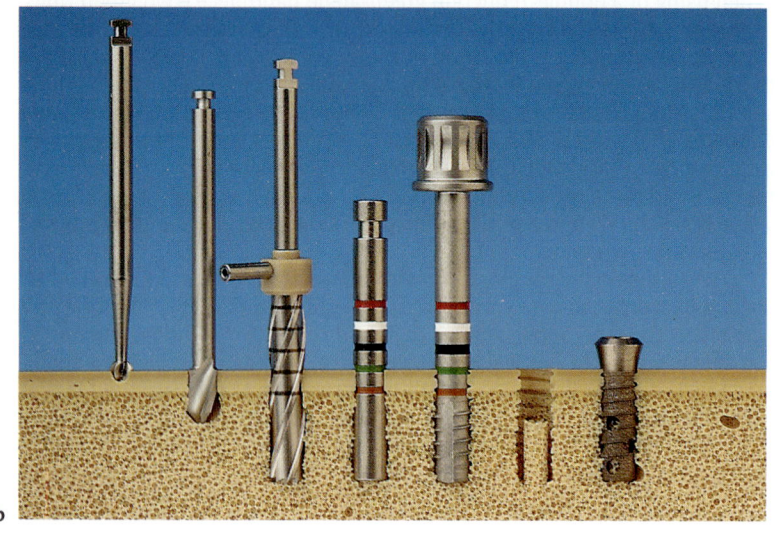

Fig. 7.**42a–c** Photographic representation of the placement procedure for ITI hollow cylinder, hollow screw, and solid-screw implants in the model

Preparation of the Implant Bed **155**

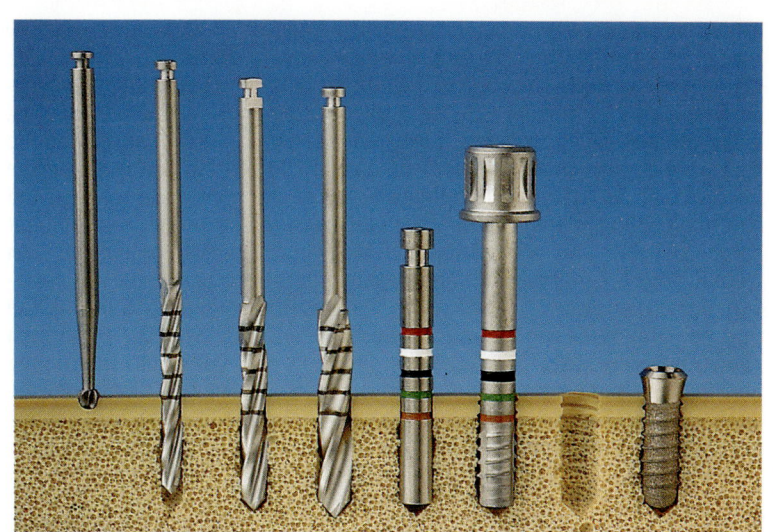

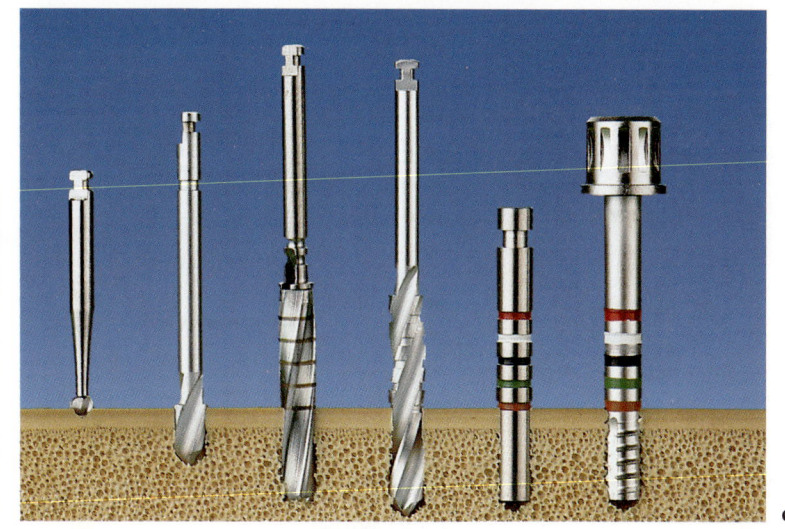

Fig. 7.**42d** Out of the instruments used for implant bed preparations, temperature measurements were performed for (from left to right): round burr, predrill, trephine and fluted drill of 3.5 mm diameter

7 The Concept of the ITI Implants

A constant initial temperature of the bone of 37 °C was attained by means of a temperature adjustable water bath. To detect the temperature changes occurring in the bone in the process of milling or drilling, two measurement probes in each case were fixed at the envisaged depth (see Fig. **7.43–7.46**). Using a drill gauge, the distance between the drill recess and the thermal elements could be exactly adjusted to 0.1 mm, so that reproducible values could be attained. Temperature rise of the bone with internal and external cooling of the instruments was measured at different instrument rotation speeds and with different temperatures of the cooling medium (p. 156–165). Wear of the drills and trephines in these experiments was established microscopically, and the service life was determined (p. 165–167). The internal cooling of the ITI instruments was ensured with the ITI system shown in Figure **7.47a–d**. The cooling fluid can pass safely into the cooling and flushing canal through an adapter ring (**a**), which is pushed onto the shaft of the standard instruments. The cutting properties of the instruments used were examined with the electron microscopic, using a dog femur.

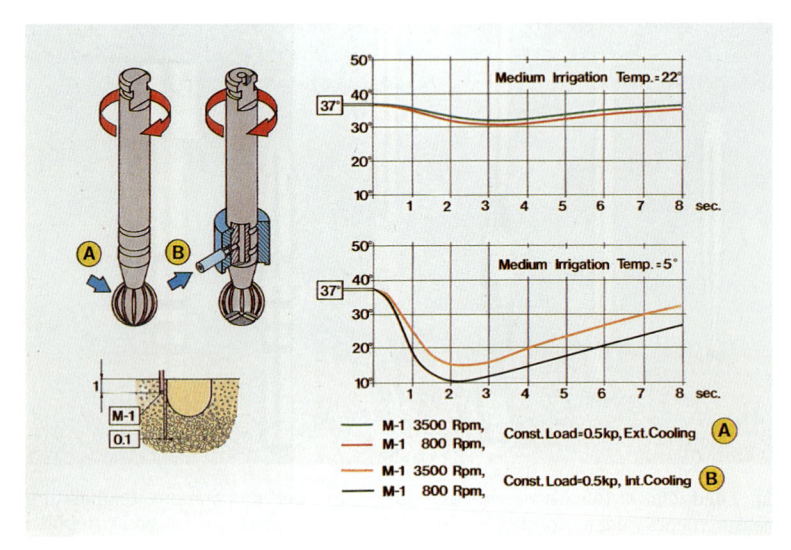

Fig. 7.**43** Results of measurements with the round bur: The curves show the temperatures of the diverse measurements (temperature of the cooling medium 22 °C and 5 °C, internal and external cooling) at 800 and 3500 rpm

The temperature curves shown in Figures 7.**43**–7.**46** demonstrate the heat curve in the region of the measurement points M-1 and M-2 determined with temperature probes in the following instruments:
- round bur; with a constant pressure of 0.5 kp, an increase in temperature was determined neither at 800 nor at 3500 rpm with the round burr. Since the depth of reaming is only about 3 mm, the temperature differences between internal and external cooling are also slight. As expected, a rapid fall of the bone temperature to about 15 °C could be detected using a cooling medium of 5 °C (Fig. 7.**32**, 7.**43**).
- predrill; a drill hole 4 mm deep is produced with this standard 3.5 mm diameter drill. The results were comparable to the temperature curves attained with the round burs (Fig. 7.**33**, 7.**44**);
- fluted drill; an enormous difference cannot be detected between internal and external cooling for this 3-grooved drill type of 3.5 mm diameter. It is important that the cooling medium reaches the depth of the drill tip (Fig. 7.**40**, 7.**45**);
- trephine mill; with a trephine mill speed (Fig. 7.**34**) of 3500 rpm, a constant axial pressure of 0.5 kp, and a temperature of the cooling medium of 5 °C, the peak values with external cooling were at about 72 °C at the deeper point of measurement M-2. The reduction of the speed of rotation to 800 rpm with the same cooling and axial pressure conditions resulted in a reduction of the bone temperature to about 42 °C (Fig. 7.**46a**). With 800 rpm, 0.5 kp load, and 22 °C cooling medium, a temperature reduction to about 48 °C could be accomplished (Fig. 7.**46b**).

158 7 The Concept of the ITI Implants

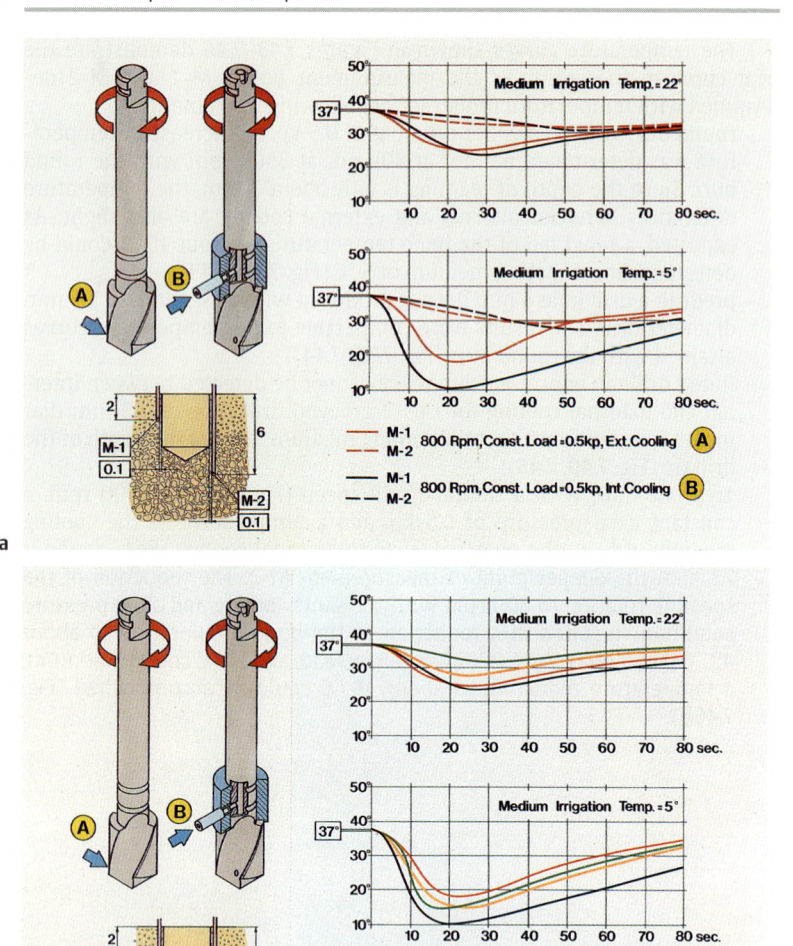

Fig. 7.**44a** Results of measurements with the predrill: The values recorded at 800 rpm roughly correspond to those of the round bur in Figure 7.**43**. The measurement point M-2 (6 mm deep) is only slightly affected in drilling

Fig. 7.**44b** Results of measurements with the predrill: Owing to the low drilling depth of only 4 mm, major temperature differences were not measured between internal and external cooling and between 800 and 3500 rpm at the measurement point M-1 (2 mm deep)

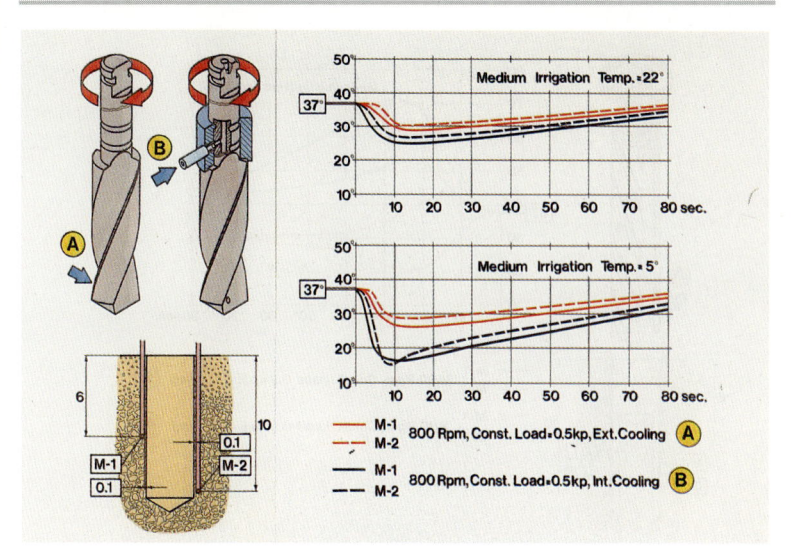

Fig. 7.**45** Results of measurement with the fluted drill: The temperature curve of the measurements with 22 °C cooling liquid temperatures shows that all temperatures tend to fall with either internal or external cooling, and that the temperature differences are slight. The differences between internal and external cooling are considerably greater with a cooling medium temperature of 5 °C

The results were substantially improved by using an intermittent up-and-down movement of the trephine instruments, as can be seen from Figure 7.**46a** and **b**. The lowering of the coolant temperature and an intermittent movement ensure temperature values in the physiological range. With internal cooling, thermal bone damage does not occur either at reduced or at normal cooling water temperature (22 °C).

160   7   The Concept of the ITI Implants

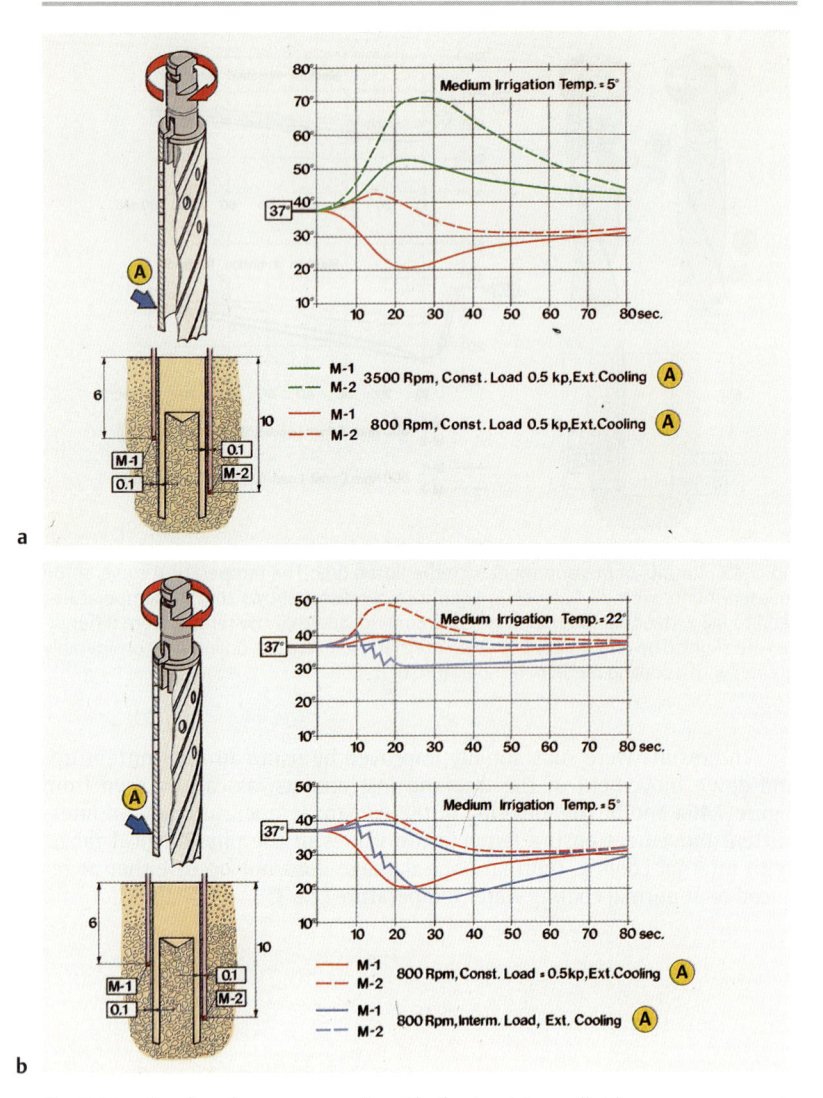

Fig. 7.**46a** Results of measurements with the trephine mill: These measurements show that a bone damaging temperature (72 °C) is induced with the trephine mills at high speed (3 500 rpm). At a speed of 800 rpm, with 5 °C external cooling and a constant load of 0,5 kg, a maximum temperature of 42 °C was determined

Fig. 7.**46b** Results of measurements with the trephine mill: These measurements attained with external cooling show that a major reduction of bone heating is achieved with intermittent movement of the trephine as compared to constant (not intermittent) load (0.5 kp)

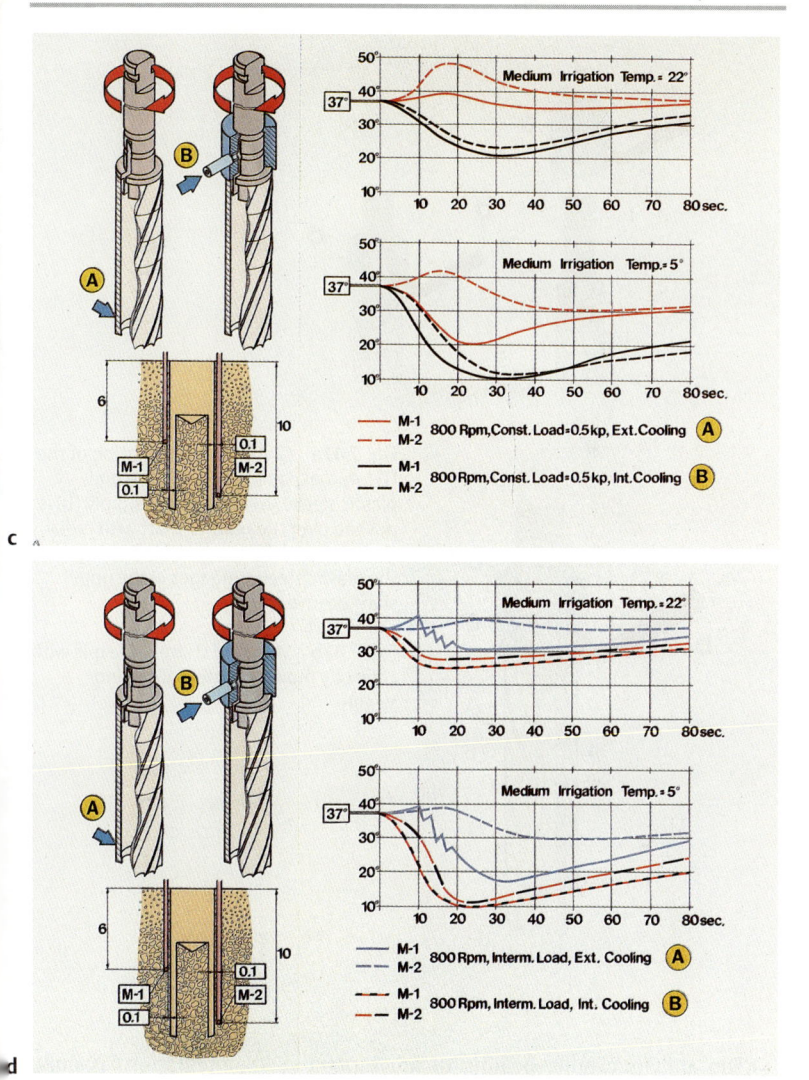

Fig. 7.**46c** Results of measurements with the trephine mill: Using the system of internal cooling shown in Figure 7.**47a–d** an immediate reduction of the bone temperature during milling could be detected due to the ideal cooling conditions resulting from the construction

Fig. 7.**46d** Results of measurements with the trephine mill: These graphs show the relatively favorable temperature curve in external cooling and intermittent pressure of the trephine, as well as the results with internal cooling under (otherwise) the same conditions

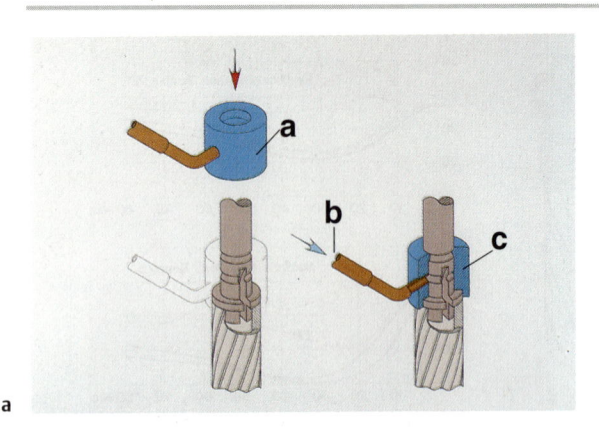

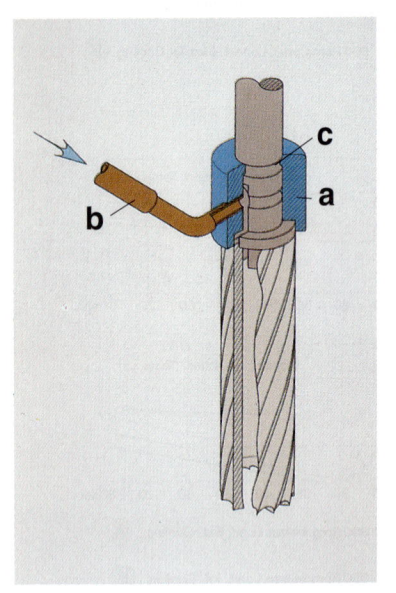

Fig. 7.**47a** Graphic representation of the ITI internal cooling system. The unit plastic sleeve (a) and coolant supply (b) is pushed over the reamer shaft with radial grooves until the torus-like inner ring of the plastic sleeve engages in the upper shaft groove (c)

Fig. 7.**47b** Standard ITI trephine mill with correctly mounted internal cooling system

The ankylotic bone healing of an implant (osteointegration) is only possible when the vitality of the bone surrounding the implant is maintained. Histomorphological investigations of Watzek et al. have shown that remodelling processes occur up to a depth of 0.5 mm during this process. Thermal damage to this area would thus endanger osteointegration. There is no doubt that thermal damage to the bone may occur in the preparation of an implant bed. Its extent depends on the nature and quality of the cutting

Preparation of the Implant Bed **163**

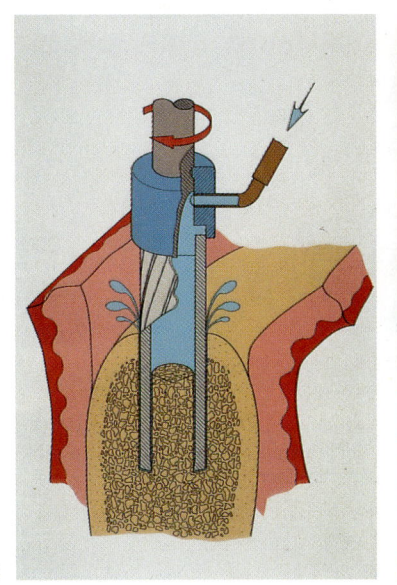

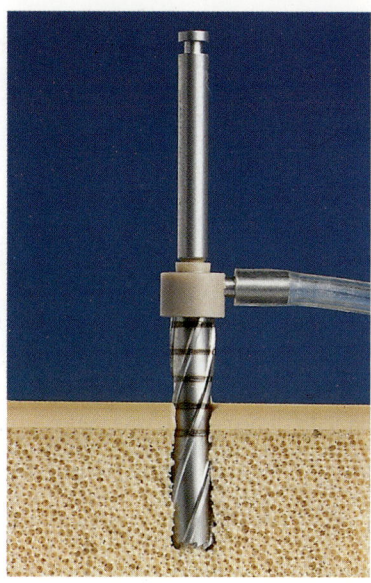

Fig. 7.**47c** Schematic representation of the process of cooling with the ITI internal cooling system. The cooling medium is directly passed to the cutting teeth at the end of the reamer during reaming. The reaming chips are flushed away continuously via the spirally arranged external grooves on the trephine mill. This prevents heating of the bone by frictional heat that occurs with obstruction of the grooves

Fig. 7.**47d** Photographic representation of the ITI internal cooling system for altraumatic preparation of the implant bed with a trephine mill

tools and their speed of rotation. By using a suitable cooling medium, it can be additionally reduced. Two methods are used. Internal cooling, which reaches the depth of the holes is the safest way. However, it must be ensured that the end of these instruments is indeed irrigated. This requires a certain form, such as that used in a canon drill or in a trephine. The coolant conveyed through the trephine instrument must be able to drain away without obstruction.

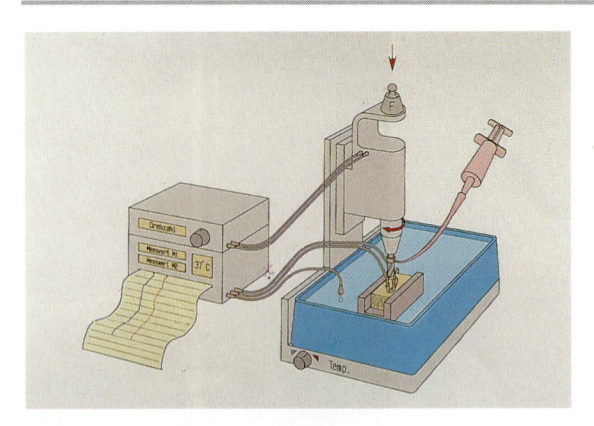

Fig. 7.**48** Schematic representation of the experimental setup to determine the temperature curve during bone preparation. Vertical drill aggregate, heat-adjustable container, measurement probes, and plotters are the essential elements

With the system of cooling fluid supplied via a syringe pump or an instrument integrated into the system, sufficient pressure can be produced to continuously flush out the bone shavings during cooling (Fig. 7.**47c**). Our measurements indicate that internal cooling for round burs and for the 3-grooved twist drills is not necessary. On the other hand, this new system of internal cooling may be very helpful for preparing the implant bed with trephine drills.

An interesting question was the service life of the drilling and milling instruments. The high quality of the material allows multiple use. Our experience has shown, that these drills can be used at least twelve times without loss of cutting efficiency (Fig. 7.**49**, 7.**50**). The cutting quality can be inferred from the fact that even very fine bone structures are still intact after preparation of the implant bed. An especially smooth by machinded surface can be attained with the trephine mills (Fig. 7.**51**). Provided there is continuous rotation at an adequate speed, this cutting quality is excellent. The implant bed produced under the same conditions with a straight-fluted drill shows none of the above mentioned excellent cutting characteristics (Fig. 7.**52**). This experimental investigation documents that these instruments of the ITI system meet the requirements for adequate bone preparation and that the introduction of internal cooling provides additional safety with regard to maintenance of bone vitality.

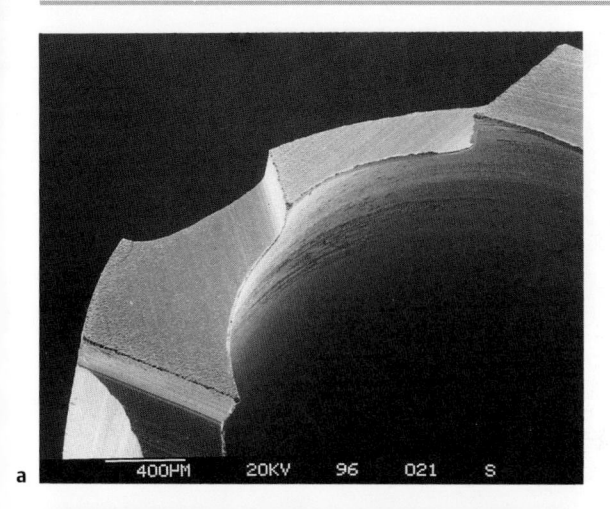

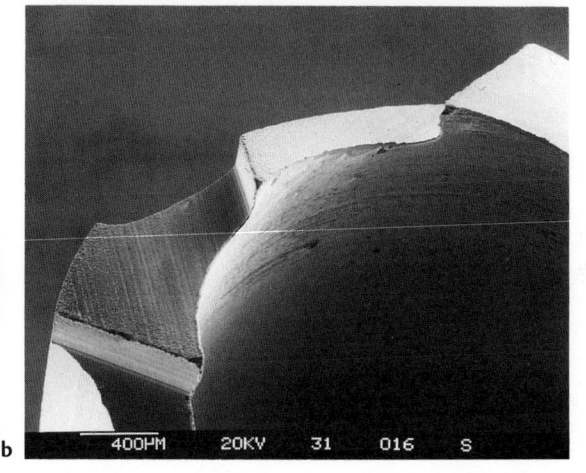

Fig. 7.**49a** and **b** Detail of the teeth of a new trephine mill and a trephine mill that has been used 18 times

166 7 The Concept of the ITI Implants

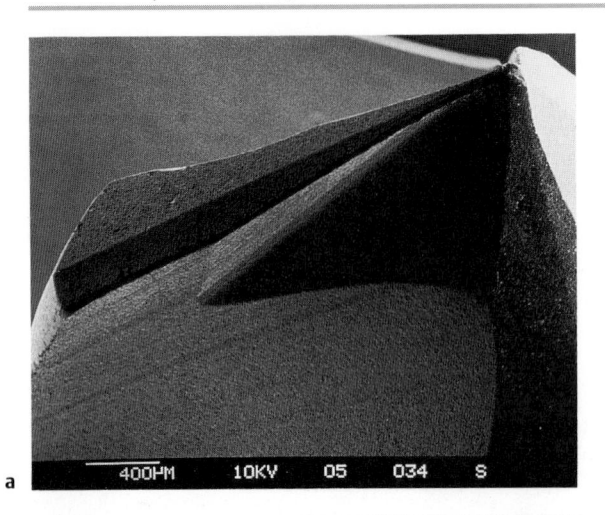

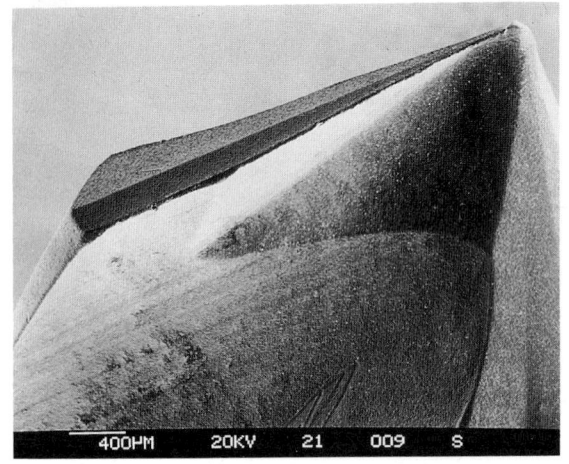

Fig. 7.**50a** and **b** Detail of a new fluted drill and a fluted drill that has been used 18 times

Preparation of the Implant Bed 167

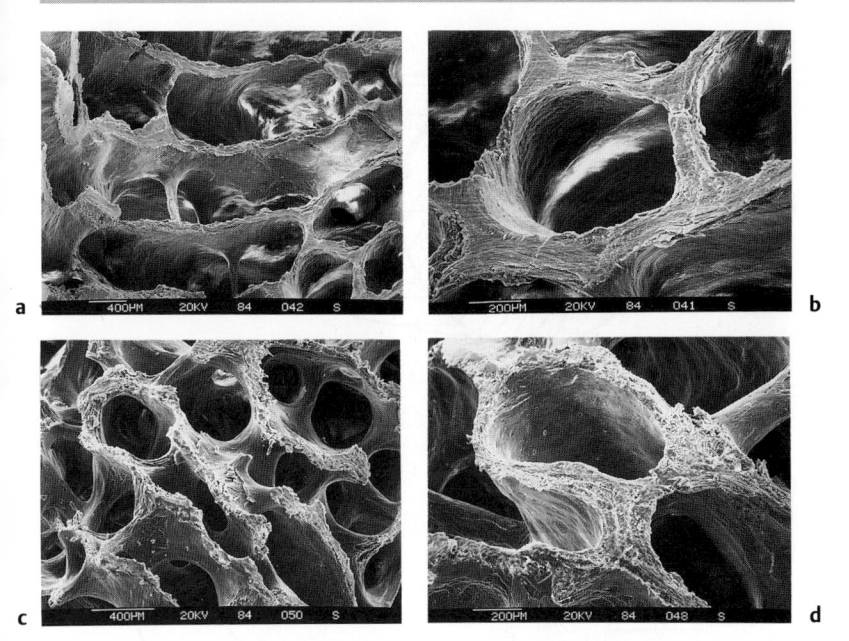

Fig. 7.**51a–d** SEM of the bone surface of the implant bed worked with a trephine mill. The holes were prepared in the distal region of a dog femur. The soft tissues of these preparations were macerated with antiformin solution at 60 °C. Figures **a** and **b** show the wall of the drillhole, and figures **c** and **d** show the surface of the bone core

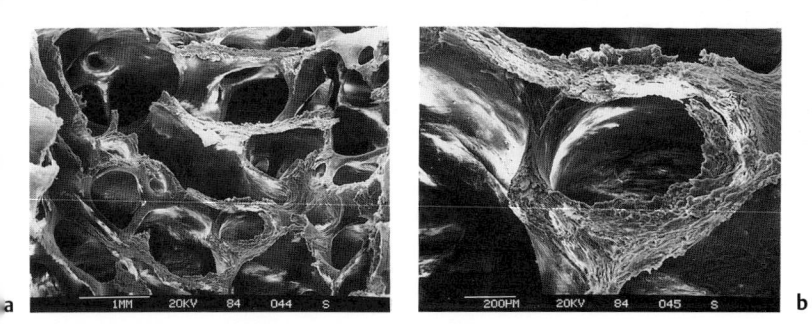

Fig. 7.**52a** and **b** These two SEM show the surface of an implant bed prepared with an internally cooled twist drill with two straight longitudinal grooves

168 7 The Concept of the ITI Implants

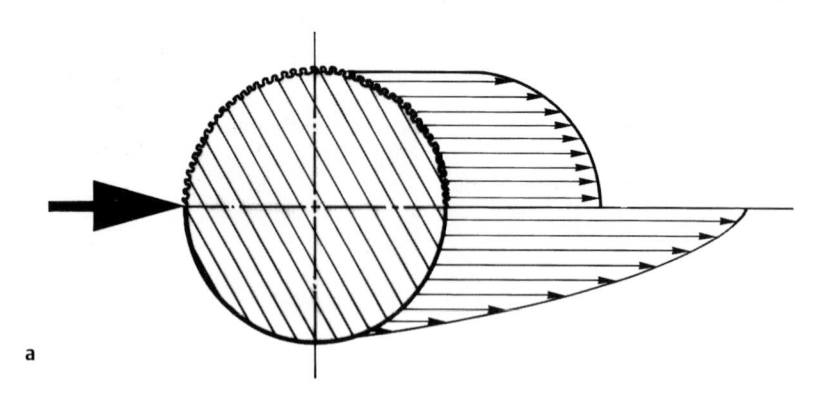

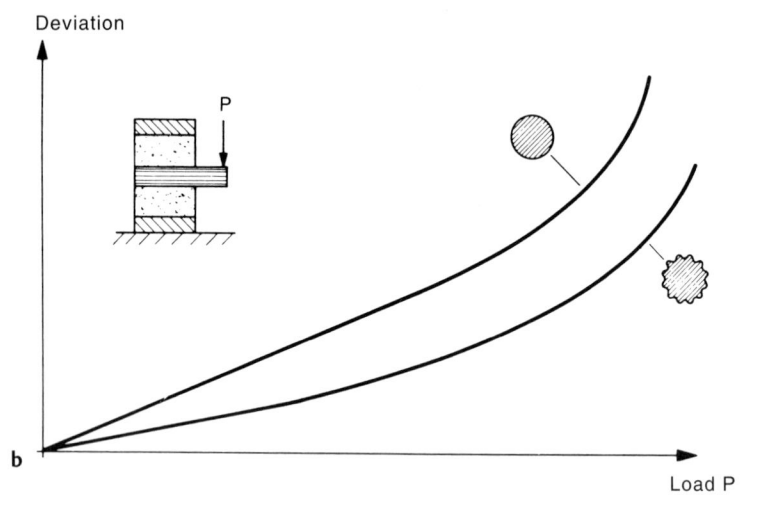

Fig. 7.**53a** and **b** Loading diagrams to illustrate the different peak pressures with a smooth and rough implant surface

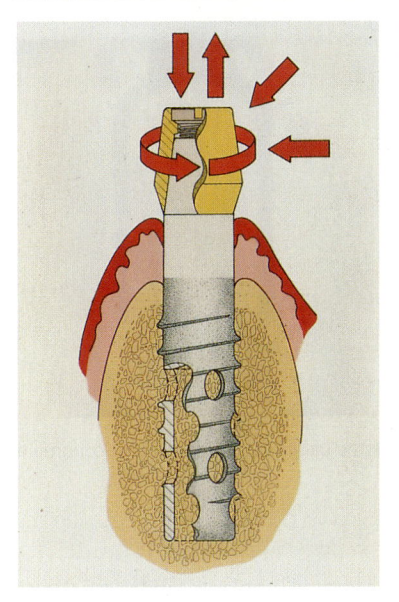

Fig. 7.**54** With a suitable implant construction and micromorphological anchoring surface, a broadly distributed force transfer without high, specific peak pressures can be attained in compression, tensile traction, torsional, and lateral loading

Biomechanics of the Implant-Bone Structural Unit

The implant design should ensure that lateral and axial forces are transmitted as evenly as possible from implant to surrounding bone when the implant is fully healed-in and incorporated in the bone. The maximum tensile, compressive, and shear stresses must lie within a certain range, i.e., the stresses or deformation produced in the surrounding bone by a fully incorporated implant should not exceed a certain level if bone resorption and implant loosening are to be avoided.

Smooth, polished implant surfaces (Fig. 7.**53a**, below the axis) either do not bond to the bone at all or bond poorly. On the other hand, an "ankylotic" bond is formed between bone and titanium plasma-sprayed surfaces (above the axis) with their rough, porous surfaces. This means that the load is spread more evenly and prevents high pressure peaks as shown on Fig. 7.**53a+b**.

The corresponding diagram is shown in Fig. 7.**56**. A photoelastic stress analysis of the situation around a Type C hollow cylinder implant by Soltész (of the Frauenhofer Institute of Materials Mechanics, Freiburg im Breisgau) confirmed these assumptions. The stress distribution around two-dimensional parallel-plane models in the surrounding (simulated) bone was measured. The goal of the measurements was to investigate the differences

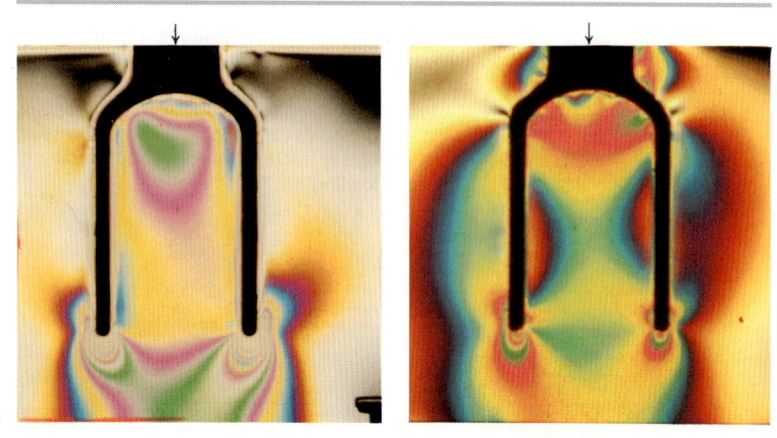

Fig. 7.55a and b Tension optical model photos under vertical loading in congruent fitting (**a**) and in glued-in model (**b**)

between smooth and titanium plasma-coated implants under axial and lateral loading, both qualitatively and quantitatively. When making the model, it was assumed that the titanium plasma-coated surface would intimately bond to the bone with no intervening connective tissue, and would thus be able to transmit both tensile and shear forces. Smooth titanium surfaces, on the other hand, would just sit in a congruent bed in contact with, (but not bonded to) the bone, a situation which transmits only compressive stresses. Other, more detailed models were made to investigate the effects of the cylinder wall perforations. The measurements were made on models, scale 10:1. The two-dimensional implant models were made of brass ($E = 95\,000$ N/mm^2) and the bone was represented by either perspex or epoxy ($E = 3500$ N/mm^2). The ratio of the moduli was thus similar to that between titanium ($E = 110\,000$ N/mm^2) and an average value for bone (cortical bone: $E \leq 20\,000$ N/mm^2, cancellous bone: $E = 1000$ N/mm^2). The ingrowth of bone into the porous titanium plasma spray coating was simulated by firmly gluing the implant model into the implant bed with an epoxy glue. Smooth surfaces were simulated by simply inserting the implant model into the congruent implant bed without gluing. The reader is referred to the articles by Soltész et al. for further details of the method and a detailed discussion of the results.

Figure 7.55a and **b** shows the stress distribution under axial loading as determined by photoelasticity for one particular model type for both methods of implant insertion. Areas of high-stress concentration can be qualitatively defined from the photographs; high stresses are mainly to be

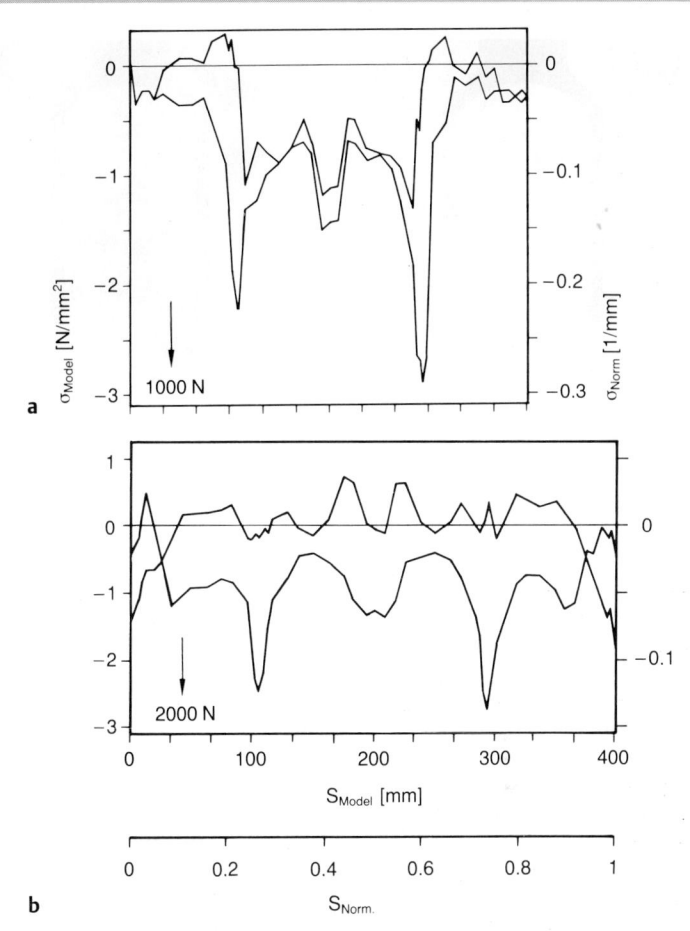

Fig. 7.**56a** and **b** Main tensions in the vicinity of the implant under vertical loading with congruent fitting (**a**) and in glued-in model (**b**) (evaluation along a contour around the implant at the interface between the implant and the bone)

found concentrated around the lower edge of the nonglued model (Fig. 7.**55a**) Stresses may be derived from photoelasticity pictures. The quantitative evaluation of the photoelastic patterns in Figure 7.**55** is given in figure 7.**56** (see, for example, Riedmüller and Soltész). The results showed that the maximum stresses in the (simulated) bone were reduced to half the value for the non glued sample compared to the glued specimen (for technical reasons

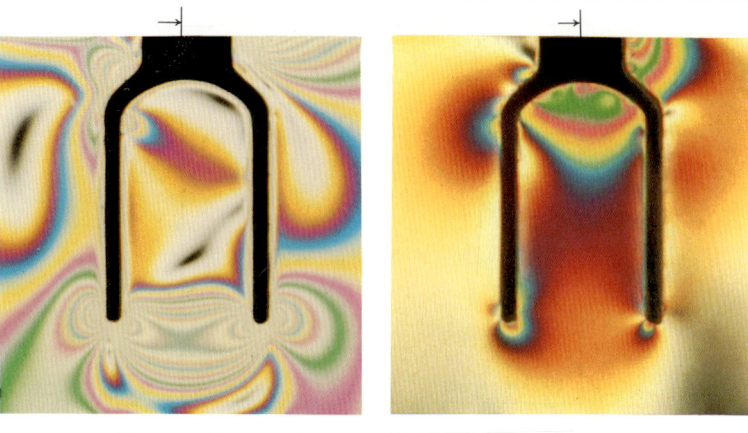

Fig. 7.**57a** and **b** Optical tension diagrams of the model type under horizontal loading with congruent fitting (**a**) and with glued-in model (**b**)

the load on the glued specimen was in fact doubled; see Figure 7.**56b**). The results for lateral loading were even better; the stresses around the glued implant (representing an akylotically incorporated implant) were reduced to a quarter of those observed around the nonglued specimen (Fig. 7.**57** and 7.**58**). For both insertion methods, when bone growth through cylinder wall perforations was simulated, is was found that this bone took part in load transmission.

These measurements, however, do not make allowances for a three-dimensional implant geometry. The level of stress concentration around the lower implant margin is expected to be lower in real life than in the model, since with rotational symmetry, the loads will be distributed over a larger area than in a two-dimensional model.

The finding that a rough, porous implant surface is better at transmitting loads from implant to bone has been confirmed by experiments on titanium plates implanted in monkey mandibles (Fig. 7.**59**). Measurements were made after a 3-month healing phase; the screw (S) was initially tightened with a torque M_a of 10 Ncm.

A moment M_t of 30 Ncm was necessary to turn plate A with its smooth surface through 2° around the screw axis. The titanium plasma-coated plate B required 60 Ncm and plate C, which was both grooved and coated, withstood 170 Ncm before it rotated through 2°.

The experimental results show that the resistance to shear and torsion loading is twice as high for the titanium plasma-sprayed coating as for a smooth titanium surface and can be increased by a factor of six with both longitudinal grooves and titanium plasma coating.

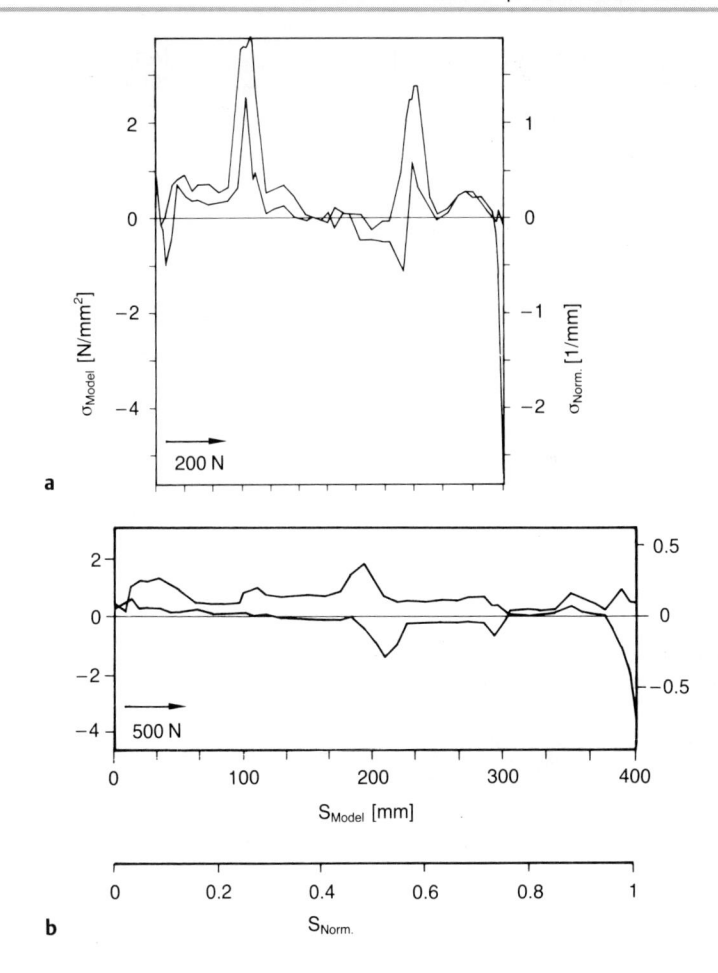

Fig. 7.**58a** and **b** Main tension lines in the vicinity of the implant under horizontal loading with congruent fitting (**a**) and in glued-in model (**b**)

	Contact surface	M_t for 2° rotation around "a"
A	smooth	30 Ncm
B	Ti plasma	60 Ncm
C	Grooved Ti plasma	170 Ncm

Screw tightening torque "M" ca. 10 Ncm

Fig. 7.**59** Comparative measurements between titanium specimens with uncoated (A), titanium plasma-coated (B), and fluted and titanium plasma-coated (C) surface under torsion (shear)

Implant Materials Considered in Terms of Their Design and the Technique of Implant Manufacture

Titanium as Implant Material
(see also section on the Basic Design of the ITI Implant System

A hollow cylinder design, with its open, perforated form (Fig. 7.**60**), is only possible when the stability of the implant material used meets the high specifications required by the design, including the high mechanical strength and the elastic modulus, which should be as low as possible. As already mentioned, the study group from which the ITI later developed,

Table 7.**1** Physical data of implant steel, titanium, cancellous, and cortical bone

	Implant grade stainless steal	Titanium	Bone cancellous	cortical
Module of elasticity (GN/m^2)	190	110	approx. 5	approx. 20
Density (kg/m^3)	7.35×10^3	4.51×10^3	approx. 1.2×10^3	approx. 1.8×10^3
Tensile strength (MN/m^2)	820–1050	750–880	approx. 12	approx. 100

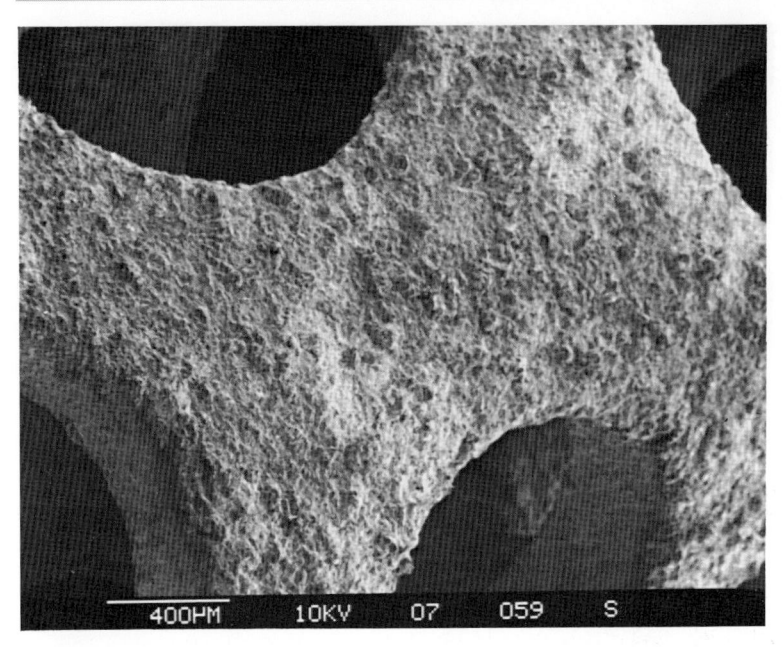

Fig. 7.**60** Surface detail of a perforated titanium plasma-coated hollow cylinder implant

decided as early as 1974 in favor of technically pure titanium as implant material and in favor of titanium plasma spraying of the implant anchoring part of the implant. The desired stability and ductility of the titanium used for the implants is attained by a choice of material and cold working. With its low elastic modular and its relatively high strength (Table **1**), titanium meets the design requirements to a large extent. Fenestrated hollow body implants with a wall thickness of only 0.5 mm were produced with titanium.

Surface Morphology of the Anchorage Element

In addition to the macroscopic form and the biocompatibility of the material, the surface characteristics of the implants are of great importance. Titanium plasma coating was used for the first time in oral implantology in ITI implants. It enables a rough porous surface with an approx. ten times greater surface (Fig. 7.**61**). This surface fosters direct bone apposition to the implant surface without a separating layer of connective tissue.

176　7　The Concept of the ITI Implants

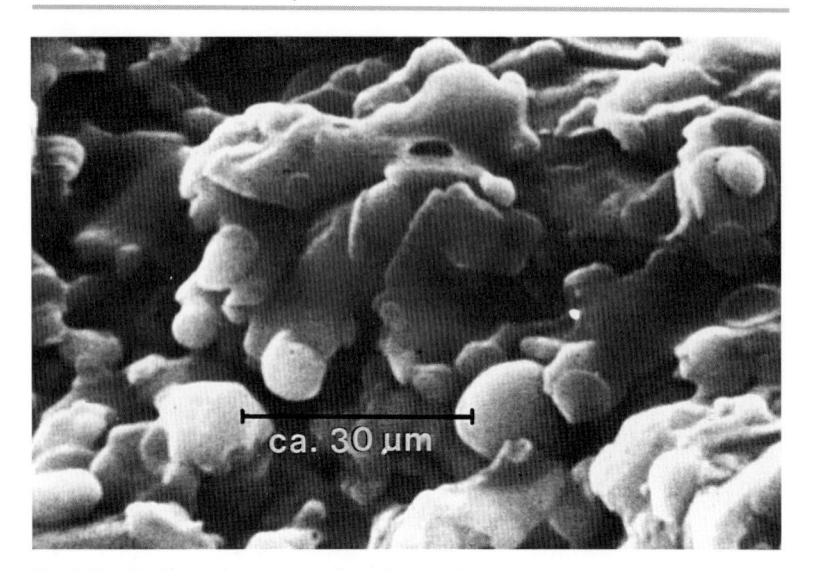

Fig. 7.**61**　Titanium plasma-coated implant surface (SEM, magnification about 5000 times)

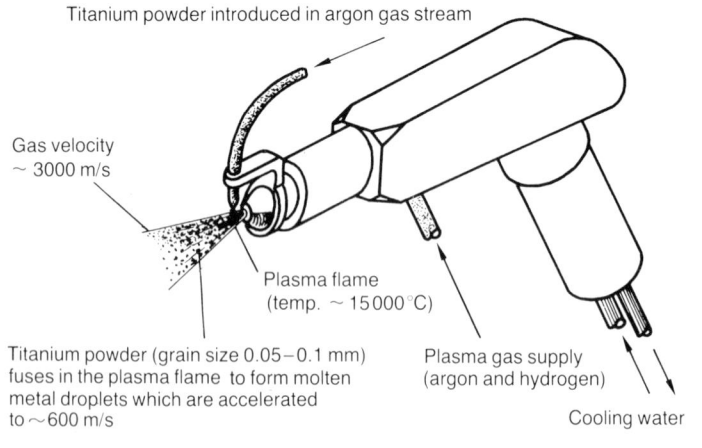

Fig. 7.**62**　Schematic representation of a plasma coating gun with the most important technical data

Implant Materials Considered in Terms **177**

The coating technique is characterized by an arc flame temperature of 15 000 to 20 000 °C and a very high gas jet velocity of more than 3000 m/s.

The titanium powder particles (conveyed to the flame tip by means of argon gas) are accelerated to about 600 m/s during the coating process, until they weld with the implant surface 15–20 cm away (Fig. 7.**62**). The coating thickness is about 30 to 40 µm. Axial pull-off experiments have shown that sufficient bonding of the coating to the implant body takes place with correct application of the titanium spray technique. A pull-off strength of 75 to 90 N/mm^2 was measured.

Implant Production Technique

Pure titanium is used as material for all ITI implants. The implants are neither cast nor sintered, but produced from the full profile to their final form. The reason for using this procedure is that the starting material is free of defects and has reproducible properties which are difficult to find with other techniques. Figure 7.**63** shows the typical microstructure of the material used.

The most important stages of the implant manufacture are:
1. Cold working of the material to the desired strength in the form of bars for implant manufacture
2. Manufacturing of the implants with very high precision and the most modern technology.

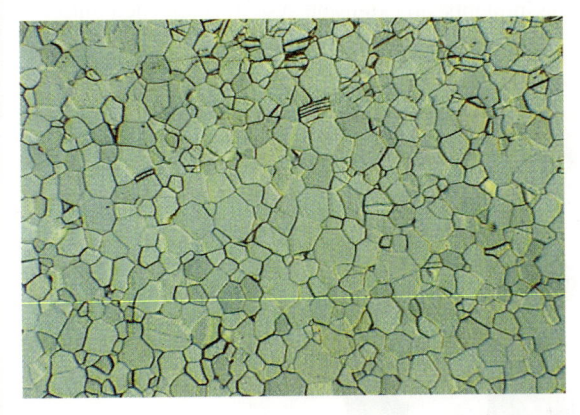

Fig. 7.**63** Typical microstructure of pure titanium with suitable granule size and deformation twins, which are used for producing implants (etched metallographic grinding, magnification x 100)

ITI Implants in Combination with Bone Grafts

In contrast to the regular implantation in the maxilla and mandible with the transmucosal ITI implants, augmentation of the alveolar ridge is necessary in the case of extreme atrophy. The simultaneous augmentation is mostly carried out with iliac bone grafts, which are fixed rigidly by means of endosseous implants and integrated into the biodynamics of the jaw.

A further main indication is the implantation into transplants in combination with functionally stable reconstrution plates as a consequence of trauma or tumor therapy. In contrast to other systems, a rigid connection between the plate and the screws is realized with the THORP reconstruction bridging system. In this way, the compact bone is relieved of strain in the region of plate support, and loosening of the screws is avoided. In addition, the perfect bone-screw surface bonding enhances the stability in the healing period, especially when using perforated, plasma-coated titanium hollow screws, which are penetrated by newly formed bone structures (Fig. 7.**64**).

Clinical experience in recent years (University clinic of Freiburg, Germany, Dir. Prof. Dr. Dr. W. Schilli and clinic of Dr. P. Asikainen, Kuopio, Finland) has shown that absolute stability of the transplanted bone segments and the implants are necessary. Early loading with physiological forces was recommended to avoid bone resorption.

As a prerequisite for the use of free bone grafts, a maximum wound closure during the healing phase is required. Accordingly, the implants in this indication should be inserted to the bone level, and the mucoperiosteal flap must cover the implants after suturing. At the second-stage surgery after osseointegration of the implants, an extension system is attached onto the

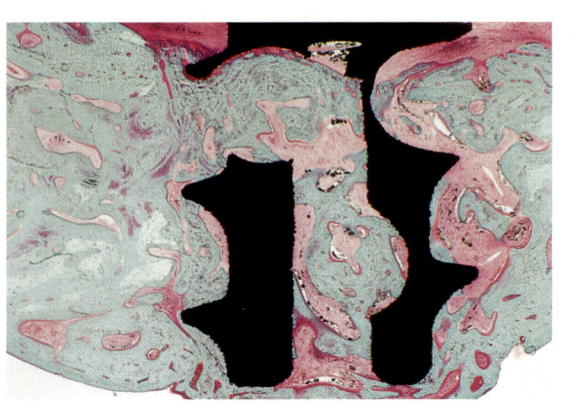

Fig. 7.**64** Detail of a human histological preparation. Ingrowth of the bone into the lateral perforations and into the lumen of the hollow screw and the direct bone-implant contact

primary implant part. Thereby, the implant is elongated and the peri-implant mucosa will adapt to the neck of the implant.

Any of the prosthetic abutments of the regular ITI dental system can be adapted on top of the elongated implant, and the suprastructure is fabricated according to standard procedures.

This extension of the indication for ITI implants in combination with bone grafts, which has been undergoing clinical tests since 1988, and the biomechanical testing of the new design (primary implant, extension parts, prosthetic abutments) is described in this chapter (Fig. 7.**65**, Table 7.**2**).

Material and Methods

Surgical Procedure

For clinical and microbiological reasons, the ITI titanium screw implants should be inserted into the transplants in a submerged manner. This requires the use of a transgingival extension sleeve, which is mounted and firmly screwed on top of the implant after the phase of primary healing (3 to 6 months) (Fig. 7.**65**, 7.**70**).

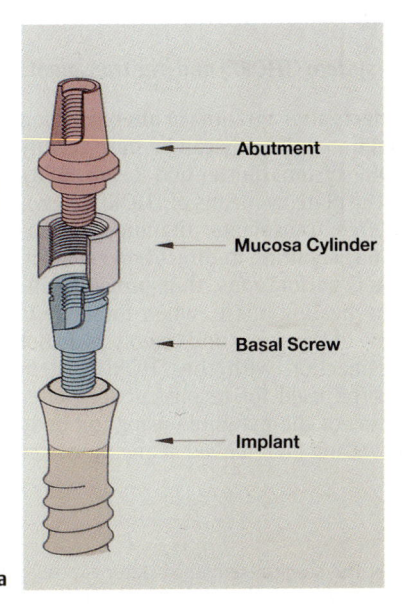

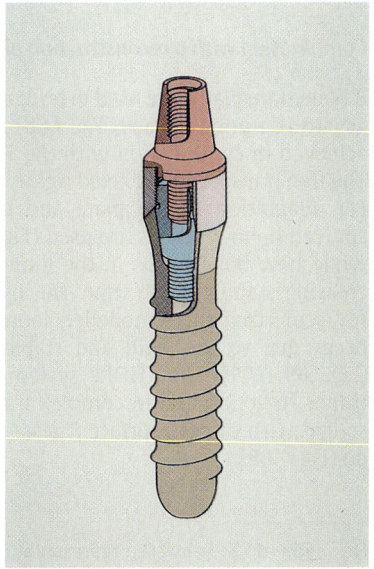

Fig. 7.**65a** and **b** Transgingival extension system shown graphically in detail and assembled

There are two main indications for the use of the ITI implants with the transgingival units:

Augmentation with bone transplants in the atrophic maxilla and mandible

Because of their V-shaped necks, the ITI screw implants function as tension screws, building up an interfragmentary compression between the natural bone bed of the jaw bone and the bone transplant (Fig. 7.**66**).

Figures 7.**66** and 7.**67** show the surgical augmentation procedure step-by-step and the implantation with ITI screw implants, as well as the use of the transgingival extension system.

First stage: The implant (ITI Type S) is inserted subgingivally, the upper end is covered with a healing cap, and the mucoperiosteal flap is positioned over the bone graft and the implant (Fig. 7.**66a–h**).

Second stage: Following a healing phase of 3 to 6 months, the implant is exposed, the healing cap removed, and the basal screw and the mucosa cylinder are screwed on to position and finally covered with a healing cap (Fig. 7.**67a–d**).

Third stage: After completion of wound healing, the prosthetic parts can be screwed on (Fig. 7.**67e**).

Combination with a reconstruction plate system (THORP) and free transplants

If bone transplants are used to bridge defects after a trauma or after resection as part of tumor therapy (Fig. 7.**68**), functional stability can be most readily achieved in combination with the THORP system (Sutter and Raveh 1988). The free transplants are fixed rigidly to the plate by means of THORP screws. For adaptation of the plate and the free transplants, titanium-plasma-sprayed hollow screws are used (Fig. 7.**64**) resulting in direct bone contact, while new bone forms in the lumen and perforations, thus providing increasing stability with time. During the healing phase, when the bone is revascularized and remodelled, loosening of the screw and osteolysis do not occur due to the rigid and stable connection with the THORP system (Fig.7.**69**, 7.**71**). The THORP system can be used for reconstructions after tumor resection and in complex fractures of the mandible using full body screws with smooth surface. These screws and be removed at any time later on (Fig. 7.**68**).

Fig. 7.**66a–d** Step-by-step representation of the surgical sequence. After exposure and augmenting the alveolar ridge with a bone transplant, the implant bed is prepared in the usual way. Marking with round burr (**a**), drilling to the desired depth with the three fluted drills (**b**), measurement of depth (**c**), and profiling of the neck portion (**d**)

ITI-Implants in Combination with Bone Grafts

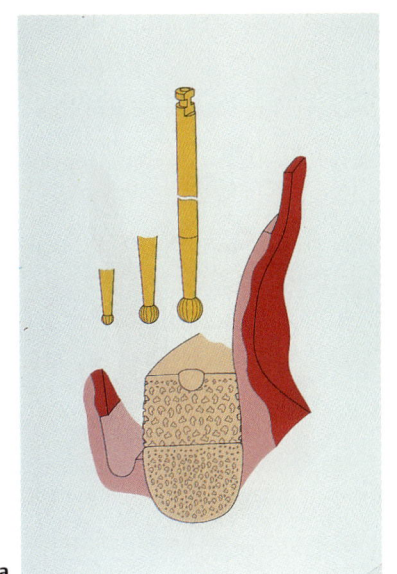

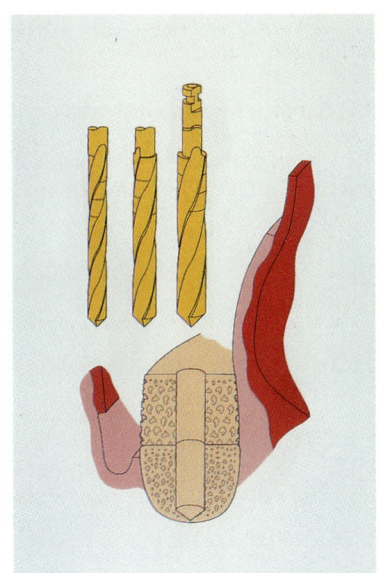

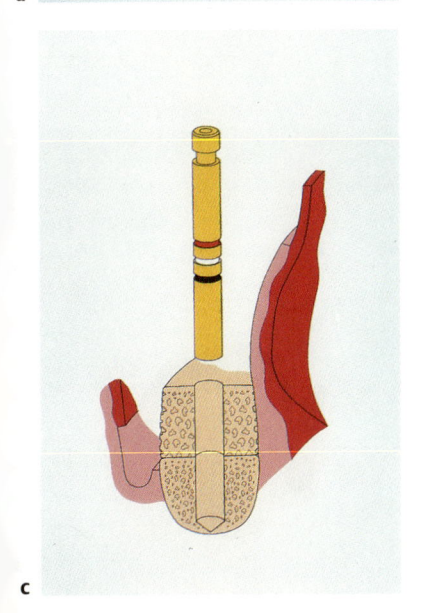

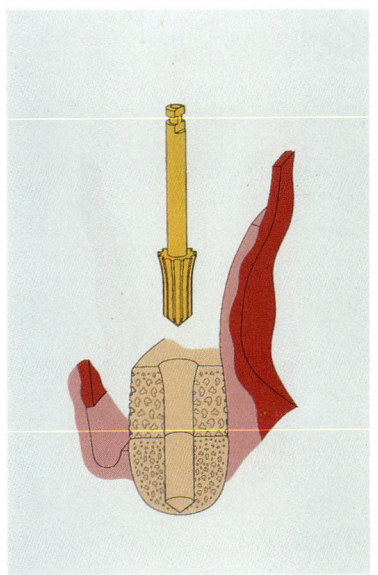

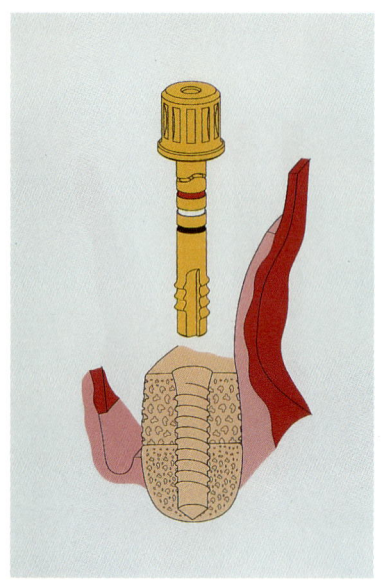

182 7 The Concept of the ITI Implants

e

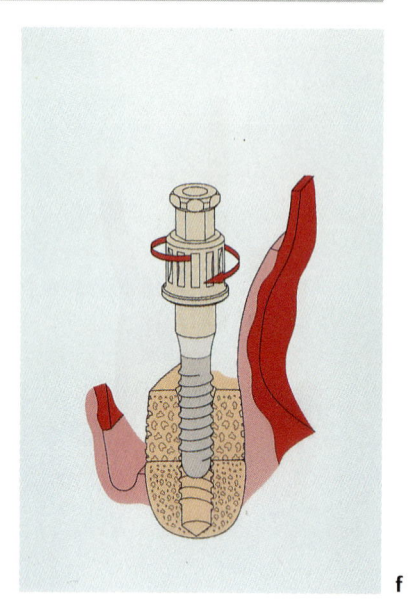

f

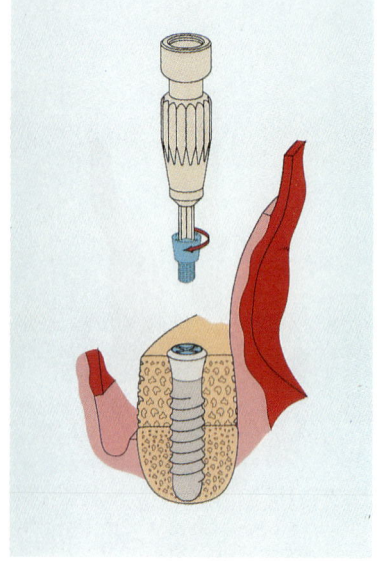

g

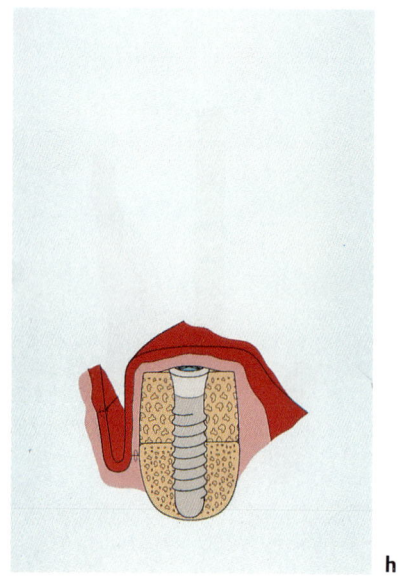

h

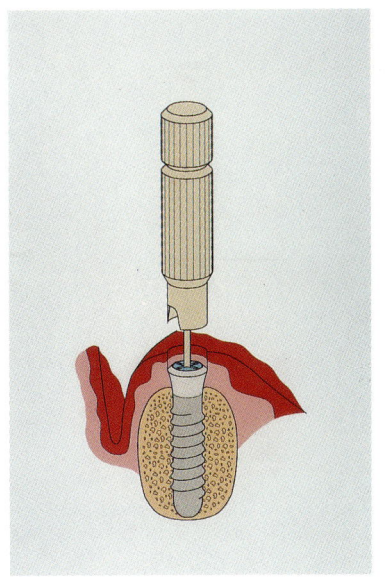

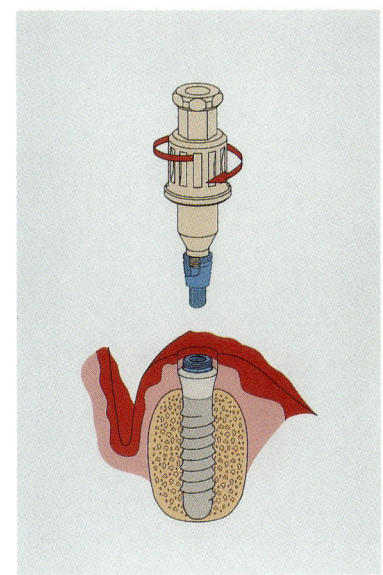

ITI-Implants in Combination with Bone Grafts **183**

Fig. 7.**67a, b**

Table 7.**2** Standard lengths of **x** and **y**

Dimension	Size-combination 1	Size-combination 2
x (mm)	3.0	5.0
y (mm)	1.5	3.5

Design and Mechanical Testing

At the second-stage surgery, the basal screw and the mucosa cylinder must always be used in corresponding pairs in accordance with the standard lengths "**x** and **y**" (Fig. 7.**65**, Table 7.**2**).

For microbiological reasons, the microgaps between the implant and the extension parts were kept as small as was technically possible (Fig. 7.**65a** and **b**).

Fig. 7.**66e–h** The next step is to pretap the thread in accordance with the depth (**e**), to insert the implant to the corect depth (**f**) with the standard inserting device, and then to insert the occlusal screw into the subgingivally positioned implant (**g**), the subgingivally positioned implant is then covered with soft tissue (**h**)

184 7 The Concept of the ITI Implants

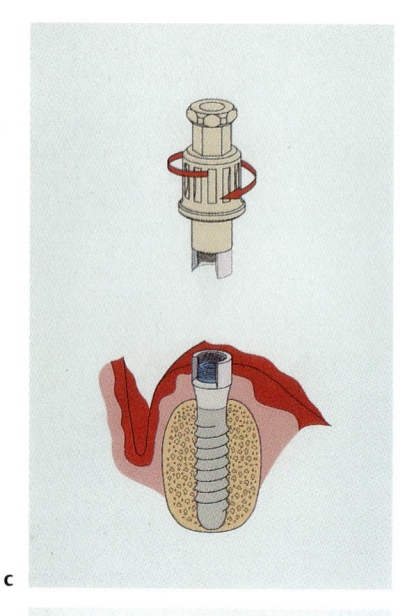

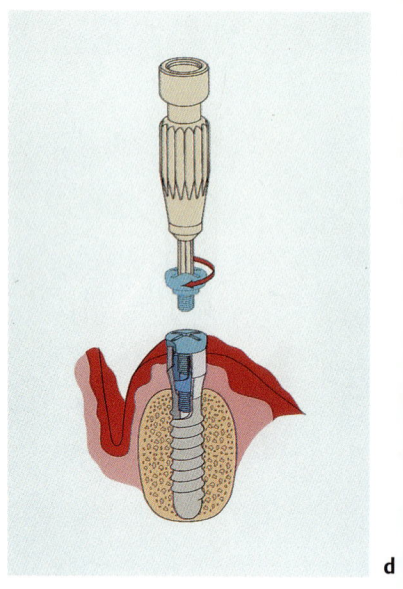

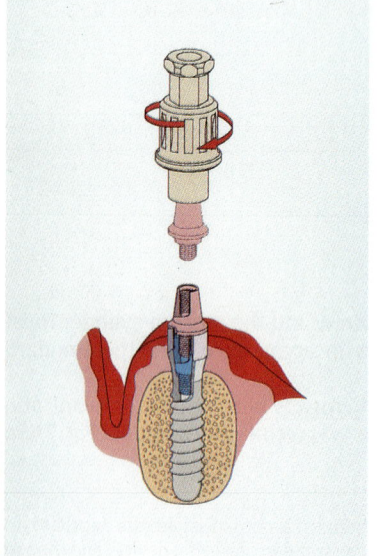

Fig. 7.**67a–e** After the healing phase, the top of the implant can be exposed either by an incision or with a punch (**a**). The next step is the insertion of the basal screw (**b**) and the mucosa cylinder (**c**) with a special screw-in instrument. Figures (**d**) and (**e**) show the insertion of the healing cap and the secondary part

ITI-Implants in Combination with Bone Grafts **185**

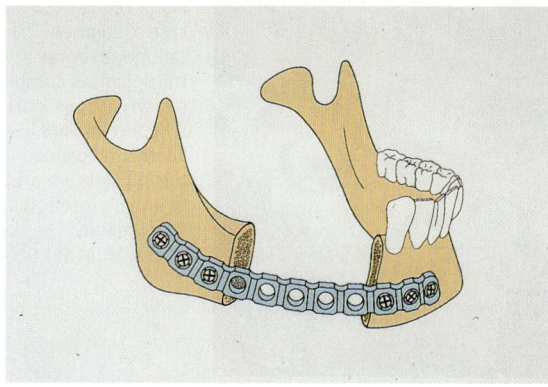

Fig. 7.**68a** Fixing of the THORP plate after description of the system and resection. In consequence of the rigid connection between the plate and the screw head, only two or three screws are necessary on both sides of the resection site

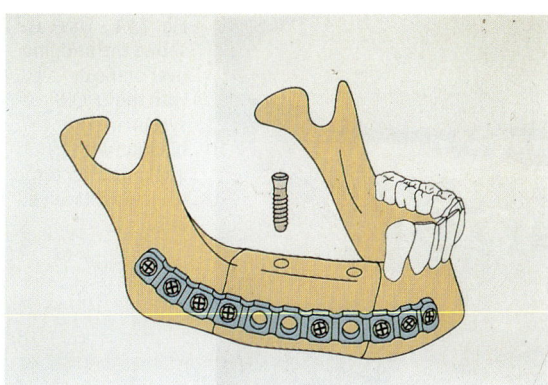

Fig. 7.**68b** The system now enables the transplant to be fitted and fixed in a stable way with the THORP screws. Implants can now be inserted Figures 7.**70** and 7.**71**

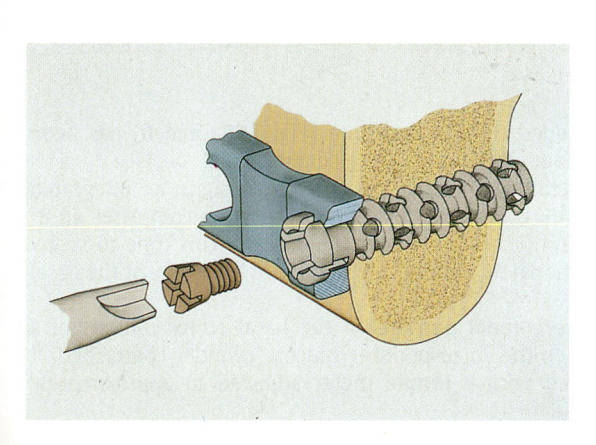

Fig. 7.**69** Graphic representation of the rigid THORP system. (Sutter et al.)

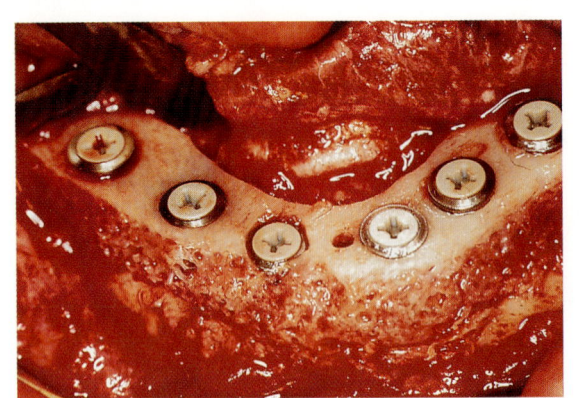

Fig. 7.70 Clinical case of augmentation with bone transplants in combination with two-part ITI screw implants. For this indication, the implants are preferentially inserted subgingivally (Weingart et al.)

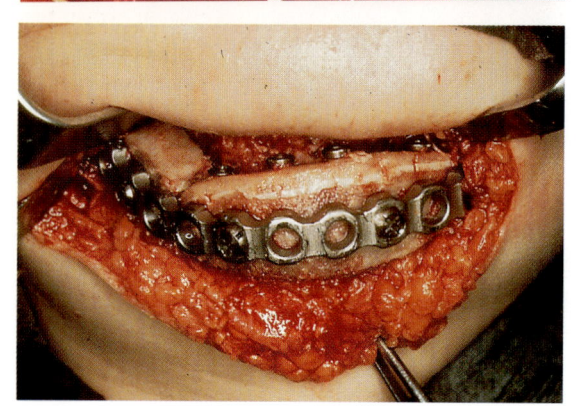

Fig. 7.71 This case shows the bridging over of the defect with the THORP system in combination with ITI implants after tumor resection (Raveh et al.)

The newly developed transgingival unit (Fig. 7.**65a** and **b**) has been mechanically tested under different loading conditions.

As a result of preliminary tests with different designs, an integrated attachment (basal screw) was chosen. The apical portion comprises an 8° cone and a 2 mm screw for attachment to the implant. This cone-to-screw design provides a frictional fit, eliminating the risk of loosening of the basal screw.

The design of the coronal portions of the basal screw consists of a threaded part, to which the corresponding mucosa cylinder is attached. It is preferably tightened with a torque meter adjusted to approximately 0.35 Nm.

With regard to their external configuration, the prosthetic parts correspond to the standard ITI implant system abutments (conus 6°, 8°, 15°, retentive anchor and octa abutment and are also manufactured from pure titanium.

Any abutment design, such as concial-, octagonal, or ball-anchor configurations can be attached to the mucosa cylinder (Fig. 7.**67**).

Discussion

Positive experience and results with endosteal implants in the field of standard oral implantology led to an extension of the indication to implantations into transplants. In these cases, the use of screw implants facilitated optimal graft adaption and fixation.

Originally, the ITI implants were designed for a nonsubmerged type of implant placement. Using bone graft procedures, it is necessary to cover the bone graft with a soft-tissue flap to get a satisfactory incorporation of the bone. These cases need a second-stage surgery and a special abutment device.

The objective of the presented new transgingival abutment design was to provide a simple method for fixed or removable suprastructures with ITI implants in combination with autogenous bone transplants. Due to the ITI implant concept, there is no additional prosthetic abutment necessary.

The advantageous combination of an 8° cone and thread connection between implant and transmucosal superstructure design created a friction lock similar to a Morse taper used in mechanical engineering and related industries. Any mated conical metallic surfaces of less than 8° in angle would create a mechanically locking friction fit.

From the design perspective, the ITI implant allows the seating of the secondary parts within its tapered coronal neck portion.

This concept is supported by the fact that the loosening moment of the cone-and-screw interface is 7–24% higher than its tightening torque compared to screws alone (loosening moment approximately 10% lower than the tightening torque).

The functional strength of the standard transgingival ITI implant designed with a conical abutment of 8° was compared to a submerged implant with a basal screw-mucosa cylinder combination and an 8° conical abutment. There is no significant difference in strength between these two designs, although the leverages and the number of parts are different.

Diameter-Reduced Screw Implants (ITI 3.3)

Use of standard implants of about 4 mm external diameter is often a problem in narrow atrophied ridges and in loss of individual teeth, since insufficient bone is available. Accordingly, diameter-reduced two-part solid screw

Fig. 7.72 Schematic representation of a diameter-reduced two-part screw implant with inserted 8° standard conical abutment

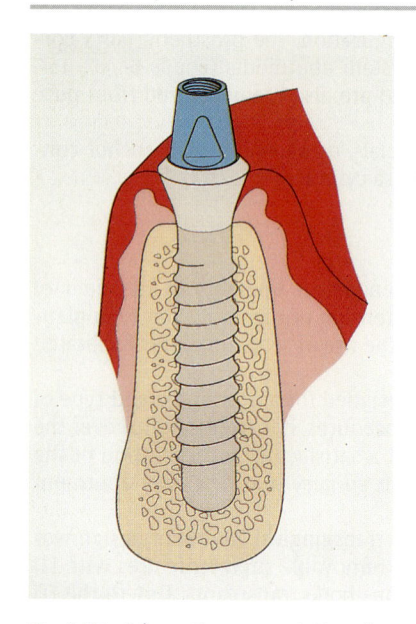

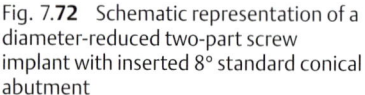

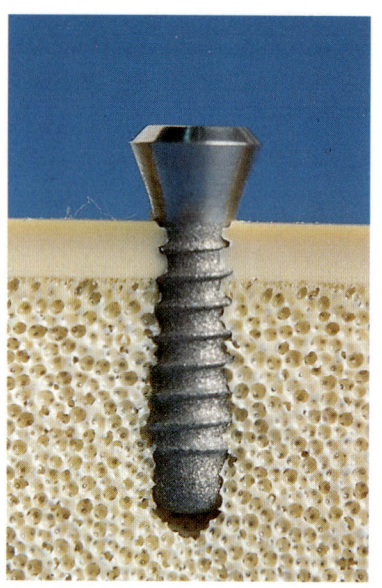

Fig. 7.73 Diameter-reduced ITI 3.3 implant

implants were developed that enabled the hole diameter to be reduced to 2.8 mm instead of the 3.5 mm standard drillholes. Since the "pilot drills" of 2.2 mm and 2.8 mm diameter are part of the standard ITI system, special drilling instruments are not required to prepare the drillholes; only these two fluted drills are used.

The ITI standard components (inserting device, ratchet, etc.) can be used to insert the screw implant, since only the dimensions of the implant anchoring element in the bone were changed. The head part was also maintained with a diameter of 4.8 mm, as with all two-part ITI implants, so that the accommodation of abutments and the basis for the prosthetic superstructure are identical with the standard implants. This means that all standard abutments can be used for these diameter-reduced implants, and the impression can be made with the same accessories (Fig. 7.72).

The ITI 3.3 special implants are available in lengths of 8, 10, 12, 14, and 16 mm anchorage depth (Fig. 7.74, 7.75). In contrast to the standard ITI system, these diameter-reduced implants are only produced in the two-part version (Fig. 7.72–7.75).

Diameter-Reduced Screw Implants

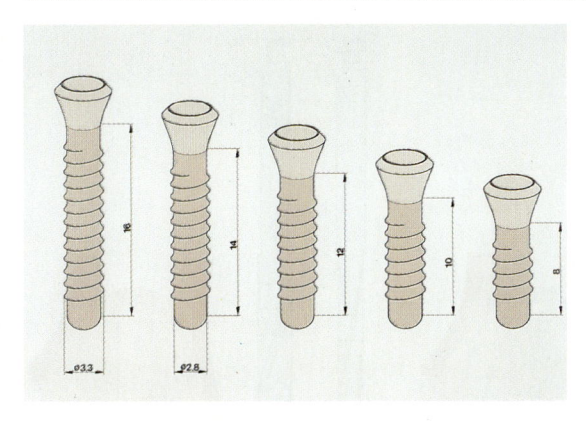

Fig. 7.**74** and 7.**75** Range of two-part ITI 3.3 implants with a core diameter of 2.8 mm, and external thread diameter of about 3.3 mm and the standard anchorage lengths of 8, 10, 12, 14, and 16 mm

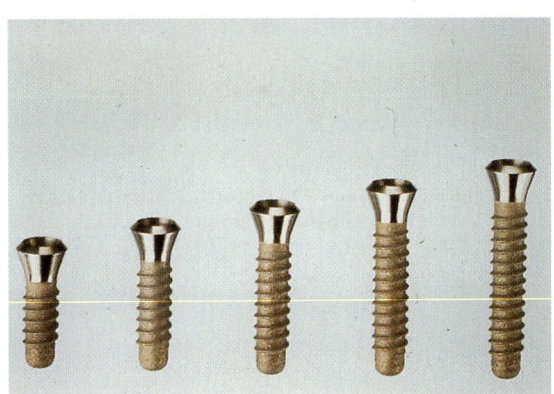

Fig. 7.**75**

The surgical procedure is explained by reference to Figures 7.**76**–7.**80** and the following descriptions:
1. The implant region is adequately exposed by a crestal incision with mesial and distal releasing incisions and elevation of the mucoperiosteal flap.
2. The marking of the envisioned implant site can now be carried out with the round burs of 1.4 mm and 2.3 mm diameter (Fig. 7.**76**).
3. As the next step, the hole is drilled to the desired depth with the 2.2 mm and 2.8 mm diameter twist drills (standard pilot drill). The radial rings (8, 10, 12, 14, and 16 mm) produced on the bits with a laser serve as depth reference.

7 The Concept of the ITI Implants

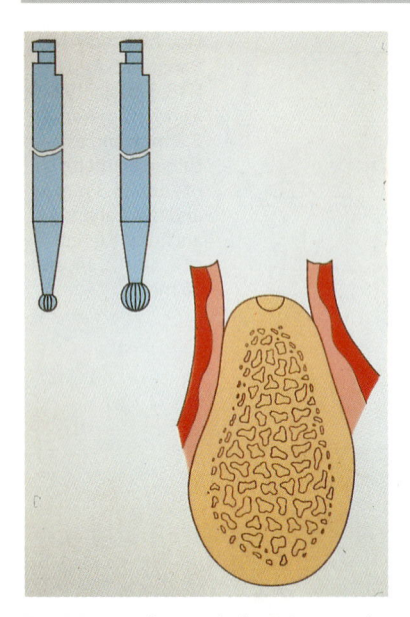

Fig. 7.**76** Marking with the 1.4 mm and 2.3 mm spherical-headed drill

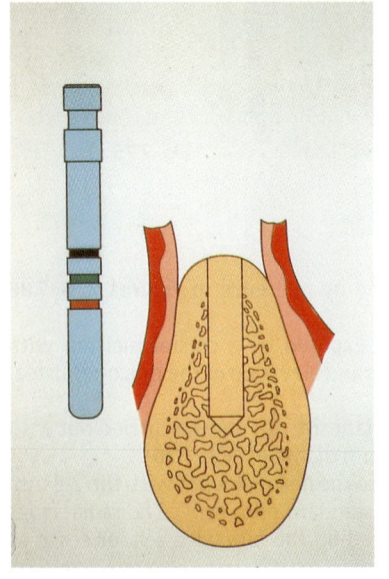

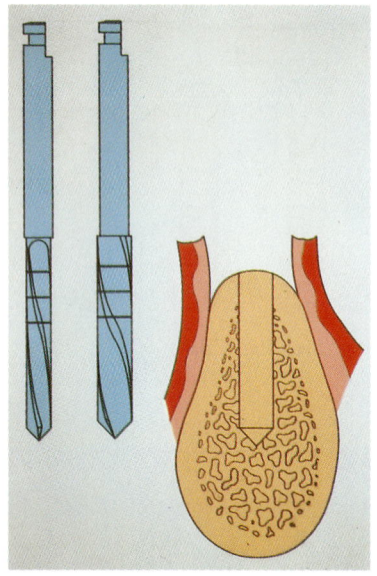

Fig. 7.**77** Preparation of the drill recess with the 2.2 mm and 2.8 mm diameer pilot drill

Fig. 7.**78** Determination of the depth with the depth gauge

Diameter-Reduced Screw Implants 191

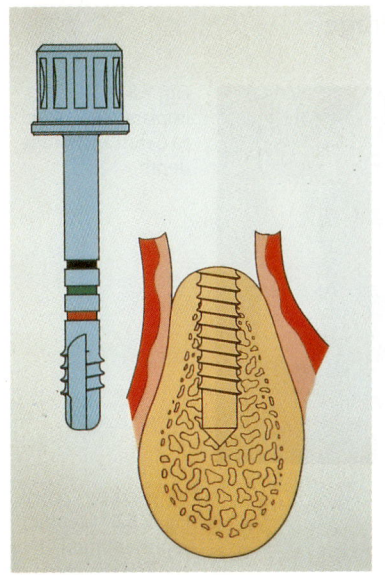

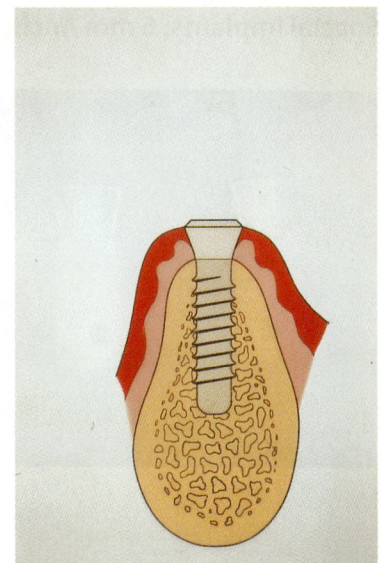

Fig. 7.**79** Precutting of the thread

Fig. 7.**80** Implant in situ

As described on page 153, the speed of the drilling instruments should not exceed 800 rpm and work should be carried out with adequate cooling. These drilling instruments are designed in such a way that a precise drill hole can be made with relatively slight axial pressure.

By use of an intermittent drilling movement, it is ensured that the bone chips are discharged automatically without getting stuck in the spiral grooves of the drill and that the cooling fluid also washes around the front part of the drill (Fig. 7.**77**).

4. After thorough flushing of the hole, the depth can be determined with the color-coded depth gauge (Fig. 7.**78**).
5. Afterward, the thread is precut to the depth determined in the usual way with the 3.3 mm thread tap (Fig. 7.**79**).
6. An appropriate implant of the confirmed length is now chosen and inserted as in the standard method (Fig. 7.**80**).

Biomechanical measurements and the results of about 4 years of clinical testing demonstrated that the range of indications can be substantially extended with these ITI 3.3 implants without reducing the recognized mechanical strength of the ITI system.

Special Implants, 6 mm Anchorage

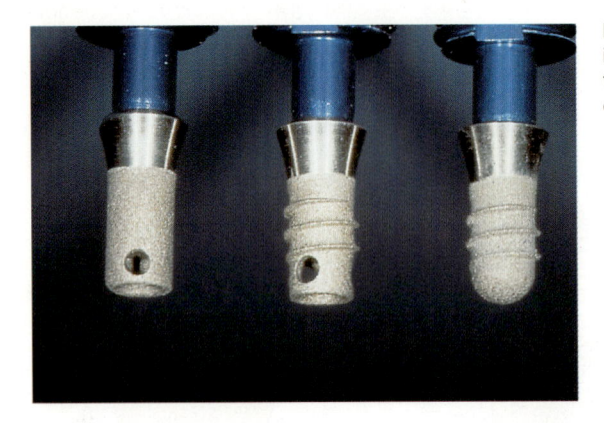

Fig. 7.**81** ITI implants shortened to 6 mm anchorage depth

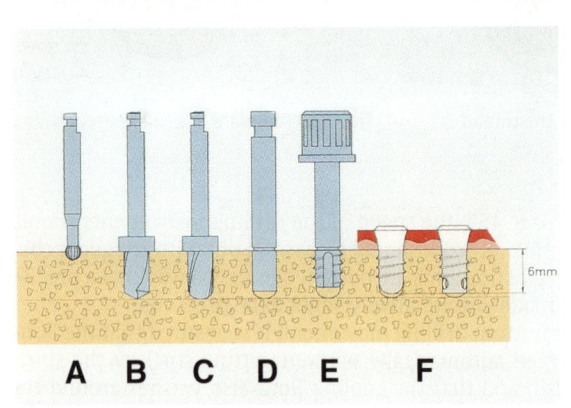

Fig. 7.**82** Graphic representation of the surgical sequence

A B C D E   F

Method of Operation

The instrumentation sequence shown graphically in figure 7.**82** comprises the following steps:
- **A** Marking with the round burs in ascending order
- **B** Full drilling to the stop with the stop drill (length 6 mm) under cooling and reduced speed of a maximum of 800 rpm
- **C** Using the 6 mm screw implant, the bone preparation is accomplished with the cylindrical stop drill
- **D** Measurement of depth with a depth gauge
- **E** Thread cutting
- **F** Inserting the implant up to the correct final position in the usual way.

Both in the mandible and in the maxilla, there is often so little bone available that implantation is no longer feasible with standard implants. Therefore, implants of only 6 mm anchorage length were developed that ensure adequate anchorage even in a greatly reduced alveolar bone height (Fig. 7.**81**).

Despite a reduced anchorage surface, complete osteointegration and adequate functional stress tolerance is made possible by the ideal macroform and the micromorphological surface characteristics of the implant anchorage element.

We recommend these implants exclusively for the following indications:
- bar supported prosthesis in the lower front (Fig. 7.**83** and 7.**84**);
- in combination with longer standard implants, for support of implant-borne fixed reconstructions (Fig. 7.**85a** and **b**) in the premolar/molar region in the maxilla and mandible.

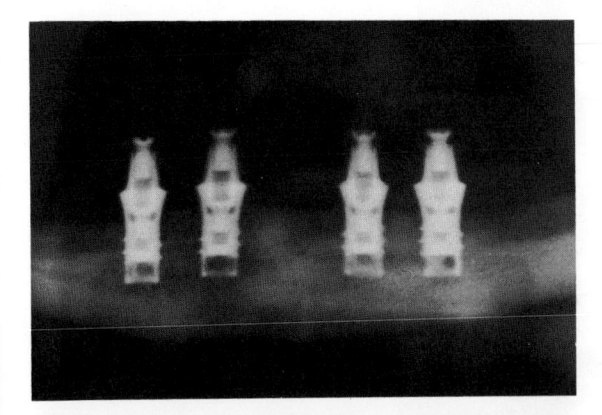

Fig. 7.**83** Four 6 mm hollow screw implants in the interforaminal region of the mandible as support for an implant-borne bar construction

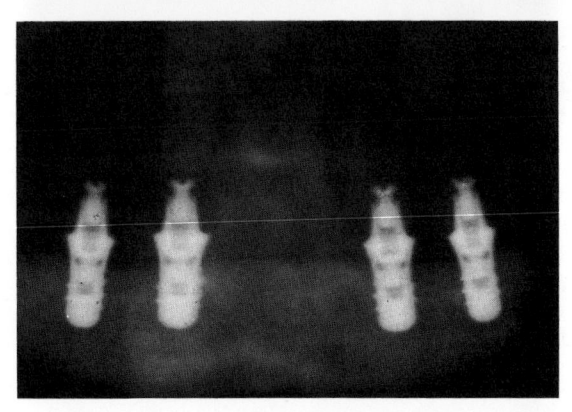

Fig. 7.**84** Four 6 mm solid screws for retention of the bar in the mandible

194 7 The Concept of the ITI Implants

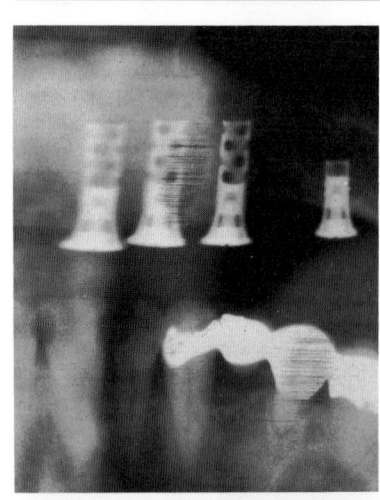

Fig. 7.**85a** and **b** As a supplementary implant in conjunction with longer standard implants to support implant-borne reconstructions in the premolar and molar region of the maxilla (X-rays from Dr. Ch. ten Bruggenkate)

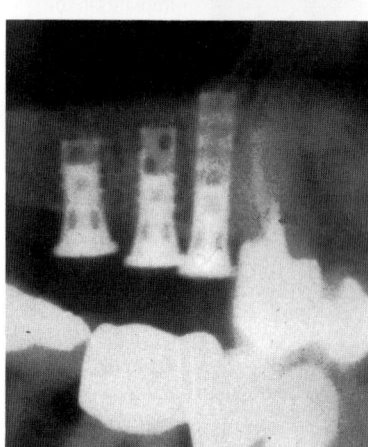

For the 6 mm implants, a special set of instruments was developed which comprises the drilling instrument with a depth stop (6 mm) as a special feature. Regular twist drills with marking at the 6 mm level are also available.

Reconstruction on Two-Part ITI Implants

The possible means of enabling a functionally and aesthetically correct solution of reconstruction of two-part ITI implants are as follows:
1. Conical abutment system
   a) cementable restorations
   b) screw-retained restorations
2. Octa-System

Depending on the type of reconstruction, the clinical and dental laboratory working steps differ.

Conical Abutment System

Cemented Restorations

The individual clinical and technical working steps hardly differ from those used in natural teeth prepared for crowns. The steps for producing the master cast implant, the die and the final restoration for cementations on the abutment device are practically identical to those for conventional crown-bridge prostheses.

The following factors prove to be advantageous in the firmly cemented version:
- the crown/bridge prosthetic abutments can be modified individually and are thus adaptable to the respective situation (Fig. 7.**86**);
- aesthetically attractive reconstructions are possible, since the entire occlusal surface can be faced (absence of screw access hole);

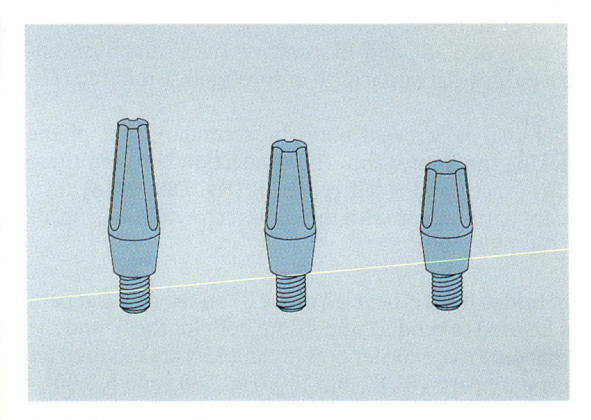

Fig. 7.**86** Standard abutments for cementable reconstructions

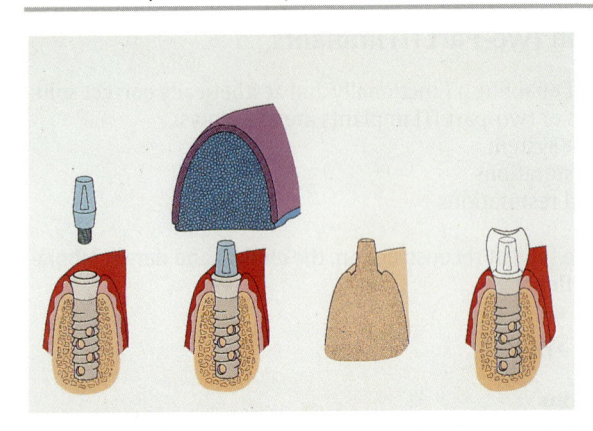

Fig. 7.**87** Step-by-step description of procedure for cemented reconstructions

- loosening of the reconstruction due to loosening of the occlusal screw is not possible;
- the technique is simpler and less expensive than the screwed version (Fig. 7.**87**).

Screw-Retained Restorations

This superstructure system (developed on the basis of the investigations of Flury and Brägger et al.) constitutes a simplification and improvement of the following transfer parts in combination with the standard conical secondary parts (Flury K., Brägger U. et al. 1991):
1. Conical secondary parts of 6°, 8°, and 15° conicity. The 6° and 8° secondary parts each have three flat surfaces to ensure against rotation (Fig. 7.**88a** and **b**)
2. Impression cylinder that is screwed onto the secondary part of the implant before making the impression. The connection between these two components fits exactly and is self-centering (Fig. 7.**89**, 7.**91a**)
3. Transfer pins that are harmonized with the conical crown/bridge heads of 6°, 8°, and 15° (Fig. 7.**89**, 7.**90**)

Since the 6° crown bridge head is beveled off by 8° on the occlusal part, the 8° transfer pin can be used to produce the stump both for the 6° and the 8° heads. This means that only two transfer pins (8° and 15°) are required for the three standard secondary parts (6°, 8°, and 15°) (Fig. 7.**89a** and **b**, 7.**90**).

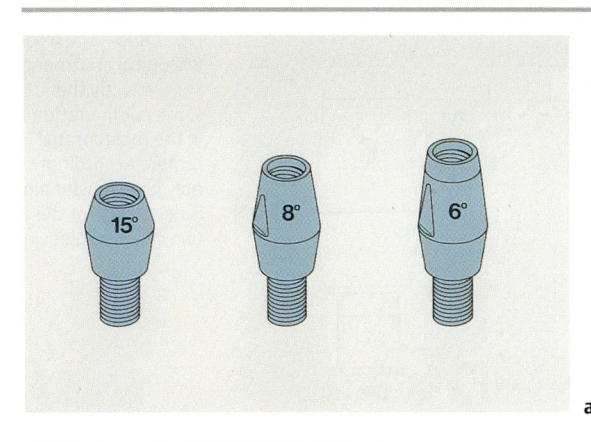

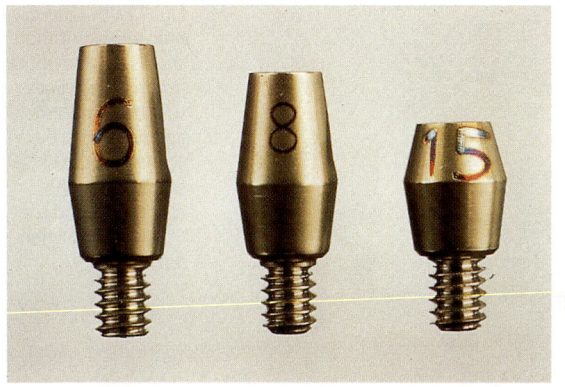

Fig. 7.**88a** and **b** The available parts for screw-retained restorations. On the right: 6° conicity for crowns and bridges. In the middle: 8° conicity for crowns, bridges, and bars. On the left: 15° conicity for bridges (only screwed version)

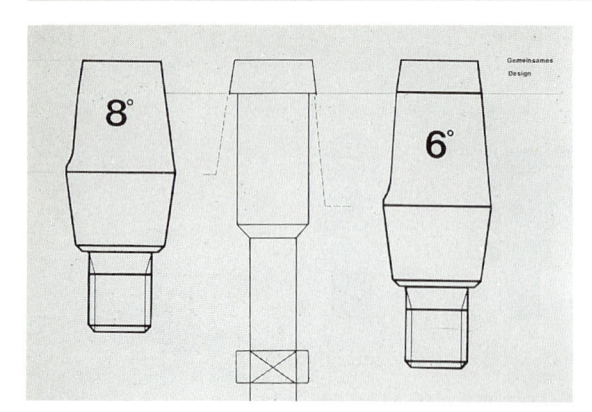

Fig. 7.**89a** The 6° or 8° conical abutments show exactly the same configuration in the mostcoronal region. Accordingly, only one transfer pin is necessary for the two conus angles

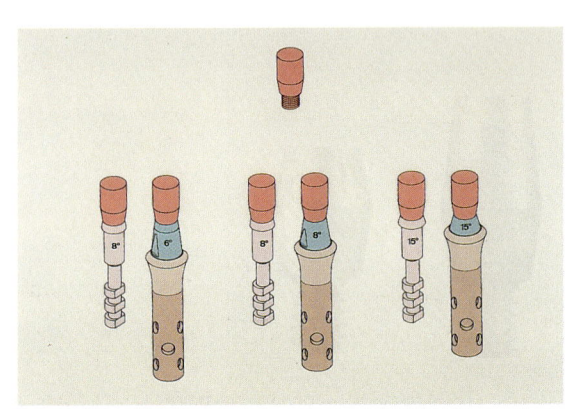

Fig. 7.**89b** This graphic representation shows the use of the impression cylinder which is standardized and which can be screwed on to fit exactly onto the abutments and the 8° and 15° transfer pins

Step-by-step Description of the Sequence of Operation

After completion of the healing phase after implantation, the healing screw is removed; the chosen secondary part (6°, 8°, or 15°) is inserted and tightened (to about 0.35 Nm) using the inserting device and the ratchet with gradually increased force.

If the secondary part is cemented in, which is not a reommended procedure but a preference of some clinicians, care must be taken that a **thin** layer of zinc phosphate cement is applied **only** in the region of the **conical** part and that the secondary part is tightened immediately.

Reconstruction on Two-Part ITI Implants **199**

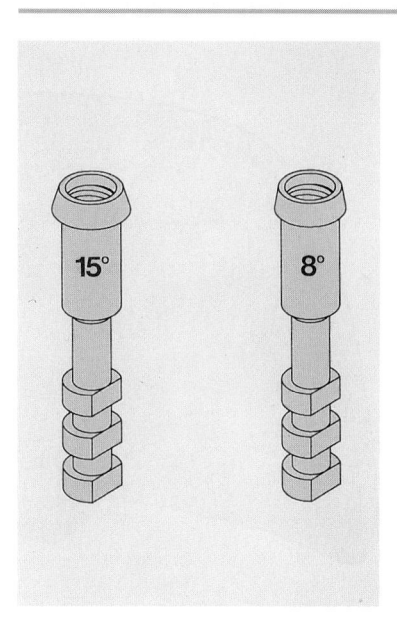

Fig. 7.**90** The two transfer pins for transfer of the occlusal thread.
On the left: 15° transfer pin.
On the right: 6°/8° transfer pin

It is possible to modify the secondary parts according to the individual situation. This also applies to the shoulder region of the implant.

Before an impression is made, the precisely fitting impression model cylinder is firmly screwed onto the secondary part (Fig. 7.**91a**).

The next step is to make an impression with an individual tray and a suitable impression material (Fig. 7.**91b**). The 15° secondary parts are mainly envisaged to deal with greater axial abutment divergences.

The impression is passed on, together with the impression model cylinders, to the dental technician for further processing after detailed checking (Fig. 7.**91c**).

Cave! The processing notes of the manufacturer should be followed precisely with regard to dimensional stability of the impression material, elastic return to shape, and time of model production.

The conicity of the secondary parts is examined and determined (7.**92b**) using the conus gauge (Fig. 7.**92a**).

The impression model cylinder is now firmly screwed onto the transfer pin up to the stop and carefully repositioned as a unit in the impression (Fig. 7.**93**, 7.**94**).

Important! If possible, always insert the same cylinder in the identical position as was used to make the impression in the patient.

200 7 The Concept of the ITI Implants

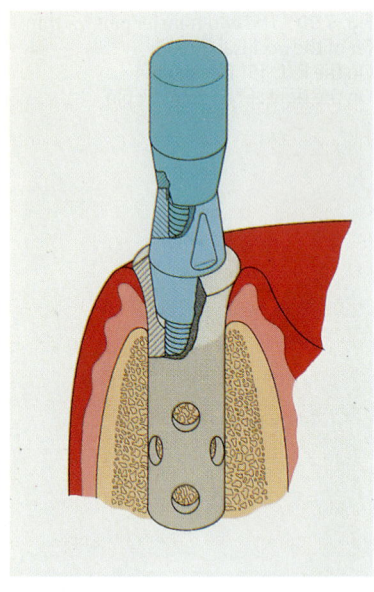

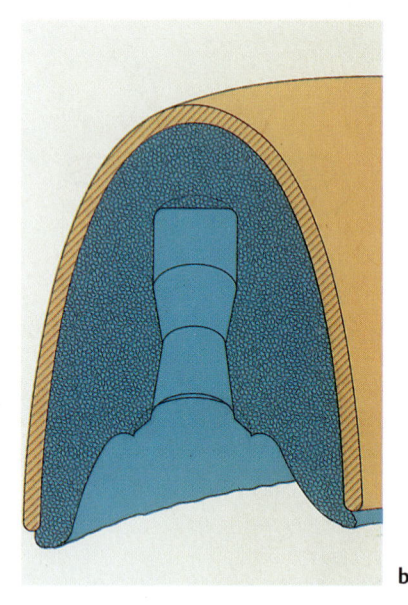

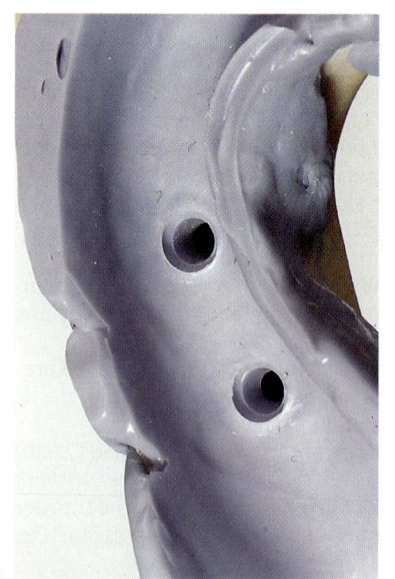

Fig. 7.**91a** Before making the impression for screw-retained superstructures, the impression model cylinder is firmly screwed onto the occlusal thread of the abutments

Fig. 7.**91b** Impression in situ, schematic representation

Fig. 7.**91c** After thorough checking, the impression is passed on for further processing to the dental technician with the original impression model cylinders used in the patient

Reconstruction on Two-Part ITI Implants

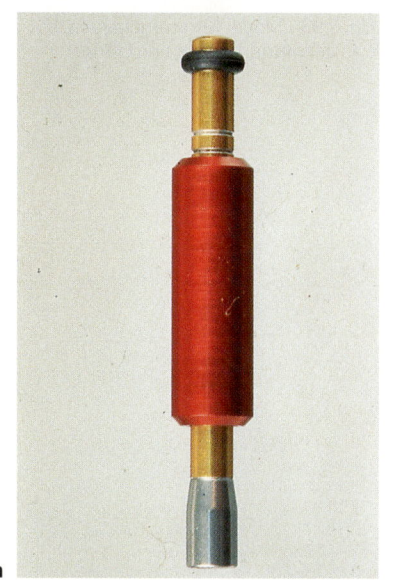

Fig. 7.**92a** Conus measuring gauge for selection of the correct transfer pins:
1st ring = 6° secondary part, 6°/8° transfer pin
2nd ring = 8° secondary part
3rd ring = 15° secondary part, 15° transfer pin

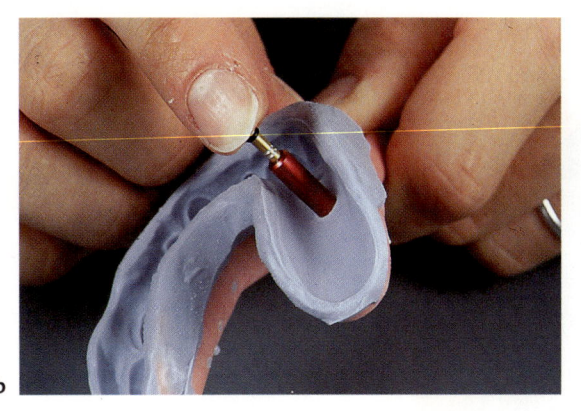

Fig. 7.**92b** Checking the conicity ensures the correct choice of transfer pins

202 7 The Concept of the ITI Implants

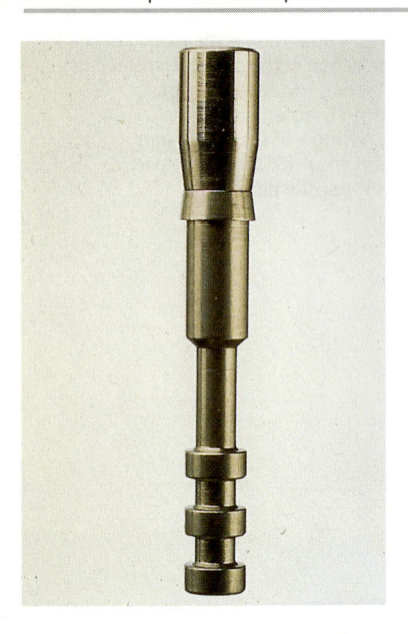

Fig. 7.**93** Model with combination of transfer pin and impression cylinder

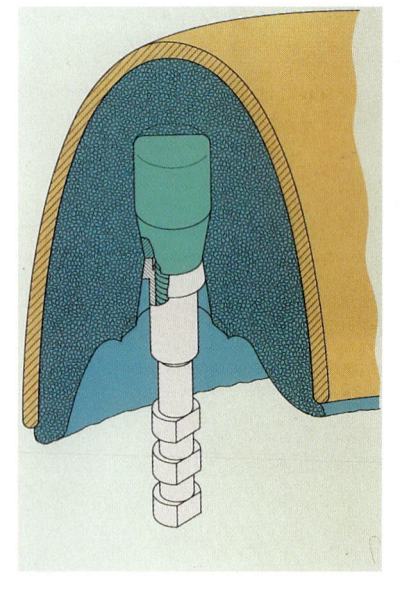

Fig. 7.**94** Schematic representation of a repositioned transfer pin

Reconstruction on Two-Part ITI Implants 203

Figures 7.**95** and 7.**96** show the working or master model produced in hard stone (die stone). In the occlusal part, the model die consists of the metal with an internal thread formed by the transfer pin. The cervical part of the die and the implant shoulder are in stone (model material).

Specific detailed dental-mechanical and constructional data concerning these operator removable fixed partial dentures are available in two publications (Flury, Brägger et al., and Scacchi/Wermuth) and in the ITI brochures and technical information (Fig. 7.**97** and 7.**98**).

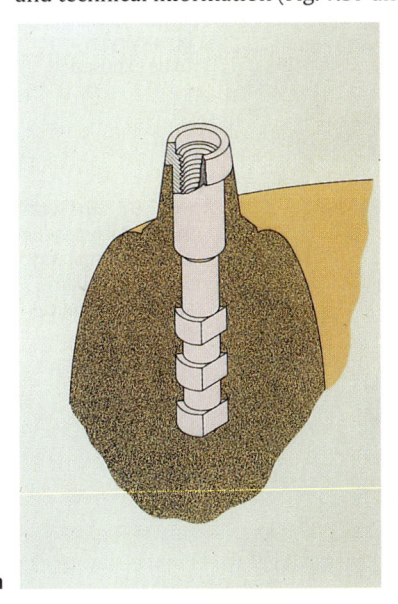

Fig. 7.**95a** and **b** Schematic representation and master model show that the abutments in the upper occlusal part have an occlusal thread on the inside. The cervical retouchable part of the conus with the shoulder is of die stone (class 4 stone)

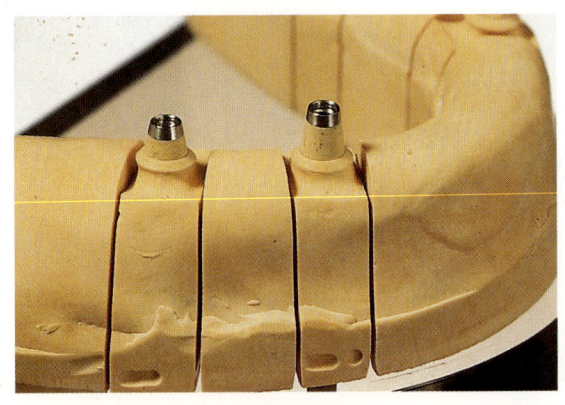

204 7 The Concept of the ITI Implants

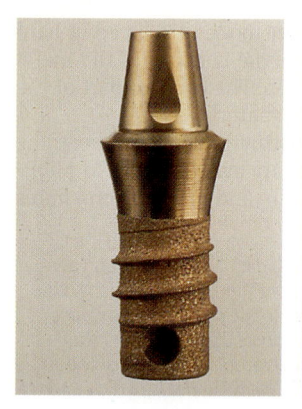

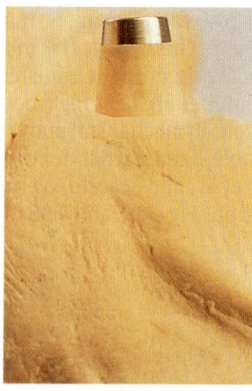

Fig. 7.**96** The conical abutment has three flat surfaces to insure against rotation.
On the left: original
On the right: precise model
The demarcation line (preparation boundary) is as yet to be exposed

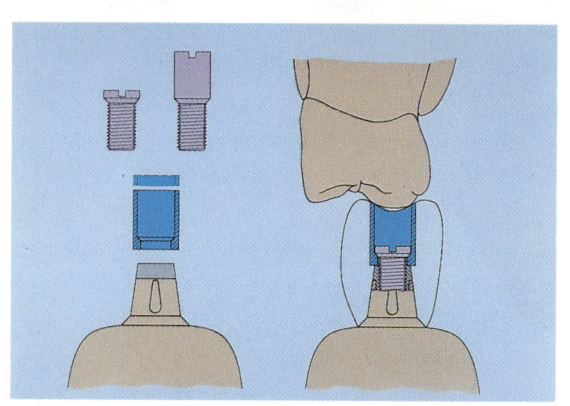

Fig. 7.**97** The working model is produced in the usual way with special hard stone (see publications)

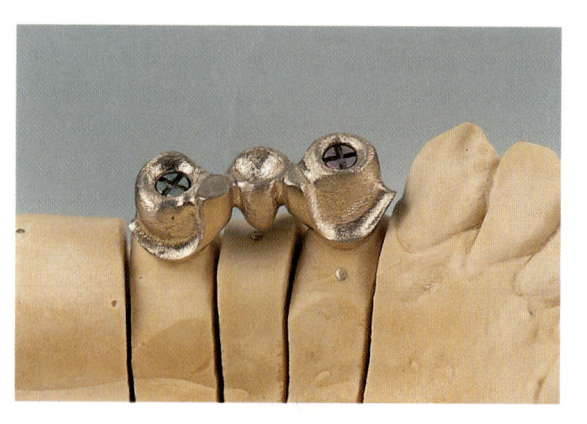

Fig. 7.**98** Check on the master model

Octa System (Screw Retained Restorations)

The Octa system was developed to create a precise transfer system for the two-part implants consisting of prefabricated parts with a transfer coping and transfer pin (analog) for transfer from the oral cavity to the master model (working model) (Sutter et al. 1992).

A decision was made in favor of the following solution based on various ideas and pretrials:
1. A secondary part with an octagonal shape of 1.5 mm height. The cervical portion (of 1.0 mm height) has parallel vertical sides, whereas the coronal upper one-third is conical (30°) (Fig. 7.**99a** and **b**)
2. For all other ITI abutments, the anchorage of the Octa abutment is achieved with an 8° conus and 2 mm screw combination
3. A nonrepositionable transfer system, i.e., a combination of a transfer coping firmly retained in the impression material, a positioning screw (guide screw), and a transfer pin (analog)

Overall, the Octa concept is conceived as a supplement for the variants described in sections one and two and has the following characteristics:
- Mechanically advantageous connection between the implant and the secondary part
- Exact impression technique modelling by use of precisely prefabricated and standardized metal parts
- Microcrevice between the implant shoulder (45°) and the transfer or gold copings can be kept very small
- Simple production of laboratory casts
- Design of the prefabricated superstructure elements to the basic Octa concept as a modular system
- Possibility for additional standardized parts, e.g., transverse screw retention for gold copings, solder base
- Improved aesthetics by easy countersinking of the implant shoulder into the soft tissue, using the transgingival healing caps available in four lengths as soft tissue shaping elements
- Safeguarding against rotation by Octa connection (e.g., single tooth implantation)
- Biomechanically favorable construction of the Octa system with regard to strain and torsional forces etc.
- Sufficient possibility to overcome divergence problems between implants

Important: Only ITI implants with 45° shoulders without bevels are to be used for reconstructions with the Octa concept.

7 The Concept of the ITI Implants

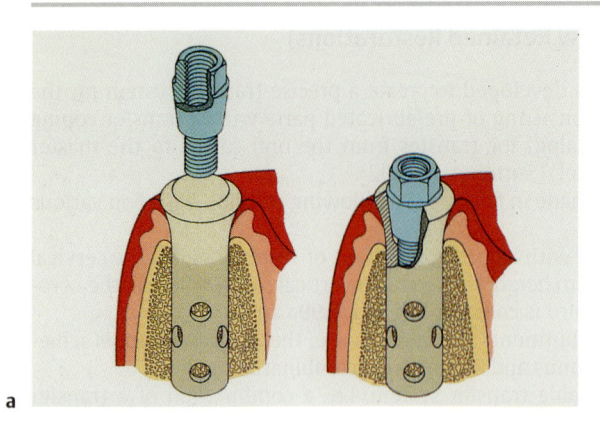

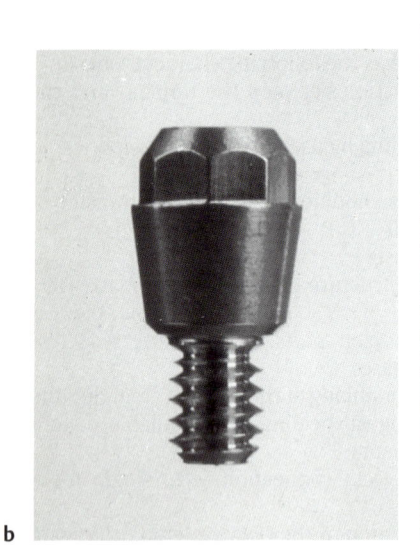

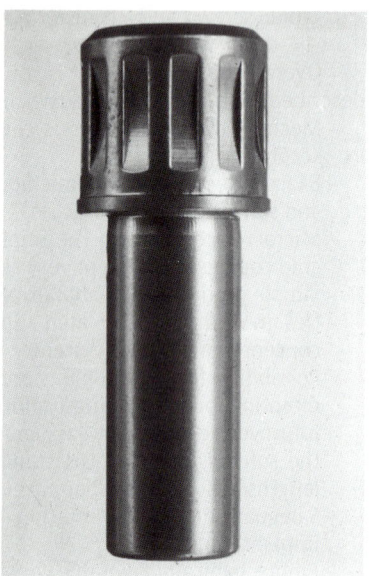

Fig. 7.**99a** Situation in the mouth: Octa secondary part is inserted after the healing phase and tightened with graduated force

Fig. 7.**99b** and **c** Pictorial representation of the abutment and the instrument required for insertion

Step-by-Step Description of the Operation

After completion of the healing phase, the healing cap is removed from the implant. The Octa secondary part is inserted and tightened with a special screw-in instrument and the ratchet, using graduated force (about 0.35 Nm).

The nonrepositionable impression coping is mounted and fixed on the implant with a guide screw (Fig. 7.**100a–c**). These guide screws are available in four different lengths (10, 12, 14, and 16 mm) and can be shortened individually.

The impression is carried out with an individual tray comprising the necessary access holes for the guide screws and with a suitable impression material (Fig. 7.**101**).

After setting of the impression material and removal of the surplus around the openings in the tray, the guide screw can be unscrewed and the impression removed from the mouth. The impression coping remains firmly anchored in the impression material (Fig. 7.**102**).

The transfer pin (analog) can now be inserted with an exact octagonal fit into the impression coping and fixed firmly with the guide screw. As described above for the impression, care must be taken that the 45° shoulder of the analog is positioned precisely and that the connection is crevice free (Fig. 7.**103a** and **b**).

The impression is now poured with a Type 4 hard stone. In the final cast, the octagon and the 45° shoulder of the transfer pin protrude. The rest of the analog is firmly anchored in the cast (Fig. 7.**104**).

208 7 The Concept of the ITI Implants

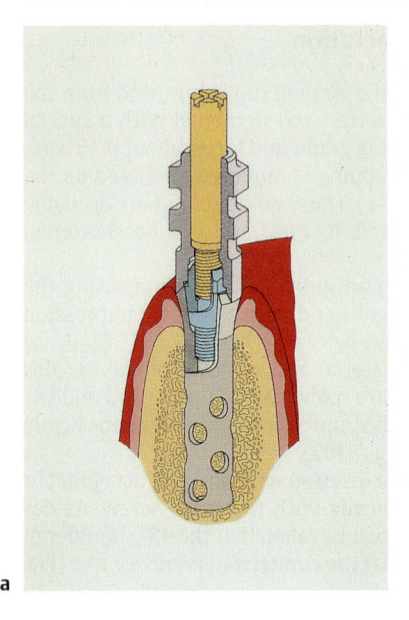

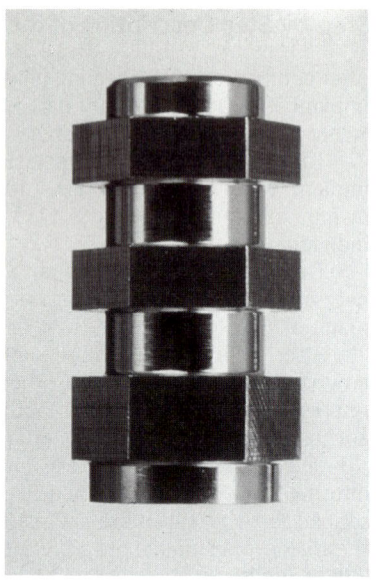

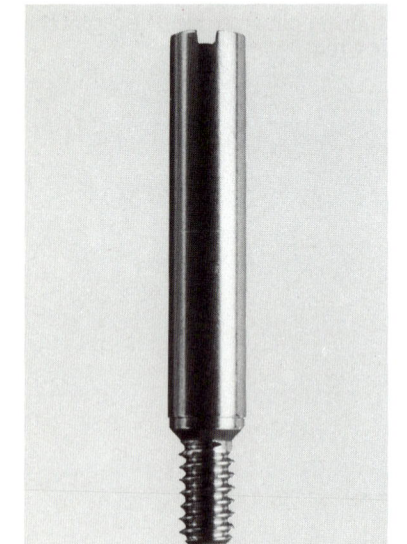

Fig. 7.**100a** The impression coping is fixed on the implant with guide screw. The shoulder and the octagon are engaged with an exact fit

Fig. 7.**100b** and **c** Pictorial representation of the impression coping and a guide screw available in lengths of 10, 12, 14, and 16 mm

Reconstruction on Two-Part ITI Implants

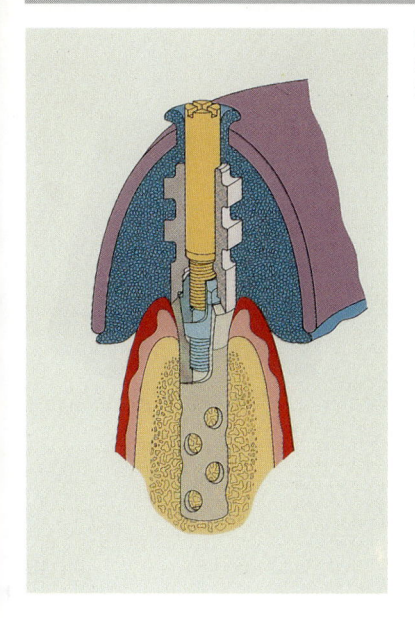

Fig. 7.**101** Making an impression by means of individual tray and a suitable impression material

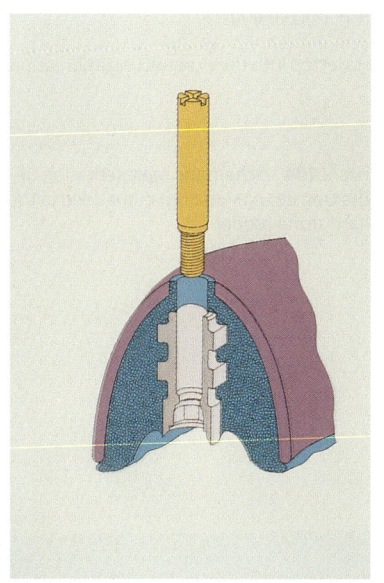

Fig. 7.**102** Guide screw is removed after setting of the impression material. The impression coping remains firmly anchored in the impression material

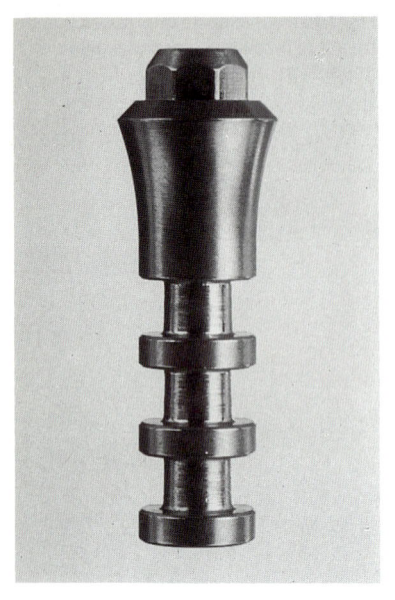

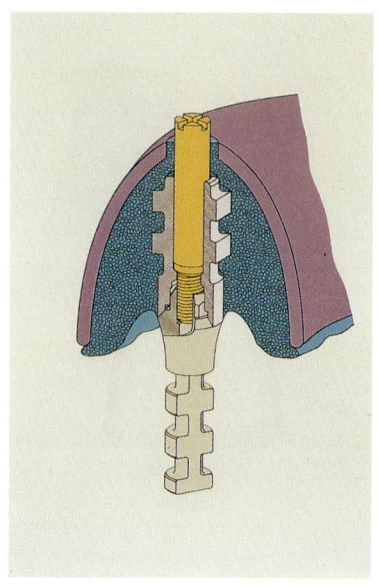

Fig. 7.**103a** Pictorial representation of a transfer pin (analog)

Fig. 7.**103b** Transfer pin (analog) can now be inserted into the exact-fitting impression coping and firmly fixed with the guide screw

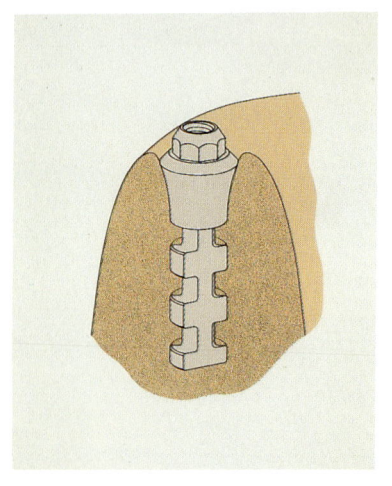

Fig. 7.**104** Schematic representation of the transfer pin (analog) embedded in the hard stone model

Base

The gold copings are fixed on the Octa abutment part by means of 2 mm titanium occlusal screws with a head of 2.5 mm diameter (Fig. 7.**105a–c**).

The 45° implant shoulder serves for centering and as a base for the gold coping (Fig. 7.**105**, 7.**108**). To meet different clinical requirements, two different internal configurations of the gold copings are available:

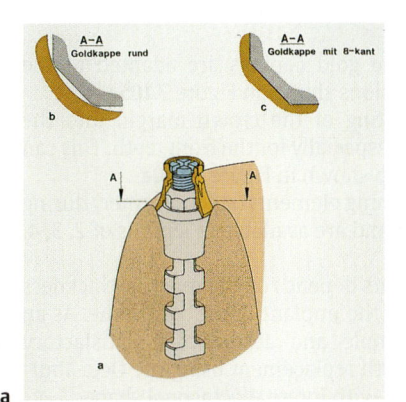

Fig. 7.**105a**
a) Master model with mounted gold coping
b) Inner configuration of the gold coping for use with fixed partial denture (bridge)
c) Gold coping with inner octagon, which fits precisely and rotation-free on the analog and the octagonal abutment. Application: single-tooth replacement

Fig. 7.**105b** and **c** Schematic representation of different gold copings

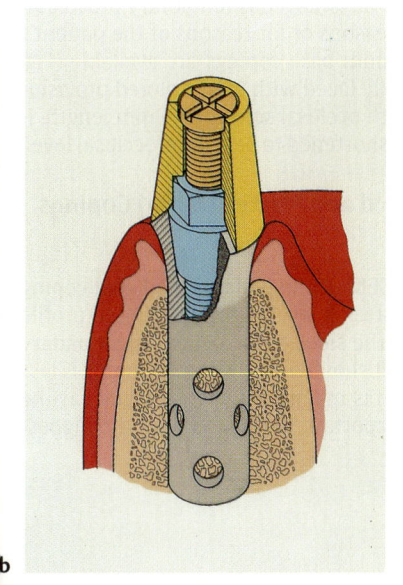

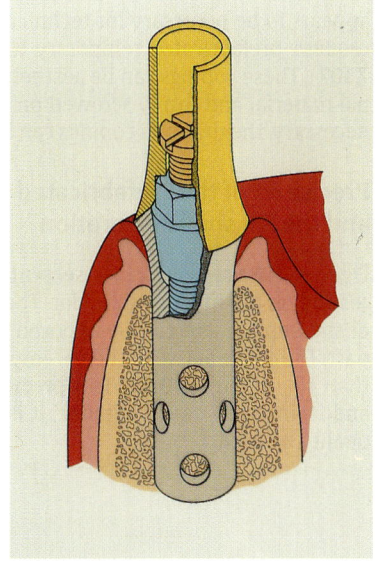

1. copings with inner octagonal profiles that fit exactly on the transfer pin (analog) or on the implant with the Octa abutment. This ensures stability and safeguards against rotation (Fig. 7.**105a** and **b**) for single crowns or other kinds of single units, e.g., under telescopic reconstructions;
2. copings with inner round profiles. The internal configuration of the round gold copings allows compensation of axial divergence due to the 0.02 mm air gap between the abutment or analog and the gold coping. These gold copings are used for the screw-retained fixed partial dentures and for cast bar constructions (Fig. 7.**105a**;Var. b).

The external configurations of the gold copings are adapted to the respective needs, e.g., the standard versions shown in Figure 7.**105a–c**.

For aesthetic reasons, countersinking of the crown margin into the sulcus may be an appropriate solution, especially for the front teeth. This can be carried out simply with a healing cap shown in Figure 7.**106a**.

These caps serve as soft-tissue forming elements (sulcus former) during the phase of healing-in of the implant and are available in lengths of 2, 3, 4, and 5 mm.

The length of the chosen components depends on the mucosal thickness and on the sinkage depth of the top of the implant in the soft tissue. As an example, Figure 7.**106b** shows a simple and aesthetically satisfactory solution of a screw-retained, single-tooth replacement using the Octa abutment and an exactly fitting gold coping with internal octagonal shape.

For cases in which an aesthetically advantageous temporary prosthesis appears to be necessary for technical reasons or for reasons of the patient's request, prefabricated temporary titanium base copings are available (Fig. 7.**107**). These copings can be aesthetically faced with tooth colored provisional material and firmly screwed on with occlusal screws of 4 mm length. If necessary, the titanium copings can be shortened to below the occlusal level.

Precise Fit of the Prefabricated Gold and Plastic (Delrin) Copings and the Finished Restoration

Figure 7.**108a** shows a cross-sectional SEM of the prefabricated gold coping resting on the implant shoulder. The latter is level with the exposed profile of the implant and closely apposed to the sides of the octagonal secondary part. The space between the 45° implant shoulder and the gold coping is less than 10 µm (Fig. 7.**108b**). This precision is maintained after integral casting and facing with dental ceramic. It is important that material of the highest quality be used.

Reconstruction on Two-Part ITI Implants 213

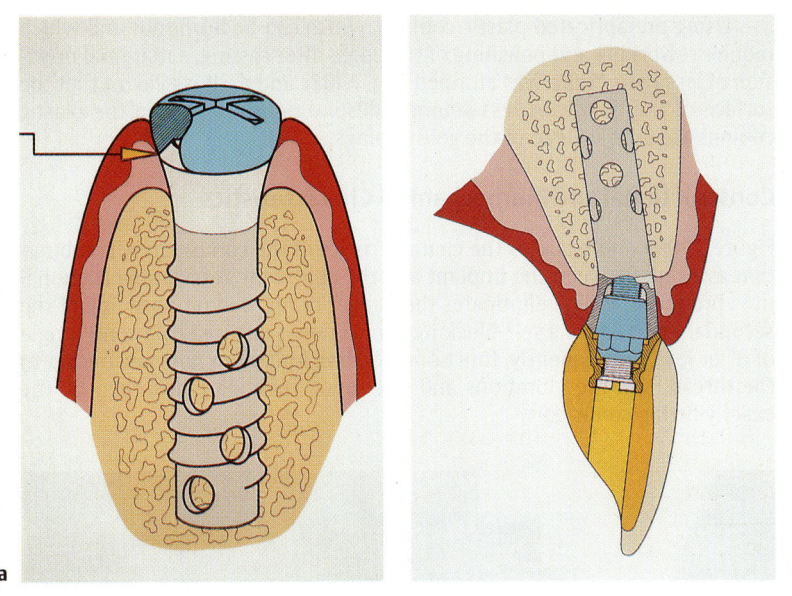

Fig. 7.**106a** Transmucosal healing caps for implants placed deeper in the surrounding tissues. Available in heigths of 2, 3, 4, and 5 mm

Fig. 7.**106b** Single-tooth restoration with the Octa system. The connection between the implant and the crown is sunk in the sulcus for aesthetic reasons

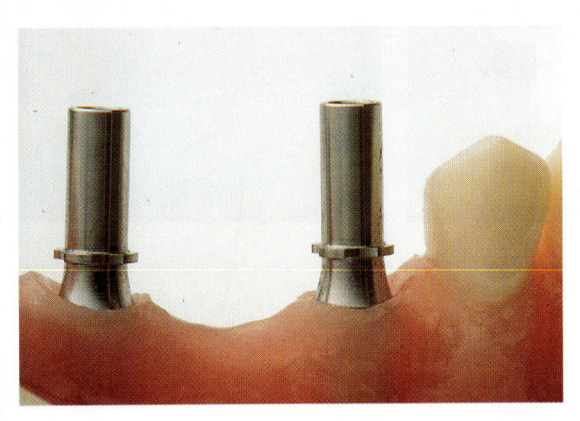

Fig. 7.**107** Temporary titanium copings are given a provisional acrylic or composite facing

Using prefabricated plastic copings, which can be burnt out and which require reworking and polishing of the edges after casting, a marginal precision of less than 15 μm was attained (Fig. 7.**108c** and **d**). It is evident that the surface of the margin is less smooth (despite polishing) when the plastic copings are used instead of the gold copings.

Constructional and Biomechanical Characteristics

Figure 7.**109a** and **b** shows the characteristics of the conus-screw combination as a link between the implant and the abutment. A favorable frictional fit is produced; which eliminates the danger of rotation or loosening of the secondary part, since a self-blocking connection is ensured by a conus angle of 8° or less. Subsequently, functional loading forces are not transmitted to the thread, and the vibrations and micromovements are absorbed by the exactly fitting conus part.

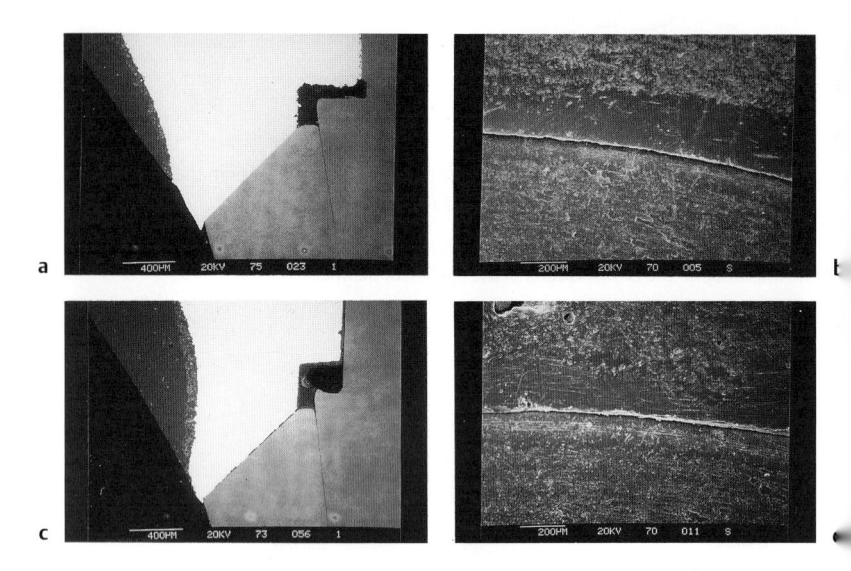

Fig. 7.**108a** Precise fit of a prefabricated gold coping on the implant shoulder and octagon after casting-on and facing with dental ceramic

Fig. 7.**108b** Edge situation of the prefabricated crown base. Marginal gap < 10 μm

Fig. 7.**108c** Machine-finished plastic coping can be burnt out and cast in a metal-ceramic alloy and veneered with dental ceramic

Fig. 7.**108d** Edge situation of the cast crown base. Marginal gap < 15 μm

Reconstruction on Two-Part ITI Implants 215

Non-rotation through mechanical lock

8°

Morse Taper: 8° or less angle will yield a mechanically locking, friction fit.

a

Cone-to-screw Precision

Less than 10μm

No micromovement in threads

Takes no functional load

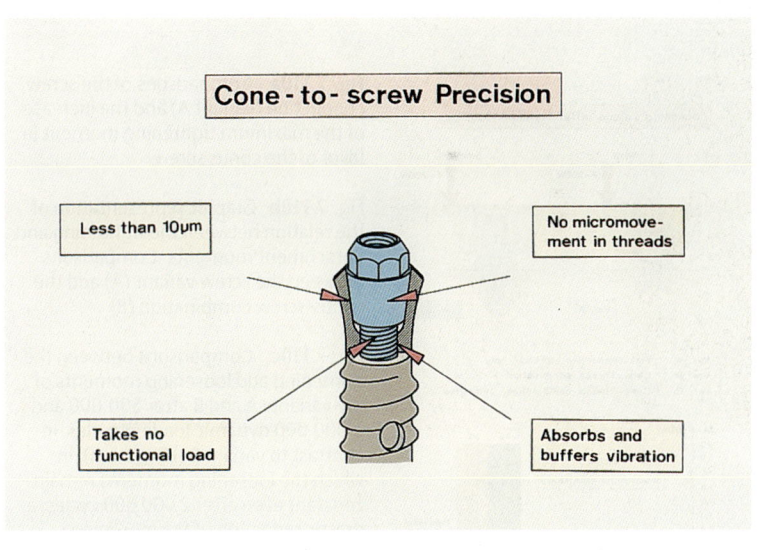

Absorbs and buffers vibration

Fig. 7.**109a** and **b** Graphic representation of the conus-screw combination as a connection between the secondary part abutment and the implant. Advantages of self-locking connection

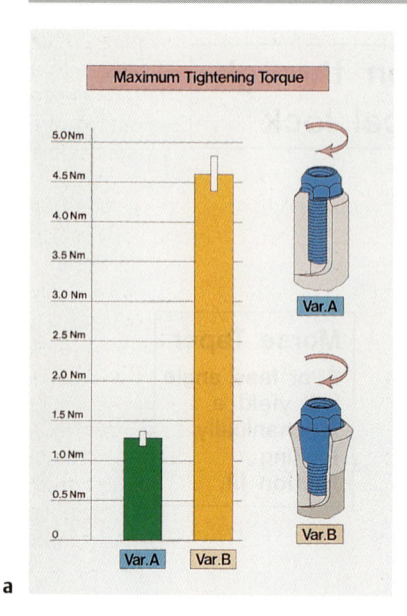

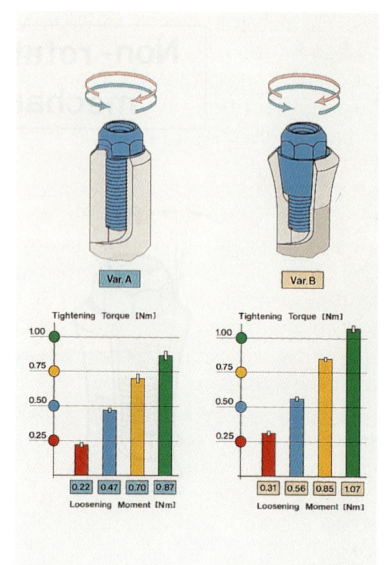

Fig. 7.110a Comparisons of the screw connection (variant A) and the increase of the maximum tightening moment in favor of the conus screw

Fig. 7.110b Graphic representation of the relation between the tightening and detachment moments. Comparisons between the screw variant (A) and the conus-screw combination (B)

Fig. 7.110c Comparisons between the tightening and loosening moments of the variants A and B after 500 000 and 2 000 000 dynamic loading cycles. In contrast to variant B (ITI system), in which the loosening moments remain constant even after 2 000 000 cycles, a drastic reduction of the loosening moment can be discerned in variant A

The different results are represented in graphical form in Figure 7.**110a** and show the advantages of the conus-screw combination compared to a standard screw connection alone (variant A). The chosen variant B proves to be about four times stronger with regard to the maximum torsional strain. Figure 7.**110b** also shows similarly positive results due to this conus-screw connection between the abutment and the implant: The loosening moments of the variant B are 10–20% higher throughout than the corresponding tightening torque, in contrast to variant A, the loosening moments of which are 8–15% lower than the tightening moments.

The results of the same series of experiments under additonal dynamic loading conditions (Fig. 7.**110c**) are interesting. The graphs show that the loosening moment after 2 000 000 cycles of variant A is reduced to almost half of the tightening moment, whereas variant B remains 10–20% higher than the tightening moment.

With regard to the connection between the implant and the prosthetic superstructure, bacterial invasions (and thus inflammation and infections) can occur when the marginal gap is too great. The construction gives rise to a favorable 45° contact surface. Besides self-centering and an advantageous stress absorption, it also brings about a reduction of the marginal gap of about 30% (Fig. 7.**111**).

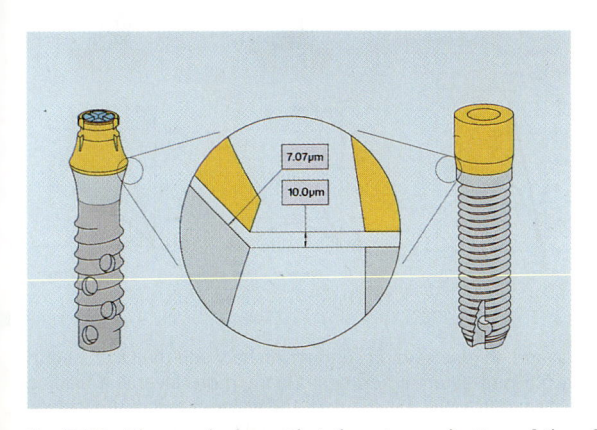

Fig. 7.**111** The graph shows that there is a reduction of the effective gap between coping and implant by about 30% due to the 45° shoulder characteristics

7 The Concept of the ITI Implants

Figure 7.**112a** and **b** show the much higher lateral and oblique stress tolerance values of the Octa system (due to its construction) compared to other commercially available solutions shown in variant A, in which the connection consists of a flat base and a hexagonal top of about 0.6 mm height.

In contrast to variant A, the loading forces are not transmitted directly to the occlusal screw in the Octa concept (variant B), but are first absorbed by the 45° implant shoulder and the vertical portion of the octagon of 1 mm height. The values of initial plastic deformation are also correspondingly higher. In all measurements, these values are increased by at least the factor 2 in the variant B (Octa system) over variant A. More detailed information in the form of publications (ITI technical information and brochures) are also available for the Octa system (Sutter et al. 1992, ITI information).

Outlook

The described Octa concept is designed as a modular system. Accordingly, further necessary components can be integrated into the system. For example, transversely (laterally) screwed-on gold copings, solder bases,

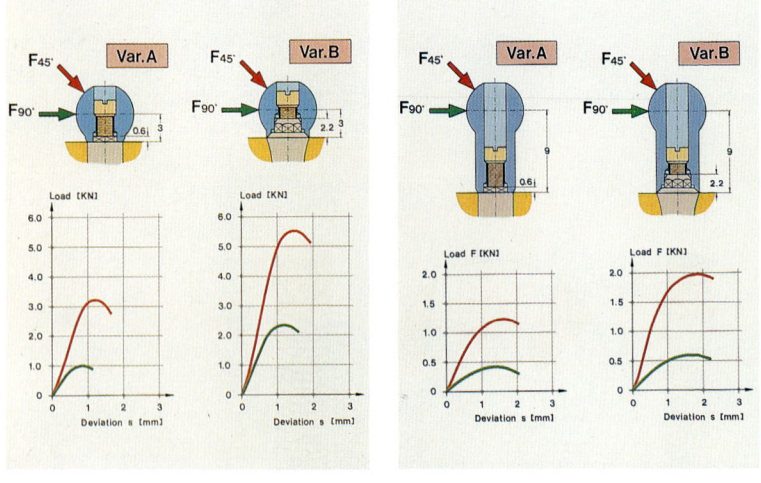

Fig. 7.**112a** and **b** Lateral and oblique loading comparison between the Octa system and the flat base with a 0.6 mm external hexagon. Clearly more favorable loading absorption in the Octa system due to the 45° shoulder, the engagement of the vertical Octagon sides, and the conus-screw combination compared to the 90° shoulder and "only" screw connection

temporary plastic caps, angular secondary parts, plastic parts as burn-out patterns, etc. are envisioned as possible extensions to the system.

This wide, but not overwhelming range of components in the ITI implant system and the different superstructures possible provide the clinician with a great scope of choices in reconstructional designs.

Further developments and improvements are a logical consequence of the approach to future work.

Sterile Packaging

Sterile packaging is the last important element in implant development.

The way in which the implants are presented for insertion into the prepared implant bed may also be a decisive factor in the efficacy of an implant system.

Our sterile packaging, in combination with the instruments required for insertion, ensures an exceedingly simple and functional handling without the need to touch the implants (Fig. 7.**113**).

All necessary designations of the implants are printed as texts on the ouer ampoule. In addition, the implant length information is colorcoded at the top of the ampoule.

A sterilization indicator is also inserted at the lower end of the ampoule to document whether the implants have been sterilized (yellow = nonsterile, red = sterile).

The outer ampoule is opened by screwing off the lid. This connection also guarantees the sterilization seal required. The sterile inner ampoule can be removed from the outer ampoule (Fig. 7.**114**).

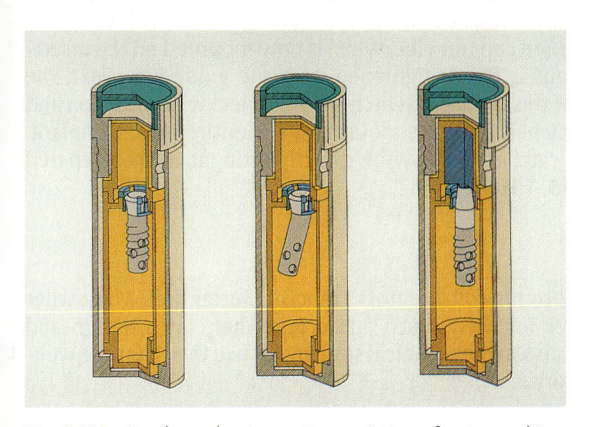

Fig. 7.**113** Sterile packaging unit, consisting of outer and inner ampoule and the two coverings, guarantees the required sterilization seal and delivery system of all ITI implants. The type, dimensions, and all further necessary data are printed in the text

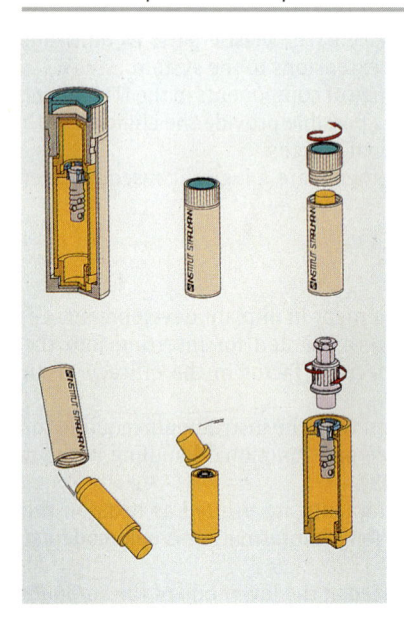

Fig. 7.**114** Exposure of the end of the implant for connection of the inserting device is shown step-by-step. The implant does not have to be touched

This inner ampoule has two different lids. The lid with the long collar can be pressed away to the side allowing the implant mounting to become visible.

The implant can be removed from the mounting with the implant inserting device. The inserting device is screwed in by hand until resistance is felt. The ratchet (turned counter clockwise) is now mounted on the inserting device. The implant is firmly tightened with the guide key. Next, the direction of rotation of the ratchet is switched to the clockwise direction and is simultaneously detached from the mounting. The entire packet implant, inserting device, and ratchet can now be directly brought to the prepared implant bed. (Fig. 7.**115**, 7.**116**).

Acknowledgement

The author is grateful to his collaborators Francis J. Sutter, Ueli Mundwiler and Reto Baumgartner for their much appreciated help with design and graphic presentation, also to the technical staff and Astrid Oesch for the well-done photographic work.

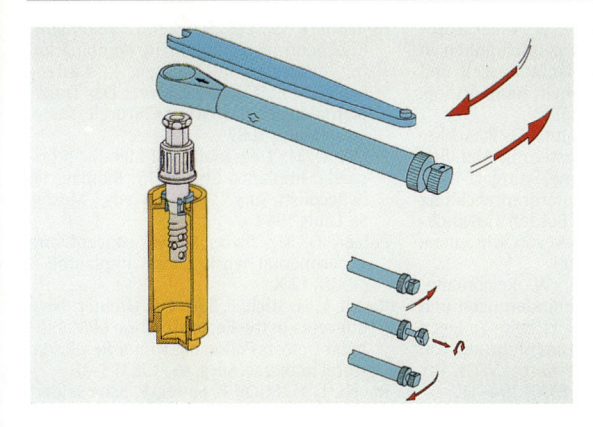

Fig. 7.**115** The ratchet, which is set in a counter-clockwise direction (see direction of the arrow at the end of the ratchet), is mounted on the inserting device already connected with the implant. The implant is now firmly tightened with the guide key

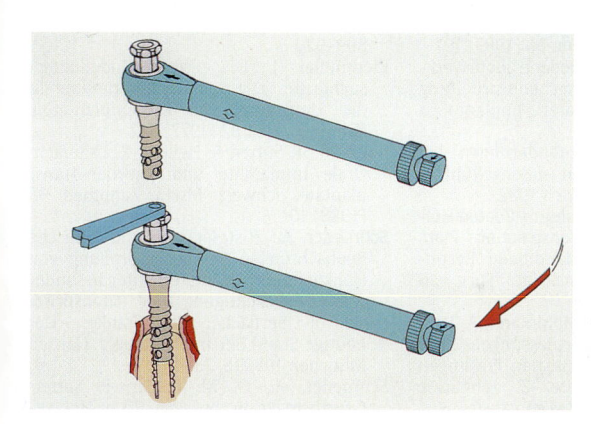

Fig. 7.**116** The ratchet is then positioned in the clockwise direction (see direction of the arrow) by 180° rotation of the bolt at the end of the ratchet. The implant can now be detached from the package mounting and inserted into the prepared implant bed without having been touched

References

Asikainen, P., F. Sutter: The New Distance System for the Submergible use of the ITI-Bonefit Implants. J. oral Implantol. 16 (1990)

Bolz, U., K. Kalweit: Vergleichende Untersuchungen zur Wärmeentwicklung mit innengekühlten und konventionellen Knochenbohrern und -fräsen. Dtsch. zahnärztl. Z. 31 (1976) 959

Brånemark, P.-I., G. A. Zarb, T. Albrektsson: Gewebeintegrierter Zahnersatz – Osseointegration in der klinischen Zahnheilkunde. Quintessenz, Berlin 1985

Breine, U., P.-I. Brånemark: Reconstruction of alveolar jaw bone. An experimental and clinical study of immediate and preformed autologous bone grafts in combination with osseointegrated implants. Scand. J. plast. reconstr. Surg. Hand. Surg. 14 (1981) 23

Claes, L., P. Hutzschenreuter, O. Pohler: Lösemomente von Corticaliszugschrauben in Abhängigkeit von Implantationszeit und Oberflächenbeschaffenheit. Arch. orthop. Unfall-Chir. 85 (1976) 155

Contzen, H., F. Straumann, E. Patschke: Grundlagen der Alloplastik mit Metallen und Kunststoffen. Thieme, Stuttgart 1967

Eichler, J., R. Berg: Temperaturentwicklung auf die Kompakta beim Bohren. Gewindeschneiden und Eindrehen von Schrauben. Z. Orthop. 110 (1972) 909

Eitenmüller, E., E. Eisen, W. Reichmann: Temperaturbedingte Veränderungen und Reaktionen des Knochens beim Anlegen von Bohrlöchern zur Durchführung von Osteosynthesen. Leitz-Mitt. Wiss. u. Techn. Bd. VII, Nr. 4–5 (1978) 104–110

Eriksson, R., T. Albrechtsson: Temperature threshold levels for heat-induced bone tissue injury. A vital-microscopic study in the rabbit. J. Prosth. Dent. 50 (1983) 101

Fuchsberger, A.: Verschiedene Bohrwerkzeuge zu spanender Knochenbearbeitung im Vergleich. Z. zahnärztl. Implantol. 3 (1987) 267–281

Hattich, Th.: Temperaturänderungen bei Knochenbohrungen mit außengekühlten Bohrern. Med. Diss. Zürich 1982

Hellem, S., J. Olofsson: Titanium-Coated Hollow Screw and Reconstruction Plate System (THORP) in Mandibular Reconstruction. J. cranio-max-fac. Surg. 16 (1988)

d'Hoedt, B., Th. Ney, H. Möhlmann, A. Lukkenbach: Temperaturmessungen mit Infrarottechnik bei enossalen Fräsungen für dentale Implantate. Z. zahnärztl. Implantol. 3 (1987) 123–130

Kirsch, A., K.-L. Ackermann: Das IMZ Manual. Die zweiphasige Implantationsmethode mit intramobilen Zylinderimplantaten. Kopf, Stuttgart 1983

Kirschner, H., U. Bolz, G. Michel: Thermometrische Untersuchungen mit innen- und ungekühlten Bohrern an Kieferknochen und Zähnen. Dtsch. zahnärztl. Z. 39 (1984) 30

Lentrodt, J., H. G. Bull: Tierexperimentelle Untersuchungen zur Frage der Knochenregeneration nach Bohrvorgängen im Knochen. Dtsch. zahnärztl. Z. 31 (1976) 115

Mühlemann, H. R.: Mikrostruktur der Implantatoberfläche. Schweiz. Mschr. Zahnheilk. 85 (1975) 97

Müller, M. E., M. Allgöwer, R. Schneider, H. Willenegger: Manual der Osteosynthese. Springer, Berlin 1977

Neukom, F. W., J.-E. Scheller, G. Feldmann: Knochentransplantation in Kombination mit enossalen Implantaten. In Kastenbauer, E., E. Wilmer, K. Meco: Das Transplantat in der Plastischen Chirurgie. Sasse, Rothenburg 1987

Pohler, O. M.: Degradation of Metallic othopaedic Implants. Chapter 15: Biomaterial in Reconstr. Surg. L. R. Rubin (eds.). Mosby, St. Louis 1983

Pohler, O. M.: Swiss screw; concept and experimental work. J. oral Implantol. 3 (1986) 12 X

Raveh, J., H. Stich, F. Sutter, R. Greiner: New Concepts in the Reconstruction of Mandibular Defects Following Tumor Resektion. J. oral max.-fac. Surg. 41 (1983) 3–16

Raveh, J., H. Stich, F. Sutter, P. Schawalder: Neue Rekonstruktionsmöglichkeiten bei Unterkieferdefekten nach Tumorresektion. Schweiz. Mschr. Zahnheilk. 91 (1981) 899–920

Riedmüller, J., U. Soltész: Modelluntersuchungen zur Spannungsverteilung in der Umgebung von Zahnimplantaten. Zahnärzt. Welt 82 (1977) 842

Roux, M., F. Sutter, S. Hellem, K. Läderach: Orale Implantate und Knochen-Transplantate. Schweiz. Mschr. Zahnmed. 98 (1988) 10

Schroeder, A.: Histologische und klinische Beobachtungen bei der Erprobung von Hohlzylinderimplantaten unter besonderer Berücksichtigung der Titanspritzschicht-Oberfläche. In Franke: Der heutige Stand der Implantologie. Hanser, München 1980 (S. 33–40)

Schroeder, A., O. M. Pohler, F. Sutter: Gewebsreaktion auf ein Titan-Hohlzylinderimplantat mit Titan-Spritzschichtoberfläche. Schweiz. Mschr. Zahnheilk. 86 (1976) 713

Schroeder, A., H. Stich, F. Straumann, F. Sutter: Über die Anlagerung von Osteozement an einem belasteten Implantatkörper. Schweiz. Mschr. Zahnheilk. 88 (1978) 1051

Schroeder, A., E. van der Zypen, H. Stich, F. Sutter: The reactions of bone, connective tissue and epithelium to endosteal implants with sprayed titanium sufaces. J. max-fac. Surg. 9 (1981) 15

Seeger, P., P. Tetsch: Tierexperimentelle Untersuchungen zur Regeneration genormter Knochendefekte bei unterschiedlichem Kühlverfahren. Dtsch. zahnärztl. Z. 33 (1978) 870

Soltész, U.: Spannungs- und interferenzoptische Modelluntersuchungen an einem Hohlzylinder-Dentalimplantat. Interner Bericht. IWM Freiburg 1980

Soltész, U., D. Siegele: Einfluß der Steifigkeit des Implantatmaterials auf die im Knochen erzeugten Spannungen. Dtsch. zahnärztl. Z. 39 (1984) 183–186

Steinemann, S.: Korrosion, Verträglichkeit und mechanische Eigenschaften von metallischen Allenthesen. In Schuchardt, K., B. Spiessl: Fortschritte der Kiefer- und Gesichtschirurgie. Bd. XIX. Thieme, Stuttgart 1975

Steinemann, S.: Characteristics of Implants for Internal Fixation. In H. K. Uhtoff: Current Concepts of Internal Fixation of Fractures. Springer, Berlin 93 (1980)

Sutter, F., A. Schroeder, D. Buser: Das neue ITI-Implantat-Konzept. Technische Aspekte und Methodik (I + II). Quintessenz 2 (1988)

Sutter, F., A. Schroeder, F. Straumann: ITI-Hohlzylindersysteme, Prinzipien und Methodik. Swiss Dent. 4 (1983) 21

Sutter, F., J. Raveh, H. Schürch, H. Stich: Titanplasmabeschichtetes Hohlschrauben- und Rekonstruktionsplatten-System (THRP) zur Überbrückung von Kieferdefekten. Chirurg 55 (1984) 741–748

Sutter, F., A. Schroeder, F. Straumann: Technische und konstruktive Aspekte der ITI-Hohlzylinderimplantate. Zahnärztl. Welt 90, 9 (1981) 50

Sutter, F., J. Raveh: Titanium-coated screw and reconstruction plate system for Bridging of lower jaw defects; biomechanical aspects. Int. J. Oral max.-fac. Sug. 17 (1988) 267–274

Tetsch, P., W. Schneider: Innengekühlte Bohrer und Fräser in der zahnärztlichen Chirurgie. Vergleichende klinische Untersuchungen. Dtsch. Z. Mund-, Kiefer- u. Gesichtschir. 1 (1977) 118

Vuillemin, Th., J. Raveh, F. Sutter: Unterkieferrekonstruktion mit dem Titanium-Hohlschrauben-Rekonstruktions Plattensystem (THORP). Schweiz. Mschr. Zahnmed. 100 (1990) 6

Watzek, G.: Vortrag GOI-Kongreß. Dresden 1990

Weingart, D., W. Schilli, J. R. Strub: Möglichkeiten der Kombinationstherapie von Knochentransplantaten und enossalen Implantaten. Vortrag 13. Wissenschaftliche Tagung der Arbeitsgemeinschaft Implantologie innerhalb der DGZMK und der Schweizerischen Gesellschaft für orale Implantologie, Zürich 1990b

Weingart, D., W. Schilli, J. R. Strub: Einfluß der Implantologie auf die präprothetische Chirurgie. Schweiz. Mschr. Zahnmed. 9 (1992b) 1074

Weingart, D., J. R. Strub, W. Schilli: Kieferchirurgisch-prothetisches Konzept zur implantologischen Versorgung bei unterschiedlichem Atrophiegrad des zahnlosen Patienten. Z. Stomatol. 3 (1990a) 137

Clinic

8 Questions Related to the Indications for ITI Implants

A. Schroeder

Contraindications

The ITI system, with its various shapes, can be utilized in a wide range of situations in endosseous dental implantology. This might lead the inexperienced to look at implants as the solution to all prosthodontic problems. Experience has shown that this very attitude leads to a high rate of failures that are not attributable to the system itself.

Therefore, it is appropriate to first give a short summary of the frequently described factors that restrict the application on *any* type of implant procedure.

According to Maeglin (1983), the following should be considered to be important *general medical contraindications:*

1. **temporary:** (e.g., transitory infections)
2. **absolute:**
   - systemic diseases of the bone, endocrine system, and hemopoetic system;
   - rheumatic diseases;
   - cardiac disease;
   - nephritises and nephroses;
   - cirrhosis of the liver;
   - allergic diseases;
   - defective immune defense;
   - suspicion of focal infection.

Feigel (1985), on the other hand, maintained that while these types of negative factors must certainly be considered, the affected patients should be considered eligible to receive implants, provided that they are kept under systematic control and supervision.

No matter which position one favors, under no circumstances may general medical findings be dissregarded in evaluating and selecting implant patients.

Unless one has been well acquainted with the patient for years, general statements, such as "I am completely healthy otherwise," should not be accepted as adequate medical history. Instead, specific medical information must be gathered, especially if the patient is elderly. This should relate not only to the physical, but also to the psychological condition of the patient.

Patients who are difficult to manage (or who are actually psychopathic) should be rejected as implant candidates, or only accepted with the greatest of reservations.

Age Limitations

Based on our experiences up until now, no clear upper-age limit can be imposed. It must be decided on a case-by-case basis whether the patient has sufficient general vigor, manual dexterity (to perform adequate oral hygiene), and the necessary mental capacity to receive implants. Equally indefinite is the lower-age limit. In principle, it is possible to place an implant (such as as a replacement for a single tooth that is congenitally absent or lost as the result of trauma) as soon as jaw growth is completed, provided the other criteria are met. This would occur after the sixteenth year, when growth has ceased in the areas where implants would be considered.

The foremost *local contraindications are:*
1. inadequate available bone. For the implant to undergo the desired integration, it must be embedded within a mass of bone that has enough bulk in all three dimensions to provide sufficient potential for regeneration and remodeling following the operation (p. 263);
2. unfavorable morphological conditions, e.g., location of the mandibular canal near the superior surface of the mandible due to extreme bone atrophy, or a maxillary sinus that is overextended;
3. difficult, complex occlusal, and articular relationships into which the implants could not be well integrated. This would call for a rehabilitation plan to change the entire situation;
4. jaw defects;
5. macroglossia;
6. limited mouth opening;
7. lack of patient motivation to perform optimum oral hygiene.

Indications

When considering the above list of contraindications, it would seem reasonable to adopt the policy of instituting no "offensive" implantation procedures immediately, but instead to think first of *conventional prosthetic* solutions. It is only after the latter have proven to have definite disadvantages for the patient from the standpoint of function, aesthetics, jeopardizing the remaining dentition, imposing a psychological (or in some cases an enonomic burden) that one should turn to implants. If this basic approach is taken and the patient is also made aware of it, any future failure that might occur will be perceived as less traumatic than in those cases where the operator has persuaded the patient to accept implantation without complete information.

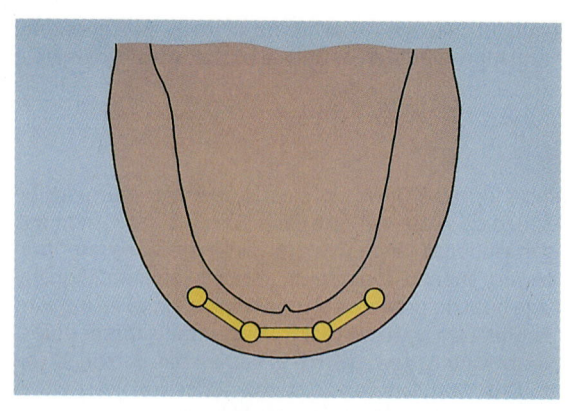

8 Questions Related to the Indications for ITI Implants

Fig. 8.1 Retention elements in an edentulous mandible: HC (hollow cylinder), HS (hollow screw), and S (screw) (one- or two-piece)

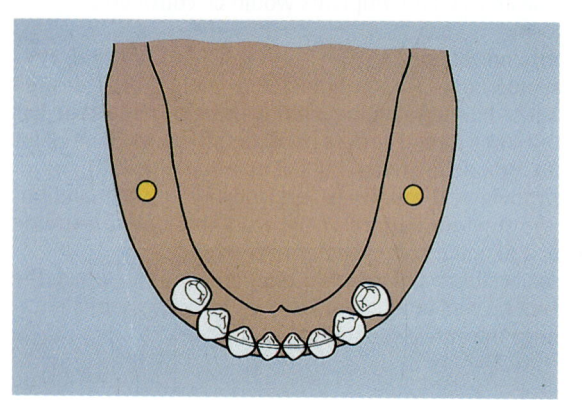

Fig. 8.2 Shortened mandibular dental arch: HC, HS, and S (sometimes one-piece, but primarily two-piece). Restoration may be solely implant-borne

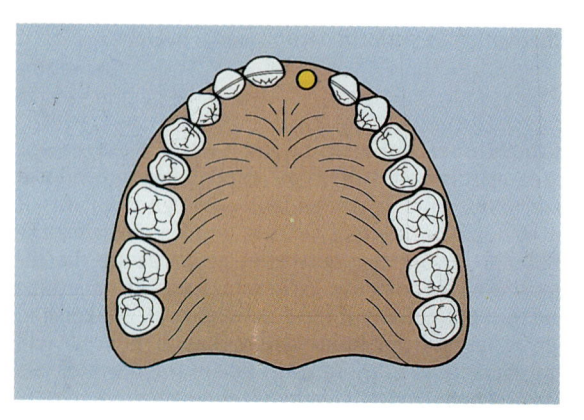

Fig. 8.3 Single-tooth replacement in maxilla or mandible: HC (two-piece)

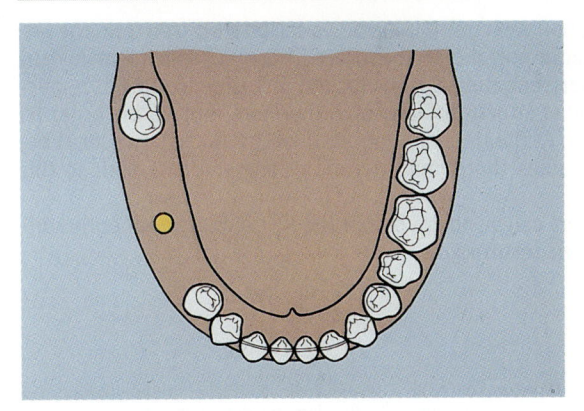

Fig. 8.4 Supporting pier-abutment implant in either jaw: HC, HS and S

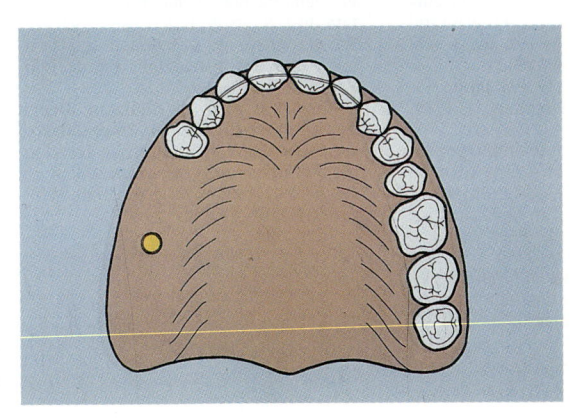

Fig. 8.5 Various indications in the maxilla: HC and HS (two-piece)

The series presented in Figures 8.1 to 8.5 was drawn up by selecting the *frequency* of the various indications as criteria.

These indications and their combinations must rule with the ITI system. The specific type of implant must be selected for each individual case according to the anatomical conditions, the availability of bone, and the prosthetic situation. The following can serve as a guide:

Indication	Type
Lower anterior	HC, HS (one- or two-piece)
Shortened mandibular arch	HC, HS
Single-tooth implant	HC (two-piece)
Pier-abutment implant	HC, HS, S
Various indications in the maxilla	

Implants of the hollow screw (HS) Type, as can be surmised from the list, could acquire greater importance in the future. This type, which was designed in 1974 and underwent clinical trials for the first time in 1981, is applicable to a wide range of situations and could therefore replace the other ITI types to some extent. At the time of publication of this book, however, there are no long-term studies that would permit a concrete statement to this effect.

In any event, there can be no doubt that the HS types are eminently suitable for implant-borne restorations.

References

Albrektsson, T., G. Zarb, P. Worthington, A. R. Eriksson: The longterm efficacy of currently used dental implants: A review and proposed criteria of success. Int. J. oral maxillofac. Implants 1 (1986) 11

Allen, W. L.: Psychological evaluation for implant patients. J. oral Implant. 11 (1983) 157

Feigel, A.: Die orale Implantologie im "deutschsprachigen Raum". Eine kritische Betrachtung. Swiss. Dent. 6, (1985) H. 5

Jacobs, K.: Implantationen in der zahnärztlichen Praxis. Ergebnisse einer Umfrage. Zahnärztl. Welt 95 (1986) 1158

Knöfler, W., B. Wetzstein, H. Hampel, W. Bethmann: Zur Indikation stomatologischer Implantate. Stomatol. d. DDR 34 (1984) 152

Maeglin, B.: Kritische Stellungnahme zur Problematik der zahnärztlichen Implantate. In J. R. Strub, B. E. Gysi, P. Schärer: Schwerpunkte in der oralen Implantologie und Rekonstruktion. Quintessenz, Berlin 1983

Schnitmann, P. A., L. B. Shulman: Dental implants: benefit and risk. Proceedings of an NIH-H Harvard Consensus Development Conference. US Department of Health and Human Services, 1980. Publication No. 81–1531

9 Preoperative Diagnosis and Treatment Planning

U. Belser, R. Mericske-Stern, D. Buser, J. P. Bernard,
D. Hess, and J. P. Martinet

Until a few years ago, the desire for implants was expressed primarily by patients with complete lower dentures whose masticatory function was severely compromised as the result of advanced alveolar ridge atrophy. Five or six endosseous implants placed between the mental foramina and splinted together by means of a fixed-detachable superstructure with bilateral distal extensions has proved, through a decade of experience, to be an excellent treatment modality for these cases (Adell and co-workers 1991). Subsequently, less invasive alternatives that are less stressful for the patient and therefore better suited to the special needs of the aged, have moved to the forefront. These are actually simple overdentures attached to two implant-borne ball attachments or to a bar attachment supported by two implants (Mericske-Stern 1992).

Based on the aforementioned excellent long-term results with implants in the anterior region of the edentulous mandible, the range of indications has recently rapidly expanded (Van Steenberghe 1990). This has led to greater involvement with partially edentulous patients. Implant-borne fixed partial dentures are now an integral part of the restorative treatment inventory and must always be considered during treatment planning as a possible alternative to conventional prosthetic procedures. As a general rule, an implant-borne prosthesis should be preferred if it is estimated that it will be less invasive, less cumbersome, and have a more favorable prognosis. In the case of a distally shortened dental arch, for example, an implant makes it possible to avoid a removable partial denture or a biomechanically unfavorable cantilever bridge. Other indications that justify at least a serious investigation into the possibilities of implants are: prospective bridge abutments that are intact or that are inadequate because of insufficient clinical crown length, tipping, root resorption, etc.; excessively long pontic spans; and single-tooth spaces that require diastemas between the replacement and the adjacent teeth.

Initial Consultation and Ascertainment of the Patient's Desires

An initial informational consultation concerning the benefits and risks of implant placement is essential prior to the medical examination (identification of possible systemic contraindications) and before an analysis of the

local conditions at prospective implant sites is undertaken. In every case, it is appropriate to record the principle desires and expectations that the patient has formulated, such as the wish to:
1. increase the stability of an existing denture;
2. avoid a removable prosthesis, or to replace an existing partial denture with a fixed bridge;
3. receive a fixed replacement for one or more missing teeth without compromising intact neighboring teeth or a previously cemented extensive restoration.

Principles of Treatment Planning

Patient Evaluation

The following points are relevant when examining a patient as a prospective recipient of endosseous implants:
- clarification of the benefits and risks of implants;
- medical, dental, and social history;
- medical examination;
- oral and dental examination;
- general aspects;
- evaluation of possible implant sites.

Selection Criteria

An analysis of the parameters listed below serves to rule out local and systemic contraindications:
- "normal" wound healing capacity;
- effective oral hygiene;
- adequate supply of sound bone in the jaws, or the potential for augmentation techniques.

The following elements fall under the category of identification of the local conditions:
- anatomy of the bony ridge (see "bone mapping");
- quality and thickness of the mucosa;
- radiographic findings;
- intermaxillary relations;
- diagnostic casts and occlusal registrations.

Systemic Contraindications

- Reduced immune defense and leukocyte dysfunctions
- Diseases treated with periodic use of steroids
- Disturbances of blood coagulation, including anticoagulation therapy

- Neoplasias that require chemotherapy
- Uncontrollable endocrine diseases
- Psychotic diseases
- Drug abuse

Local Contraindications

- Inadequate oral hygiene
- Retained roots
- Local inflammatory processes
- Diseases of the mucosa
- Prior radiation therapy
- Inadequate width and height of bone
- Inadequate bone quality (compare "Type IV")

Many of the contraindications listed above are now viewed more as conditional than as absolute contraindications (Smith and co-workers 1992).

In the following pages, the factors listed above will be evaluated within the framework of an overall treatment plan. After the goal of prosthetic treatment has been defined, the type, number, and distribution of implants are determined, taking into consideration the biomechanical principles specific to dental implants.

Treatment Planning for Implant-Borne Overdentures in Edentulous Jaws

The presurgical evaluation of an overdenture patient has the following goals:
1. to avoid interference between the prospective positions of the implants, the attachments, and the denture base;
2. to optimize placement of the implants in relation to bone mass and anatomical structures;
3. to distribute the implants so that the attachment devices are reasonably arranged.

Planning Steps

According to the conditions in each case, it is important to perform one or more of the planning steps described below:
- Clinical intraoral inspection
- Radiographic examination
- Bone mapping (bone profile)
- Evaluation of the old dentures
- Planning the provisional prosthesis for the healing phase
- Diagnostic set-up in wax

A thorough clinical inspection of the oral cavity to evaluate the soft tissues and bony structures is the first step (Fig. 9.**1**). In the mandible, the form of the alveolar ridge and the basal bone can be determined fairly well by palpation because the mucosa is mostly thin. However, problems can be encountered in the anterior area, where fiber bundles of the orbicularis oris muscle can lead to the false impression that the vestibular bony contours are favorable, and the floor of the mouth cannot always be displaced sufficiently.

In the palatal region, it is not possible to determine bone thickness by digital palpation because the mucosa here is very thick. Labially, there are concavities in the apical region of the basal bone that can be seen or palpated. In the maxilla, better information can be gained through bone mapping than by palpation.

Various radiographic techniques are available. As a rule, computer tomograms are not necessary for the planning of implant-retained removable prostheses. An overdenture attachment allows a certain latitude for decisions to be made during the surgery relative to the location and number of implants.

An orthopantomogram (OPG), in combination with metal position markers of known diameter, allows for calculation of the actual bone height (Fig. 9.**2**). At the same time, the position of the mental foramen can be determined. Finally, the quality of the bone and pathological structures can be interpreted to some extent with the OPG (Fig. 9.**3**). With the information from the OPG markers, a template can be made to be used during surgery to transfer the desired implant locations to the jaw.

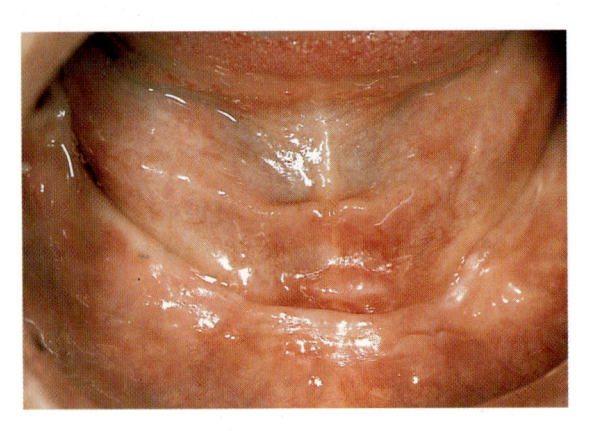

Fig. 9.**1** Atrophic edentulous mandible

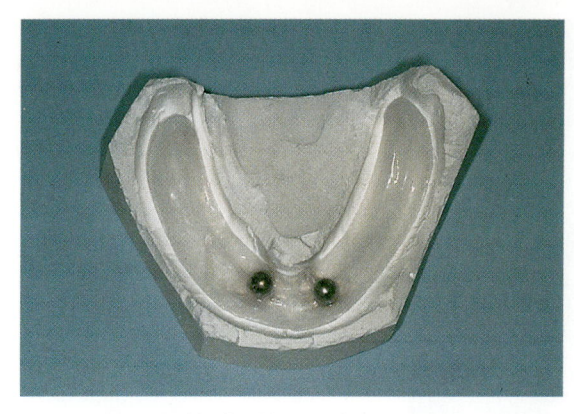

Fig. 9.**2** Two metal balls of known diameters to be used as markers for radiographic measurement attached to a plastic shell on the diagnostic cast

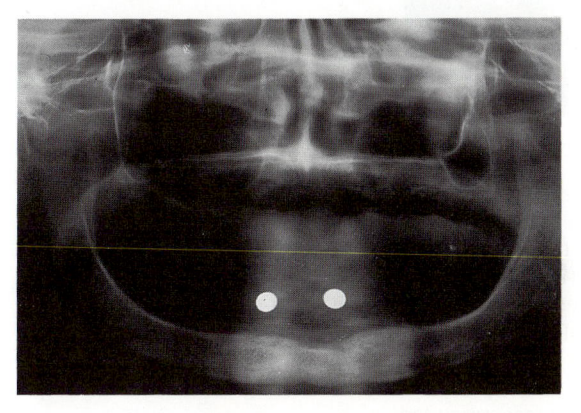

Fig. 9.**3** Orthopantomograph with images of the corresponding measurement markers

A cephalometric radiograph permits distortion-free measurements and is useful for obtaining more information on the shape of the bone in the lingual area of the mandible. It also allows the available bone to be accurately evaluated in the maxilla, where it often reveals the presence of only a thin shell (Fig. 9.**4**).

Measurements from cephalometric radiographs of patients with implants in the maxilla have shown that as a rule, the axes of the implants are inclined toward the vestibule, corresponding to the original position of the alveolar process. Cephalometric radiographs of dentate individuals clearly show the ventral inclination of the axes of the natural teeth. In the

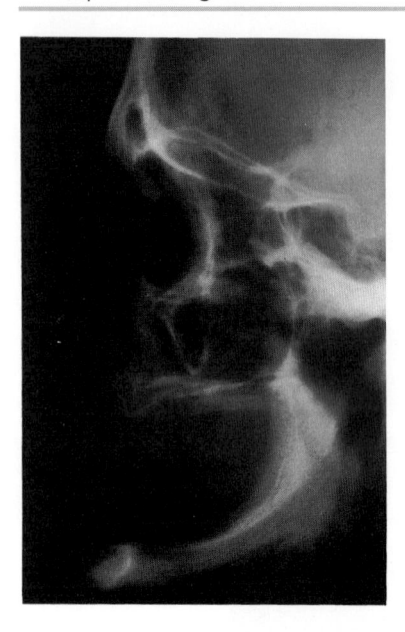

Fig. 9.4 Lateral cephalometric radiograph of the patient in Fig. 9.3

mandible (depending on cephalometric and morphologic characteristics of the alveolar ridge) a lingual inclination of the implants risks restricting the tongue space when the bar is connected and the denture inserted.

Bone mapping (bone profile, Figs. 9.**5**–9.**8**) is useful in planning an overdenture in the upper jaw, but it is a step that can be dispensed with in the mandible. It is usually impossible to examine the critical lingual surface of the ridge accurately enough because of the floor of the mouth. Palpation of undercuts, with the aid of a periodontal probe during the surgery, is a simple procedure that can be recommended.

Inspection of the old denture can provide information about the original position of the natural teeth, especially if it was the patient's first complete denture or a modification of a partial denture. A desirable implant site is at or slightly mesial to the canine region, especially when only two implants are to be placed. When multiple implants are placed, an effort is made to space them equally in the ridge segment lying between the mental foramina, where the mandibular nerves exit the bone.

A preoperative intraoral inspection of the old denture is important because it reveals whether or not fabrication of the new prosthesis will require any changes in, for example, the vertical dimension, the position of the posterior teeth, the amount of lip support, and the esthetics of the anterior teeth.

Treatment Planning for Edentulous Jaws **237**

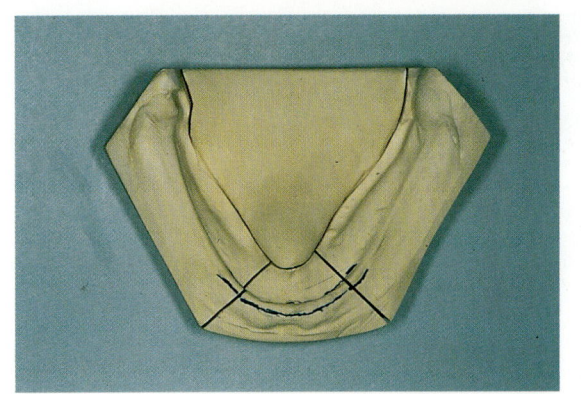

Fig. 9.**5** Split cast of an edentulous mandible

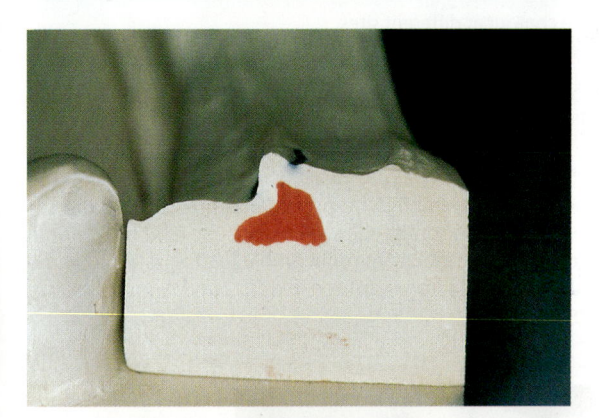

Fig. 9.**6** Bone mapping (transverse section of bony ridge drawn on cast)

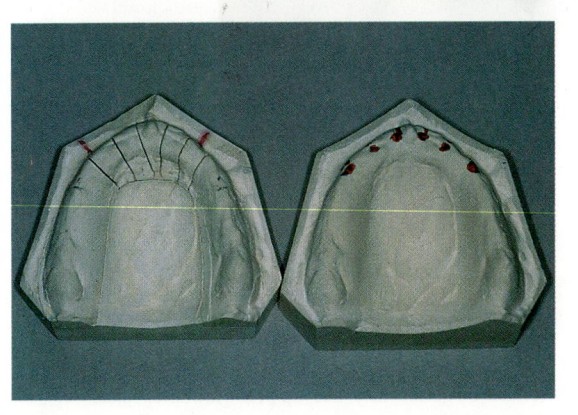

Fig. 9.**7** Split cast of an edentulous maxilla

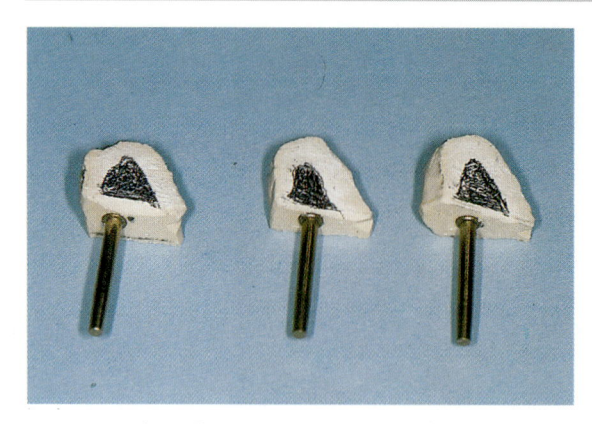

Fig. 9.8 Outline of bone contour at different sites

Finally, it must be decided whether or not the old denture will be suitable as a provisional denture during the healing phase (Fig. 9.9).

The provisional denture is very important during the healing phase. While the transmucosal healing is taking place, the implantation, i.e., the osseointegration process, is vulnerable. The provisional prosthesis can present a problem, especially in the totaly edentulous patient. The provisional prosthesis must protect the implants from unfavorable loading, should allow speech and mastication, if only to a limited extent, and should satisfy minimal cosmetic demands.

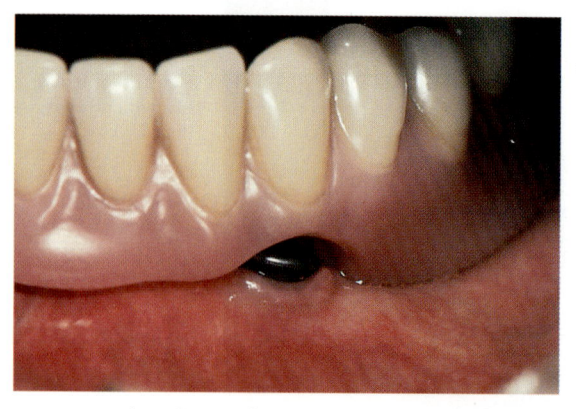

Fig. 9.9 Healing phase: either an existing or a newly fabricated denture may be used as a provisional restoration. it must be generously relieved over the implant sites

The provisional prosthesis must be precisely supported on the portions of the alveolar ridge that do not carry implants and receive additional stabilization from the occlusion. If this cannot be assured through the fit of the existing denture, it is appropriate to fabricate a new one before implant placement. This complete denture can later be transformed into an implant-anchored overdenture.

There are various other factors in favor of making a new denture prior to implant insertion:

1. a better provisional can be provided;
2. patients who seek implants are usually wearing poorly fitting dentures;
3. patients often do not realize the necessity of a new denture, thinking that inadequate function is caused solely by lack of anchorage;
4. problem patients (those who fail to comprehend our explanations, "know-it-alls," hypercritical, and mistrustful patients) can (with the preliminary prosthetic treatment) become better prepared for the eventual implant procedure; the operator becomes acquainted with the patient and this makes the evaluation of indications and contraindications for implants easier.

The provisional denture set-up in wax (Fig. 9.**10**, Fig. 9.**11**) on the articulator is usually not necessary in the planning of overdentures, but it can be of help in difficult cases, such as following jaw resection, cases with extreme interalveolar relationships, e.g. vertical dimension, problems with available space, mismatches in the courses of the two alveolar ridges, when the patient has special wishes concerning tooth position, and when a decision must be made between a fixed restoration or an overdenture.

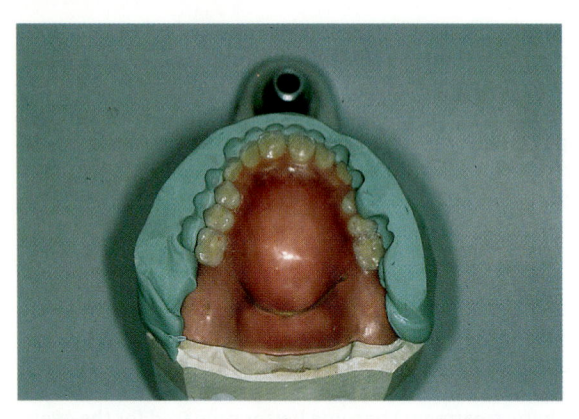

Fig. 9.**10** Set-up of an upper denture in wax with silicone index

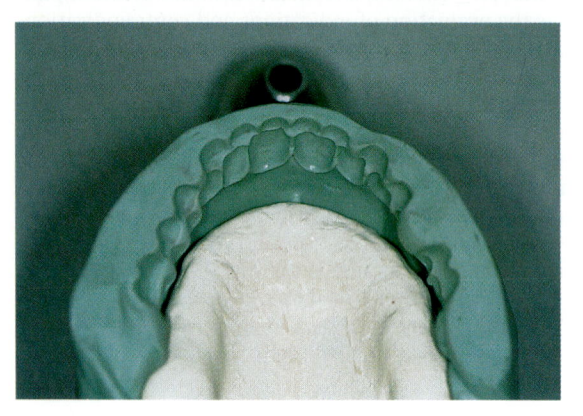

Fig. 9.**11** Maxillary cast with silicone index repositioned. The spatial relations of the prospective implant sites to the alveolar ridge and to the desired position of the anterior teeth can be clearly seen

Number of Implants

Today, two to four implants are usually used to anchor an overdenture. There is an increasing tendency to place only two implants, especially in the mandible. Many reasons for this can be cited:
- economic considerations, i.e., reduction of the total expenditure for planning and treatment;
- consideration of the general condition of the patient;

- simplification of the surgical procedure to the necessary minimum;
- clinical experience indicating that two implants provide enough retention.

So far, there have been few long-term studies of overdentures with any of the implant systems used, and the retrospective investigations that have been done include only small numbers of patients. Our own work with a group of patients with an average age higher than that in any other studies found a high success rate ($\geq 90\%$) for overdentures supported by only two implants after more than 5 years.

The number of implants and their arrangement is decided by local factors and technical considerations.

Evaluation Criteria

Local findings include the size of the jaws (extent of the interforaminal region in the mandible, extent of the sinus in the maxilla), the inclination and curvature of the alveolar ridges, the degree of resorption in the vertical and buccolingual dimensions, and the resorption pattern.

Technical aspects include the choice of retention elements (separate individual attachments or bar connector), the retention mechanism (mobile or rigid anchorage), and the bar connection (need for bar to run straight between implants for mobile denture anchorage versus rigid anchorage where this requirement is not as critical).

Requirements

1. The distance between bar-connected implants must be no less than 8 to 10 mm, so that the lengths of the bar segments between implants are sufficient for proper placement of the retention clips
2. The arrangement of the implants should be as symmetrical as possible
3. The points of emergence of all implants should lie at the same height
4. In the mandible, two implants may be sufficient
5. In the maxilla, more than two implants are recommended

In the mandible, optimum results can be realized with only two or three implants regardless of which type of attachment is used. Investigations to date with various implant systems show that in the maxilla, there is a significantly higher rate of failure and frequently, more rapid bone resorption than in the mandible. Therefere, four implants are recommended combined with a bar construction in the upper jaw because of the pronounced anterior curvature. Ball attachments should not be used here because the axes of the implants are often divergent (Fig. 9.**12a–c**).

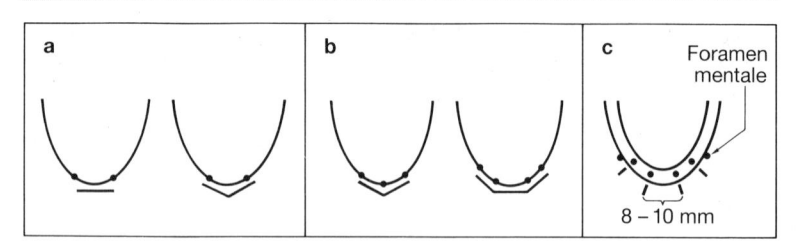

Fig. 9.**12**
a Course of bar between two implants in an edentulous mandible: straight and V-shaped configurations
b Course of bar with three or four implants in either maxilla or mandible
c The distance between the individual implants should permit bar segment lengths of at least 8 mm

Implant-Specific Planning Principles for the Partially Edentulous Jaw

Premolar Units

The 5-mm cervical diameter of two-part ITI implants in the shoulder region corresponds to the approximate mesiodistal dimension of natural premolars (Fig. 9.**13**). In correctly contoured prosthetic superstructures, the diameter at the height of contour is approximately 7 mm (Fig. 9.**14a** and **b**). To accommodate this, the involved edentulous segment should optimally be 8 mm wide mesiodistally at the level of the shoulder of the inserted implant for an implant-borne single tooth replacement. If it is less wide, there will not be enough space for correctly formed papillae, or for interdental spaces that are easily accessible for cleaning. In the opposite situation, i.e., excessive space, the consequence will be unfavorable contours accompanied by food impaction.

Based upon the concept of designing premolar units for posterior restorations (Buser et al. 1988, Brägger et al. 1990), the following distances should be observed (Fig. 9.**15a–c**):
1. from center of the implant to the cervical region of an adjacent natural tooth: *5 mm*;
2. between the centers of two adjacent implants: *7 mm*;
3. between two implants connected by a pontic (measured from the center of each implant): *14 mm*;
4. from the center of an implant to the cervical region of a natural tooth, where the plan is to place a pontic as either a connector between implant and tooth, or as a cantilevered pontic: *11 mm*.

Implant-Specific Planning Principles **243**

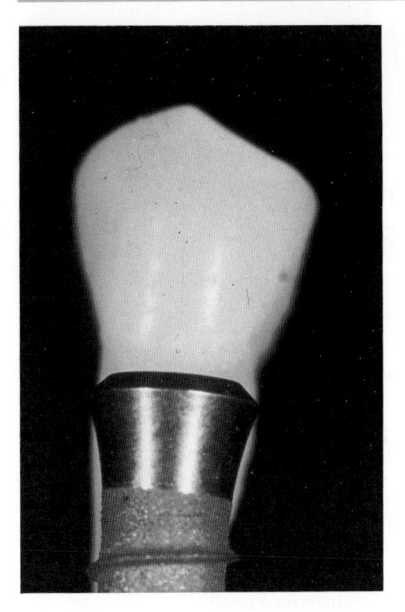

Fig. 9.**13** Comparison of the mesiodistal dimension of a natural upper premolar with the diameter of an ITI implant in the shoulder region

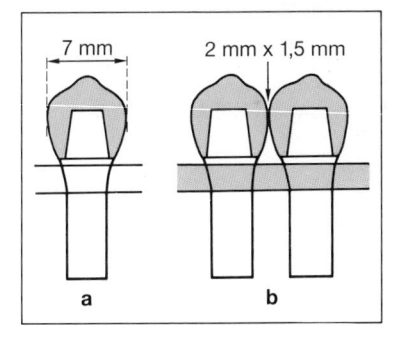

Fig. 9.**14**
a Correctly sized for an ITI implant
b Optimum distance of adjacent implants for maintaining an easily cleanable interproximal space

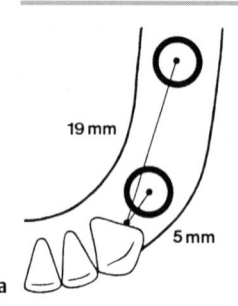

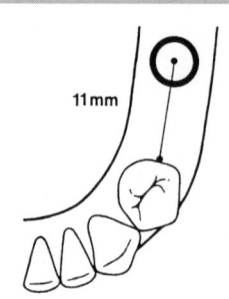

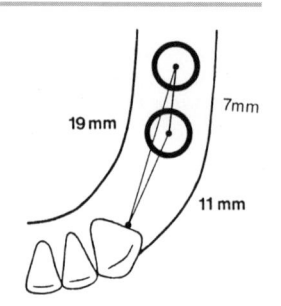

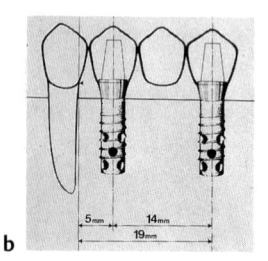

Fig. 9.15
a Distances are measured at the bone level from the distal surface of the most distal tooth to the implant sites, which are then marked with a small bur. In the case of a purely implant-borne prosthesis, distances of 5 and 19 mm are selected. For the variation with support from both tooth and implant, the mark is made with its center at 11 mm. The mesial cantilever requires punches centered at 11 and 19 mm (Brägger and co-workers 1990)
b The allowed distances for a totally implant-borne three-unit fixed partial denture are shown (Buser and co-workers 1988)
c The allowed distance for a combined tooth- and implant-borne three-unit fixed partial denture is 11 mm (Buser and co-workers 1988)

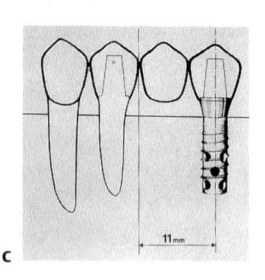

Biomechanical Guidelines

From the preceding paragraphs, it can be concluded that during the planning phase, edentulous jaw segments must be partitioned into premolar units. In determining the location and number of implants to be inserted, the solution that has the surest biomechanical foundation should be selected from the following list (Fig. 9.**16a–d**):
1. Immediately adjacent single-tooth implants, either unsplinted or splinted, depending upon implant length and bone quality
2. Fixed partial dentures with terminal implant abutments at both ends

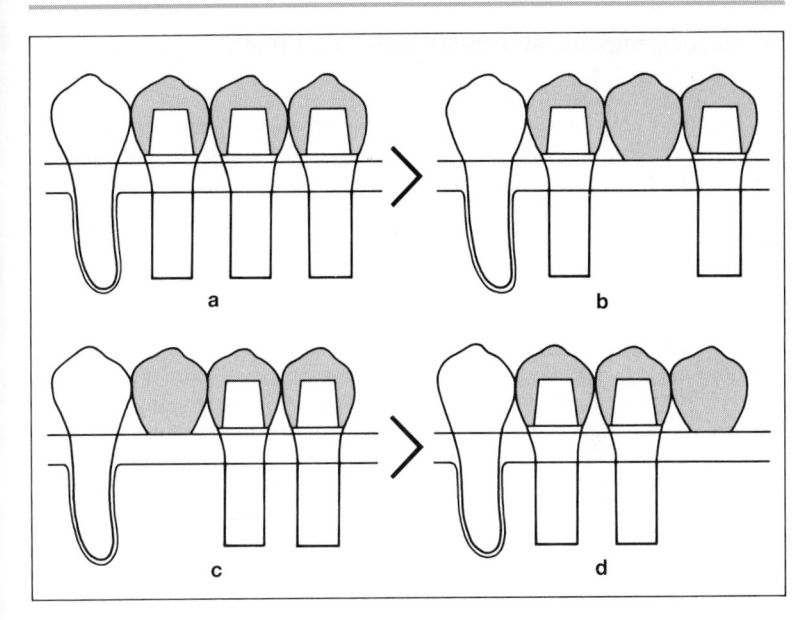

Fig. 9.**16**
a Directly adjacent single-tooth implants: Depending on implant length and bone quality, the superstructures may be either left unconnected or splinted together
b Three-unit fixed partial denture with an implant abutment at each end
c Adjacent implants splinted together by the superstructure with a *mesial* cantilever pontic
d Adjacent implants splinted together by the superstructure with a *distal* cantilever pontic

3. Splinted implants, either immediately adjacent to one another or connected by a pontic, supporting a *mesial* cantilever pontic, the latter to be limited to one pemolar unit
4. The same as 3, except with a *distal* cantilever pontic. Based upon the unfavorable leverage and negative experiences reported in the literature for similarly configured conventional prostheses (Strub et al., 1989), this variation should be avoided whenever possible

Connecting Implant Abutments to Natural Teeth

From purely theoretical considerations, the splinting of osseointegrated ("functionally ankylosed") implants to natural teeth that are suspended by a periodontal membrane with a certain degree of mobility is not rational. Because the two types of attachment are basically different (Picton 1969, Brånemark and co-workers 1969, Schroeder and co-workers 1976) it is possible that while functioning, the involved implant abutment is the primary recipient of the load, comparable to a cantilever bridge abutment (Weinberg 1993). Whether or not this has any effect on the prognosis is still unclear at the present time (Ericsson and co-workers 1986, Astrand and co-workers 1991, Gunne and co-workers 1991, Gunne and co-workers 1992). The benefit of incorporating viscoelastic elements or "stressbreakers" cannot yet be conclusively judged (Kirsch and co-workers 1983). In general, it seems advisable to avoid connecting natural teeth to implant abutments whenever possible.

Fixed-Detachable Implant-Borne Superstructures

Constructing the fixed implant-borne superstructure so that it can be detached by the dentist is indicated in the following situations:
- Foreseeable necessity for repeated interventions
- Reduced interocclusal space
- "Mixed" reconstructions, i.e., splinting of natural teeth and implant abutments (detachable precision attachment between natural abutment and implant abutment)
- Extensive, complex implant-borne superstructures

Practical Planning Procedure

From a theoretical point of view, endosseous implants can be placed anywhere (within certain limitations). Cases can be classified as either primary or secondary indications for implants, based on the suitability and frequency of implant use, as follows:

Primary indications

- Shortened mandibular dental arch (distal extension base situation)
- Single tooth gap in the maxilla (traumatic loss of an anterior tooth, congenitally missing incisor etc.,)
- Edentulous mandible

Secondary indications

- Shortened dental arch in the maxilla (distal extension base situation)
- Single tooth gap in the mandible
- Extended edentulous spaces in either jaw
- Edentulous maxilla

Apart from the obvious aspects these indications have in common, they each require a specific planning protocol adjusted for the respective indication.

Single-Tooth Space in the Maxilla

This indication is often encountered in young patients with traumatic tooth loss or congenitally missing lateral incisors (Fig. 9.**17a** and **b**). Because the adjacent teeth are frequently intact, an implant-supported replacement that

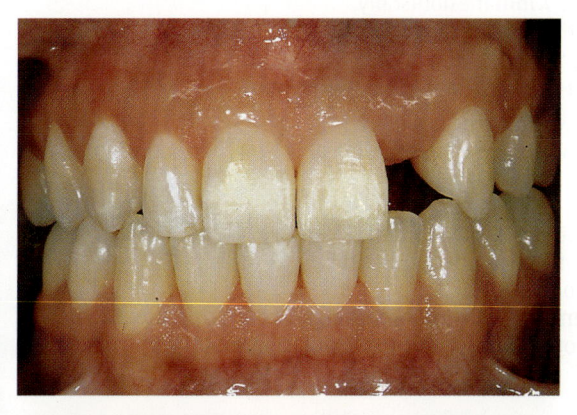

Fig. 9.**17**
a Frontal view of a dentition with congenitally missing left lateral incisor

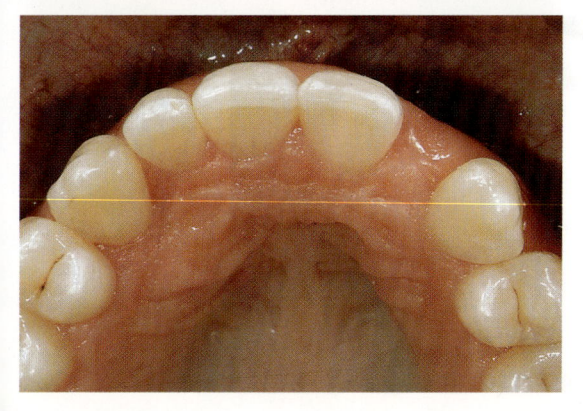

b Palatal view of the same dentition

does not involve natural teeth as abutments is at the top of the list of treatment choices. It is important to note that in these cases, the amount of transverse bone present is often a limiting factor, and as a rule, no implant should be placed before the age of 16–18 years (until growth has been completed!). In cases of this type, conventional prosthetic alternatives, such as resin-bonded bridges must also be included in the list of therapeutic alternatives.

In cases of single-tooth gaps in the upper anterior region, placement of a hollow cylinder implant is advantageous. First, because the bone quality in the anterior maxilla is usually firm and allows for good primary stability of a press-fit implant, and second because of the availability of the HC implant with a 15° angle in its neck portion.

Furthermore, it is important to keep in mind the diameter of the bone anchoring part of the implant (3,5 mm), as well as the shoulder width of 5 mm, which means there must be at least 5.5 mm of bone in the orofacial direction and at least 7 mm mesiodistally.

This dictates the following diagnostic and planning steps:

Single-Tooth Gap in the Maxilla–First Appointment

- Analysis of the width of the space
- Evaluation of the adjacent teeth (clinical crown, periodontium, endodontium)
- Palpation of the bony ridge
- Evaluation of the smile line
- Evaluation of soft-tissue configuration
- Interarch relationships
- Radiographic findings; vertical bone height, bone structure, anatomy of the adjacent roots, space relative to the adjacent roots (in extreme cases, CT scan)
- Diagnostic casts

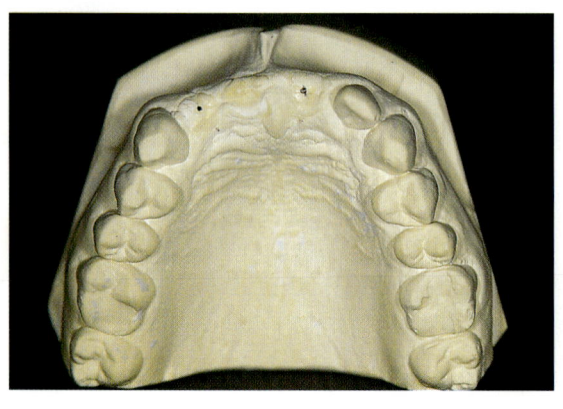

Fig. 9.**18a**
Maxillary cast of a patient with traumatic loss of both central incisors and the right lateral incisor

Implant-Specific Planning Principles **249**

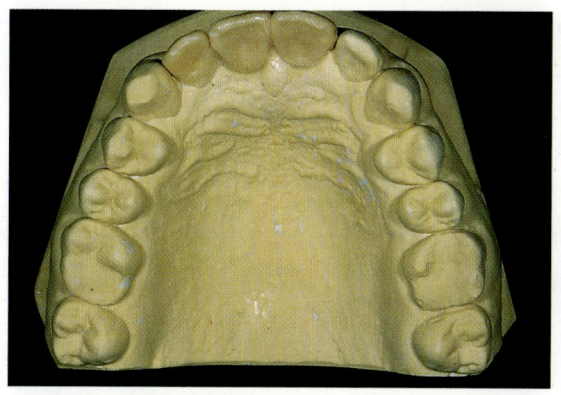

Fig. 9.**18**
b Diagnostic wax-up replacing the three missing incisors on the diagnostic cast

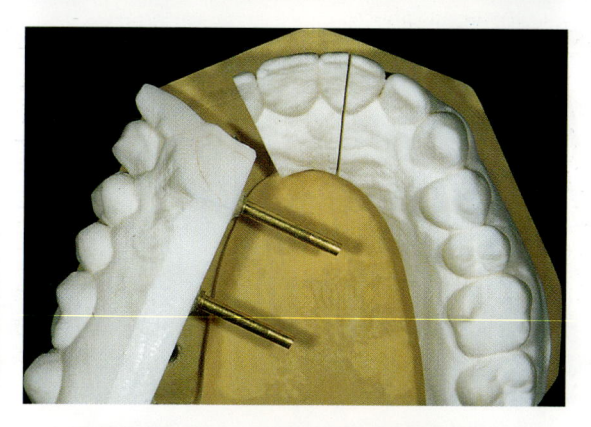

c Sectioned duplicate of the diagnostic cast and wax-up

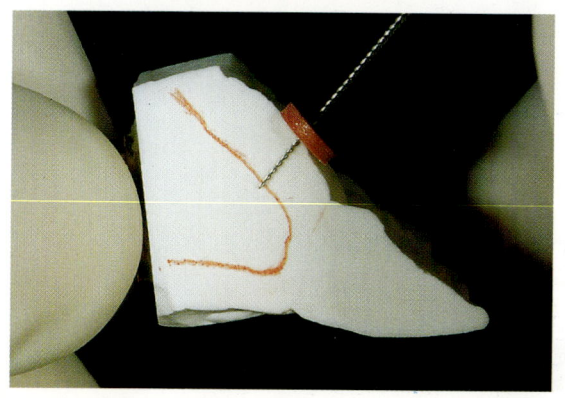

d The sagittal bone outline is drawn on the sectioned cast using the "bone mapping" procedure

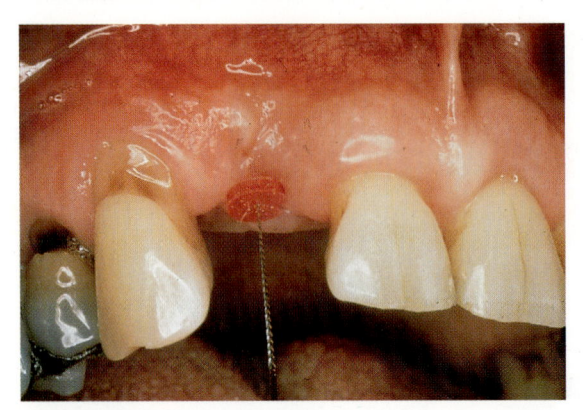

250 9 Preoperative Diagnosis and Treatment Planning

Fig. 9.**19**
a Determination of the mucosal thickness in the region of the missing right lateral incisor

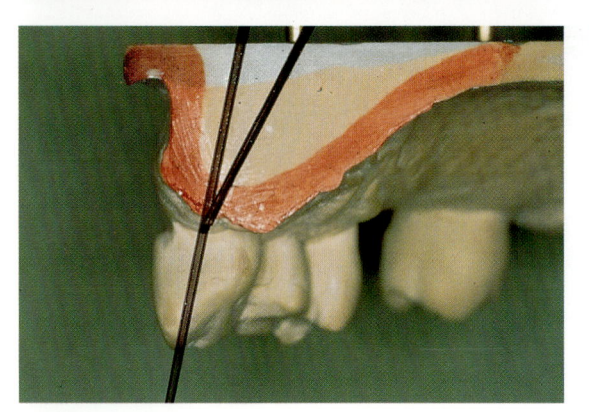

b Sectioned cast with drawing of the bone outline, long axis of the adjacent canine, and the axis of the alveolar ridge

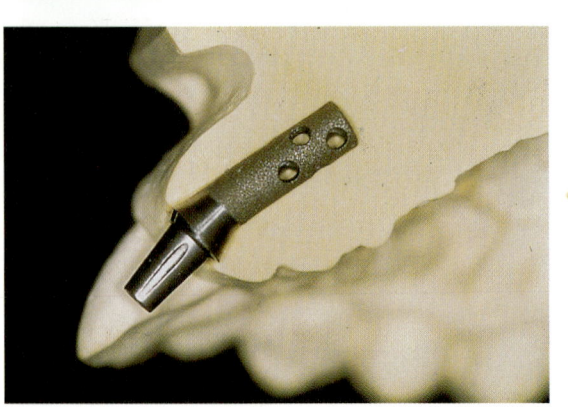

Fig. 9.**20** Saw-cut cast with 15° hollow cylinder implant attached

Single Tooth Gap in the Maxilla–Second Appointment

- Mounting the diagnostic casts for detailed analysis of the interarch relationship
- Precise determination of the transverse bone dimension according to the bone-mapping method, by means of intraoral measurement of the mucosal thickness (Fig. 9.**18a–d**, 9. **19a** and **b**). This leads to the final selection of the type of implant (e.g., hollow cylinder 15°), as well as to the decision whether or not some type of augmentation procedure is indicated (Fig. 9.**20**).

Shortened Mandibular Dental Arch

For this indication, the two-part hollow screw (HS) and solid screw (SS) are the preferred implant types.

Shortened Mandibular Dental Arch–First Appointment

- Palpation of the ridge width and undercuts. Bone mapping is done only if clinical palpation reveals marginally acceptable conditions. This differs from maxillary denture cases, where it is usually difficult to determine the thickness of the mucosa by palpation alone
- Condition of the remaining teeth
- Panoramic radiograph
- Impressions and jaw relation records
- Articulation of the diagnostic casts

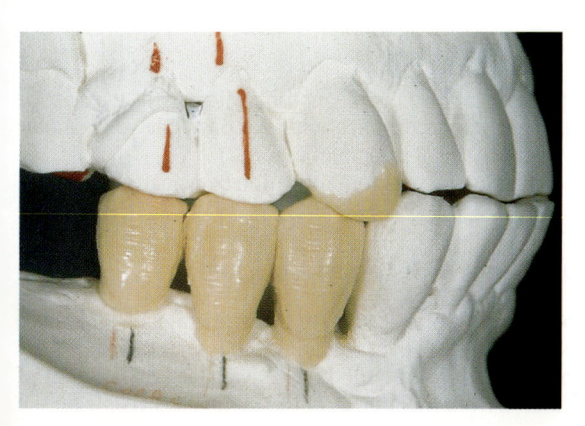

Fig. 9.**21** Determination of the desired implant position by means of a diagnostic wax-up utilizing premolar units

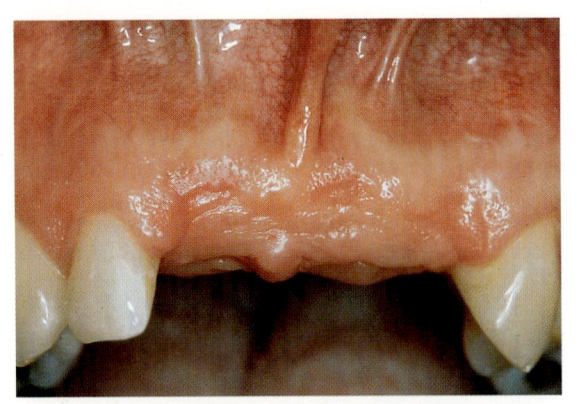

Fig. 9.**22**
a Frontal view of a maxilla following the loss of three upper incisors

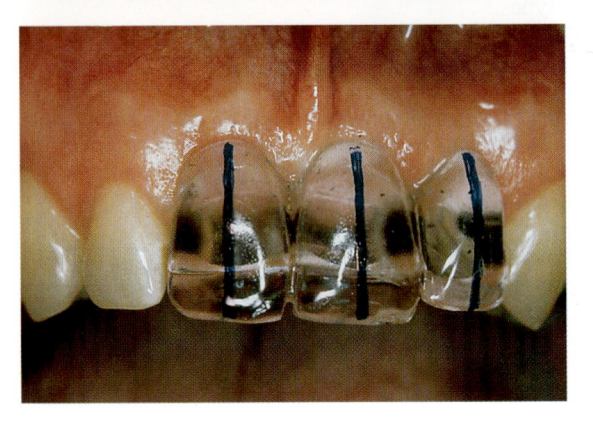

b Same case with a removable plastic template in place to serve as a surgical template

- Selection of implant locations by means of a diagnostic wax-up or setting of denture teeth in accordance with the principle of premolar units and sound biomechanical principles (Fig. 9.**21**)
- Duplication of the diagnostic casts for fabrication of a clear plastic shell
- Split cast, if indicated

Shortened Mandibular Dental Arch–Second Appointment

- Panoramic radiograph with plastic shell in place; metal balls of known diameters are fixed to the shell over the proposed implant sites
- Determination of the amount of bone height available (the amount of distortion is calculated from the images of the metal balls visible on the

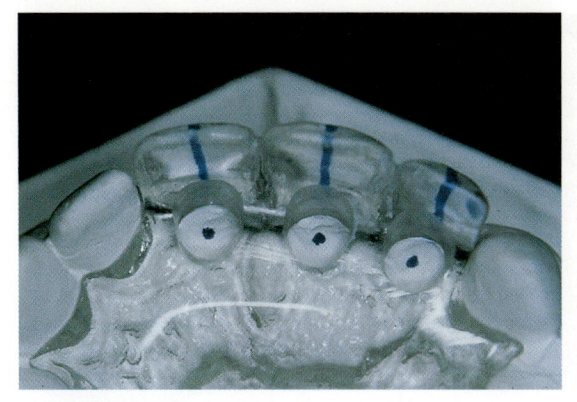

Fig. 9.**22**
c Palatal view of the surgical template on the diagnostic cast with perforations over the planned implant sites.

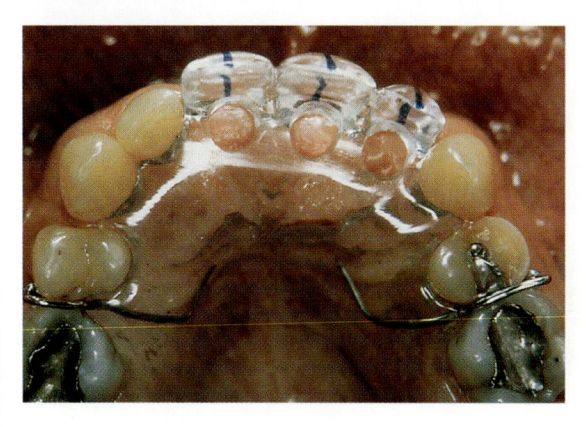

d Clinical palatal view with surgical template in place

radiograph). Note: any bone contouring that might be necessary must be included in the calculation so that there will still be a minium safe distance from the mandibular canal of 1 mm *after* the surgery.
– Definitive establishment of the implant positions, lengths, and type.
– Possible fabrication of a template for use during the surgical procedure (Fig. 9.**22a–d**).

Shortened Maxillary Dental Arch

– The procedure is the same as in the mandible except in unusual cases, in which information from the panoramic radiograph is inconclusive. In these cases, a computer tomogram may be indicated (Fig. 9.**23a–c**).

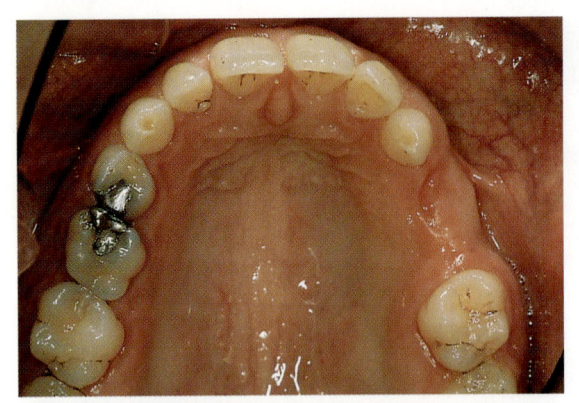

254   9 Preoperative Diagnosis and Treatment Planning

Fig. 9.**23**
a Maxillary occlusal view. Teeth 4, 5, 6, 11, 12, and 13 (ADA numbering system) are congenitally absent. Primary teeth are retained in areas 15, 14, 13, and 23

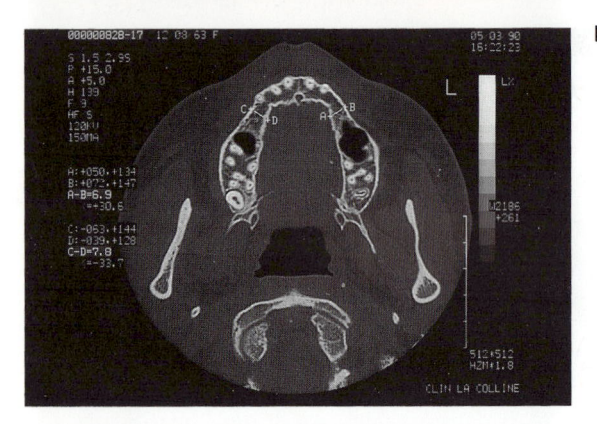

b Computer tomogram of the maxilla for determination of the transverse bone volume in the buccal segments

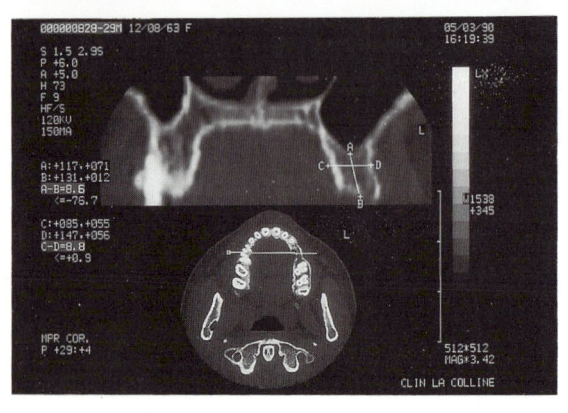

c Computer tomogram for analyzing the vertical bone volume at the prospective implant sites

References

Adell, R., B. Eriksson, U. Lekholm, P. I. Brånemark, T. Jemt: A long-term follow-up study of osseointegrated implants in the treatment of totally edentulous jaws. Int. J. oral max.-fac. Implants 5 (1991) 347–59

Astrand, P., K. Borg, J. Gunne, M. Olsson: Combination of natural teeth and osseointegrated implants as prosthesis abutments: a 2-year longitudinal study. Int. J. oral max.-fac. Implants 6 (1991) 305–312

Brägger, U., D. Buser, N. P. Lang: Implantatgetragene Kronen und Brücken. Schweiz. Mschr. Zahnmed. 100 (1990) 731–740

Brånemark, P.-I., U. Breine, R. Adell, B. O. Hansson, J. Lindström, A. Ohlsson: Intraosseous anchorage of dental prostheses. Scand. J. plast. reconstr. Surg. 3 (1969) 81

Buser, D., U. Brägger, N. P. Lang: Implantologie. Schweiz. Mschr. Zahnmed. 98 (1988) 747–757

Gunne, J., P. Astrand, K. Ahlén, H. Borg, M. Olsson: Implants in partially edentulous patients. A longitudinal study of bridges supported by both implants and natural teeth. Clin. oral. Impl. Res. 3 (1992) 49–56

Kirsch, A., K. L. Ackermann: Das IMZ-Implantationssystem: Indikation – Methode – Langzeitergebnisse. Dtsch. zahnärztl. Z. 38 (1983) 106

Mericske-Stern, R.: Implantate im zahnlosen Unterkiefer. Schweiz. Mschr. Zahnmed. 102 (1992) 1215–27

Picton, D. C. A.: Vertical movement of cheek teeth during biting. Arch. oral Biol. 8 (1963) 109–118

Schroeder, A., O. Pohler, F. Sutter: Gewebereaktion auf ein Titan-Hohlzylinderimplantat mit Titan-Spritzschichtoberfläche. Schweiz. Mschr. Zahnheilk. 86 (1976) 713–27

Smith, R. A., R. Berger, T. B. Dodson: Risk factors associated with dental implants in healthy and medically compromised patients. Int. J. max.-fac. Implants 7 (1992) 367–72

Strub, J. R., H. Linter, C. P. Marinello: The rehabilitation of partially edentulous cases with cantilever bridges: a retrospective study. Int. J. Periodont. Restorat. Dent. 9 (1989) 364

Van Steenberghe, D., U. Lekholom, C. Bolender, T. Folmer, P. Henry, I. Herrmann, K. Higuchi, W. Laney, U. Lindén, P. Astrand: The applicability of osseointegrated oral implants in the rehabilitation of partial edentulism. A prospective multicenter study on 558 fixtures. J. oral max.-fac. Implants 5 (1990) 272–81

Weinberg, L. A.: The biomechanics of force distribution in implant-supported prostheses. Int. J. oral. max.-fac. Implants 8 (1993) 19–31

Zarb, G., F. Zarb, A. Schmitt: Osseointegrated implants for partially edentulous patients. Dent. Clin. N. Amer. 31 (1987) 457–72

10 Surgical Procedure with ITI Implants

D. Buser and B. Maeglin

Anyone wishing to perform endosseous implant procedures should have surgical training and practical experience in the field of dentoalveolar surgery. An experienced surgeon is able to operate low-traumatically and quickly–important prerequisites for surgical procedures on bone. Every surgical intervention demands consideration of the basics of asepsis and sterility, and the placement of endosseous implants is certainly no exception. Although conditions in the oral cavity of a healthy person are generally excellent for the healing process, every effort must be made to prevent infection by foreign organisms. Not all of the demands that are imposed in a modern hospital operating room can be met in the daily dental practice. Nevertheless, the dentist who wishes to be active in implant surgery must invest in a more extensive infrastructure than that required for his or her "normal" professional activities. The goal is to insert implants under the most hygienic conditions possible and with as little trauma to the tissues as possible. With this goal in mind, we begin this chapter by discussing the infrastructure and preoperative preparations that are recommended for achieving the optimum conditions for a successful practice with implant surgery.

As has already been mentioned, from a surgical point of view, ITI implants require only a one-stage procedure. In a standard situation, they are inserted transmucosally and therefore are not covered by soft tissue during the wound healing phase. A closed healing procedure is indicated only in special situations, such as in combination with membranes utilizing the guided bone regeneration (GBR) technique (p. 319) or in combination with iliac crest grafts, which will not be further elaborated upon here. From a clinical point of view, a transmucosal healing offers many advantages (Table 10.**1**). Of these, the avoidance of a second surgical procedure is doubtless the most important one.

The concept of transmucosal healing has a direct influence on what is necessary concerning surgical technique and postoperative treatment to

Table 10.**1** Clinical advantages of transgingival healing of ITI implants

– Avoidance of a second surgical procedure
– Good healing of the soft tissue
– Maintenance of the preoperative width of keratinized ridge mucosa
– Insertion of the prosthetic abutments under clinically clean conditions

achieve a predictable tissue integration of ITI implants. For this reason, the surgical procedures for main indications will be described in detail, with a discussion of general surgical principles for endosseous implantation in edentulous lower jaws. At the end of the chapter, soft tissue surgery and the use of the GBR technique with ITI implants will be presented with case reports.

Infrastructure and Preoperative Preparations

Equipment

The prerequisites for successful tissue integration mentioned above can be fullfilled much more easily with a suitably equipped operating room. This includes the installation of a special sterilizable rotary handpiece system (with detachable sterile hoses) to provide an abundant flow of physiologic saline for effective cooling during the bone preparation. In addition, the handpiece should be powerful enough to allow a precise bone preparation at approximately 500 RPM utilizing a speed-reducing gear (1:7 to 1:64). In recent years, various drilling units with these capabilities have appeared on the market in various price ranges. In addition, a digital RPM indicator is advantageous, in that the operator can continuously monitor the rotational speed as the bone is being cut. A strong operating light with a sterilizable hand grip (Fig. 10.**1**) is also useful. With this, the surgeon can adjust and refocus the light during the operation without contaminating the sterile gloves. If no such light is available, the same result can be achieved by placing a sterile towel or sterile aluminum foil around the hand grip.

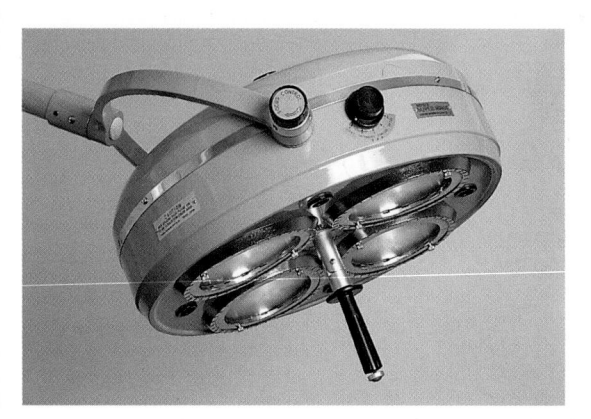

Fig. 10.**1** Operative lamp with a sterilizable handle that allows the surgeon to adjust the light during the surgery without breaking the chain of sterility

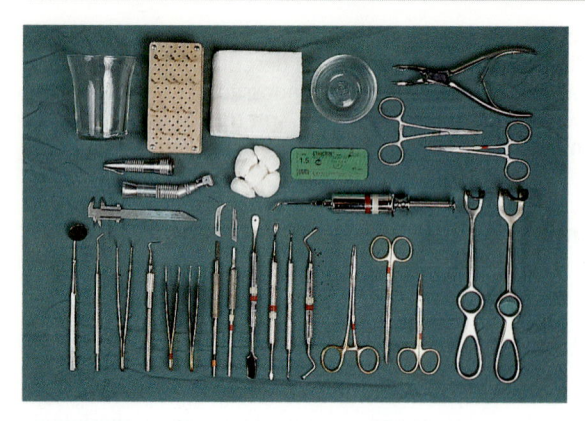

Fig. 10.2 Surgical tray with instruments for an implant surgery:
Dental mirror
Dental probe
Cotton pliers
Periodontal probe
Fine tissue pliers, flat
Fine tissue pliers with "teeth"
Two scalpel handles with No 15 and 12b blades
Two fine bone files
Double-ended excavator
Sharp double-ended curette
Needle holder
Dissection scissors
Suture scissors
Small and large cheek and lip retractors
Two hemostats
Bone ronguer
Small glass cup for bone graft material
Atraumatic suture material
Irrigating syringe
Gauze sponges and compresses
Dental drill kit
Glass for irrigating solution
Straight handpiece and special contra-angle handpiece
Caliper

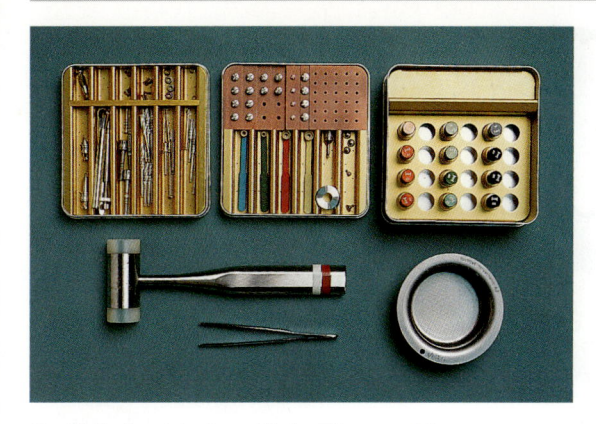

Fig. 10.**3** Special setup with the ITI surgery kit
Set of various ITI instruments
Set of various ITI closure screws
Set with preselected ITI implants
Mallet
Titanium forceps
Metal cup for used ITI instruments

The sterile surgical instruments include a flap setup and the special implantation set. The instruments are laid out in plain view on a sterile towel. Because the soft tissue must be handled as gently as possible, especially delicate surgical instruments are used. The instrument kit from Hu-Friedy (Chicago, IL 60618) was especially created for implant and membrane surgeries and has proven itself in clinical use. (It is available through Institut Straumann AG, CH-4437 Waldenburg, Switzerland.) The instruments in a standard surgical kit for endosseous implantation (that also includes the special Hu-Friedy instruments) are shown in Fig. 10.**2**.

For the sake of good visibility, all of the instruments that are directly associated with the actual implantation procedure are placed on a sterile towel on a specially designed instrument table so that they are readily available (Fig. 10.**3**).

To avoid contamination with fabric fibers, the implants and instruments that come into direct contact with the bone are not allowed to come into contact with the drape. Such contact could cause fibers to be transferred into the implant bed, thus causing a foreign body reaction. For the same reason, implants should not be handled or touched with talcum-treated rubber gloves. Instead, the implant must be removed from its sterile ampule and inserted directly into the prepared site in the bone using the appropriate instruments.

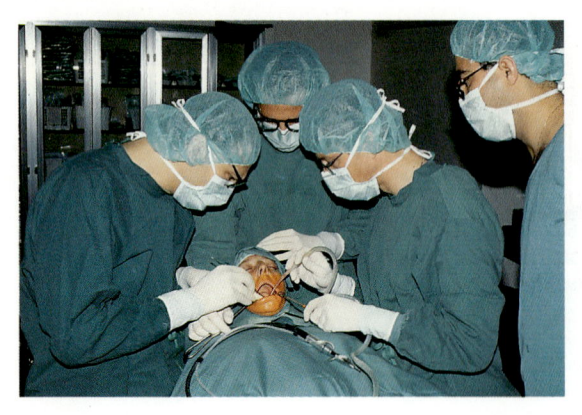

Fig. 10.**4** The surgery in progress with sterile surgical gowns, sterile gloves, head coverings, face masks, and protective eyewear for the operators

Preparation of the Surgical Team

The surgeon and assistants wear surgical caps, face masks, and protective eyewear. Hand disinfection follows the standard surgical procedure; finally, sterile surgical gowns and rubber gloves are put on (Fig. 10.**4**). During the entire operation, special attention is given to the relationship between the operating team and the surroundings. There should be no break in the chain of asepsis, such as through refocusing the operating light.

Premedication and Disinfection

Premedication with atropine (0.5 mg IM) to reduce salivary flow has proven to be useful because it substantially reduces the risk of the operative field becoming flooded with saliva during the operation. Premedication of the anxious patient with a sedative may also be indicated. After the removal of any dentures and before the operation, the oral cavity is rinsed with a 0.12 –0.2% chlorhexidine solution for one minute to reduce the bacterial count. Finally, the perioral area of the face is disinfected with a skin disinfectant, and a sterile drape is placed on the patient, leaving the mouth accessible (Fig. 10.**5**).

Anesthesia

The surgical placement of dental implants is usually carried out under local anesthesia. For this, a long-acting local anesthetic agent is recommended. Depending upon the clinical situation, a nerve block, infiltration, or both may be used.

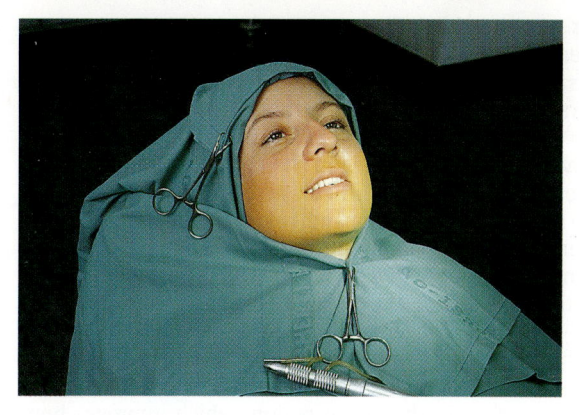

Fig. 10.**5** The patient draped with sterile towels following disinfection of the perioral area

Surgical Procedure for Main Indications

The Edentulous Mandible

Two to six implants are placed in the edentulous mandible according to the treatment plan. Most frequently, implants are placed only in the anterior portion between the mental foramina because the alveolar process in the posterior region is offen too severely atrophied to receive implants. When local anesthesia is used, it is usually administered as bilateral nerve block with additional local infiltration in the anterior region to reduce bleeding during surgery.

In these indications, either one-piece or two-piece ITI implants can be used. The one-piece implant is a further development of the TPS screw designed exclusively for treatment of edentulous mandibles with bar attachments. Two-piece implants provide greater flexibility in prosthetic treatment because they can be combined with various abutments. However, the two-piece implants, unlike one-piece implants connected by a bar, do not gain stability by being splinted together during the initial healing phase. Therefore, threaded implants are preferred in these situations at the Department of Oral Surgery University of Bern, because the screw threads provide excellent primary stability.

In regard to the length of the implant, only about two-thirds of the available vertical bone height is utilized. For example, if the remaining bone height is 15 mm, implants with 10 mm in length are selected, so that the inferior cortical bone is intentionally left intact. This concept is unlike that of other implant systems, in which a bicortical stabilization with the longest implants possible is recommended. The concept of using shorter implants and leaving the inferior cortical plate intact can be used with ITI implants with no clinical disadvantages because the TPS surface permits a significantly better bone anchorage than do fine textured or smoothly machined titanium surfaces (p. 91). This concept reduces the risk of undesirable complications such as overheating of the bone in the apical region of the recipient site because of the increasingly difficult access of the cooling fluid or–in the worst case scenario–the risk of mandibular fracture if there should be an early circumferential peri-implant infection (p. 472).

A choice must now be made between screw-type (S) or hollow screw (HS) implants, and this depends on the implant length selected preoperatively. If implants of 10 mm and longer can be used, S implants in lengths of 10, 12, or 14 mm are preferred. For bone heights of less than 10 mm, HS implants 6 mm or 8 mm long are preferred because the hollow implants have a greater macroscopic surface in the apical region, which improves bone anchorage.

Treatment with Two ITI Implants

When the treatment plan calls for the placement of two implants to be fitted with either a bar or two ball anchors, the first step is to expose both implant sites by making two small trapezoidal mucoperiosteal flaps in the areas formerly occupied by the canine teeth (Fig. 10.**6a** and **b**). For this, the mucoperiosteum is sharply separated with a No. 15 scalpel blade. Next, the mucoperiosteal flap is separated from the bone that is to be exposed with a fine periosteal elevator such that good visibility and access to the operative field is provided. The mucoperiosteal flap is held back with a suture instead of retractors to avoid traumatizing the soft tissues. If the alveolar ridge has a narrow crest, it can be carefully shortened and smoothened with a large round burr to create a flat, broad surface of bone (Fig. 10.**6c**). The alveolar ridge should not be shortened more than 2–3 mm, and the spongiosa should not be exposed to any great extent because this would create a risk of greater than average postoperative bone resorption . The standard ITI implants have endosseous diameters of 3.5 to 4.1 mm. The width of the alveolar ridge should consequently be at least 6 mm (Table 10.**2**) so that a bone wall of at least 1 mm thickness will remain on both the facial and lingual side of the implant. This is important for the long-term success of endosseous implants. When the width of the alveolar ridge is between 5 mm and 6 mm, screw implants of a reduced diameter of 3.3 mm are used. When the alveolar ridge is less than 5 mm in width, the GBR technique is used to reconstruct the lost alveolar ridge width (see p. 318).

The preparation of the implant bed is done exclusively with the standardized drills and burrs furnished with the selected implant. The bone is cut using a rotational speed of approximately 500 rpm, intermittent light

Surgical Procedure for Main Indications 263

Table 10.2 Selection of the implant depending upon the width of the alveolar ridge

Ridge width	Implant choice
> 6 mm	Standard ITI implant (3.5 mm and 4.1 mm)
5–6 mm	Reduced diameter S implant (3.3 mm)
< 5 mm	Membrane technique

Table 10.3 Precautions for avoiding heat necrosis during preparation of the implant channel

– Reduced rational speed (500–800 rpm)
– Cooling with chilled, sterile physiologic saline (from the refrigerator)
– Use of sharp drills and burrs
– Avoidance of excessive force during preparation
– Intermittent drilling technique

hand pressure, and a *continuous* flow of cooling solution (Table 10.**3**). Heating of the bone carries the risk of damage and must be avoided at all costs. Heat necrosis of the bone around an implant occurs after heating to above 47 °C (117° F) for prolonged periods. *Sterile* physiologic saline or Ringer's solution that has been precooled to approximately 4 °C (39° F) in a refrigerator serves to cool the site and to flush away debris. A rotary handpiece that has a foot-controlled automatic dispenser to deliver coolant to the surgical field and the drill site is an ideal and practical setup. With round burrs, pre-drills, pilot drills, and spiral drills, the coolant is applied externally and in copious amounts. With the trephine mill, internal cooling is possible in which the cooling fluid is fed through an attached inner cooling system to the inside of the mill. A bottle (from which the coolant flows through a hose and out of a dull canula) can also be hung high on an infusion stand to serve as a coolant delivery system that intermittently flushes the implant bed being drilled in the bone. Sterile syringes that are repeatedly filled are another possible solution for cooling. The use of the spray or water stream that comes directly from the dental unit for cooling while cutting bone is *contraindicated* because the system of tubes and hoses in the unit is always contaminated with microorganisms, some of which may be pathogenic.

The first step in preparing the implant bed for an S implant is to determine the desired implant location with a caliper (Fig. 10.**6d**) and mark it in the center of the ridge with the smallest round bur (Fig. 10.**6e**). Next, the first preparation is cut under constant coolant flow with the small pilot drill (2.2 mm ø) to the desired depth (Fig. 10.**6f**). The depth can be easily read on the laser-marked rings placed at 2 mm intervals. In the edentulous mandible, the drill depth is usually selected so that the superior boundary of the TPS layer is located just below the surface of the bony ridge. After the implant cavity is rinsed, it is carefully widened to 2.8 mm with the second pilot drill (Fig. 10.**6g**). When S implants of reduced diameter are used, the preparation of the implant bed is completed except for cutting the threads with the thin tapping instrument. For the standard S implant, the bone cavity is further widened with a spiral drill to 3.5 mm (Fig. 10.**6h**). After checking the sink depth with the depth gauge (Fig. 10.**6i**), the second implant bed is prepared while the depth gauge remains in the first preparation to serve as a guide pin (Fig. 10.**6j**) to create the best possible parallelism between the two implants. The next step is the cutting of the threads with the tapping instrument, which is guided slowly into the depths of the bony implant bed using the hand ratchet and the guidance key (Fig. 10.**6k** and **l**). An alternative is the preparation with the hand-piece adaptor allowing a cutting speed at 15 RPM. In normal bone structure, the threads are precut along the entire length of the bone cavity (Table 10.**4**).

In bone that is more cancellous than average, threads are precut only in the coronal part of the bone cavity so that the implant is inserted in the apical region as a self-tapping implant. In this way, good primary stability can be achieved in spite of the spongy structure of the bone. After flushing out the completed implant bed one more time (Fig. 10.**6m**), the corresponding S implant is mounted tightly to the inserting device and removed from its sterile ampoule, while avoiding contamination. Finally, with the help of the hand ratchet and the guide key under constant cooling, the implant is slowly inserted into the bone (Fig. 10.**6n** and **o**). When the bottom of the bony cavity is reached, resistance increases perceptibly. At this point, the insertion is completed and the inserting device is removed by loosening the set screw with a counter-clockwise rotation. If the procedure has been carried out correctly, the implant should exhibit excellent primary stability; the coronal boundary of the TPS layer should be located slightly below the bone surface (Fig. 10.**6p**).

Before wound closure, a closure screw of the correct size is selected and screwed onto the implant. The large closure screw, which measures 6 mm in diameter, is usually selected for the edentulous mandible (Fig. 10.**6q**). The wound margins are closely adapted with atraumatic sutures, such as size

Fig. 10.**6** Implant procedure on an 84-year-old patient with two two-part ITI implants in the edentulous mandible
a Preoperative appearance of the edentulous mandible
b Elevation of a small trapezoidal mucoperiosteal flap that will be held out of the way with a retraction suture
c Careful smoothing of the alveolar ridge with a large round bur

Surgical Procedure for Main Indications

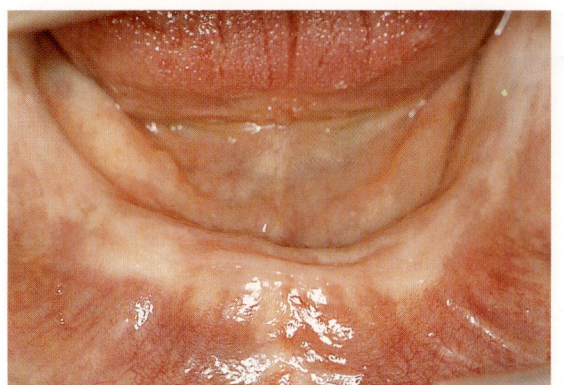

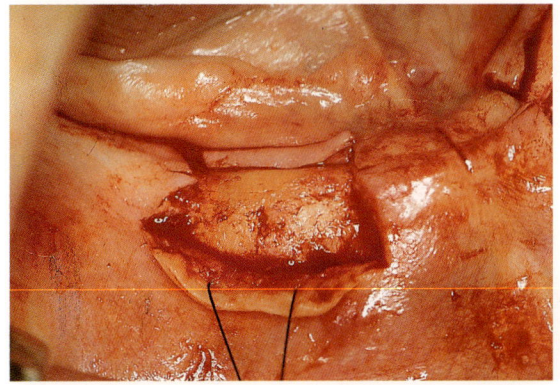

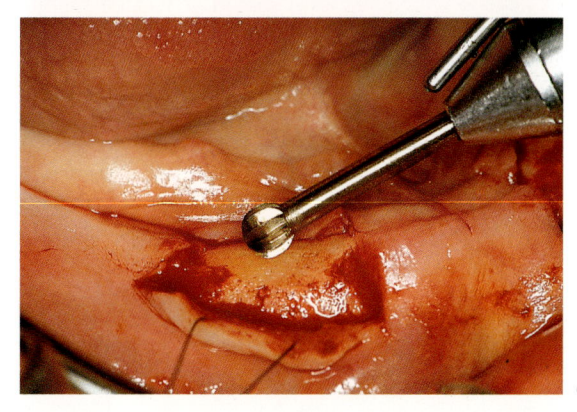

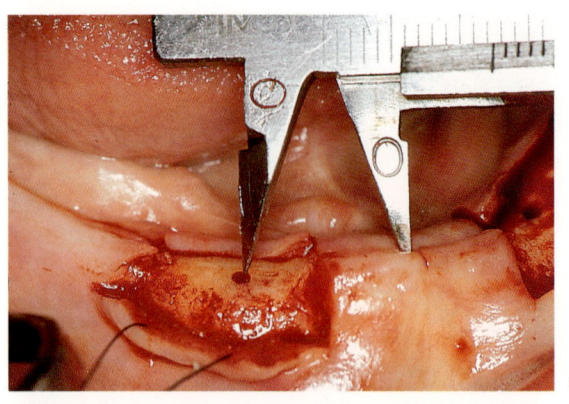

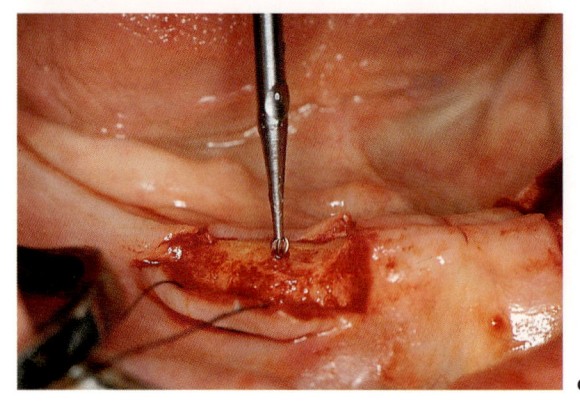

d Determination of the desired implant sites with a caliper
e Marking the implant sites with the smallest round bur

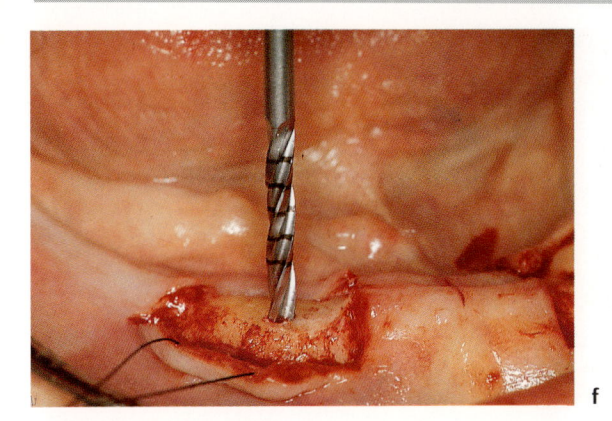

Surgical Procedure for Main Indications **267**

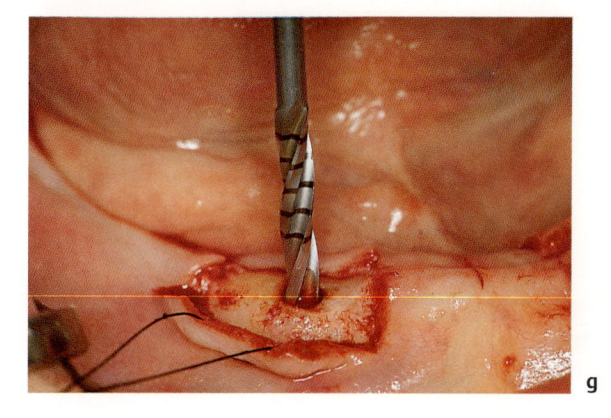

f Preparation with the first pilot drill (2.2 mm Ø) to a depth of 12 mm
g Excavation of the implant cavity with the second pilot drill (2.8 mm Ø)

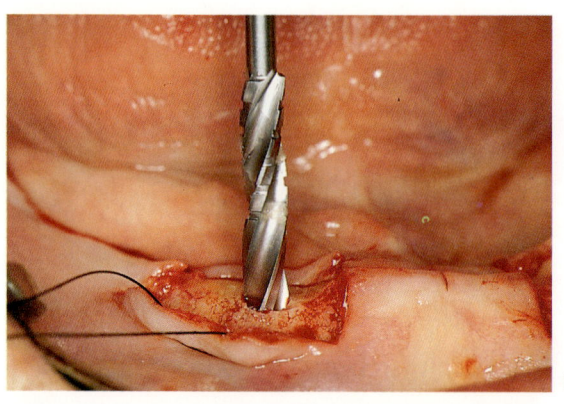

268 10 Surgical Procedure with ITI Implants

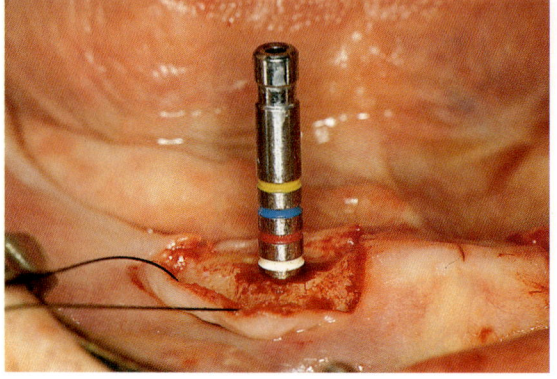

h Enlargement of the implant bed with the spiral drill (3.5 mm Ø)
i Confirming the depth of the preparation with the depth gauge

Surgical Procedure for Main Indications **269**

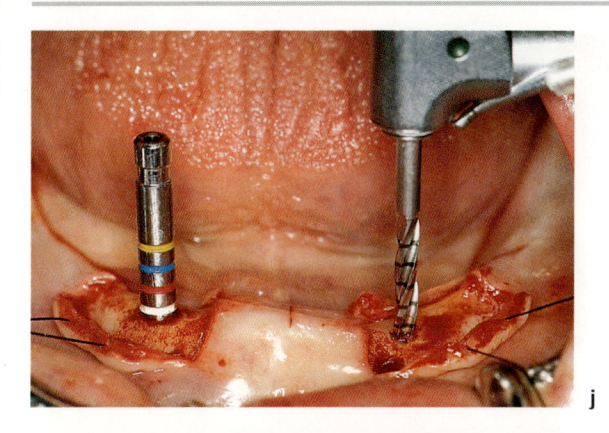

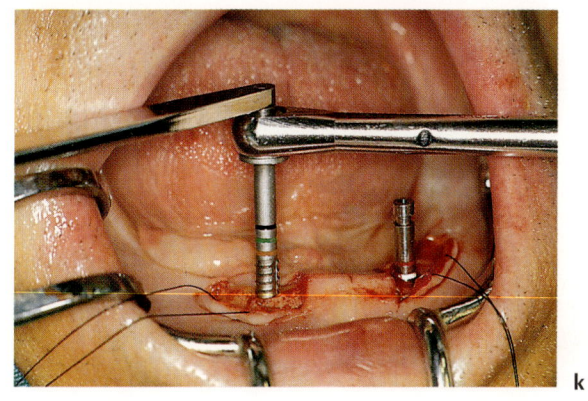

j Preparation of the second implant channel. The depth gauge in the right canine region serves as an orientation guide
k Precutting threads in the channel using a thread cuter (tap), hand ratchet, and guidance key

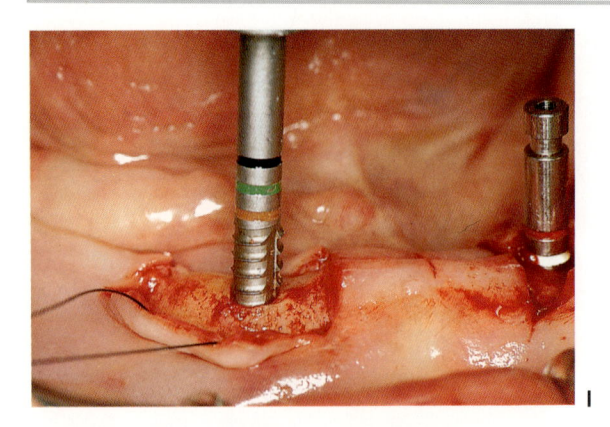

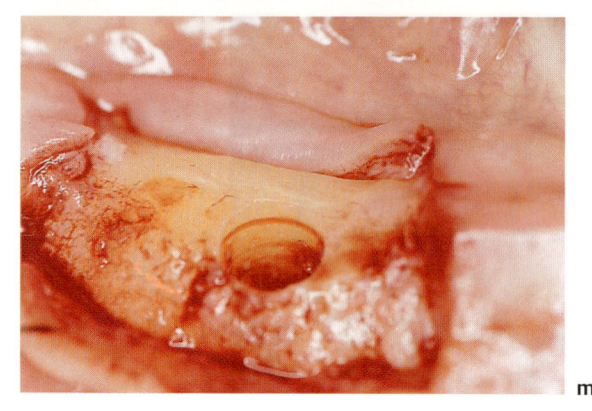

l Closer view of the color-coded thread cutter (tap)
m Completed implant bed with the screw threads clearly visible in the bony wall

Surgical Procedure for Main Indications **271**

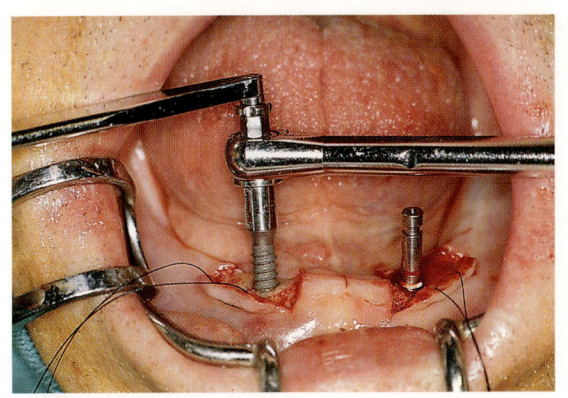

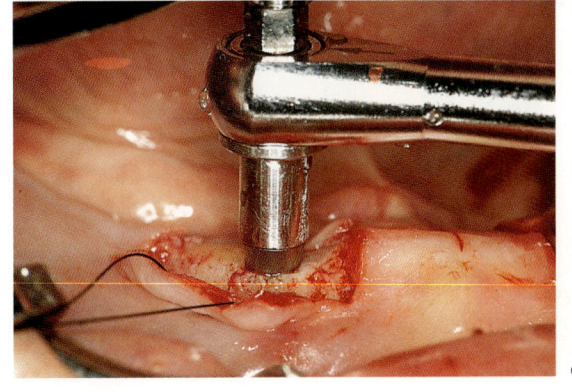

n The implant being screwed in place using the inserting device, hand ratchet, and quidance key
o Insertion procedure completed and insertion tool ready for removal

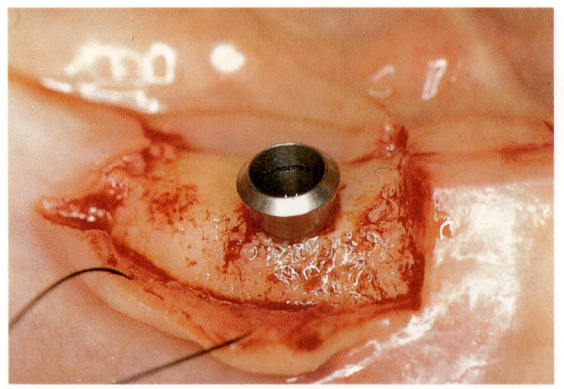

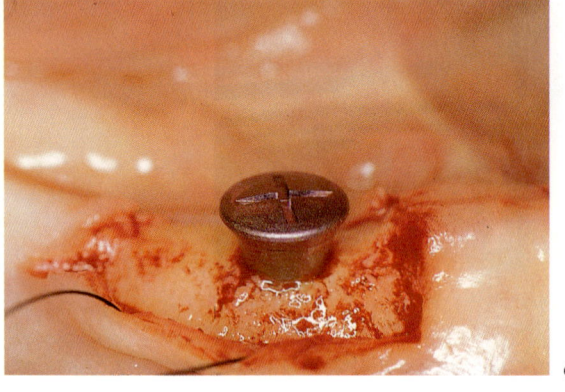

p The implant has on optimal buccal bone wall and exhibits excellent primary stability
q Insertion of a large closure screw that will hold the soft tissue apically during the healing period
r Precise, tension-free adaptation of soft tissue to the implant post; wound closure with interrupted sutures that are not tied too tightly
s Status around both implants following wound closure
t Condition three months after implantation with Octa abutments in place

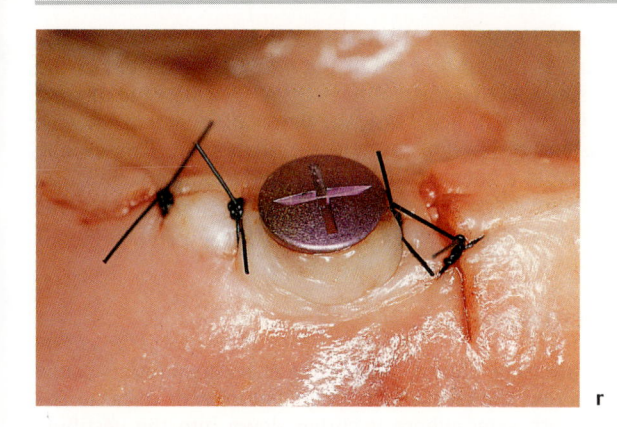

Surgical Procedure for Main Indications **273**

r

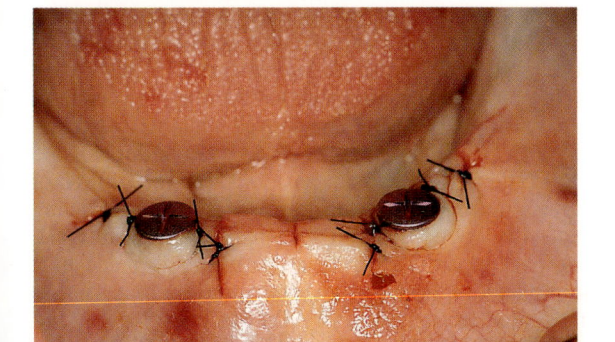

s

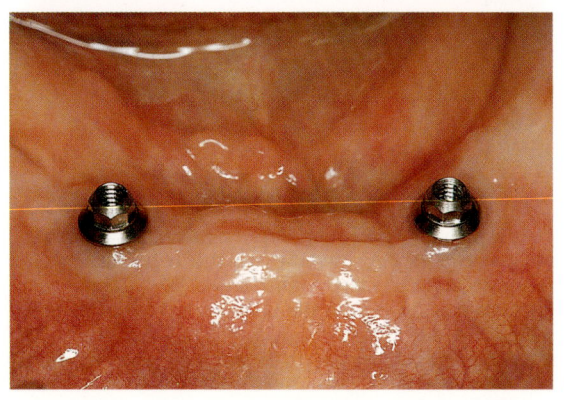

t

4–0. To avoid necrosis at the margin of the wound, these should not be tied too tightly. One suture is placed on each of the two proximal sides of the implant and closure screw so that the wound margins are closely adapted to the implant (Fig. 10.**6r** and **s**). If necessary, the flaps can be mobilized with small releasing incisions to provide tension-free adaptation. This usually makes it possible to avoid a gingivectomy that would sacrifice keratinized mucosa. The large closure screw also serves as a vertical stop that prevents the wound margins from slipping over the shoulder of the implant as the soft tissues swell during the first days following surgery.

Treatment with Four ITI Implants

When four implants are to be placed, a large mucoperiosteal flap is made. Again, the incision follows the crest of the ridge, but extends distal to the mental foramina on both sides where it curves down into the vestibule (Fig. 10.**7a**). It is sometimes also necessary to make a vertical releasing incision into the vestibule in the median line to obtain good exposure of the surgical field. After the facial and lingual mucoperiosteal flaps have been reflected, both mental foramina are exposed (Fig. 10.**7b** and **c**). The extent of available bone is now easy to determine and the desired implant sites can be marked in accordance with the treatment plan (p. 261). Smoothing of the alveolar ridge, marking of the desired implant positions, and preparation of the implant beds is done with the usual instruments (Fig. 10.**7d**). Following insertion of the implants, the wound is closed with interrupted sutures (Fig. 10.**7e** and **f**). When one-part implants are used, an impression is made after the surgery using impression copings and a custom tray, so that the bar attachment can be fabricated in the laboratory. On the following day the completed bar is inserted and attached with occlusal screws after its exact fit has been confirmed (Fig. 10.**7h**).

Fig. 10.**7** A case treated with four one-part ITI implants in the edentulous mandible ▶
a Ridge incision between the two second premolar regions. A primary anterior vestibuloplasty with free mucosal grafts was performed previously
b Reflection of mucoperiosteal flaps to expose the bony ridge. To provide better exposure, a releasing incision was also made in the midline
c Identification of the mental nerve (arrow) in order to determine the area available for implant insertion

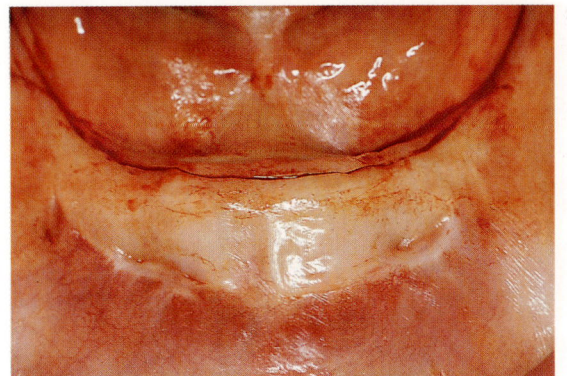

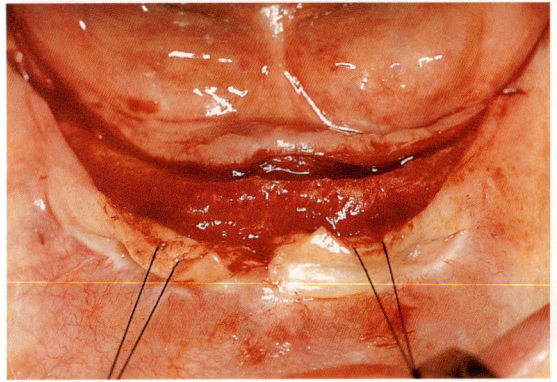

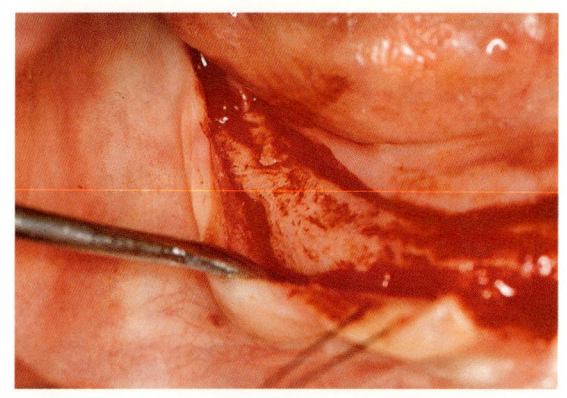

Surgical Procedure for Main Indications 275

a

b

c

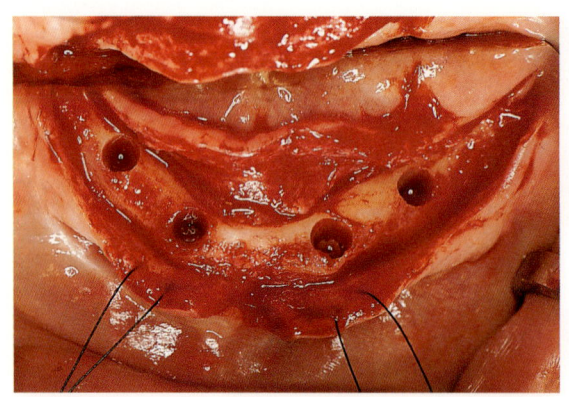

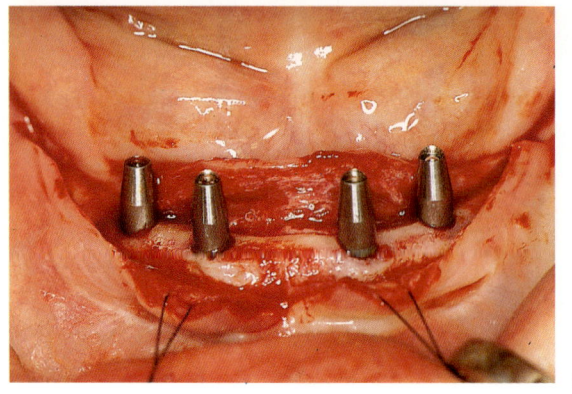

d Situation following preparation of the symmetrically spaced implant sites
e Four one-part ITI implants inserted
f Status following wound closure
g One day after implantation, the bar that was fabricated in the interim is inserted after appropriate fit has been verified
h Four weeks after implantation, the peri-implant soft tissues are healed so that (due to the splinting effect of the bar) the prosthetic treatment can be started

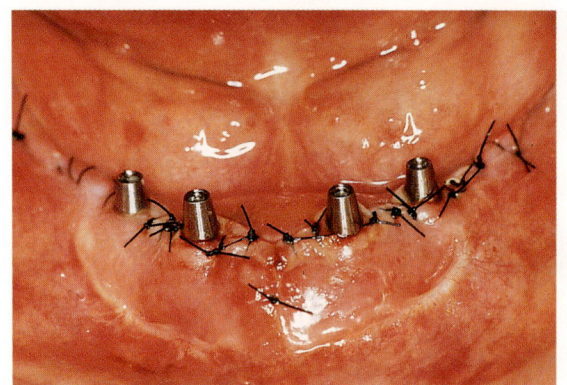

Surgical Procedure for Main Indications 277

f

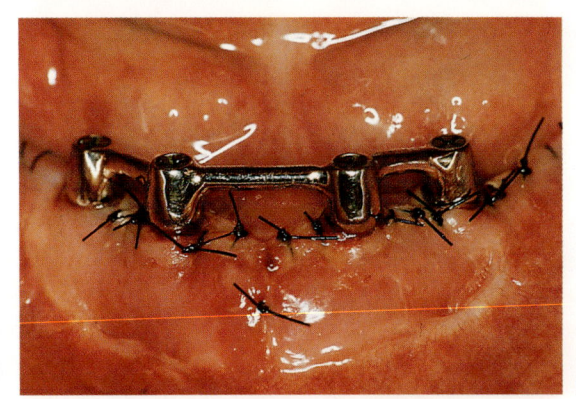

g

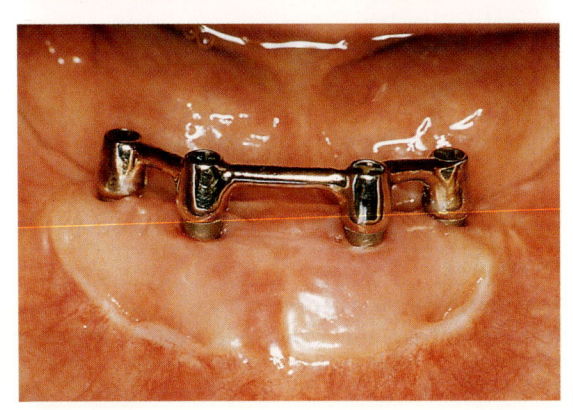

h

278 10 Surgical Procedure with ITI Implants

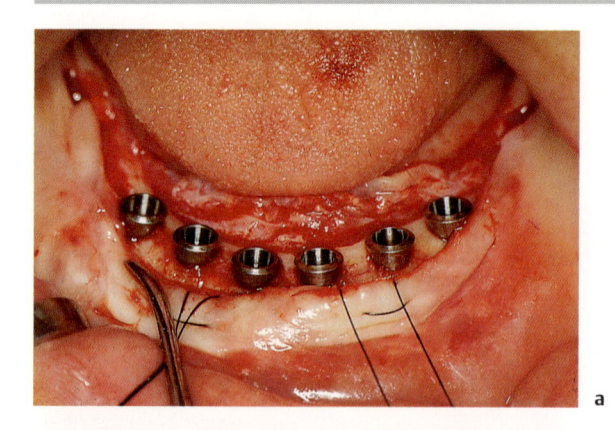

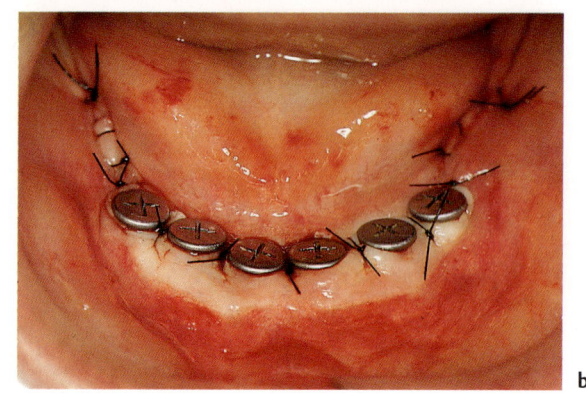

Fig. 10.8 Implant placement of six ITI implants
a Insertion of six two-part ITI implants
b Status following wound closure

Table 10.4 Cutting of threads depending upon the bone structure at implant site

Bone structure	Surgical procedure
Normal	Precutting of threads in the entire bone cavity
Spongy	Precutting of threads only in the coronal portion of the bone cavity (For insertion of the implant as a self-tapping implant to improve primary stability)

Surgical Procedure for Main Indications 279

Treatment with Six ITI Implants

When an edentulous patient is to be treated with an implant-borne fixed partial denture in the mandible, six implants are inserted if possible. The surgical technique is the same as for four implants (Fig. 10.**8a** and **b**).

Postoperative Treatment

Rapid, low-trauma surgery has a positive influence on the postoperative course. In the optimum situation, one can expect the following sequelae: a low level of pain, little or no swelling, low incidence of infection, and uncomplicated wound healing. The prescription of antibiotics is recommended in some cases. This is especially true for operations of long duration in the mandible. Short-term perioperative antibiotic coverage (e.g., 500 mg amoxycillin 3 or 4 times daily) may be prescribed, beginning 2 hours before surgery. However, antibiotic coverage must never be used as a substitute for careful attention to sterile surgical technique.

The patient must be informed of the possibility of complications and what to expect during the postoperative phase. Printed information forms that are given to patients are useful for this purpose. Cooperative, prudent patient behavior can have a positive influence on the course of healing. Regular application of ice packs or cold compresses to the external soft tissues during the first 2 postoperative days will contribute substantially to the prevention of swelling. An additional prescription for a nonsteroidal anti-inflammatory drug, such as 50 mg diclofenac t.i.d., has proved to be effective in reducing swelling and pain. Continuance of normal oral hygiene in combination with chlorhexidine mouth rinses (0.1–0,2% solution for one minute t.i.d.) helps to prevent wound infection. Sutures will be removed after 7 days.

In the edentulous mandible, wearing of the existing denture during the soft-tissue healing phase is generally avoided. Healing is thus not unnecessarily disturbed. The patient is informed of this necessity at the preoperative consultation, and if it is explained properly, it will be accepted by the patient without complaint. After 2 or 3 weeks, the soft tissues are usually sufficiently healed to allow the existing denture to be worn after it has been relieved and relined with a soft material.

Healing Period for Osseointegration of ITI Implants

When ITI implants are placed, the time allowed for healing does not depend upon the location of the implant; i.e., no distinction is made between the maxilla and mandible. The decisive criterion for establishing the length of the healing period is the type of bone structure at the implant site determined during placement of the implant. If the implant site exhibits

Table 10.5 Healing periods as determined by the bone structure

Bone structure	Healing period
"normal"	3 months
spongy	4 months

Table 10.6 Criteria for successful tissue integration of an ITI implant

– No subjective complaints by the patient
– Absence of a periimplant infection with suppuration
– A stable, ankylosed implant that emits a sharp sound on percussion
– Absence of a continuous peri-implant radiolucency
– Implant position that allows prosthetic restoration

"normal" bone structure, i.e., firm, cortical bone, a three-month healing period with no functional loading is observed (Table 10.5).

When there is predominantly soft, cancellous bone, as it is frequently the case in posterior areas of both jaws, at least 4 months are recommended before the prosthetic treatment begins.

Because there is mostly a firm bone structure in the anterior edentulous mandible, a three-month healing period is usually sufficient in these cases. This rule does need to be followed for implants splinted with a gold bar for overdenture retention. These can be functionally loaded earlier, as has been verified by many years of clinical experience with the TPS screw implant (Ledermann 1986, Krekeler and co-workers 1991). Therefore, when four one-part implants are used in combination with a bar, fabrication of the final prosthesis can be started as soon as the soft tissues have healed (Fig. 10.**7h**). When free-standing two-part implants are used, the normal integration phase of 3 months has to be observed. After the healing period is completed (Fig. 10.**6**). the implants are evaluated clinically and radiographically. If the implants fulfill the criteria of successful tissue integration (Table 10.**6**), the abutments can be attached (Fig. 10.**6**) and the definitive prosthesis produced.

The Distal Extension Situation in the Mandible

In these cases, a thorough clinical and radiographic preoperative examination must be performed to establish a detailed treatment plan with the aid of articulated casts (p. 251). In this region of the mouth, threaded implants are preferred so that these free-standing implants, unsplinted during the healing phase, can achieve good primary stability in the often spongy bone. The choice between Type S and Type HS implants depends upon the hight of bone available above the mandibular canal. Because the alveolar process in the posterior region is often somewhat atrophied with 10 mm or less of vertical bone height, HS implants are often used in these cases.

In the following, the placement of an HS implant in the lower right quadrant distal to a shortened dental arch is described (Fig. 10.**9a**). Ordinarily, anesthesia is achieved with an inferior alveolar nerve block supplemented by infiltration of the buccal nerve. Some authors have recommended not using a nerve block in the lower posterior region, so that if the implant preparation comes too close to the mandibular canal, the operator will be alerted by the patient's pain reaction. Today this recommendation can be ignored when using cylindrically shaped ITI implants if the amount of bone present above the mandibular canal is precisely determined before surgery (Fig. 10.**9b**).

The next step is the incision of the soft tissues over the ridge (Fig. 10.**9c**). The flap is extended generously mesiodistally for optimal view of the surgical field and to facilitate the possible need for a correcting of a previously determined implant position without reaching the borders of the mucoperiosteal flap. If possible, the ridge incision is placed so that the mucoperiosteal flap will have keratinized ridge mucosa on both, the buccal and lingual margins. If the zone of available keratinized ridge mucosa is too narrow, the incision is made more toward the buccal aspects so that the keratinized mucosa will be on the lingual margin. If a plastic surgical procedure to restore keratinized mucosa needs to be done, this would be relatively simple on the buccal side. A lingual grafting procedure, however, would be much more diffucult. Mesial and distal releasing incisions may be made, depending upon the situation, so that the surgical field will be well exposed after the mucoperiostela flap is reflected. The mucoperiosteal flap is lifted with a special fine, double-ended periosteal. (Hu-Friedy, Chicago IL 60618) to minimize trauma to the soft tissues. For the same reason, the use of tissue retractors within the flap is avoided. Instead, the mucoperiosteal flap is held back with retraction sutures to provide good access and a good view of the implant site (Fig. 10.**9d**). The alveolar ridge is inspected and smoothed if necessary to create a flat bone surface. The anatomy of the lingual bone surface is also explored with a Lukac curette so that any undercuts that might be present can be avoided during preparation of the implant bed. Concerning the width of the alveolar ridge and selection of implant type, the same rules stated previously apply (Table 10.**2**).

The desired implant position is determined with a caliper and marked with a round bur. In doing so, the use of three round burs with increasing diameter is recommended (Fig. 10.**9e**) so that after the position has been marked with the smallest bur, it can be verified again. If necessary, the position can be corrected in the desired direction with the next larger bur. This procedure allows precise positioning of the implant in the mesiodistal direction, which is important for the later prosthetic treatment. Exact positioning in the faciolingual direction is also important so that a bone wall of at least 1 mm thickness will remain on both the lingual and buccal aspects of the implant. Next, the preparation of the implant bed is begun with the pre-drill (Fig. 10.**9f**).

If the implant is to be inserted in the standard way, i.e., with the upper border of the TPS layer just beneath the crest level of the alveolar ridge, the pre-drill must be sunken into the bone all the way to its shoulder. The final direction of the implant is determined by the pre-drill, and for that reason, the three-dimensional positioning of the pre-drill must be well controlled during this step. It is recommended that the operation be carried out with an assistant who can, among other tasks, monitor the faciolingual orientation of the pre-drill, while the surgeon controls its mesiodistal direction. In a posteriorly edentulous case with the canine also missing, a surgical template fabricated before the operation is very useful for aligning the implants appropriately. Next, the preparation is continued with the trephine mill (Fig. 10.**9g**). The depth of the preparation can be easily monitored because the various depths are marked with rings at 2-mm intervals. The effective depth of the implant bed is checked with the depth gauge. If two implants are to be placed, the mesial implant bed is prepared first, including excavation with the trephine mill. The depth gauge is then placed in the mesial cavity to serve as a guide pin for preparing the second, distal implant bed. Finally, threads are cut into the wall of the bony cavity (Fig. 10.**9h**), but the entire length is pretapped only if the bone is of "normal" density. It is not uncommon in mandibular distal extension cases, and even more common in maxillary distal extension cases, that threads have to be pretapped only in the coronal portion of the implant bed because of the spongy nature of the more apical bone. Better primary stability will be achieved if the implant is self-tapping in the apical region. After thorough rinsing, the prepared bone cavity is inspected once more (Fig. 10.**9i**). If the central bone core should be fractured, as evidenced by its eccentric position, it is removed with a probe. The cap is broken off the sterile ampoule of the selected HS implant; the inserting device is attached and tightened to the implant; the implant is then removed from the ampoule and slowly inserted into the implant bed using the hand ratchet and guidance key, avoiding contamination as far as possible. As alternative, the hand-piece adaptor can be utilized with 15 RPM.

Fig. 10.**9** Insertion of a HS implant in the first molar position of a posteriorly edentulous mandible
a Preoperative marking of the intended implant site
b Panoramic radiograph to determine the vertical bone height available in the first molar area, which measures approximately 14 mm
c Widely extended incision along the crest of the ridge from first premolar area to second molar area, with mesial and distal releasing incisions

Surgical Procedure for Main Indications

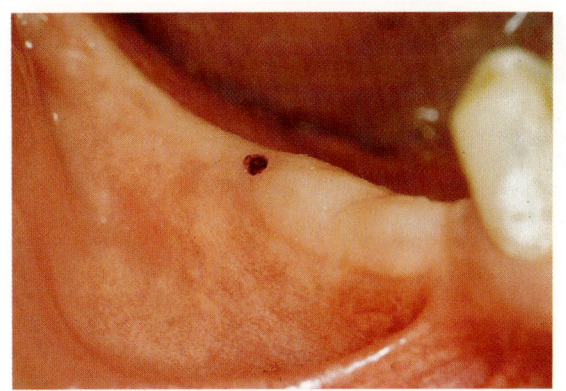

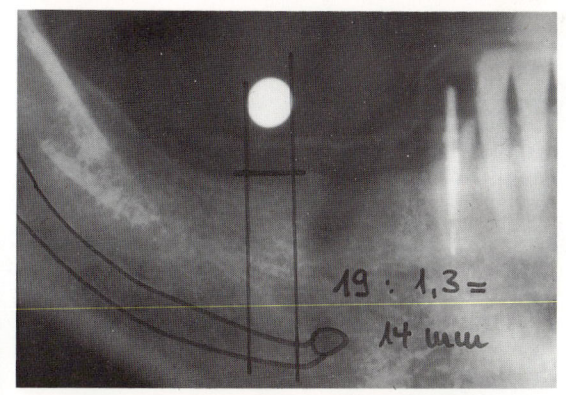

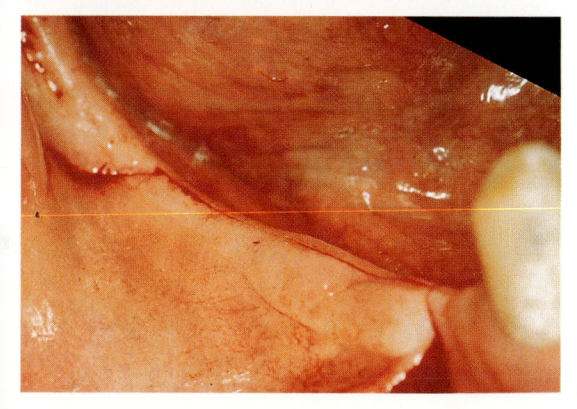

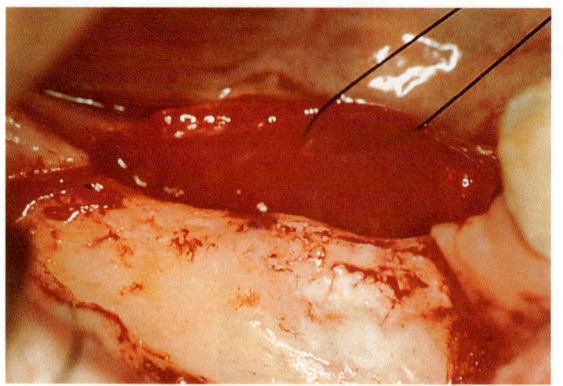

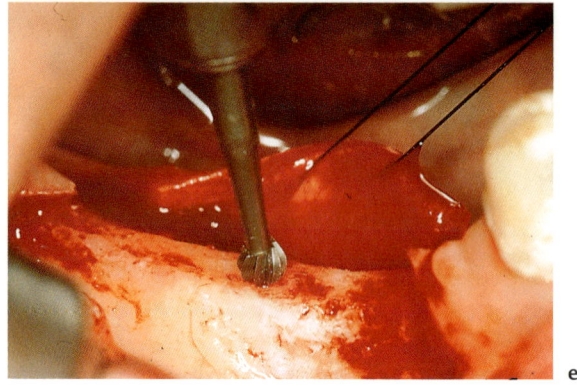

d Reflection of vestibular and lingual mucoperiosteal flaps. Both flaps are held in position with retraction sutures
e Marking the implant site with a round bur
f Preparation with a pre-drill that is sunk up to its shoulder into the bone
g Preparation with the trephine mill. The depth can be easily monitored by the circles of perforations
h Precutting of screw threads with the color-coded tap

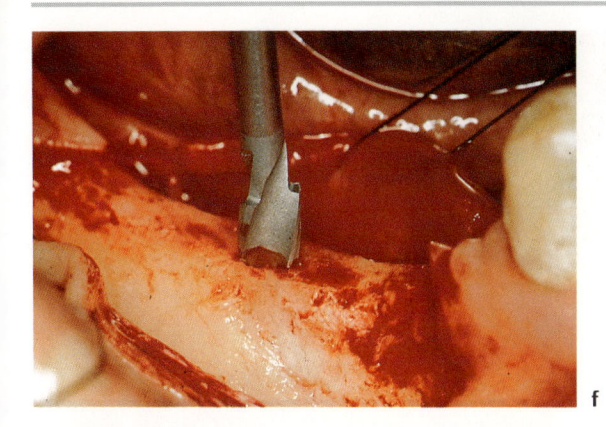

Surgical Procedure for Main Indications

f

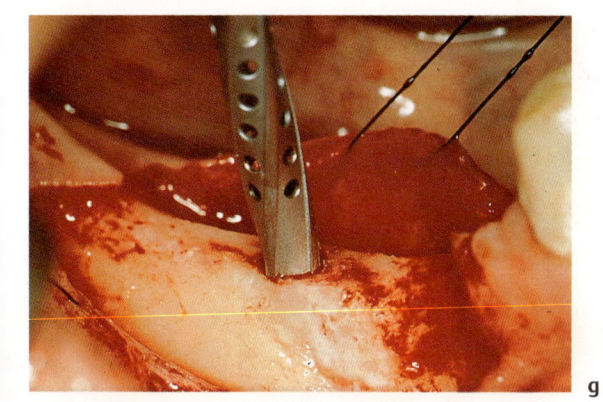

g

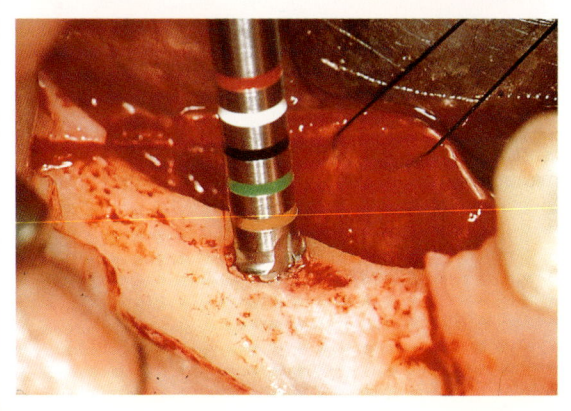

h

286 10 Surgical Procedure with ITI Implants

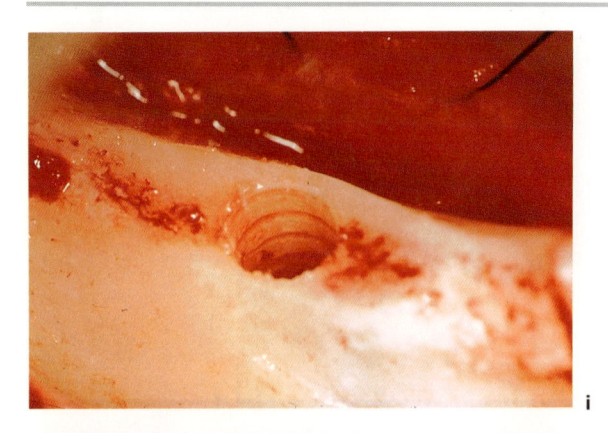

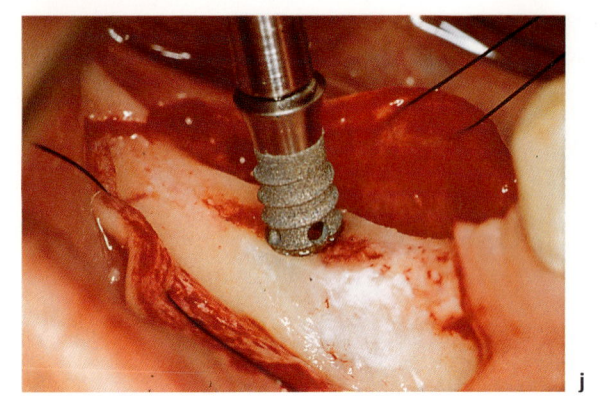

i
j

- **i** Completed implant bed
- **j** Insertion of the HS implant with the inserting device
- **k** The HS implant has excellent stability, and a sufficiently thick bone wall is present buccally
- **l** After placement of a large closure screw, the wound margins are adapted to the implant post without tension, and the wound is closed with interrupted sutures
- **m** Postoperative panoramic radiograph (OPG) showing the long axis of the implant to be in good alignment

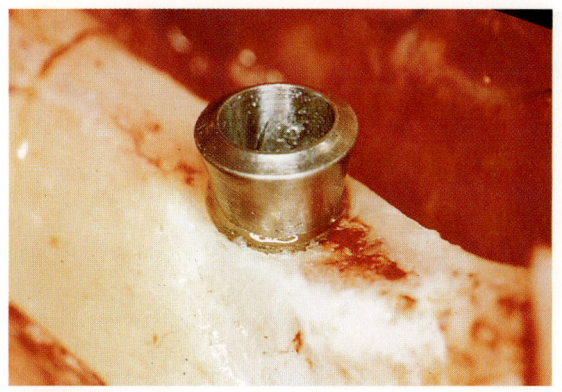

Surgical Procedure for Main Indications 287

k

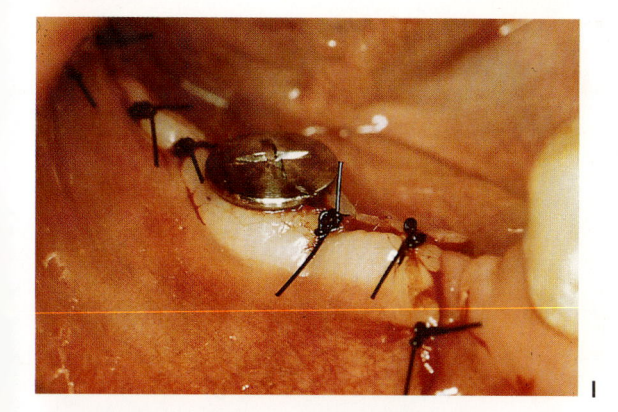

l

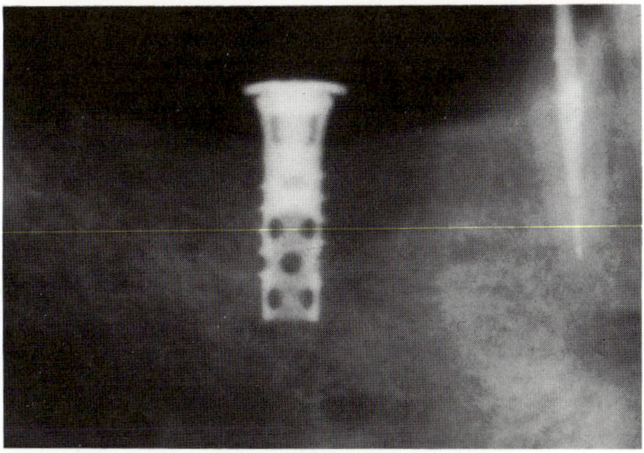

m

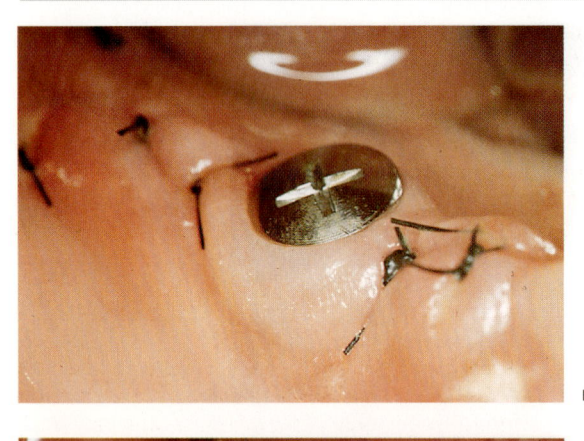

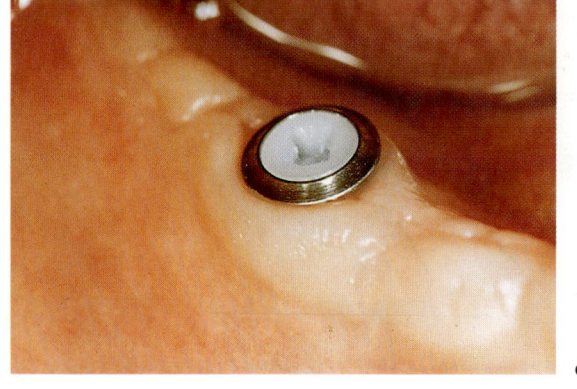

n Clinical status one week following implantation and prior to suture removal
o Clinical appearance 3.5 weeks following implantation. The large closure screw has been replaced with a small one

When the bottom of the bone cavity is reached, increased resistance will be felt and the implant is turned no further. The insertion tool is then removed by loosening the locking screw. At this point, the primary stability of the implant is tested. If bone structure is good and the procedure is carried out precisely, HS implants achieve excellent primary stability. If slight mobility of an implant placed into cancellous bone can be detected, the implant may be tightened with the hand screwdriver after the corresponding healing cap is screwed into place. This final adjustment can achieve primary stability because the hand screwdriver can be removed without extering any destabilizing force on the implant.

The next step is to select the proper closure screw. If, as in the case presented here, the implant has been inserted so that the upper layer of the TPS layer is even with the surface of the bony ridge (Fig. 10.**9k**), the wound margins will almost coincide with the shoulder of the implant. As a rule, the large closure screw is selected in this type of situation, as was previously discussed for totally edentulous mandibles. In cases where the implant is placed 1 mm −2 mm deeper, the implant shoulder will be positioned submucosally, especially in the approximal areas, and for these cases, a transgingival extension healing cap that extends the implant through the soft tissue is chosen (Fig. 10.**10a**). In closing the wound, high prioritiy is given to maintaining the zone of keratinized ridge mucosa that was present preoperatively. When, as in this case, the implant is at some distance from the adjacent natural tooth, the wound margins can be widely mobilized through the extended (in this case distal) incision, allowing them to be closely adapted around the implant post without tension and fixed with interrupted sutures (Fig. 10.**9l**). If the implant is placed directly adjacent to the next tooth, wound closure must be modified somewhat. In this case, the first step is the exact adaptation of the adjacent papilla with a single suture. Next, small releasing incisions are made distal to the implant (Fig. 10.**10b**) so that the wound margins can be rotated and thereby adapted accurately and without tension at the distal aspects of the implant (Fig. 10.**10c**).

Frequently, a minimal gingivectomy must be performed mesial to the implant to achieve precise adaptation of the wound margins. When two implants are inserted directly adjacent to each other in a posteriorly edentulous situation, wound closure is facilitated if the implants are not too close together. If the earlier mentioned distance of 7 mm between centers of implants can be increased to 8 mm, it will leave a broad interimplant space of approximately 3 mm, which will allow for good adaption of the two margins of the wound after they are mobilized and rotated forward from the distal. In this way, a gingivectomy can usually be avoided. A somewhat more difficult situation presents itself when two implants are placed in a tooth-bounded edentulous space (Fig. 10.**11a**). In such a situation, the mesial papilla is first adapted with a single suture (Fig. 10.**11b**). Finally, using a double-edged, sickle-shaped scalpel blade (No. 12b) a wedge-shaped

290 10 Surgical Procedure with ITI Implants

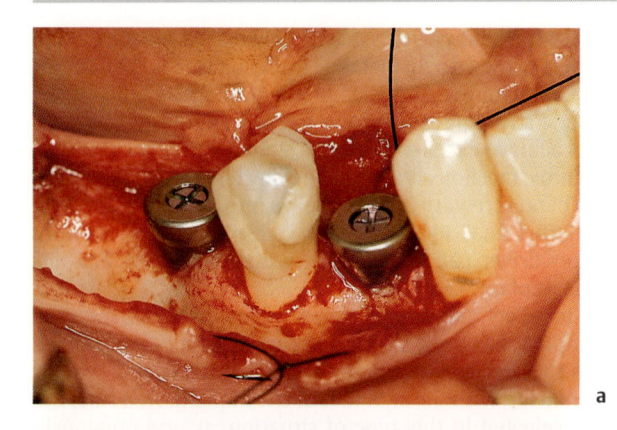

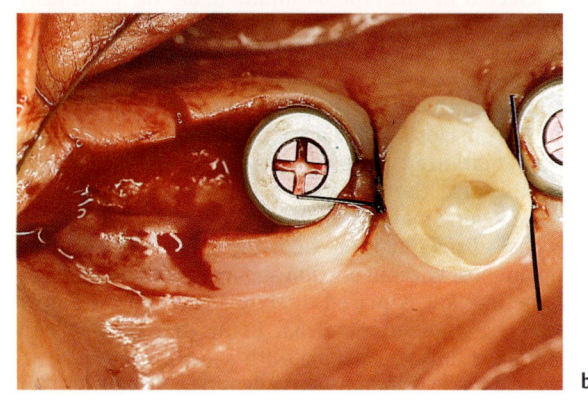

Fig. 10.**10** Implantation of a normal S implant in the lower right molar region and a reduced diameter S implant in the first premolar area
- **a** After insertion of both implants, 2-mm-high transgingival healing caps are screwed into place
- **b** After a single suture is placed through the mesial papilla, two small releasing incisions are made distal to the implant
- **c** The two free edges of the wound are rotated and fixed with interrupted sutures
- **d** Three weeks following implantation, healing is already well advanced
- **e** Three months following implantation, there is no clinical evidence of soft tissue inflammation. The zone of keratinized ridge mucosa has been well preserved

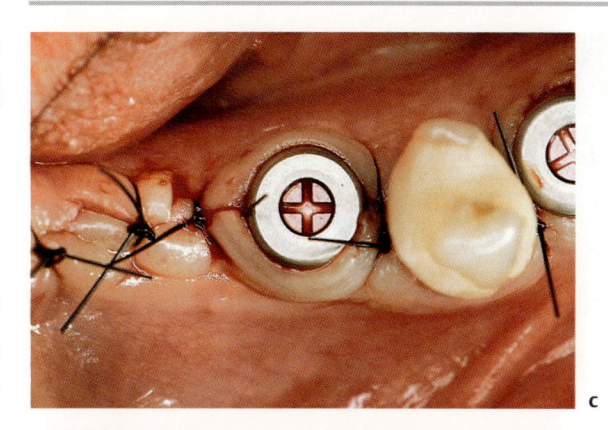

Surgical Procedure for Main Indications

c

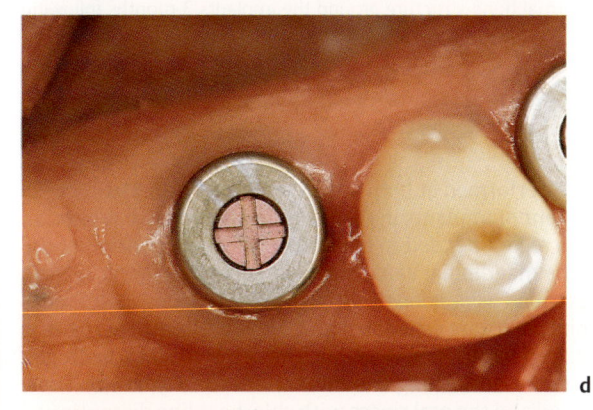

d

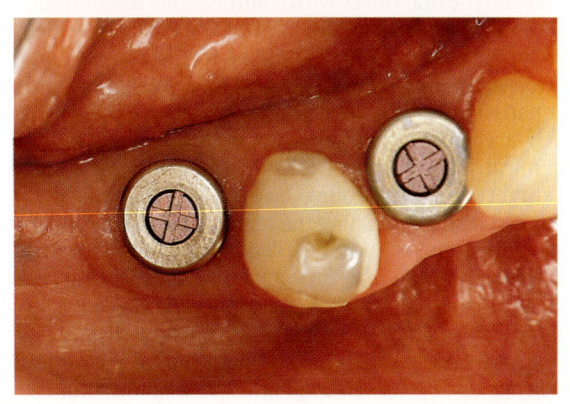

e

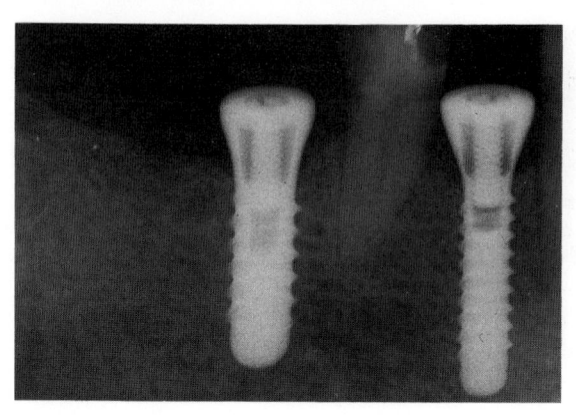

f Radiograph shows normal bone structure around the implants 3 months following implantation

gingivectomy must be performed at both implant posts (Fig. 10.**11d**).

Following placement of implants in the mandibular posterior region, an orthopantomogram is recommended to document the exact position of the implants relative to the mandibular canal for forensic purposes (Fig. 10.**9m**). Medications are prescribed as previously discussed.

Follow-up appointments are scheduled at 7, 14, and 21 days. At the first recall appointment after 7 days, the wound is cleaned with 0.1% hydrogen peroxide, and the progress of healing is monitored. Normally, at this time, the sutures are removed and the oral rinses with chlorhexidine discontinued (Fig. 10.**9n**). In their place, a chlorhexidine gel (Plak Out Gel, 0.2%, Hawe Neos AG, Gentilino, Switzerland) is prescribed to be applied by the patient to the surgical site with a cotton swab three times daily for 1 to 2 weeks. The gel is more pleasant for the patient than the mouthwash because its side effects are less pronounced. If a chlorhexidine gel is not available (e.g., federal approval lacking), chemical plaque control is continued with the rinses. Fourteen days after surgery, wound healing has usually progressed far enough that the patient can resume brushing the areas around the implants with a soft toothbrush. The patient is given detailed instructions on how to use the toothbrush in the area of the implants. At the 21-day checkup, the patient's oral hygiene is evaluated for the first time. If a large closure screw was used, it is now replaced with a small titanium closure screw (Fig. 10.**9o**). The large closure screw must not be replaced too soon, because a certain amount of force is exerted during its removal, and the implant could be loosened from its initial bony anchorage. The transgingival healing caps placed on implants inserted deeper, as outined above, are left in place during the entire healing period (Fig. 10.**10d**). If clinical inspection reveals deposits of soft calculus or chlorhexidine stains on the healing cap, these can be removed with a rubber cup and a fine abrasive paste.

As discussed previously, the duration of the bone healing phase of 3–4 months depends on the bone structure at the implant site (Table **10.5**). If, after the healing phase, the implant meets the criteria for success as outlined in Table 10.**6** (p. 280), the closure screw (healing cap) is removed and an appropriate abutment is selected in accordance with the prosthetic treatment plan. The abutment is inserted using the respective inserting tools (Fig. 10.**10e** and **f**, Fig. 10.**11e–g**). The prosthetic treatment can now be initiated.

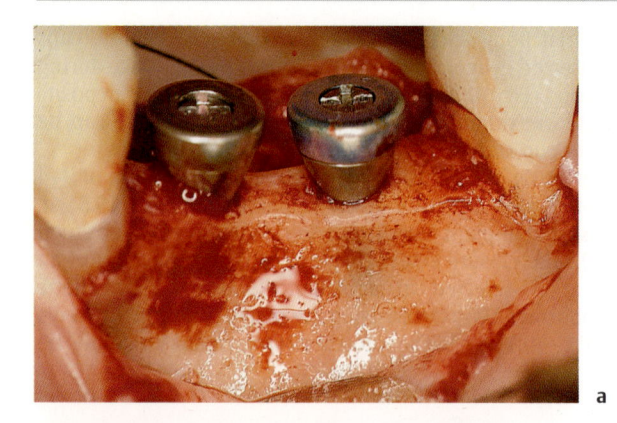

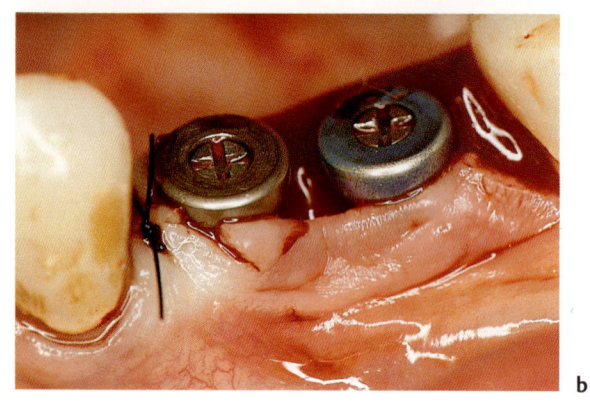

Fig. 10.**11** Edentulous space in the lower left quadrant: treatment with two reduced-diameter S implants
a Two reduced-diameter S implants placed in the premolar region
b After placement of a single suture through the mesial papilla, a wedge of tissue is excised in the region of the implant posts
c Adaptation of the margins following tissue excision
d Wound closure with interrupted sutures
e Clinical appearance 3 months following implant placement

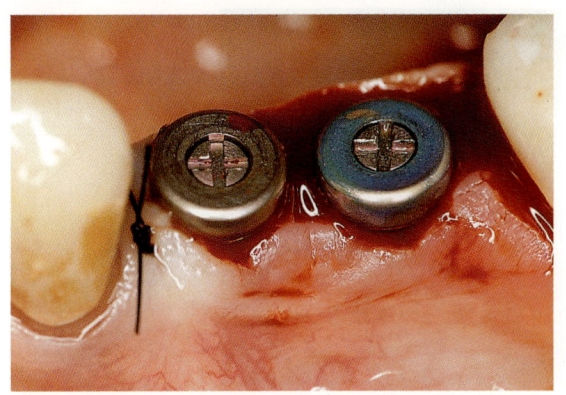

Surgical Procedure for Main Indications 295

c

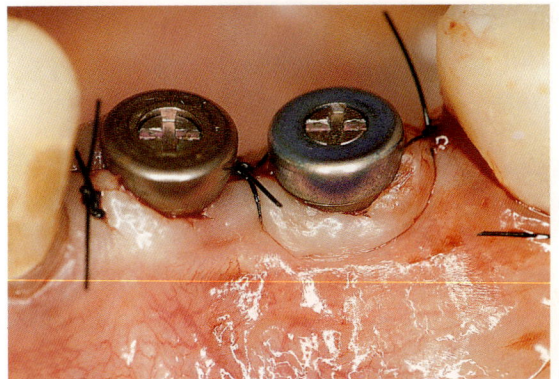

d

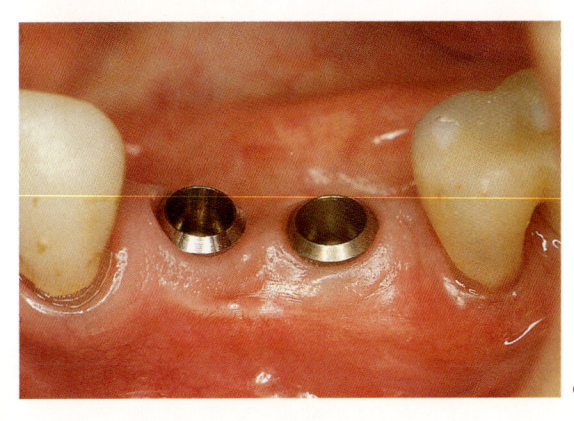

e

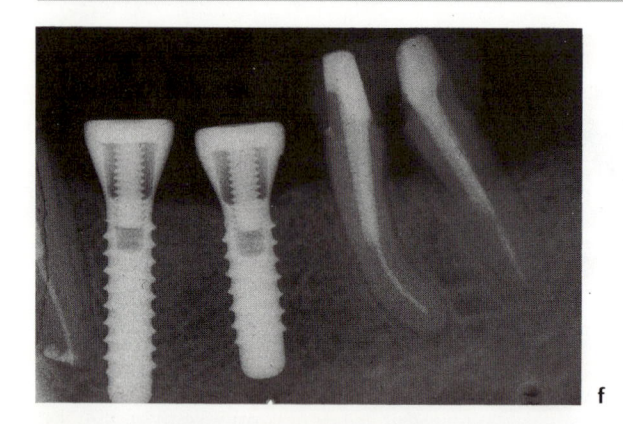

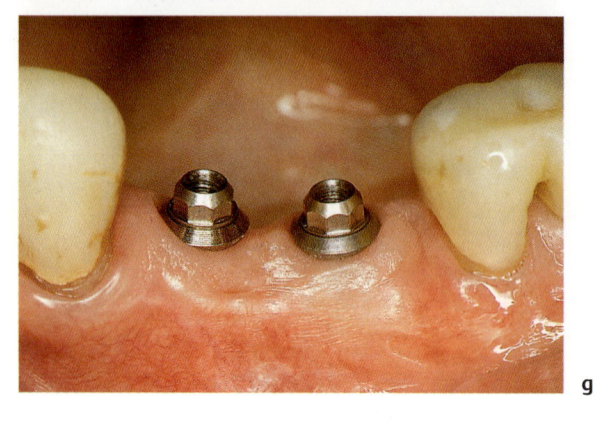

f Follow-up radiograph 3 months after surgery shows normal bone structure
g Insertion of two Octa abutments for a screw-retained restoration

The Single-Tooth Gap in the Maxilla

The single-tooth gap in the maxilla presents a difficult challenge from an esthetic point of view and demands a special surgical technique to meet the increased esthetic demands. To achieve an esthetic implant-borne restoration, several conditions must be established prior to and during surgery (Table **10.7**). First, no metal of the implant shoulder should show after healing, which means that the implant must be inserted deeper into the bone as in standard sites. Furthermore, to ensure that a metal margin does not become visible at a later date, stable soft tissues must be established around the implant to avoid a later gingival recession. In addition to meticulous plaque control for the prevention of peri-implant inflammation, the presence of sufficient bone wall of 1 mm or more on the buccal aspect of the implant is critical for long-term support of the soft tissues. This bone wall is extremely important, and in this regard, no compromises may be made. The contours of the peri-implant mucosa are also important for a good esthetic result. Special attention must be given to maintaining the interdental papillae. As a final point, we must mention the positioning of the implants, which must be optimal not only mesiodistally but also faciolingually to make a suitably esthetic replacement for a single tooth. The Octa System (p. 205) is recommended for this type of restoration. Therefore, it requires close attention to not only placing the implant in the correct position vertically and horizontally, but also to orienting the long axis of the implant so that no difficulty will be encountered with the screw access canal for the future screw-retained crown.

Single-tooth gaps are frequently caused by trauma, which can lead to a collapse of bone in the vestibular region. This makes it difficult to properly align the axis of the implant because the implant must be anchored palatally in the remaining bone. To circumvent possible problems with the orientation of the long axis, the HC implant is frequently chosen because it is available not only in the straight form, but also in a 15° angled version (p. 118). This offers a sophisticated solution to axis angulation problems in most cases. Today, if the direction of the axis must be corrected by more than 15°, the guided bone regeneration (GBR) technique is used to reliably correct fenestration defects in the apical region of an implant that has been placed

Table 10.**7** Surgical requirements for an esthetic implant-borne restoration

- Subgingival implant shoulder (so there will be no visible metal collar)
- Prosthetically favorable implant position (to allow the restoration to have a natural emergence profile)
- Favorable soft tissue contours (to maintain the papillae)
- Stable peri-implant soft tissue (to avoid later gingival recession)

at the correct angulation (p. 322). Even when the width of the alveolar ridge is reduced to less than 5 mm by atrophy on the labial aspect, a sufficiently wide layer of labial bone can still be achieved by using the GBR technique.

The surgery is carried out under local anesthesia. In the maxilla, a highly concentrated local anesthetic solution is used for a profound anesthetic effect (e.g. Ultracain D-S Forte, Hoechst AG, Germany; Carticaine Hydrochloride 4 %). Next, an incision is made slightly palatal to the midcrest (Fig. 10.**12a–c**). Finally, the incision is extended into the sulci of the neighboring teeth toward the vestibule and palate. In standard sites, no vestibular releasing incisions are made. After the two small mucoperiosteal flaps are elevated, they are held back with sutures (Fig. 10.**12d**). The potential implant site is then inspected; the width of the alveolar ridge and the anatomy of the facial surface of the bone under the mucoperiosteal flap is explored with a fine periosteal elevator. In cases where a pronounced undercut is present and a fenestration defect seems likely, it is advisable to make buccal releasing incisions and to reflect a trapezoidal mucoperiosteal flap. This provides an excellent view of the facial surface of the bone, which is necessary in this exceptional situation. As mentioned previously, the implant should be inserted deeper into the bone than usual to keep the implant shoulder submucosally. The vertical position of the implant shoulder is guided by its relation to the adjacent teeth. If the periodontium around adjacent teeth is intact, the implant shoulder should be placed just apical to an imaginary line joining the cementoenamel junctions of the two teeth (Fig. 10.**12e**). If the surface of the ridge lies too far coronally, the ridge must be shortened (Fig. 10.**12f**). As this is done, the approximal bone next to adjacent teeth is not touched, as its presence is important for maintaining the papillae.

Finally, preparation of the implant bed is initated by first marking the center of the selected implant site with the smallest round bur (Fig. 10.**12g**) and then enlarging the hole with the two successively larger round burs (Fig. 10.**12h**). This procedure allows the position of the implant bed to be adjusted in any direction, if necessary. The preparation is continued with the pre-drill, bringing the shoulder about 2 mm deeper into the bone than in standard sites (Fig. 10.**12i**). The final direction of the implant must be established with

Fig. 10.**12** Treatment of a single-tooth gap in the upper right canine region with a HC implant
- **a** Single-tooth space, upper right canine with adjacent teeth that are poorly suited as abutments for a conventional bridge
- **b** Radiographic view of the space and adjacent teeth
- **c** Incision slightly palatal to the midcrest

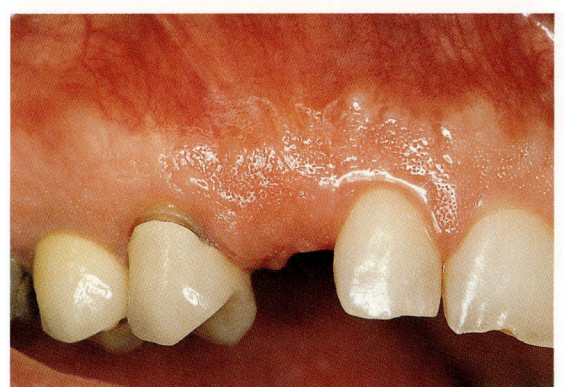

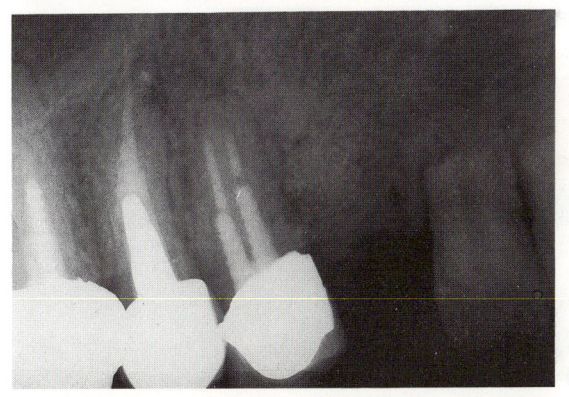

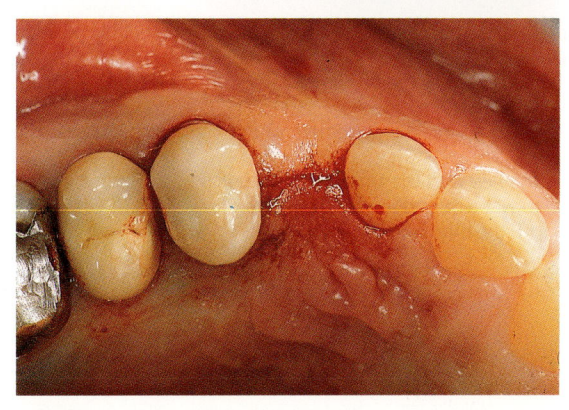

The Single-Tooth Gap in the Maxilla

300 10 Surgical Procedure with ITI Implants

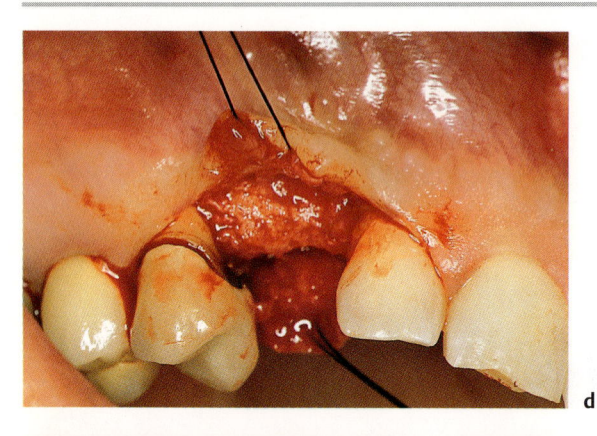

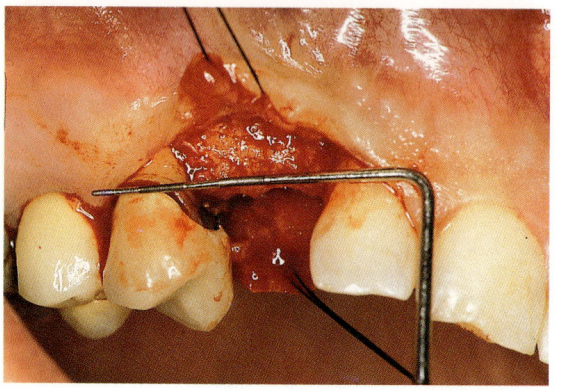

d Two small mucoperiosteal flaps have been reflected and are being held in position with retraction sutures
e A periodontal probe held in line with the cementoenamel junctions of the adjacent teeth determines the reference height
f Reduction of ridge height to permit the placement of the implant shoulder at the correct vertical position
g The implant location is marked with the smallest round bur. The location is slightly too far to the facial and must be moved toward the palate
h Corrected mark made with the third round bur

The Single-Tooth Gap in the Maxilla

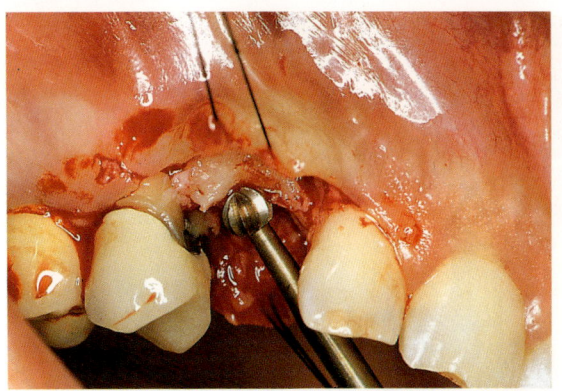

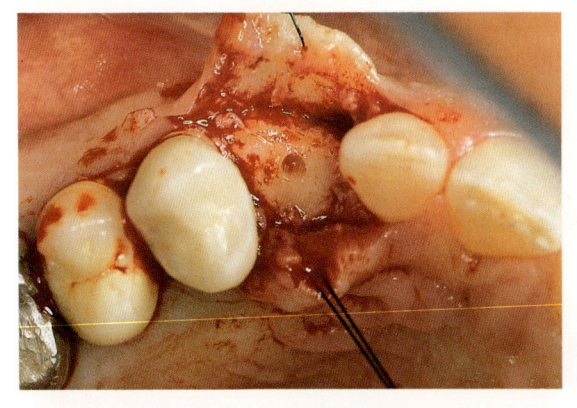

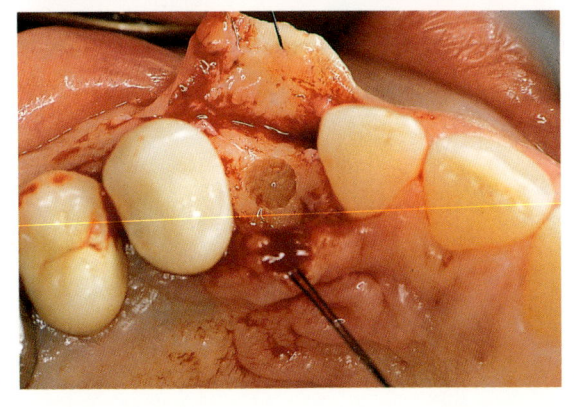

302 10 Surgical Procedure with ITI Implants

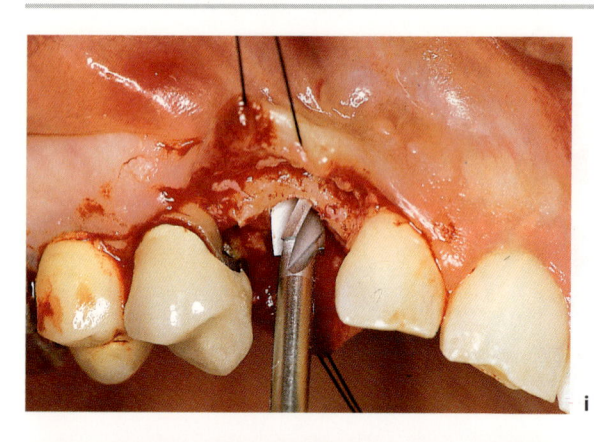

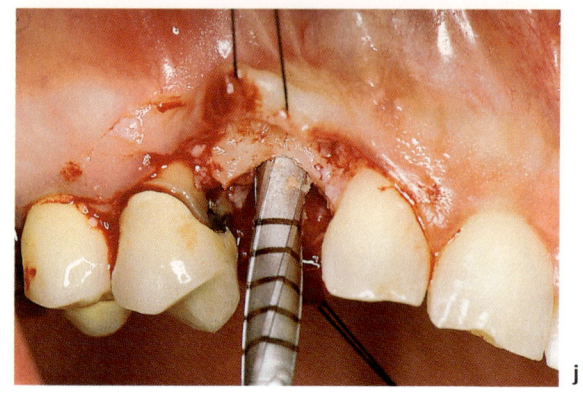

i Preparation with the pre-drill
j Preparation with the trephine mill to a depth of 14 mm. The depth is monitored by the laser-marked rings
k Occlusal view of the implant bed with a well-centered core of bone
l Depth gauge in place (facial view)
m Depth gauge in place (occlusal view)

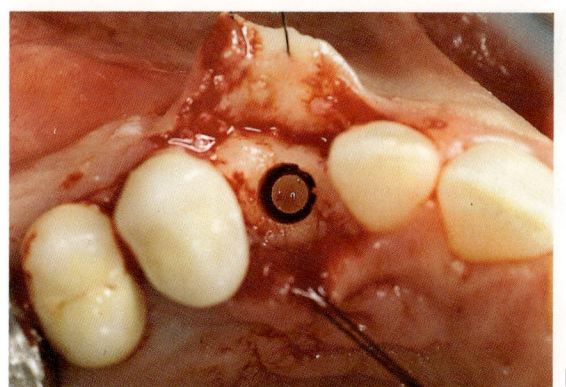

The Single-Tooth Gap in the Maxilla

k

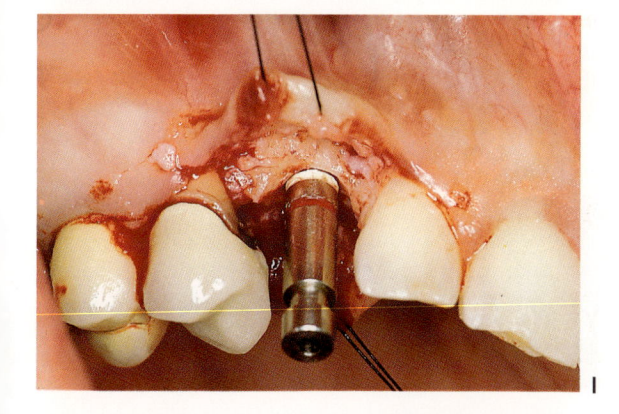

l

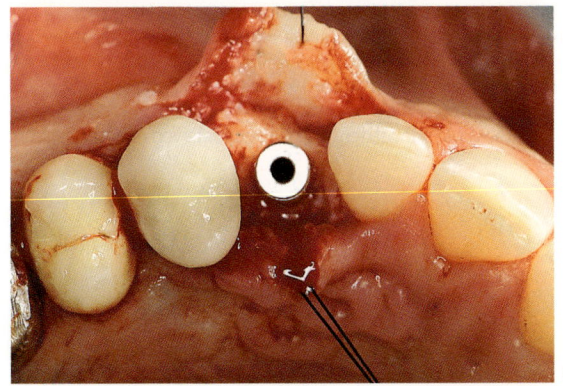

m

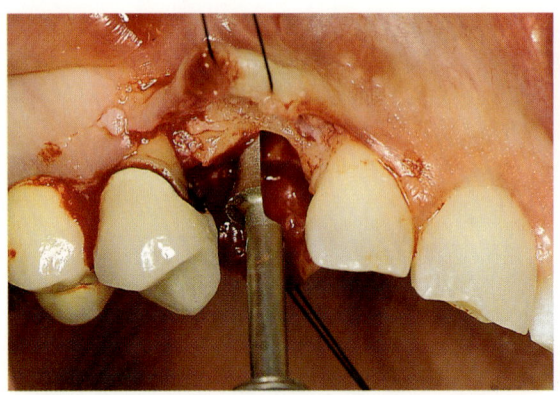

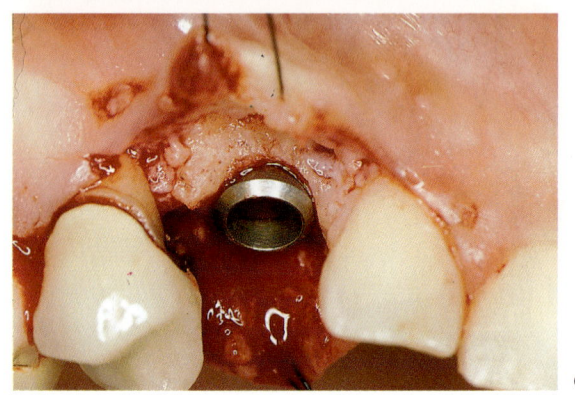

n Preparation the entrance of the cavity with a profile drill (prototype)
o This HC implant has excellent primary stability, and its shoulder lies slightly above the bone crest on the facial aspect
p A 2 mm transgingival healing cap has been placed for the healing phase
q Wound closure with two interrupted sutures
r The existing provisional removable partial denture has been relieved over the implant and reinserted

The Single-Tooth Gap in the Maxilla

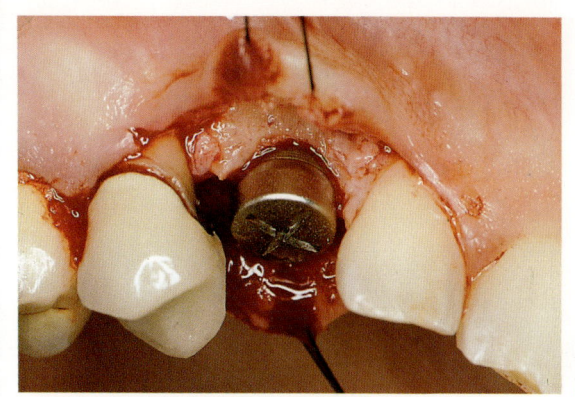

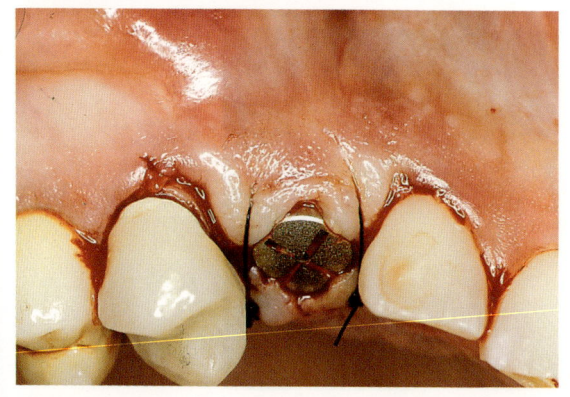

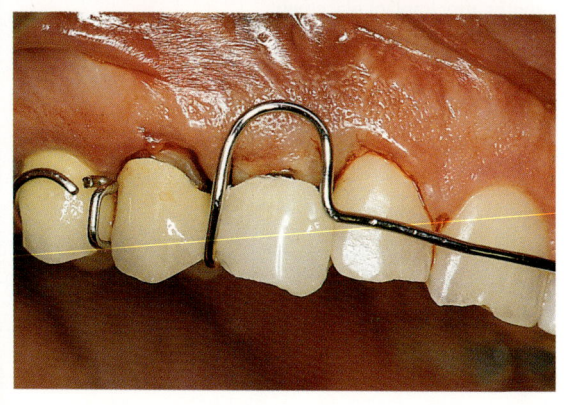

306 10 Surgical Procedure with ITI Implants

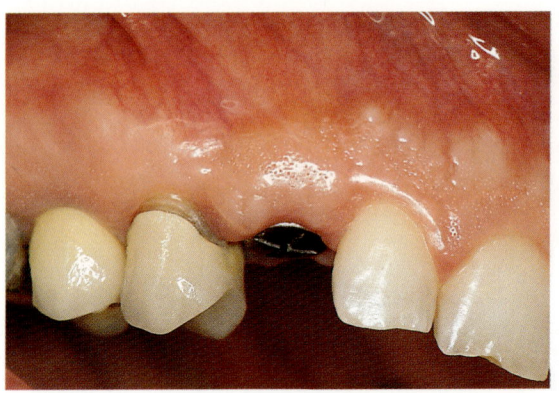

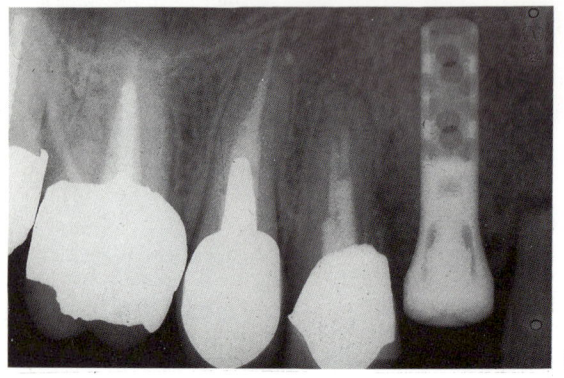

s Clinical appearance 3 months after implant placement
t Radiographic appearance 3 months after implant placement

the pre-drill because any subsequent change of direction can only be made with difficulty. The next step is the preparation with the trephine mill, which is placed approximately 2 mm deeper into the bone than usual (Fig. 10.**12j**). With this technique, it is possible to place the shoulder of the implant in the desired subgingival position. After rinsing the implant bed, the sink depth is measured with the color-coded depth gauge, and at the same time the oro-focial direction of the implant axis is reevaluated (Fig. 10.**12k–m**). This guides the decision of whether a straight or angled HC implant should be used. Because the implant will be inserted deeper into the bone, the entrance of the bone cavity must be slightly beveled with a profile drill (Fig. 10.**12n**). This beveling accommodates the tulip-shaped widening in the shoulder region of the implant, and is easily accomplished. With this final preparation step, the implant bed is completed and is ready to receive the corresponding HC implant. The HC implant is taken directly from its sterile ampoule using the inserting device and pushed into the bone cavity until resistance is distinctly felt from contact of the implant with the walls of the implant bed. The inserting device is removed. Using the insertion mallet, the implant is then carefully driven deeper until it reaches the bottom of the prepared bone cavity. This is immediately recognized by the change in sound. Ideally, the facial aspect of the implant shoulder should be located approximately 1 mm above the bony crest (Fig. 10.**12o**). After primary stability is verified, a transgingival healing cap is screwed into place (Fig. 10.**12p**). Mostly, a 2 mm-high cap is used. During wound closure, special attention is given to maintaining the interdental papillae, as these are of tremendous importance to the esthetic result. Therefore, the papillae are repositioned as precisely as possible and held with interrupted sutures that are not tied too tightly (Fig. 10.**12q**, Fig. 10.**13a** and **b**).

Postoperatively, the existing provisional partial denture is relieved so that there is no direct contact with the surface of the wound (Fig. 10.**12r**). To fasten healing, Solcoseryl Dental Adhesive Paste (Solco Basel AG, CH-4000 Birsfelden, S.) is prescribed to be applied by the patient three times daily for 2 to 3 weeks.

Sutures are removed after 1 week. Additional checkups take place after 14 and 21 days. Patients are recalled again after approximately 2 months for evaluation of the condition of the soft tissue. If it is necessary to improve the contour of the labial mucosa, a gingivoplasty is performed at this time. As a rule, a 3-month healing period is sufficient in single-tooth replacement cases because the bone structure is usually of normal density. Patients are recalled once again after this healing period and evaluated both clinically and radiographically. If this examination indicates successful tissue integration of the implant (Fig. 10.**12s** and **t**) the healing screw is removed and the proper abutment screwed into place (Fig. 10.**13c**). The prosthetic treatment can now be initiated.

Both cases demonstrated (Fig. 10.**12** and 10.**13**) were treated in 1991 and 1992, respectively. Since then, the wound closure technique has been modified to improve the predictability for optimal soft tissue contours. Currently, a semi-submerged healing is preferred with a partial coverage of the healing cap by the buccal wound margin. Details of this technique are presented in a videotape on "Esthetic Implant Dentistry" (Buser + Belser 1995).

Fig. 10.**13** Single-tooth space, upper right first premolar
a Wound closure with two interrupted sutures not tied too tightly
b Precise adaptation of the papillae
c Clinical appearance after completion of the healing phase and placement of an Octa abutment. The papillae have been very well preserved

The Single-Tooth Gap in the Maxilla

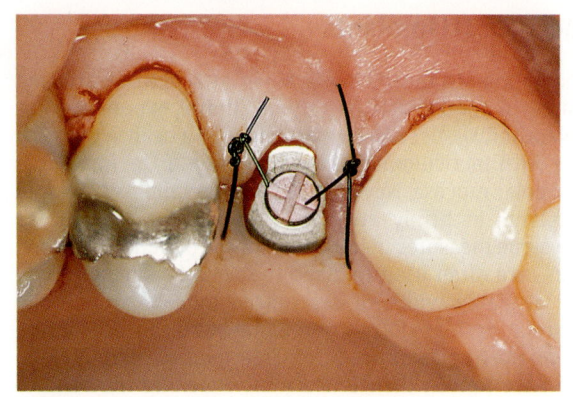

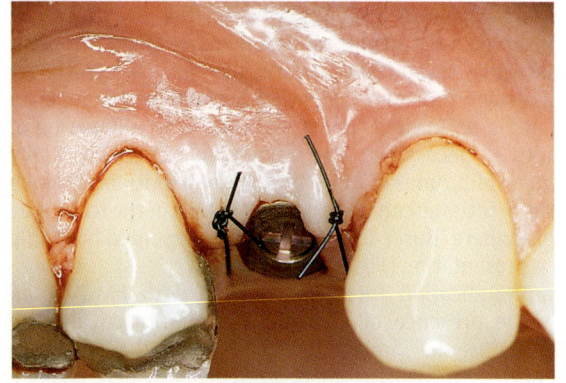

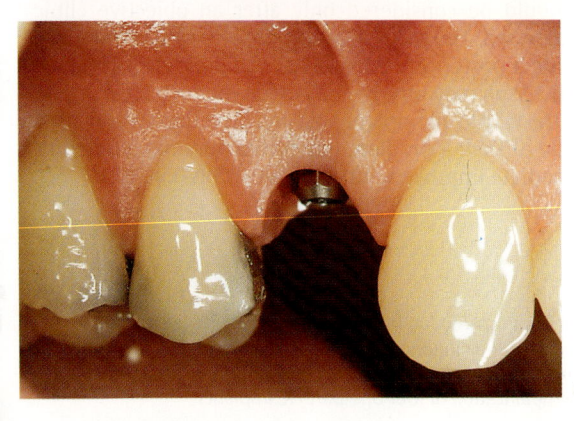

Soft-Tissue Surgery for ITI Implants

The requirement that implants must be placed in attached, keratinized mucosa is still debated in the current literature. Clinical experience has shown that peri-implant soft tissues can be maintained in a healthy state for a long period of time with meticulous oral hygiene, even if the implant is located in movable alveolar mucosa. Nevertheless, it is certainly advantageous to have the implants in firmly attached keratinized ridge mucosa because this makes hygiene measures much easier for the patient. Therefore, plastic-surgical "tricks" are often used to avoid the need for gingivectomy and to maintain the available width of keratinized mucosa around the implant. If anatomic relationships do not permit this, the mucosa can be corrected with appropriate surgical procedures. Free-mucosal grafts (FMG) from the hard palate have proven their efficacy for widening the band of attached keratinized mucosa in both periodontal and preprosthetic surgery. Problems resulting from a zone of attached mucosa that is too narrow (or nonexistent) are observed most frequently around mandibular implants. In the edentulous mandible, the missing keratinized mucosa can be re-established with a two-stage procedure. First, an anterior vestibuloplasty with free-mucosal grafts is performed (in combination with a lowering of the floor of the mouth if necessary). The vestibuloplasty is especially indicated in the presence of fibromas induced by denture irritation, in which case the condition of the soft tissue can be improved. Details of the technique have been published elsewhere (Buser 1987) and will be presented here only in the context of a case presentation (Fig. 10.**14**).

The most common indication for a mucoplasty with FMG in an edentulous patient is the presence of movable, nonkeratinized alveolar mucosa lying directly against the implant in a patient who has difficulty performing good oral hygiene measures. The point to be made here is that a corrective surgery should be considered only after an objective clinical problem has been diagnosed. The surgical procedure will be presented with a clinical case involving a posteriorly edentulous mandible (Fig. 10.**15**). Re-contouring of the soft tissue may also be indicated when a buccal or labial frenulum extends all the way to an implant post and produces tension on the margin. The correction of such a problem represents minimal intervention and produces an immediate improvement of the situation (Fig. 10.**16**).

Fig. 10.**14** Primary soft tissue correction in an edentulous mandible
a An edentulous mandible with an inadequate soft tissue situation
b Condition following an anterior vestibuloplasty with two free mucosal grafts
c Wound closure after implantation of four one-part HC implants

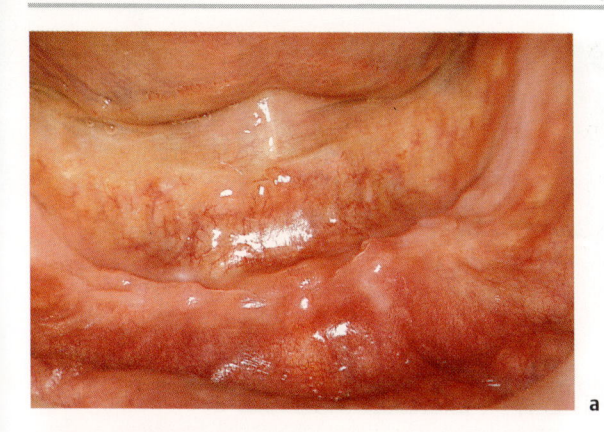

Soft-Tissue Surgery for ITI Implants 311

a

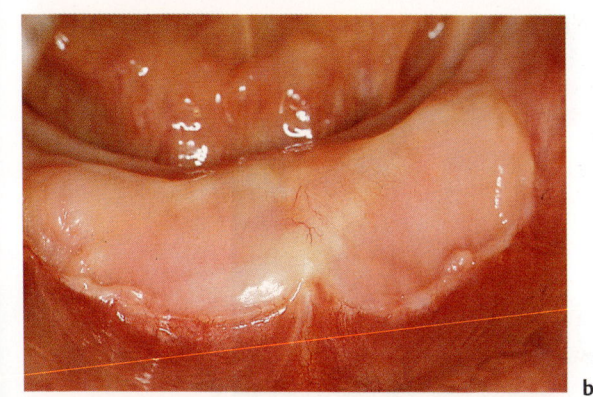

b

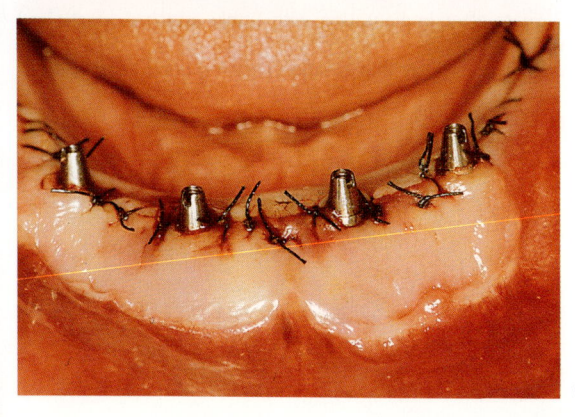

c

312 10 Surgical Procedure with ITI Implants

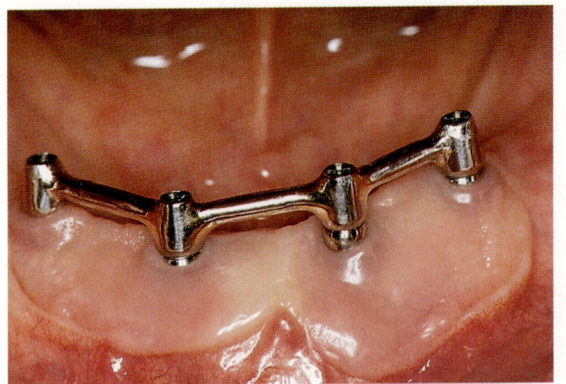

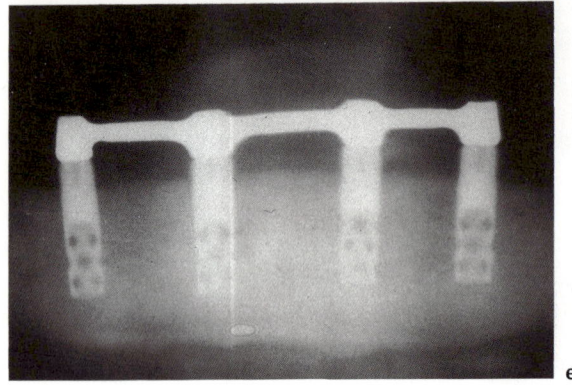

d Clinical appearance 7 years after implantation with firmly attached keratinized mucosa around the implants
e Radiographic appearance 7 years after implantation showing good adaptation of bone

Soft-Tissue Surgery for ITI Implants **313**

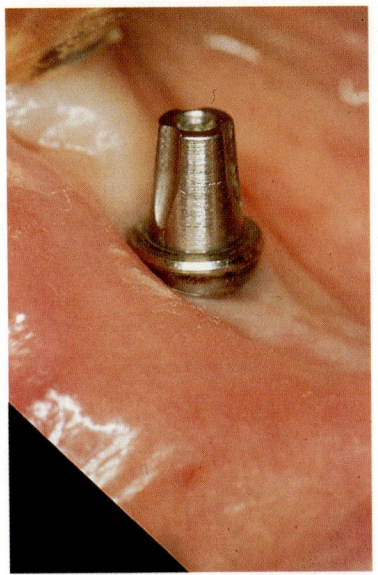

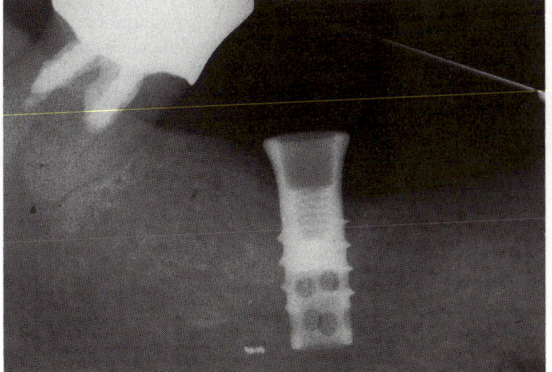

Fig. 10.**15** Recontouring of the mucosa around a HS implant in the lower right first molar area
a Clinical condition 3 months following implantation. Alveolar mucosa extends right up to the implant post, causing the patient problems with daily oral hygiene
b A radiograph made 3 months after implantation shows signs of bone resorption in the crestal area mesially

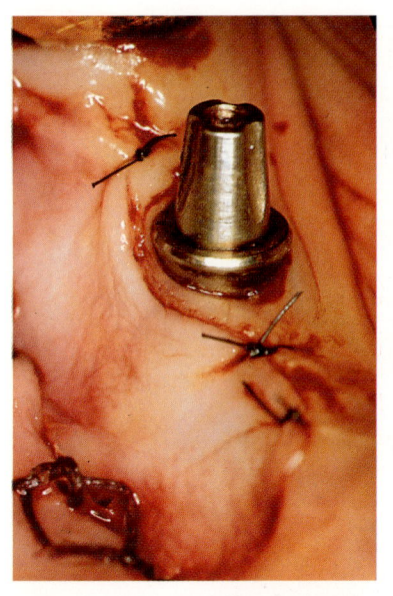

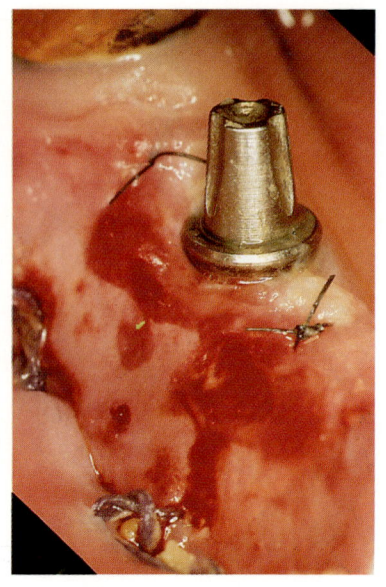

Fig. 10.15c–g

c A 12-mm-wide free-gingival graft has been taken from the palate and sutured over the surgical site

d Appearance 5 days after the corrective surgery

e Clinical appearance 2 months after the operation. The zone of keratinized ridge mucosa has been greatly increased

Soft-Tissue Surgery for ITI Implants 315

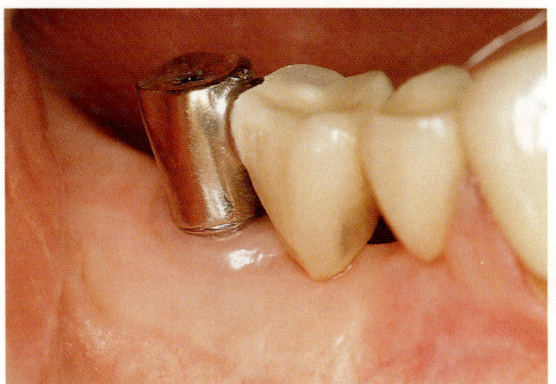

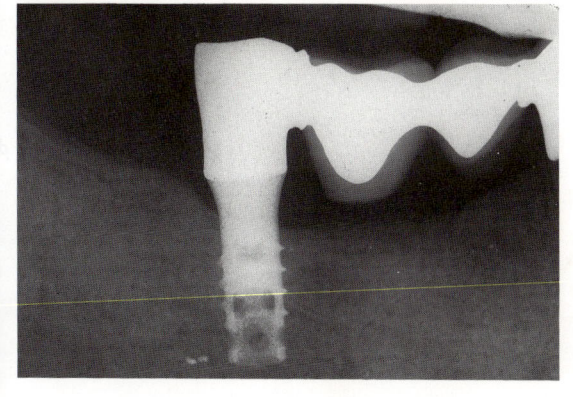

f Clinical appearance 5 years after implantation
g Radiographic appearance 5 years after implantation. The area of bone resorption mesially has been remineralized, and the bone crest level is stable.

316 10 Surgical Procedure with ITI Implants

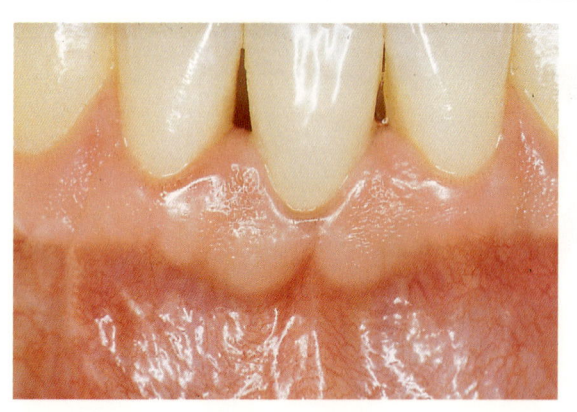

Fig. 10.**16** Corrective soft tissue surgery for high insertion of a labial frenulum near a single-tooth implant replacing the lower left central incisor

a High frenulum insertion labially

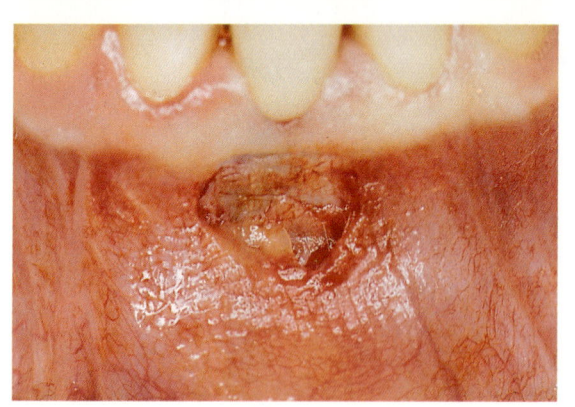

b The muscle fibers have been cut and an epiperiosteal preparation made

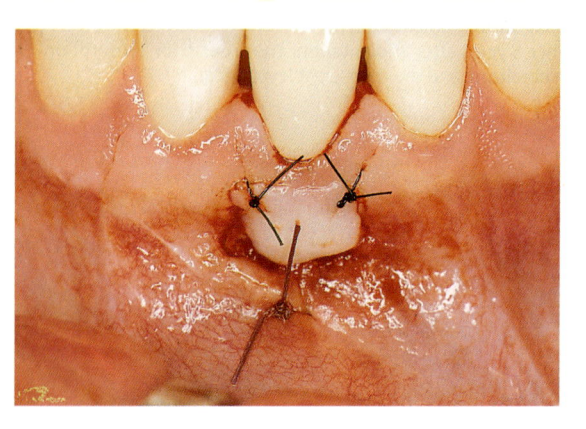

c A small free-mucosal graft has been placed and stabilized with fine sutures

Soft-Tissue Surgery for ITI Implants 317

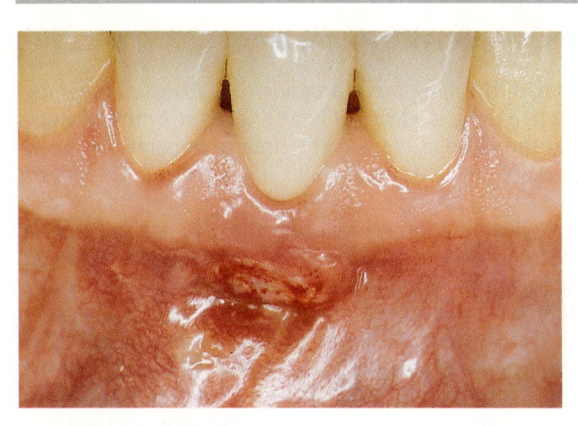

d Appearance 1 week after the transplantation

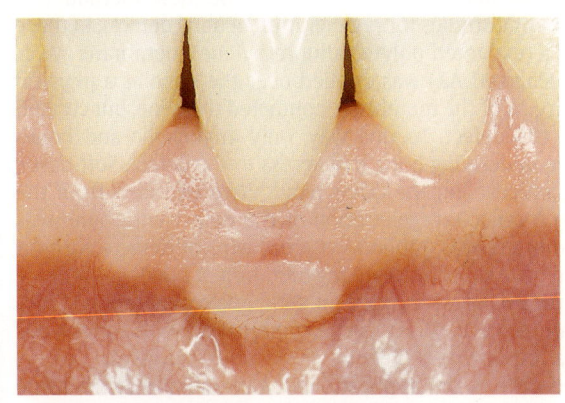

e Appearance 3 months after the procedure

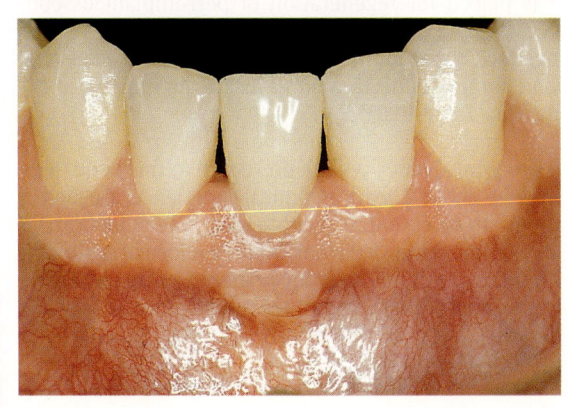

f A wider view of the area with a resin provisional crown on the implant

Use of the GBR Technique with ITI Implants

As previously mentioned, the long-term prognosis of an osseointegrated implant is improved when there is a layer of bone of at least 1 mm thickness around the implant at the alveolar crest at the time of implant placement (Lekholm and co-workers 1986, d'Hoedt 1986, Dietrich and co-workers 1993).

If the preoperative examination reveals that the alveolar ridge is too narrow (less than 5 mm), this deficiency of bone should be corrected through a suitable surgical procedure before the implant is placed. A new surgical technique, which uses alloplastic membranes, has been developed over the past 7 years. This technique is based upon the principle of guided tissue regeneration, which was developed at the beginning of the 1980s for regeneration of the tooth-supporting apparatus in advanced cases of marginal periodontitis (Nyman and co-workers, 1989). This new method was tested next in experimental studies for regeneration of bony defects. In these tests, a bioinert e-PTFE (expanted polytetrafluorethylene) membrane (W. L. Gore and associates, Flagstaff AZ) was applied over the bone as a physical barrier so that the margins of the membrane contacted the bone, but created secluded space over the defect. In this way, only angiogenic and bone-forming cells from the underlying bone had access to the defect. Soft tissue cells of the covering mucosa, on the other hand, were excluded from the regenerative process. A reliable regeneration of the defect with bone was found when the membrane was applied, whereas control defects without membranes exhibited only an incomplete regeneration of bone.

This membrane technique, also called guided bone regeneration (GBR), has been used clinically since 1988. For use in combination with endosseous implants, two applications are possible:
1. A one-stage procedure is the application of a membrane at the same time the implant is placed for regeneration of peri-implant osseous defects (Table 10.**8**).
2. In a two-stage procedure, a membrane is placed for localized ridge augmentation. A second surgery is performed to insert the implant in the newly augmented ridge (Table 10.**9**).

Only two examples of typical cases will be presented in this book (Figs. 10.**17** and 10.**18**). Based upon about 7 years of clinical experience, the factors listed in Table 10.**10** appear to be essential for obtaining predictable results with the GBR technique in implant dentistry. For detailed information on this new technique and its fundamentals, we refer the reader to a comprehensive textbook (Buser and co-workers, 1994), and other publications (Buser and co-workers, 1990, 1992, 1993, 1995a, 1995b, 1996a, 1996b; Schenk et al. 1994).

Use of the GBR Technique with ITI Implants 319

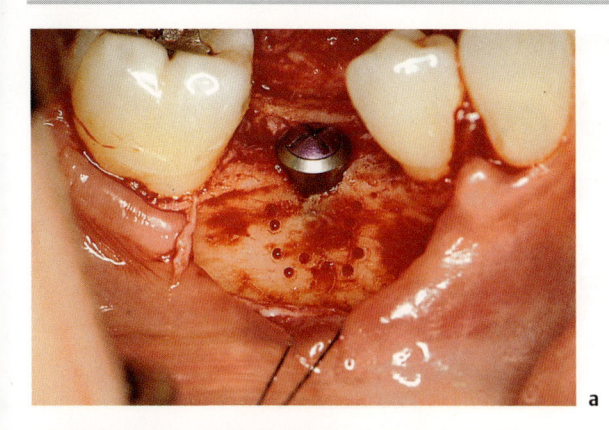

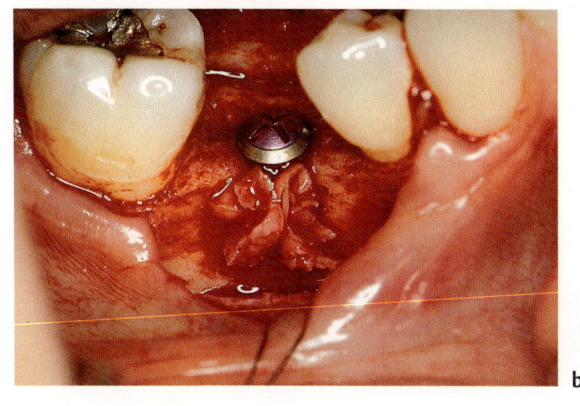

Fig. 10.**17** One-stage procedure for a single-tooth gap in area 29 (ADA numbering system)
a Implantation of an 8-mm HS implant to a depth of approximately 10 mm. There is a thin plate of bone with a buccal dehiscence defect
b Application of autogenous bone grafts to support the membrane

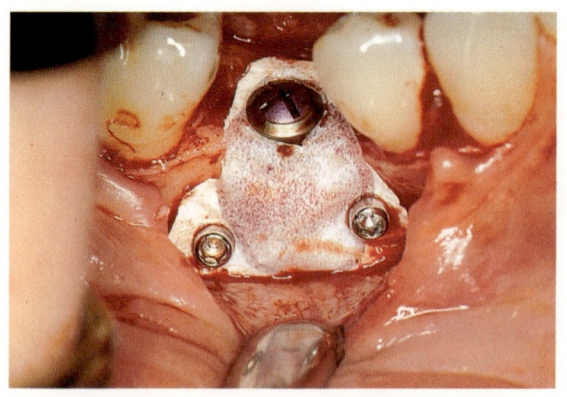

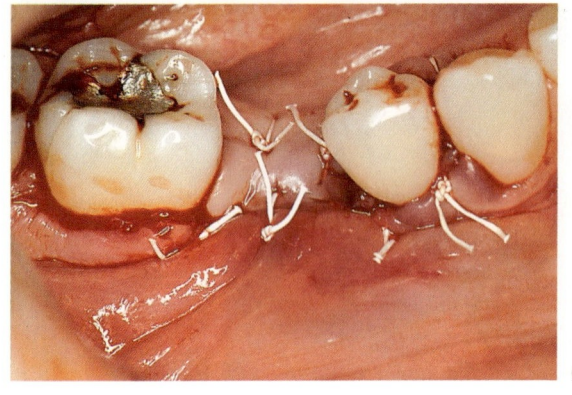

c A GTAM membrane has been applied and secured with two Memfix fixation screws
d Primary closure with Gore-Tex sutures. The implant is covered to protect the membrane from bacterial contamination
e Appearance 6 months after complication-free wound healing
f Condition upon reentry: the membrane and fixation screws can be clearly seen
g The operation has resulted in a broad, thick buccal bone wall. A transgingival healing cap is in place

Use of the GBR Technique with ITI Implants 321

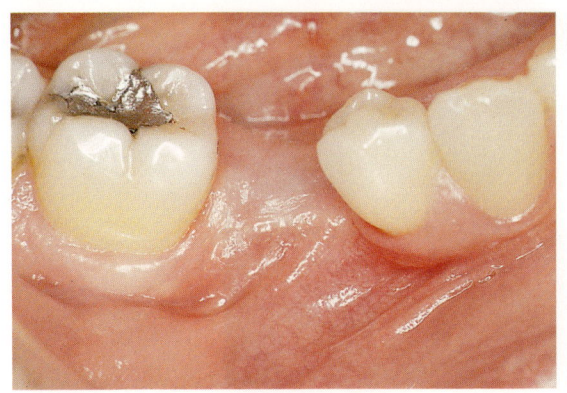

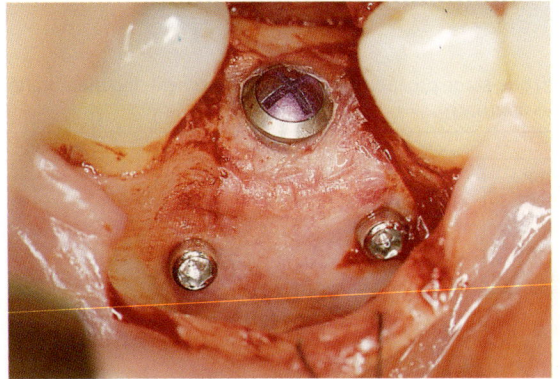

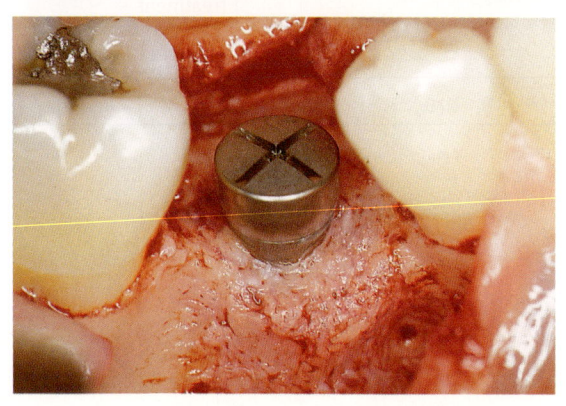

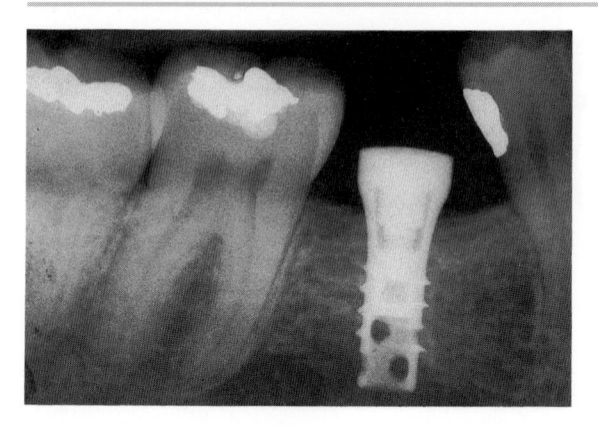

h Radiographic appearance after the second operation

Table 10.**8** Schedule with one-stage procedure for implant placement and membrane application (simultaneous approach)

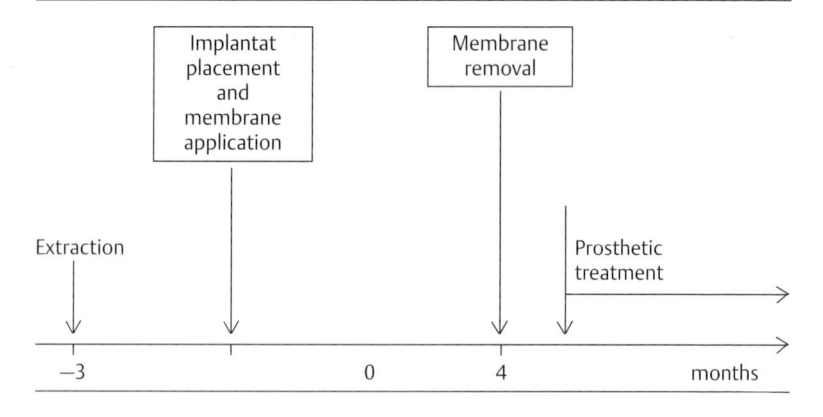

Table 10.9 Schedule with two-stage procedure for membrane application and implant placement (staged approach)

Extraction	Membrane application		Membrane removal and implant placement	Prosthetic treatment
−3	0		7	10 months

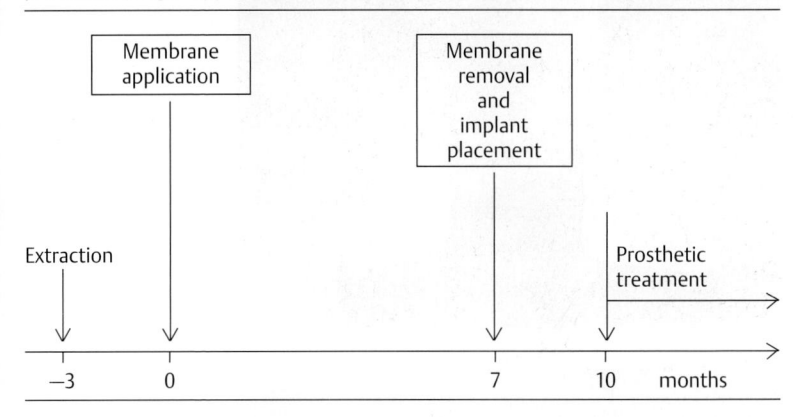

Table 10.10 Surgical requirements for predictable success with the GBR technique

– Utilization of a GTAM membrane
– Close adaptation of the membrane to the bone and stabilization of the membrane with Memfix fixation screws
– Creation and maintenance of a membrane-protected space with an autogenous bone grafts
– Primary wound closure and healing
– Sufficiently long healing period (4–9 months) depending on defect size

324 10 Surgical Procedure with ITI Implants

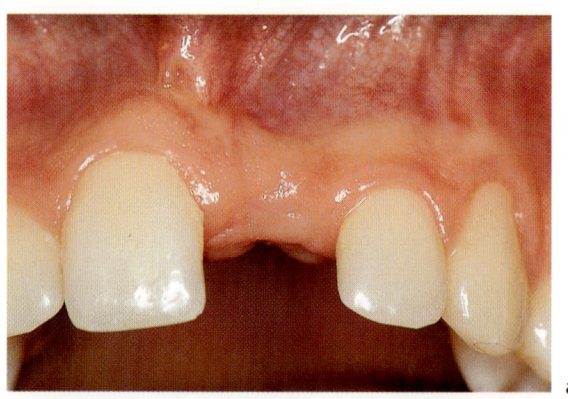

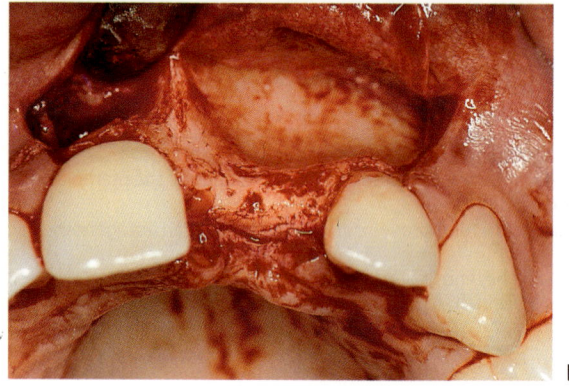

Fig. 10.**18** Staged approach for localized ridge augmentation in the area of a missing upper left central incisor
a Clinical view of the single-tooth space with intact adjacent teeth
b During surgery, an inadequate ridge width and a distinct labial undercut have become apparent
c Placement of an autogenous block graft
d A GTAM membrane has been applied and fixed with a Memfix fixation screw
e Primary wound closure with Gore-Tex sutures

Use of the GBR Technique with ITI Implants

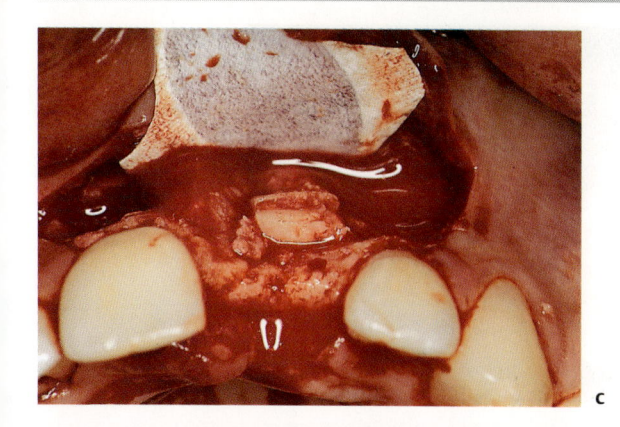

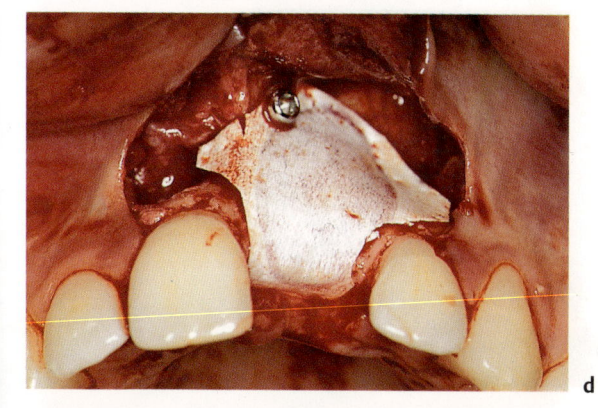

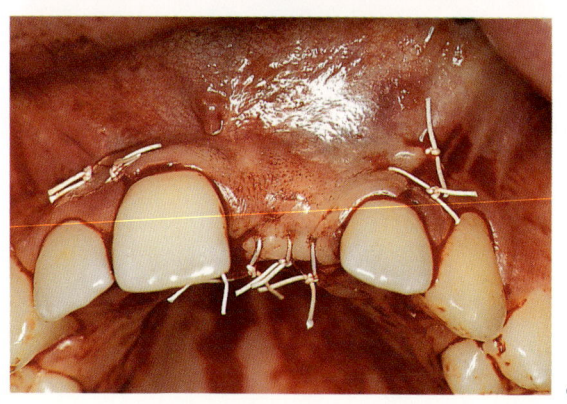

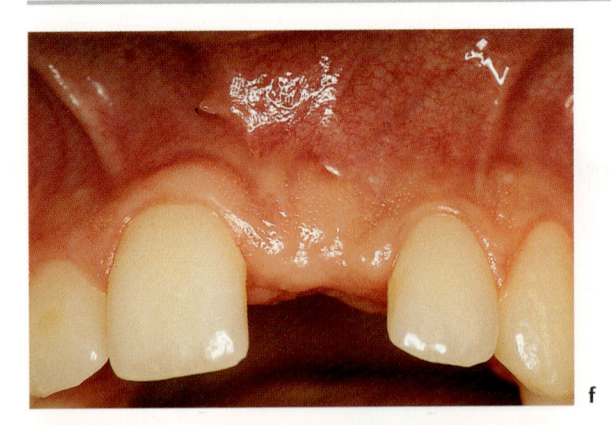

f Condition after 9 months of uncomplicated healing
g Appearance at reentry with the membrane in place
h The augmentation procedure has resulted in a ridge width of more than 7 mm
i Status after insertion of a HC implant with a transgingival healing cap
j Wound closure with interrupted sutures

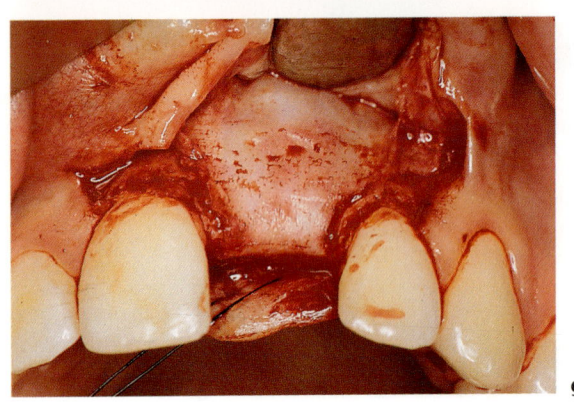

Use of the GBR Technique with ITI Implants

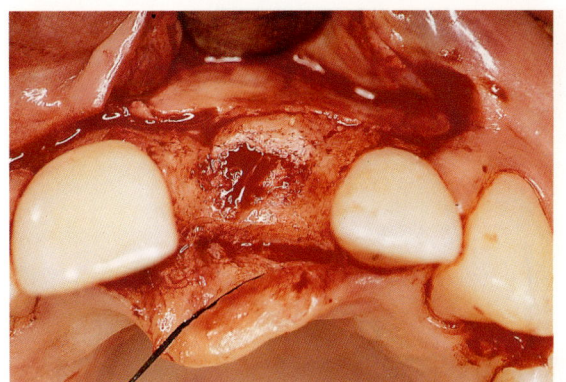

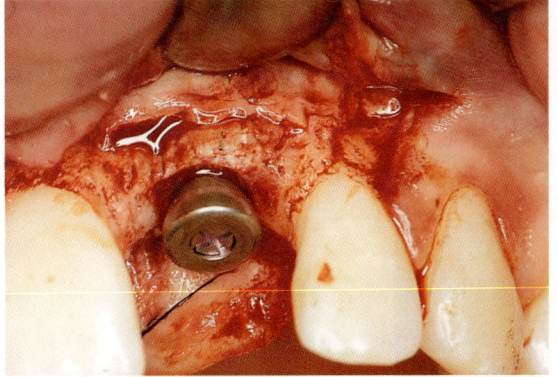

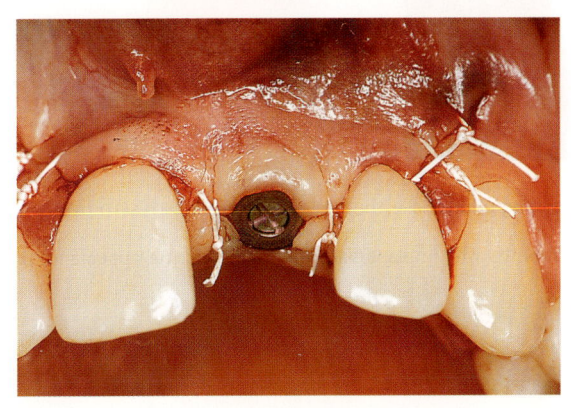

328 10 Surgical Procedure with ITI Implants

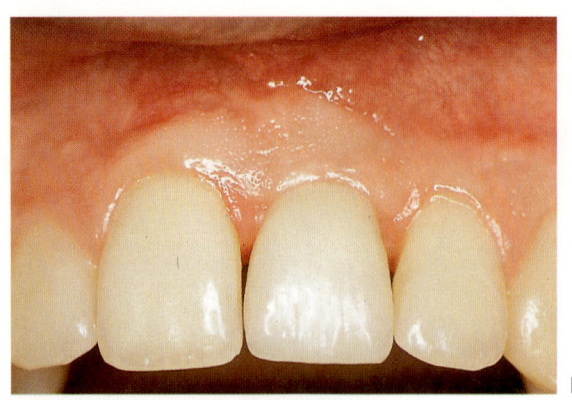

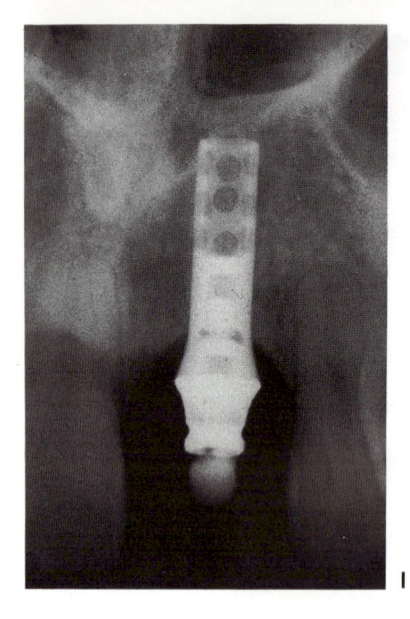

k After conclusion of the integration phase, the implant is fitted with a resin provisional crown
l A radiograph made 6 months after implant placement shows normal appearance of bone

References

Buser, D.: Die Vestibulumplastik mit freien Schleimhauttransplantaten bei Implantaten im zahnlosen Unterkiefer – Operationsmethode und vorläufige Ergebnisse. Schweiz. Mschr. Zahnmed. 97 (1987) 766

Buser, D., H. P. Weber, U. Brägger: The treatment of partially edentulous patients with ITI hollow-screw implants: Presurgical evaluation and surgical procedures. Int. J. oral. max.-fac. Implants. 5 (1990) 165–174

Buser, D., U. Brägger, N. P. Lang, S. Nyman: Regeneration and enlargement of jaw bone using guided tissue regeneration. Clin. Oral. Impl. Res. 1 (1990) 22–32

Buser, D., H. P. Hirt, K. Dula, H. Berthold: GBR – Technique/Implant Dentistry. Simultaneous application of barrier membranes around implants with periimplant bone defects. Schw. Monatsschr. Zahnmed. 102 (1992) 1491–1501

Buser, D., K. Dula, U. Belser, H. P. et al.: Localized ridge augmentation using guided bone regeneration. I. Surgical procedure in the maxilla. Int J Periodont Rest Dent 13 (1993) 29–45

Buser, D., C. Dahlin, R. K. Schenk (Eds.): Guided Bone Regeneration in Implant Dentistry. Quintessence Publishing, Berlin, Chicago, Tokyo (1994)

Buser, D., K. Dula, U. Belser, et al.: Localized ridge augmentation using guided bone regeneration. II Surgical procedure in the mandible. Int J Periodont Rest Dent 15 (1995a) 13–29

Buser, D., J. Ruskin, F. Higginbottom, et al.: Osseointegration of titanium implants in bone regenerated in membrane-protected defects. A histologic study in the canine mandible. Int. J. Oral Maxillofac. Implants 10 (1995b) 666–681

Buser, D., K. Dula, H. P. Hirt, R. K. Schenk: Lateral ridge augmentation using autografts and e-PTFE membranes. A clinical study in 40 partially edentulous patients. J. Oral Maxillofac. Surg. (1996a) in press.

Buser, D., K. Dula, N. P. Lang, S. Nymann: Longterm stability of osseointegrated implants in bone regenerated with a membrane technique. 5-year results of a prospective study with 12 implants. Clin. Oral. Impl. Res. (1996b) in press.

Dietrich, U., R. Lipphold, Th. Dirmeier, N. Behneke, W. Wagner: Statistische Ergebnisse zur Implantatprognose am Beispiel von 2017 IMZ-Implantaten unterschiedlicher Indikation der letzten 13 Jahre. Z. zahnärztl. Implantol. 9 (1993) 9–18

d'Hoedt, B.: 10 Jahre Tübinger Implantat aus Frialit – Eine Zwischenauswertung der Implantatdatei. Z. zahnärztl. Implantol. 2 (1986) 6

Hardt, N., G. W. Paulus: Vestibulumplastik im Oberkiefer mit palatinalen Spaltschleimhaut-Transplantaten. Dtsch. zahnärztl. Z. 38 (1983) 785–789

Krekeler, G.: Parodontale Probleme am Implantatpfeiler. Schweiz. Mschr. Zahnmed. 95 (1985) 847–852

Krekeler, G., W. Schilli, H. Geiger: Das TPS-Implantat, ein zuverlässiges Retentionselement. Z. zahnärztl. Implantol. 6 (1991) 229–234

Ledermann, Ph.: Kompendium des TPS-Schraubenimplantates im zahnlosen Unterkiefer. Quintessenz, Berlin 1986

Lekholm, U., R. Adell, J. Lindhe et al.: Marginal tissue reactions at osseointegrated titanium fixtures. (II) A cross-sectional retrospective study. Int. J. Oral. max.-fac. Surg. 15 (1986) 53–61

Nyman, S., J. Lindhe, T. Karring: Reattachment-new attachment. In Lindhe, J.: Textbook of clinical periodontology. 2nd edition. Copenhagen, Munksgard 1989 (S. 450–476)

Schenk, R. K., D. Buser, W. R. Hardwick, C. Dahlin: Healing pattern of bone regeneration in membrane-protected defects. A histologic study in the canine mandible. Int. J. Oral. Maxillofac. Implants 9 (1994) 13–29

11 Overdentures Supported by ITI Implants

R. Mericske-Stern

Patient Selection (Indications and Contraindications)

An individual's psychological reaction to the loss of teeth or to becoming totally edentulous is determined largely by his or her cultural background and social group affiliation. The success of primary and secondary measures to prevent caries and periodontitis in the last 20 years has led to a significant reduction in the loss of teeth. The evolution of better restorative methods and reparative techniques has resulted in higher patient expectations regarding chewing comfort, function, cosmetics, and aesthetics. The overall effect of all these developments is evidenced by the fact that today, edentulousness is more prevalent in people of advanced age. This tendency is further reinforced by the increasing life expectancy. Therefore, we are more often faced with patients who became totally edentulous only in

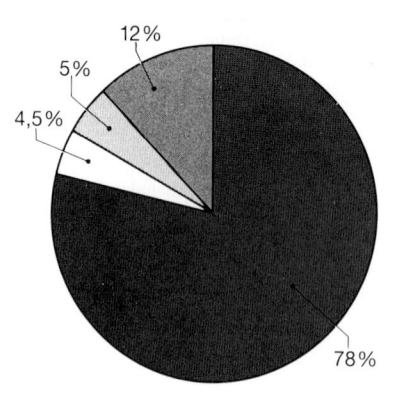

Fig. 11.**1** Percentages of various types of implant-supported restorations utilized in patients over 65 years of age. The implant-supported overdenture is the most frequently used type of prosthesis

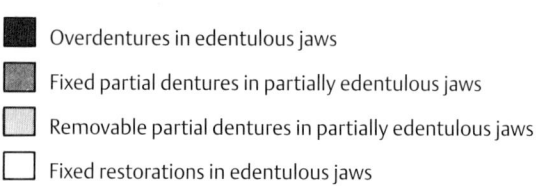

- Overdentures in edentulous jaws
- Fixed partial dentures in partially edentulous jaws
- Removable partial dentures in partially edentulous jaws
- Fixed restorations in edentulous jaws

advanced stages of their life. On the other hand, there are and always will be patients who, for one reason or another, became edentulous while still young. These patients have been able to function for a lifetime with complete dentures with relatively few problems. They have either long ago forgotten the experience of chewing comfortably with their own natural teeth, or it was never implanted in their consciousness. When patients becomes endentulous, in their old age, when skill and motor abilities are waning, they become aware of the denture as a foreign body, and the wearing of complete dentures is experienced as a disturbing limitation of comfort. It is also striking that a high percentage of complaints are associated with lower dentures. Thus, there are two groups of edentulous patients who can profit from simple implant procedures:
1. Denture wearers who lost their last teeth at advanced age and are not able to adapt well to complete dentures
2. Long-time denture wearers who have gradually lost the ability to cope easily with complete dentures

Today, both of these groups represent candidates for implant-supported overdentures.

Figure 11.1 shows the percentages of the various types of implant-supported restorations in patients over age 65 treated at the Clinic for Dental Prosthetics in Bern (Stand 1992).

Indications

It is suggested that the decision to use implants should be based primarily on strict selection criteria related to both general (patient specific) and local (quantity and quality of bone) factors.

Specific criteria used for patient selection are:
– Adequate age;
– High interest and motivation on the part of the patient;
– Good general health;
– Good quality and quantity of bone;
– Long-term cooperation for maintenance care;
– Economic situation.

These selection criteria are important prerequisites in treatment planning for patients with high expectations and demands regarding the prosthetic restoration, i. e., cases that will require a long treatment time and extensive preparatory phase, high cosmetic and esthetic demands that must be met, and technical problems that are difficult to solve.

These selection criteria, however, would often exclude older edentulous patients. The indications must be enlarged and applied selectively on an individual basis.

Indications for Implant-Supported Overdentures

1. Atrophic ridge, therefore objective improvement cannot be expected by fabrication of new conventional dentures.
2. Edentulous patients who are no longer able to wear complete dentures.
3. The patient is basically satisfied with complete dentures but wants the security of increased retention (psychological and social aspects).
4. The patient's general health allows only a short surgical procedure.
5. The residual ridge will permit the insertion of at least two implants.
6. The patient has no exaggerated, unrealistic expections for success.
7. The patient has worn removable dentures previously.
8. Economics: The patient is either unwilling or unable to bear the expense of a fixed reconstruction.

The patient's financial situation has an influence on the formulation of a treatment plan for implant-supported overdentures and in most cases must be taken into account.

A few comments on the previously listed indications:
1: Clinical experience indicates that placement of implants is preferable to all other surgical procedures for improving the ridge.
2: Elderly, long-term denture wearers lose their ability to function well with dentures because of impaired motor skills.
If, in addition, the remaining few natural teeth should be lost after the patient has become elderly, the chances for rapid, successful adaptation to complete dentures is very slim. In the future, we will be confronted with this even more frequently.
3: Satisfied denture wearers who accept a removable prosthesis as the final treatment should not be convinced to have fixed reconstruction. Changes in the morphology of the intraoral space can lead to significant impairment of speech and mastication. This type of patient will consider the removable denture with the additional retention provided by implants to be the optimum in comfort.
4: The general condition of a high percentage of older patients is impaired. It is important that the patient believes him or herself capable of undergoing surgery. This is especially true in cases of cardiovascular disease. Consideration must be given to the patient's momentary sense of well-being for a surgical operation, and stressful situations must be avoided as far as possible. Consultation with the patient's physician, preferably in written form, is the most reasonable solution, and will the concerned patient. Long-term planning is neither reasonable nor possible with aged, health-impaired patients. The surgical operation must take place soon after the planning, at a time when the general health condition of the patient allows it, and should be of short duration.

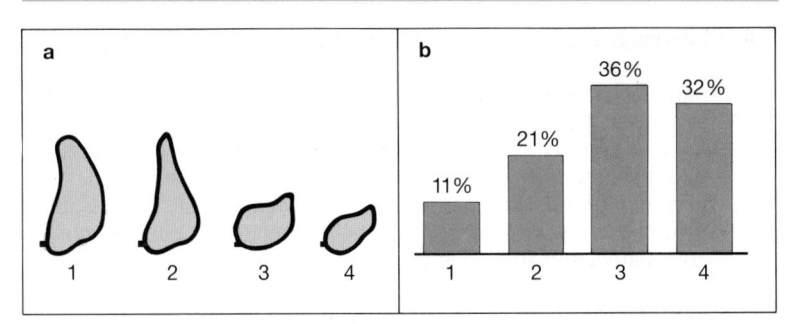

Fig. 11.**2a** Classification of degrees of atrophy of the mandible, adapted from Atwood and co-workers. Only four of their six groups are represented here:
1 *High, well rounded;* slight atrophy of the alveolar ridge, and bone height is only slightly reduced.
2 *Knife-edge;* advanced atrophy, predominantly in the faciolingual dimension with a narrow ridge. Often unfavorable for implantation in spite of the bone height.
3 *Low, well rounded;* more advanced atrophy of the alveolar ridge with severe reduction of bone height. Usually a favorable configuration for implantation.
4 *Depressed;* total resorption of the alveolar ridge with advanced atrophy in all dimensions and greatly reduced bone mass. Often unfavorable for implantation.

b Distribution of the classes of atrophy (1–4) by percentage

5: There are no exceptions to the requirement that the implant be surrounded by an adequate layer of healthy bone, both circumferentially and vertically. Procedures for building up the alveolar ridge (such as the conventional technique of bone grafting or the newer method of guided bone augmentation by the use of membranes) exist, and used in combination with implants, are very promising. However, they are seldom used in older edentulous patients for the reasons mentioned above. So-called clinically "poor ridge conditions" do not always imply an unfavorable ridge form. Often, resorption up to grade three or four is preferable to grade two resorpiton. Experience over the past 9 years indicates that it is not so much the lack of ridge height, but rather the form of atrophy that causes problems (Fig. 11.**2a** and **b**).

6: Patients should be told that there will always be some movement with any removable denture. Aesthetic conflicts rarely occur and can usually be resolved because the complete denture allows a certain amount of freedom in setting the teeth. The denture base compensates for the loss of alveolar bone and provides support for the lips and cheeks. The complete denture wearer, no longer accustomed to cleaning the natural teeth, must not underestimate the importance of daily home care necessary for implants.

7: The prognosis is favorable if the patient has already had experience with wearing a removable denture, regardless of whether it was a partial denture, complete denture, or overdenture. The patient will not be confronting an entirely new situation with the insertion of an implant-supported overdenture. However, the transition to the edentulous condition is very difficult for patients when the natural dentition or fixed restorations are lost suddenly due to advanced periodontal disease or caries. When the need for complete dentures is anticipated, implants can be recommended as an aid to adaptation.

Patient selection for implant-supported overdentures is best established on the basis of the following exclusion criteria:

Exclusion Criteria

1. Reduced intellectual capacity to the point that communication is difficult or impossible.
2. Mental disorders or unresolved emotional problems.
3. Abuse of medications and drugs.
4. Inadequate bone substance for placement of at least two implants.
5. Systemic conditions that are absolute contraindications to any surgical procedure.

There is no generally binding treatment protocol to be observed, as with patients who have specific medical problems, since specific measures have to be taken individually. The oral surgical procedure is not different from other surgical procedures that are carried out on older patients in regard, for example, to anesthesia, duration of treatment, analgesics, antibiotics, and the healing phase.

The major risk factor during surgery is cardiovascular disease, which can suddenly cause problems, especially during a stressful situation. It bears no direct relationship to implants; however, since dental implantation is still regarded as an elective surgical procedure, all risk factors should be considered carefully and, as far as possible, eliminated.

General medical contraindications that are unfavorable for the surgery and healing phase, and especially for the long-term prognosis, are listed below:

Absolute

- Chemotherapy
- Uncontrolled metabolic disorders
- Long-term antibiotic therapy
- Long-term steroid therapy
- Immunosupression
- Intolerance of adrenaline in local anesthetics

Relative

- Diabetes
- Prior radiation therapy
- Anticoagulation therapy

Table 11.1 gives the percentage distribution of general medical conditions detected prior to surgery in approximately 65% of all patients treated with implant-supported overdentures in edentulous mandibles (1992 figures).

Table 11.1 Various medical conditions. These were found in 65% of patients wearing implant-born overdentures

Cardiorascular system	61%	**Rheumatic disease**	9%
– hypertension		– hip joint surgery	
– heart attack		– lameness	
– pacemaker		– impaired manual dexterity	
– coronary bypass			
– thrombosis, embolism		**Malignant tumors / cancer**	7%
– cerebrovascular insult		– oral	
– anticoagulant therapy		– other body areas	
		– radiation therapy	
Respiratory system	8%		
– asthma		**Parkinson's disease**	2%
Diabetes	8%	**Other**	5%

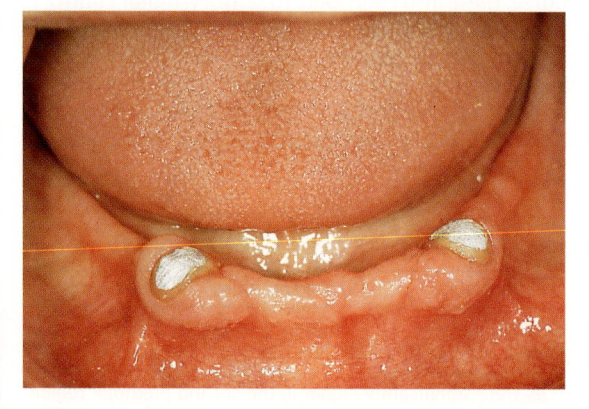

Fig. 11.3 Simplest case of overdenture with two natural roots

Prosthetic Procedures

Many different prosthetic designs fall under the category of overdentures for restoring the severely reduced ridge with a few remaining tooth roots. The overdenture has combined support (both periodontal and gingival) but as a rule, the outer appearance is that of a complete denture.

There are various reasons for retaining the roots of teeth in poor ridge dentitions:
1. The ridge atrophy that begins soon after the extraction of teeth is avoided. This is especially important in the mandible, which offers poor support for a complete denture in its atrophic form.
2. Maintaining roots in an almost edentulous jaw serves to enlarge the support base for the prosthesis.
3. Sensory feedback is maintained through the remaining periodontium. This can be important for the transmission of force and muscular control during chewing and biting.
4. Retained roots can also be used in combination with single attachments or bar splints.

Function of the Overdenture

With the insertion of osseointegrated implants into an edentulous jaw for denture anchorage, we create a clinical situation similar to an overdenture supported by natural tooth roots. From the histological and morphological point of view, the situations are different, since the connection between implant and bone is an ankylotic one with no periodontal membrane around the implants. Sensory feedback is provided by other structures, such as receptors in the mucosa, the bone, the temporomandibular joint, and in muscle spindles. Of course, these also contribute to sensory-motor control in dentate and partially edentulous individuals. The subjective evaluation of implant-supported overdentures by patients indicates that they represent the optimum treatment as far as function and comfort in chewing are concerned. Patients report that they feel as if they are chewing with their own natural teeth. This leads to the conclusion that firm fixation of the

Table 11.2 Maximum biting force (average values, in Newton)

Region	First premolar		Second premolar		Molar
Root	112.1	↔	131.2	↔	119.1
Implant	130.0	↔	142.6	↔	135.5

The maximum biting forces were significantly higher in the second premolar regions with roots and implants.

denture is of greater importance than is the presence of periodontal receptors. Stability of the denture with the assurance that there will be no noticeable movement is seen by edentulous patients as being equivalent to a natural dentition. Studies comparing wearers of overdentures over natural roots with wearers of overdentures over implants have shown that tactile discrimination is reduced with implants. The patients with implants made significantly more errors in detecting thin (10–100 μm) metal strips between the denture teeth. This means that the active oral sensibility is reduced. Still more noticeable was the difference in passive tactile sensibility, that is, direct touching of the natural root or the implant. Patients with roots could detect forces averaging between 1g and 4 g, while with implants, forces had to be about 100 times greater to be detected. This discovery that force perception is reduced in implant patients suggests that implants might be subjected to overloading. Measurements comparing maximum biting forces showed considerable variability within both groups, with a statistically insignificant tendency toward higher maximum forces with implants (Table 11.**2**). Apparently, factors other than the presence of a periodontium play a role in the control of maximum-force exertion in prosthesis wearers.

Design of the Overdenture with Implants

The design of overdentures anchored to tooth roots must take into account the vestibular bone contour of the remaining roots. Since no bone resorption has occurred in this region, the alveolar bone around the roots will usually not be covered by the denture base. In the edentulous jaw, with implants designed to support an overdenture the design of the overdenture resembles a complete denture. Only the border extensions of the base will be different because of the relative immobility of the overdenture. Complete dentures move within the envelope of muscle movements and must have a good border seal to preclude the ingress of air under the denture base that can occur with even the slightest movements. With overdentures, on the other hand, a suction effect is not desired, and the borders should be made somewhat shorter. As with a complete denture, the implant-supported overdenture must replace lost supporting tissues and recreate the facial and lingual morphology. The location of the implants and mechanical attachments must not interfere with this function.

Fabrication of the Implant-Supported Overdenture

In the following, a step-by-step description of the clinical and laboratory procedures for the fabrication of overdentures will be presented. Two variations are designated as A and B. The series of illustrations (Fig. 11.**4**–11.**12**) show variations A and B through examples of two mandibular implant cases and the Octa-System.

Variation B is usually preferred, particularly when only two implants are placed, even though it requires one more appointment for a trial insertion of the bar. This can sometimes be avoided if a provisional splint is used to verify the accuracy of the master cast.

There are two main advantages of variation B: First, the shape of the bar will harmonize with the curvature of the ridge and the arrangement of the anterior teeth. Second, a two-stage impression makes it possible to record the resilient mucosal area with a material that is made specifically for this purpose. In this case, a zinc oxide paste is used. It is even more important to avoid overcontouring the denture base in the area of the vestibular fold. This can easily occur when a firm elastomeric impression material is used. This pushes the unattached mucosa laterally, resulting in a denture base with open borders that encourage food trapping.

Refer to the series of illustrations in Figures 11.**4**–11.**13**.

Prosthetic Procedures

Table 11.3 Step-by-step prosthetic procedures

Variation A	Variation B
1. – Alginate impression for custom tray – Impression for bar fabrication (full arch or quadrant) Lab: custom tray, bar	1. – Alginate impression for custom tray Lab: custom tray with openings over implants
2. – Bar try-in – Full arch impression in custom tray with bar in place Lab: master cast with implant analogs and bar, wax rim	2. – Two-stage impression with custom tray (altered cast technique) Lab: master cast with implant analogs, wax rim
3. – Jaw relation records, tooth selection if applicable Lab: mounting of casts, tooth setup if applicable	3. – Jaw relation records, tooth selection if applicable Lab: mounting of casts, tooth setup if applicable
4. – Verify occlusal records, try-in – Corrections in wax – Complete try-in Lab: corrections, prepare for processing	4. – Verify occlusal records, try-in – Corrections in wax – Complete try-in Lab: corrections, prepare for processing
5. – Laboratory procedures for completion of the dentures – Fabrication of the cast framework utilizing the master cast and plaster index – Processing the denture – Equilibration on articulator	5. – Laboratory procedures for fabrication of the bar and completion of the dentures – Orientation index: bar fabrication
6. – Delivery of the denture with bar	6. – Bar try-in Lab: fabrication of the metal framework with plaster index – Processing the denture – Equilibration on articulator
	7. – Delivery of the denture with bar

Steps 3 and 4: usually three appointments are necessary

11 Overdentures Supported by ITI Implants

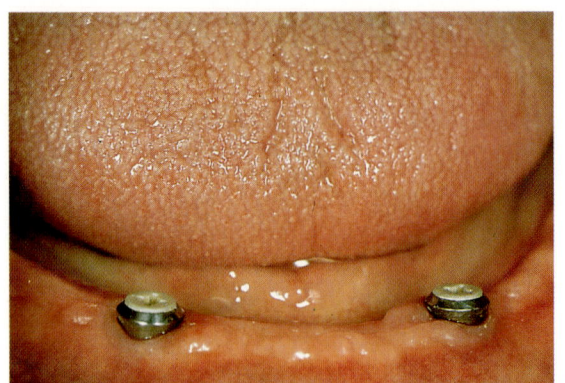

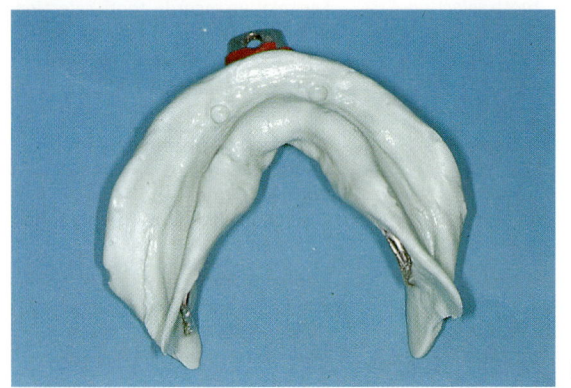

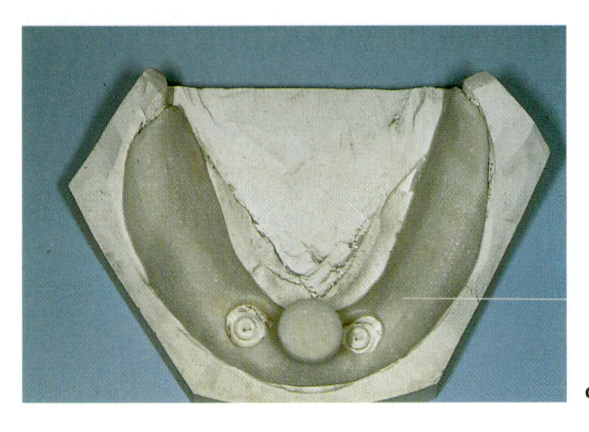

Prosthetic Procedures **341**

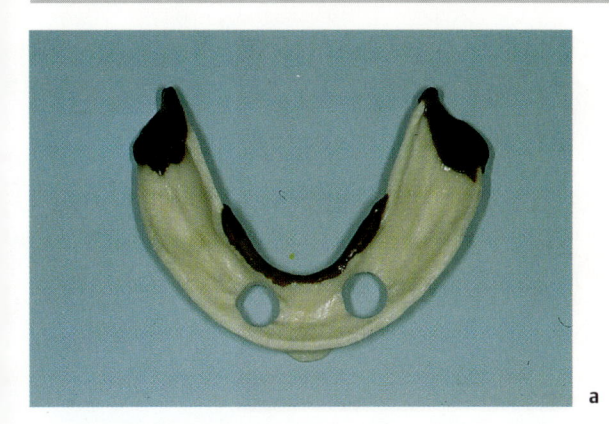

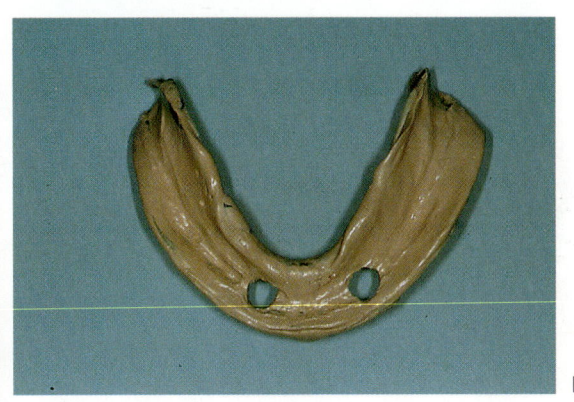

Fig. 11.**5a** The functional borders of the custom tray are formed with Kerr impression compound
b The impression of the ridge with its resilient mucosa is made with a zinc oxide-eugenol impression paste

Fig. 11.**4a** Two ITI implants in an edentulous mandible after a 3-month healing period
b Alginate impression
c Custom tray on the cast with openings over the two implants

11 Overdentures Supported by ITI Implants

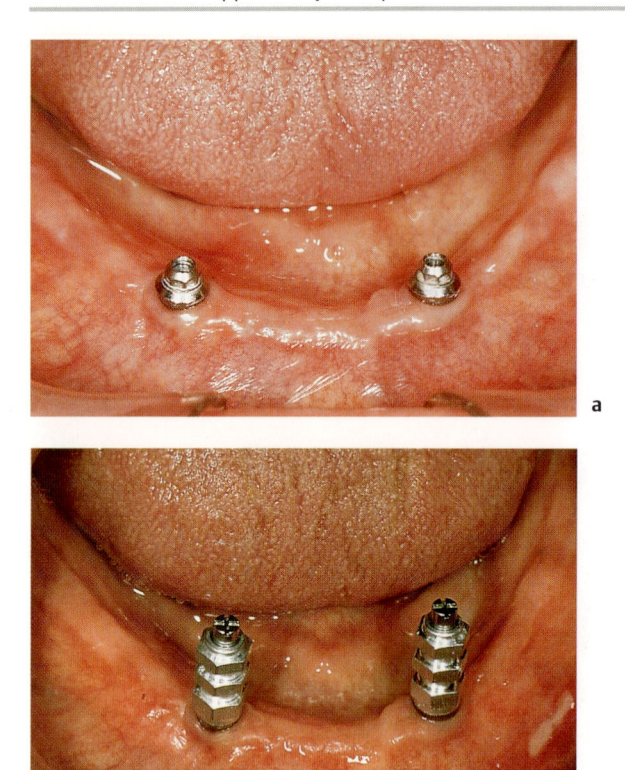

Fig. 11.**6a** The cover screws have been removed and the Octa abutments inserted in their place
b Transfer copings mounted
c Custom tray replaced
d A stiff elastomeric material is injected around the transfer copings. The screws remain exposed
e The screws are disengaged and the impression removed from the mouth

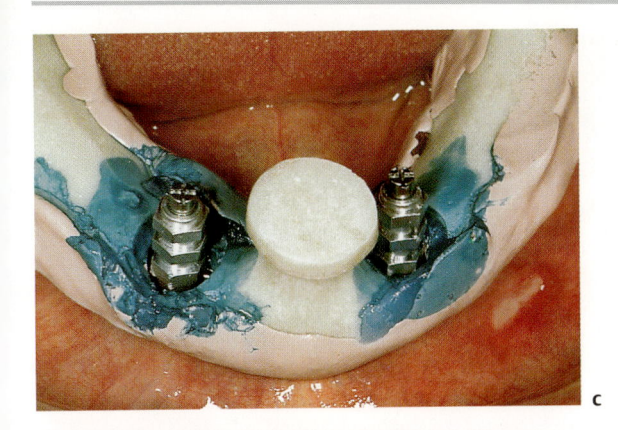

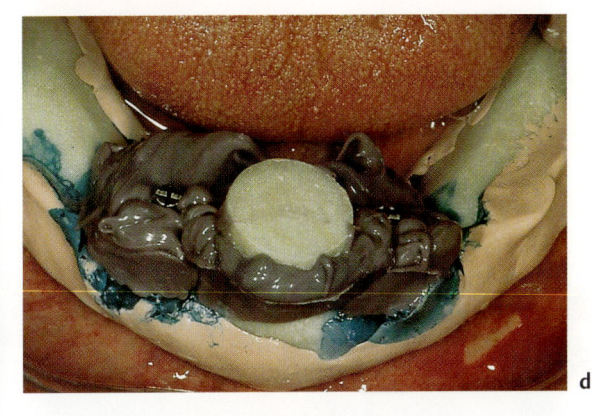

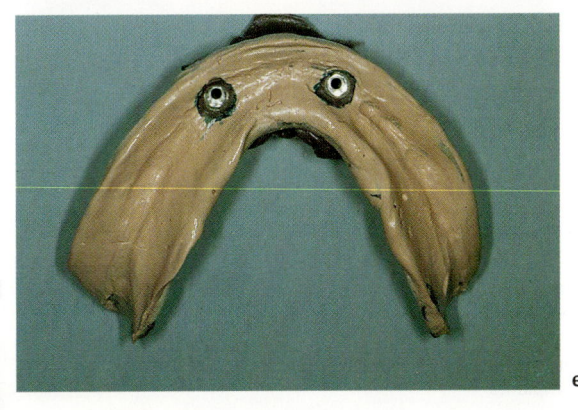

Prosthetic Procedures 343

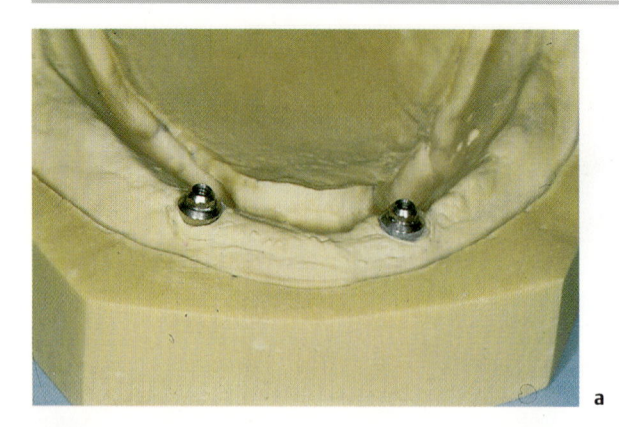

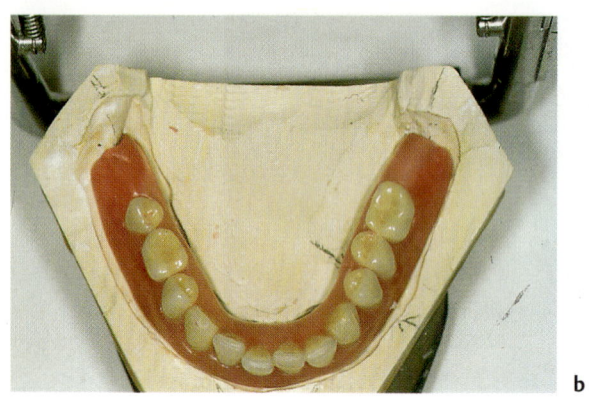

Fig. 11.**7a** Master cast with the implant analogs in place
b Prosthetic procedure: completion of the denture by a teeth set-up

Fig. 11.**8a** Facial and lingual orientation indexes are made of the completed denture set-up to be used in later fabrication steps
b Facial index
c Facial index in place on the master cast revealing the spatial relationships of the lower anterior teeth to the implants

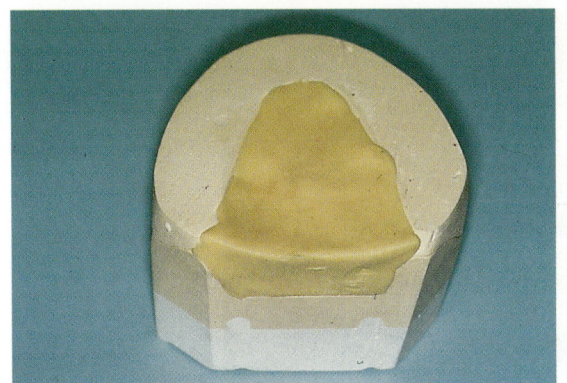

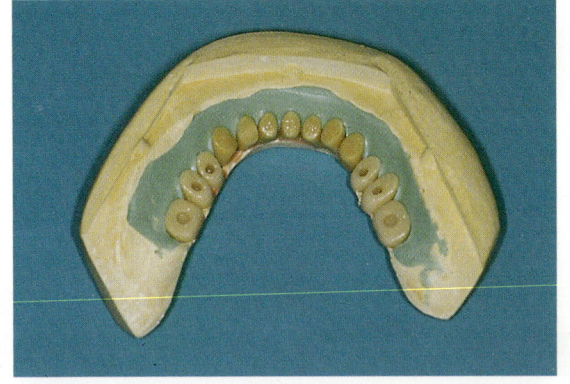

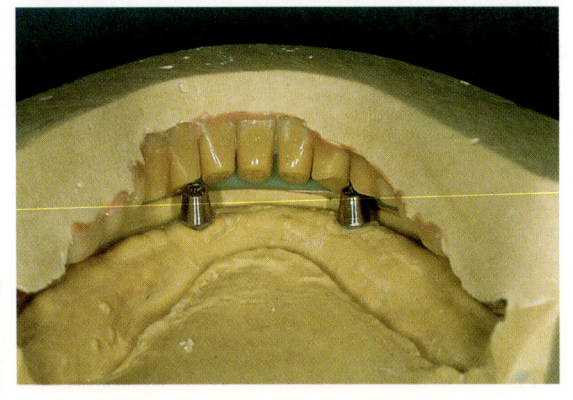

Prosthetic Procedures

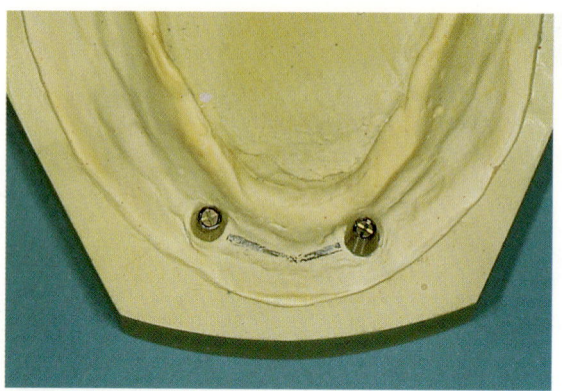

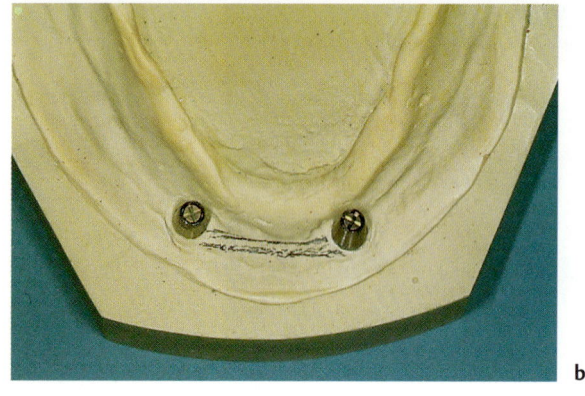

Fig. 11.9 Bar variations drawn on the cast
a angled bar design
b straight bar design positioned slightly to the labial side

Prosthetic Procedures

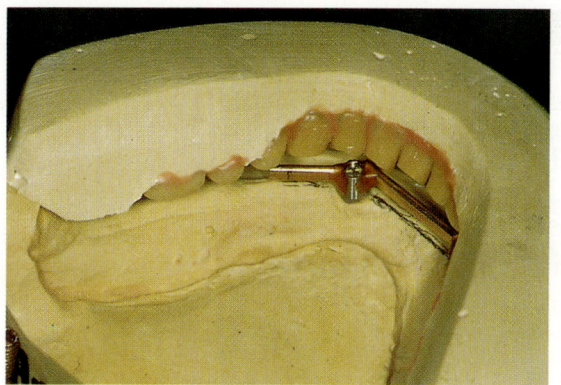

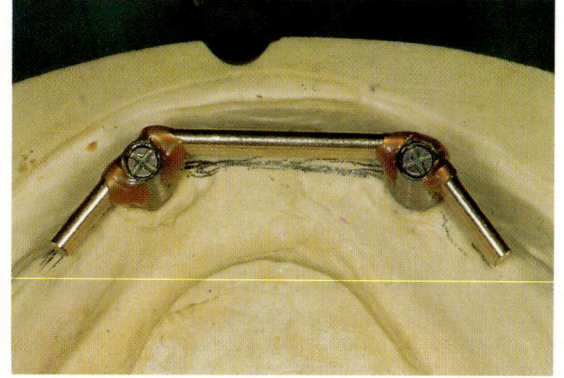

Fig. 11.10a U-shaped, rigid bar and extensions fixed in place with sticky wax. Interference with the position of the anterior teeth is prevented
b Bar in place on the master cast

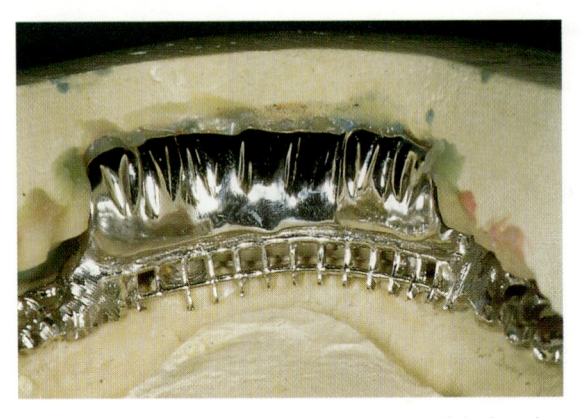

Fig. 11.**11** After completion and trial insertion of the bar, the cast metal framework is fabricated on the master cast

Insertion of the Overdenture

Clinical and technical aspects that must be considered at the final insertion of an implant-anchored overdenture are similar to those encountered at the delivery of a complete denture, with the addition of special considerations relating to the anchorage devices. The denture must first be tried in before the female parts of the attachments are activated so that the border extensions and shape of the base can be properly adjusted. The best method is to make a diagnostic impression of the borders and saddles with a low-viscosity silicone material. The same procedure can be repeated after the bar clips have been activated. In the same way, the occlusion is evaluated and adjusted before and after activation of the clips. Mounting the bar clips or other female retainers can lead to a slight increase in vertical dimension in the anterior area. With the use of only two implants, an intrusion of the posterior denture base into the mucosa cannot be prevented, especially with ball anchors and round bars. The prosthesis must therefore be tested for rocking and tipping movements after it is attached to the implants. In some cases, the clips must be removed and reattached to the denture directly in the mouth because of small changes that occurred when the denture was being completed in the laboratory. The attachment of the bar clips to the base must not interfere with their activation. This means that the lateral strips must not be embedded in acrylic resin. The resin of the denture base must not be allowed to touch either the implant or the resilient parts of the attachment devices.

Prosthetic Procedures **349**

Checklist for Delivery of the Prosthesis

- Shape of denture base and its borders
- Occlusion
- Changes caused by attachment of retentive devices
- Rocking movements over retentive devices
- New fixation of the bar clips, if necessary
- Can the clips or other attachments be activated?
- Relief of the resin base over the implants

Anchorage Device and Retention Mechanism

When selecting the anchorage device, the biological and mechanical aspects must be taken into consideration. *Biological* means that the attachment of the prosthesis to the implants will not create unfavorable conditions that could lead to failure of the osseointegration of the implants. *Mechanical* means that the attachment achieves a level of stability, comfort, and security that is acceptable to the patient. The question of whether, and to what extent, these two aspects may be combined cannot be answered currently. The load that implants are subjected to under various clinical conditions must be investigated further.

A basic principle of overdenture treatment is that the dimension of retention desired depends upon various factors.

Retention

- Numer of abutments (implants and/or roots)
- Distribution of abutments within the ridge segment
- Curvature of the ridge segment
- Size and type of the anchorage device
- Length of the bar attachment and number of clips
- Degree of jaw atrophy

There are now many varieties of bars and individual attachments available that can be used to anchor overdentures to ITI implants. The available Dalla Bona type anchors (retentive anchors) provide a movable retention mechanism, while bars can provide either a rigid or movable retention mechanism depending on their design.

Therefore, choices must be made as to type of attachment device (individual anchor vs. bar attachment) and function (movable vs. rigid).

The issue of rigid versus movable retentive mechanism is controversial and opinions are based upon empirical results. There are no scientifically based facts to unequivocably support either type of attachment. In the case of implants, it is argued that a movable retention mechanism could protect

11 Overdentures Supported by ITI Implants

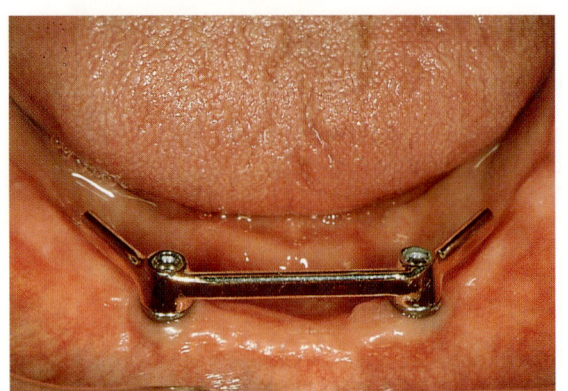

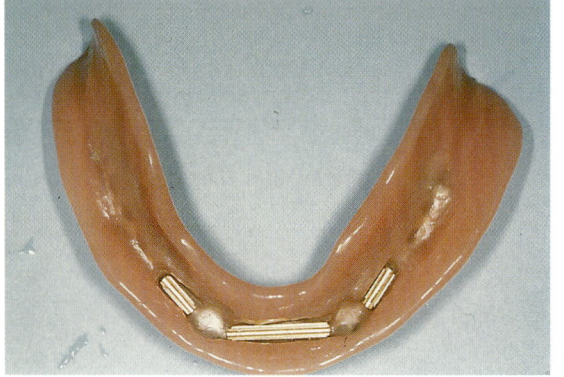

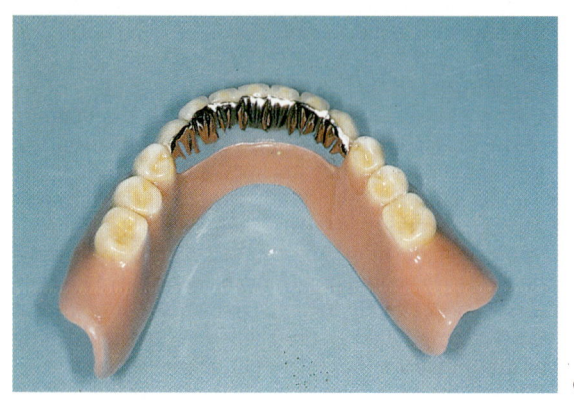

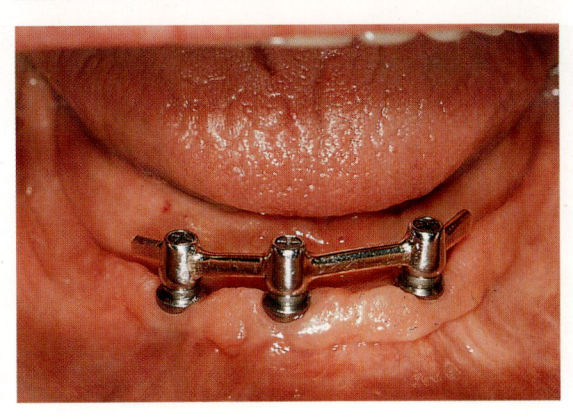

Fig. 11.**13** For comparison: a sliding attachment bar on three implants with conical abutments

the implant from overloading (stress breaking function) because more force is transmitted to the posterior edentulous ridge segments. One could also argue that forces acting upon the implant are very uncontrolled with movable retention mechanism. With rigid retention, it is possible that forces are increasingly directed onto the implant. Splinting bars, regardless of their design, do not flex along with the elastic deformation of the mandible that occurs during jaw movement, and this could therefore lead to overloading. This especially seems to be the case with long multiple segmented bars. In this respect, individual anchors might be prefered. However, it must also be considered that the denture itself has a splinting effect when it is in place. The number of implants is reduced, the load on each implant is obviously greater. Otherwise, more load might be transmitted by the denture to the posterior jaw segments.

Fig. 11.**12** Delivery of the prosthesis
a Bar is inserted in the mouth
b Tissue side of the denture showing the clips
c Outer surface of the denture. The concave lingual portion of the metal framework can be relined. This is advantageous if pressure areas should appear

352 11 Overdentures Supported by ITI Implants

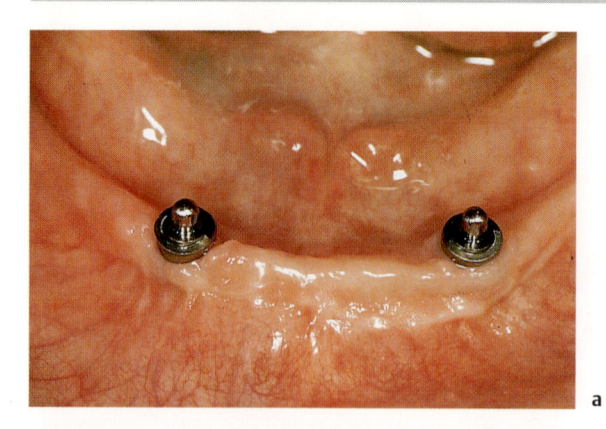

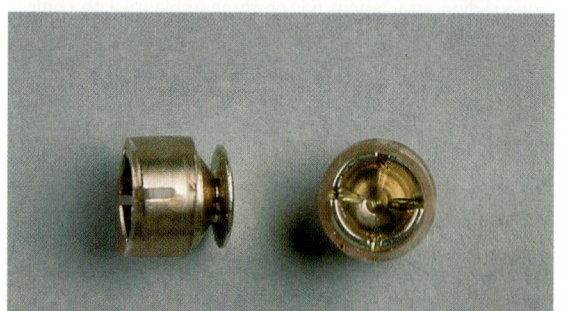

Fig. 11.**14a** Ball anchors as individual attachments. The two implants have been placed parallel to each other
b These metal female elements with adjustable leaves are currently preferred

Fig. 11.**15** Slightly resorbed lower ridges
a Two ball anchors offer good retention for a denture
b Ball anchor combined with cast gold copings and soldered retention elements on natural roots
c Same case as **b** with denture in place

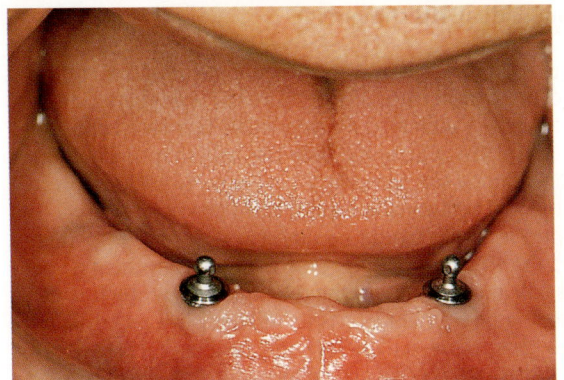

Prosthetic Procedures 353

a

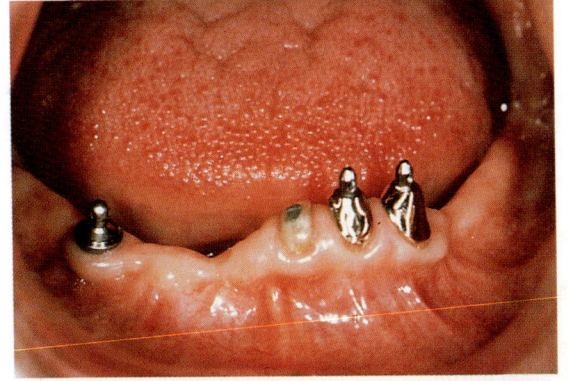

b

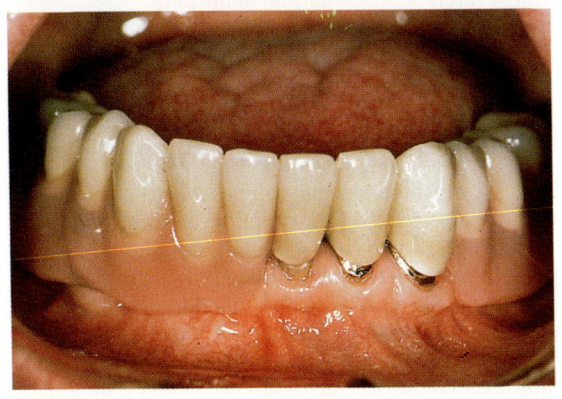

c

Retention Devices: Individual Attachments

The individual single attachment is the most economical and technically most simple way of connecting a complete denture to ITI implants. Individual attachments are especially indicated if a previously fabricated denture is to be attached to the implants. Currently, only the ball-shaped Dalla Bona type anchor is available. Since the secondary part is screwed into internal threads in the implant, only rotationally symmetrical bodies can be used as individual attachments (unless it would be possible to set the implants in absolute parallelism). Controversial discussions took place in the past over the usefulness of this ball anchor because the retention frequently proved to be unsatisfactory. The female element exerts its full retentive potential only when it encirles and grasps the ball below the height of contour. This requires that two or more implants be placed as parallel as possible to one another so that their heigths of contour lie on the same plane (Fig. 11.**14a**). Ball anchors, therefore, are no remedy for unfavorably aligned implants. In the maxilla, the implants are usually labially inclined with diverging axes. Ball attachments are therefore a poor choice for retentive elements here. In addition, the loose bone structure in the maxilla seems to demand a rigid anchorage to preferably more than two implants.

In the mandible, individual anchors are satisfactory, especially if the ridge morphology presents a good foundation for the denture base. The ball anchor is a movable retentive mechanism. There are no rigid attachments available as attachments to ITI implants.

Indications for Ball Anchors

- Mandible with good ridge contours
- Provisional restoration during prolonged prosthetic therapy
- In combination with severely reduced natural dentition
- When a movable retention mechanism is desired

(Fig. 11.**15a–c**)

Retention Devices: Bar Variations

Due to the availability of prefabricated gold copings that can be combined with prefabricated bar segments, the fabrication of bar attachments is technically simple. It is not necessary to custom mill the bars.

Those unfamiliar with bar attachments frequently (through misunderstanding) attribute them not only with the function of anchoring a prosthesis, but also with the function of splinting the remaining roots. In implantology, the only purpose of the bar is to anchor the prosthesis. The extent to which mechanical and biological factors are in conflict is unknown.

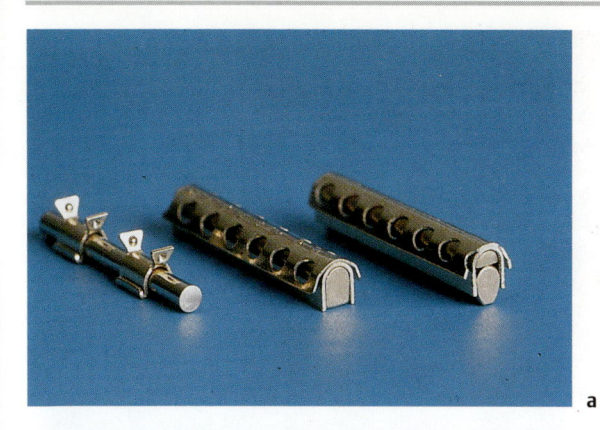

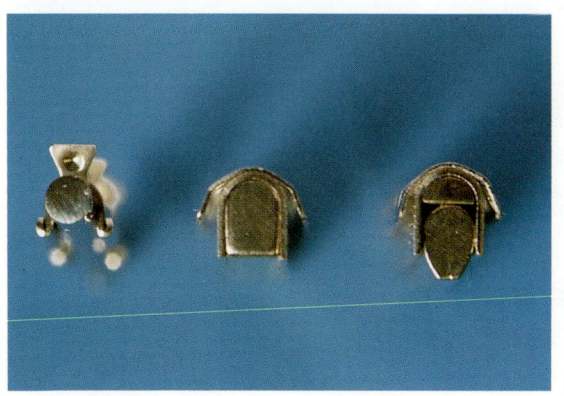

Fig. 11.**16a** Left to right: round bar, rigid sliding attachment bar, Dolder joint bar
b Cross-sectional view of the three bar types

Movable retention mechanism of bars include the round bar and the egg-shaped bar by Dolder (bar joint). *Rigid* bars are U-shaped (sliding attachment bar). (Fig. 11.**16a, b**)

The round bar and the Dolder bar allow the denture to rotate around the bar's axis provided the bar connects two implants in a straight line via the shortest path (Fig. 11. **17a, b**). Therefore, the posterior ridge segments become loaded by the denture. The rigid sliding attachment bar provides better retention and is advantageous when ridge resorption is advanced

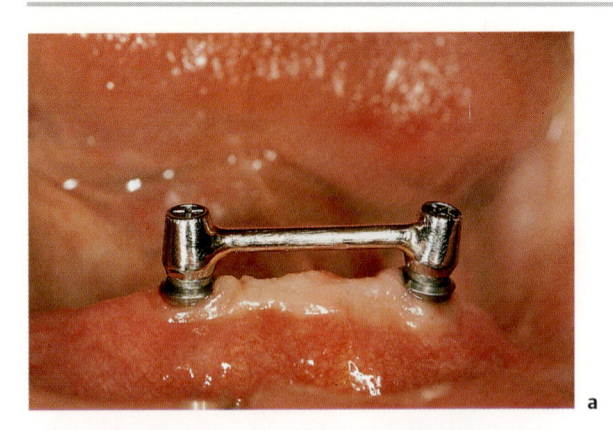

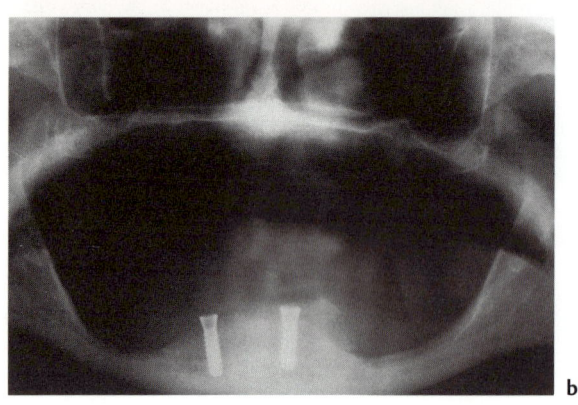

Fig. 11.**17a** Straight round bar with a ridge contour that falls off sharply posteriorly
b Orthopantomogram of the same case; the use of the round bar in a case with unfavorable ridge atrophy will result in relatively poor denture retention (rotation of the denture around the bar)

(Fig. 11.**18**). If a round bar is bent between two implants or if multiple implants are connected with round bar segments, two or more axes of rotation result, which (together) prevent rotation (Fig. 11.**19**). The sliding attachment bar is a rigid attachment regardless of the number of implants. Figures 11.**20a** through **g** show a rehabilitation case with four ITI implants in the maxilla and three in the mandible using the Octa-System and rigid sliding attachment bars with extensions. The posterior ridge segments remain virtually unloaded. It can be assumed that when rigid attachments

Prosthetic Procedures 357

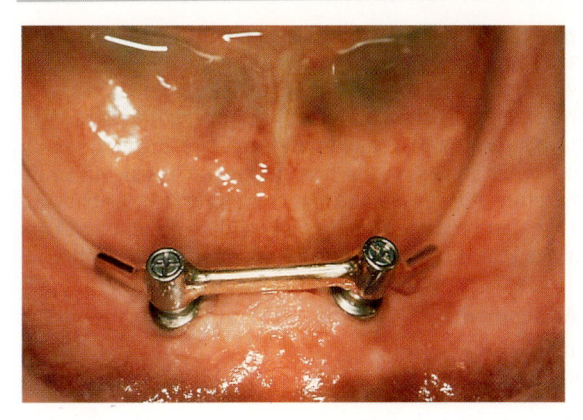

Fig. 11.**18** A similar situation with a sliding attachment bar and extensions over a ridge that is severely resorbed in the posterior regions; retention is better than in the preceding case

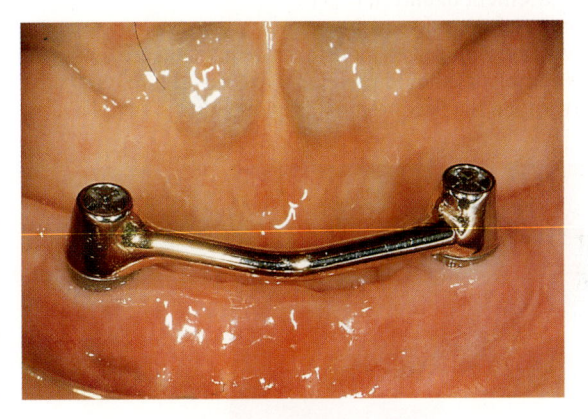

Fig. 11.**19** A round bar that is slightly bent to follow the ridge

are used, more load must be borne by the implants. The question of whether or not this results in excessive loading has not been answered. The highest concentration of stress will always occur at the cervical portion of the implant where it emerges from the bone.

When the bar itself is short and straight, short cantilevered extensions distal to the last implants can act to prevent lateral shifting and thereby contribute to further stabilization of the prosthesis. Generally, no clips are placed on the extensions. From experiences with prostheses that are firmly screwed to the implants, we have learned that the distal implants are subjected to increased loads, and extensions should not exceed 1.5 cm in length. When only two implants have been placed, they both function as end abutments. Therefore, extensions should always be short. With overdentures, in vivo studies have indicated that maximum forces are encountered on the second premolars, while forces on the first premolars are significantly lower (Table 11.**2**). Therefore, it is reasonable to recommend that the bars not be extended beyond the first premolar region. Only sliding attachment bars present a contact surface that is broad enough for adequate solder joints.

Indications for Bar Attachments
- Maxilla and mandible
- Severely atrophied ridge

Recommendations for Placing Bar Attachments
- Do not impinge on the tongue space.
- Allow space for placement of anterior teeth.
- Follow the curvature of the ridge.
- With sharply curved and wide ridges, more than two implants are suggested.
- Distance between implants should preferably exceed 10 mm.
- Add extensions through the first premolar region only.

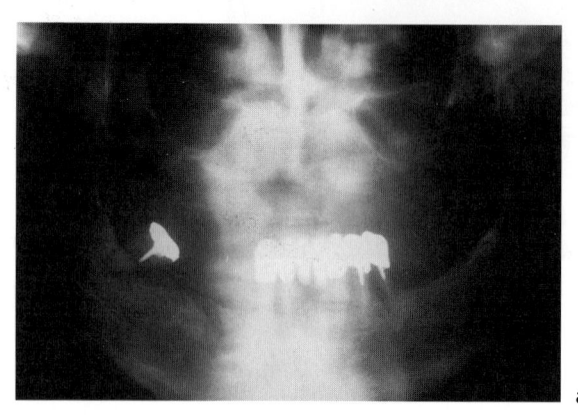

Fig. 11.**20** Example of a case:
a Orthopantomogram before treatment. All lower teeth must be extracted
b Maxilla with 4 ITI implants and Octa abutments
c Mandible with 3 ITI implants and Octa abutments. No implant could be placed in the lower right incisor region because of inadequate bone substance 4 months after extractions
d The maxillary prosthesis in place

Prosthetic Procedures 359

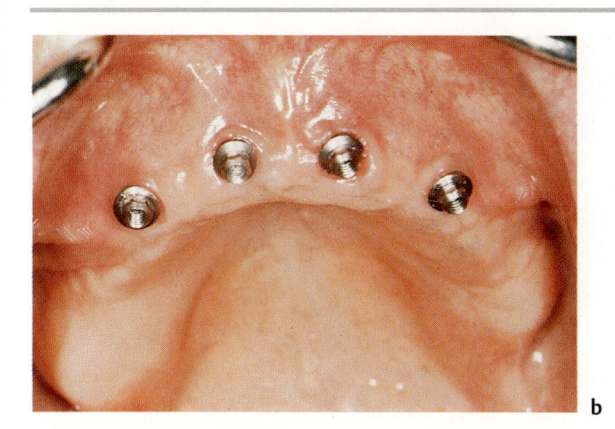

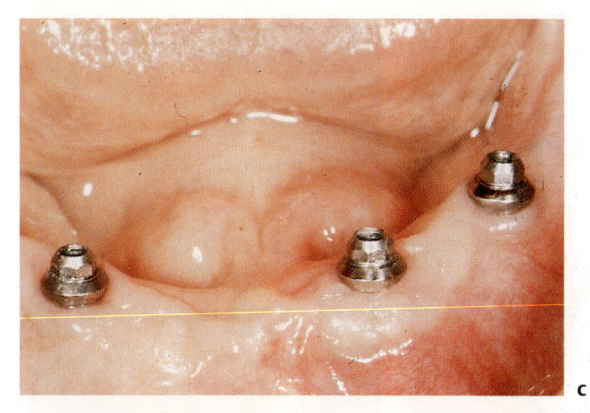

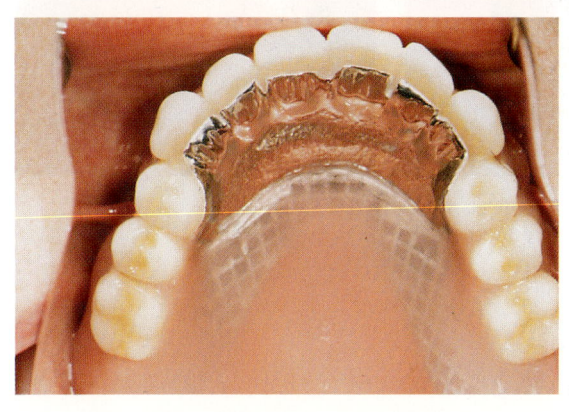

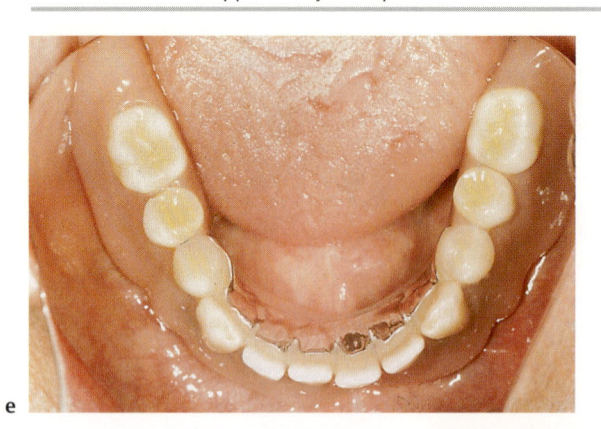

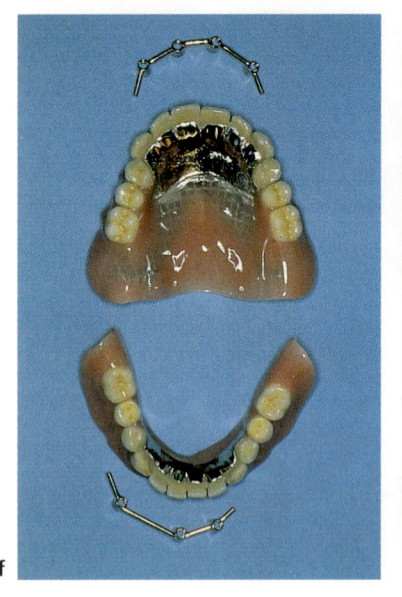

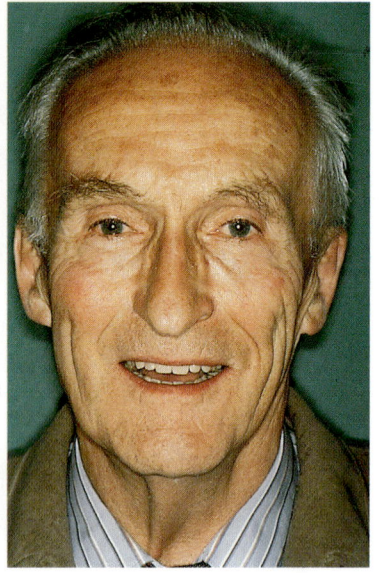

e The mandibular prosthesis in place
f Dentures and bars before insertion
g The 83-year-old patient

Prosthetic Procedures **361**

Figure 11.**21a–g** shows a screw-attached, retrievable denture as a variation of the conventional overdenture in a young woman with congenital absence of the permanent dentition. All remaining deciduous teeth had to be extracted. For financial reasons, only the lower arch was treated at this time. The treatment required 14 months to complete. The screw-retained prosthesis is similar in concept and design to an overdenture, but could also be regarded as a variation of a fixed denture. Due to of the small amount of available bone, solid screw implants of reduced diameter were used.

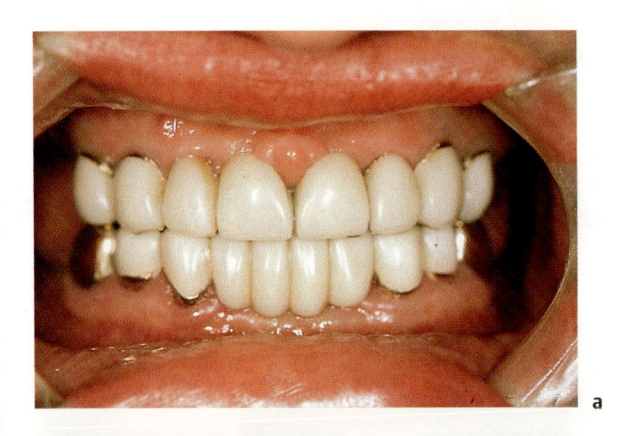

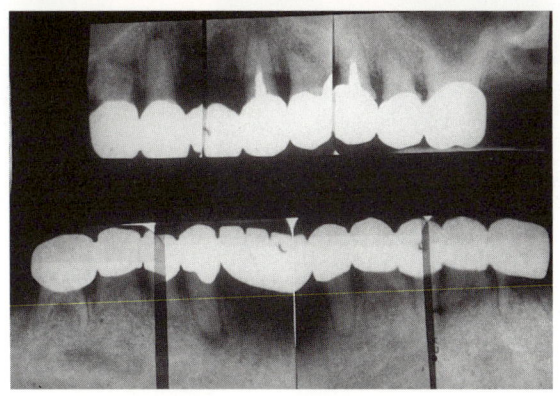

Fig. 11.**21** Example of a case:
a Presenting condition
b Radiographic appearance

362 11 Overdentures Supported by ITI Implants

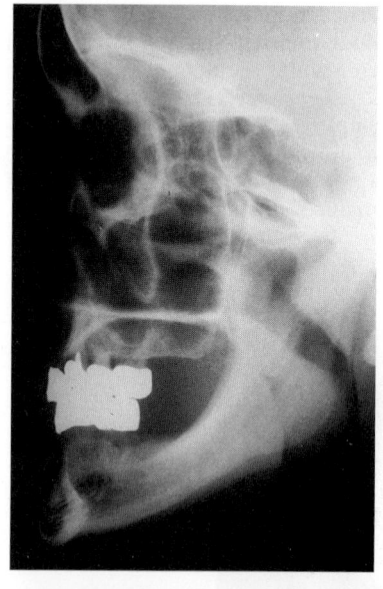

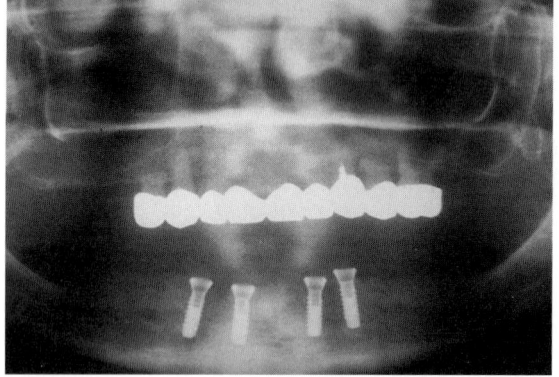

c Cephalometric radiograph. Note the spongy bone structure
d Orthopantomogram with the four ITI implants (3.4 mm diameter)
e Screw-attached implant prosthesis
f View of the prosthesis
g The patient

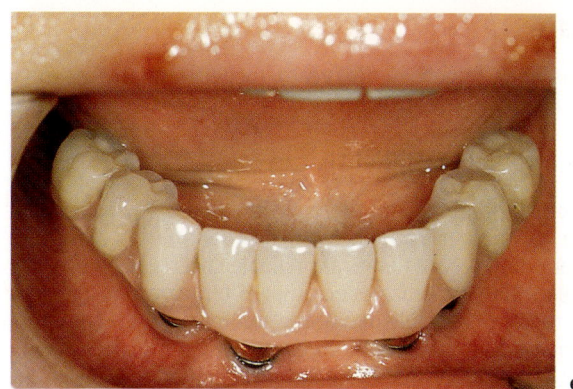

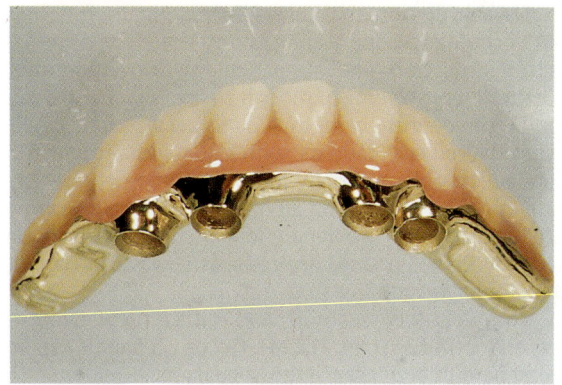

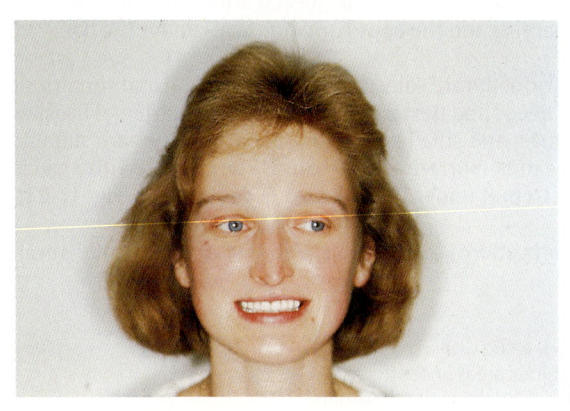

Prosthetic Procedures

Maintenance Care

Maintenance care is very important in regard to peri-implant marginal tissues and prosthetic follow-up care.

Hygiene and Peri-implant Marginal Tissues

The same basic recommendations and prerequisites that apply to implant patients apply also to implant patients with overdentures. It has been debated whether periodontal parameters are reliable criteria to be used for evaluating peri-implant tissues. As far as no other criteria are available, our maintenance care program is established in the same way as the program designed for prevention and early recognition of disease in patients with conventional dental reconstructions. Plaque-induced inflammation of the marginal tissues may be controlled and eliminated with a good oral hygiene program. Wearing a removable denture that covers the marginal soft tissues creates conditions that encourage plaque accumulation. Therefore, a special effort must be made to instruct and motivate patients with overdentures. Marginal inflammation produces swelling of the soft tissues that in turn can lead to traumatization by the denture base, thus initiating a vicious circle. We must also remember that elderly patients, with visual impairment and reduced dexterity, may not be able to strictly follow our instructions. The cleaning aids, therefore, must be selected on an individual basis. It may be difficult for the edentulous patient to use dental floss or superfloss because one hand must be used to hold the lips and cheek out of the way. The patient is instructed to clean the implants at home in two steps:
1. First, removal of gross debris is recommended with a regular toothbrush or a child-sized toothbrush (Fig. 11.**22a**). The brush handle can be warmed and slightly bent to better reach the lingual areas.
2. Second, fine cleaning is accomplished. Special attention must be given to the implant margins and the approximal surfaces under the bar.

The cleaning instruments are selected according to local oral conditions and to the individual needs and dexterity of the patient. Interdental brushes with or without handles, and small single-tufted toothbrushes are suitable (Fig. 11.**22b** and **c**). The undersurface of a bar can also be cleaned with a gauze strip, which is easier to pull under the bar than is dental floss (Fig. 11-**22d** and **e**).

The following procedure is recommended for the patient's recall appointment:

Fig. 11.**22a** Preliminary cleaning with a toothbrush
b Spiral brush for approximal areas under the bar
c Single-tufted toothbrush for the gingival margins

Maintenance Care **365**

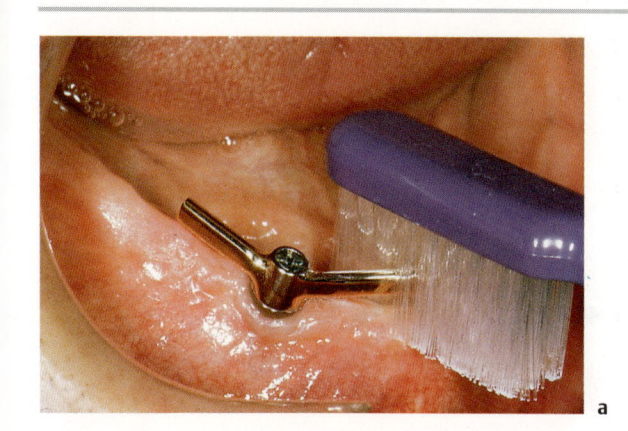

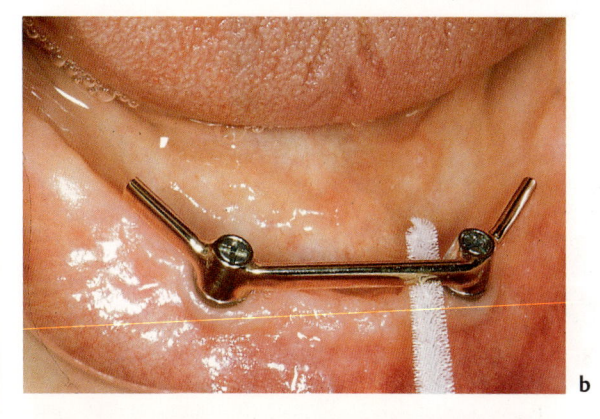

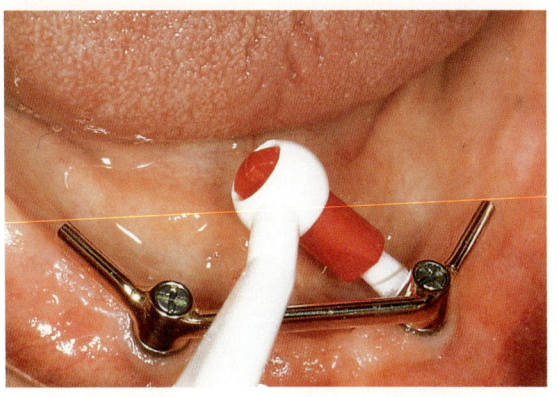

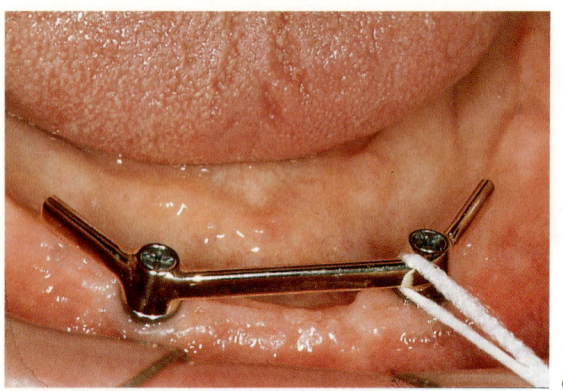

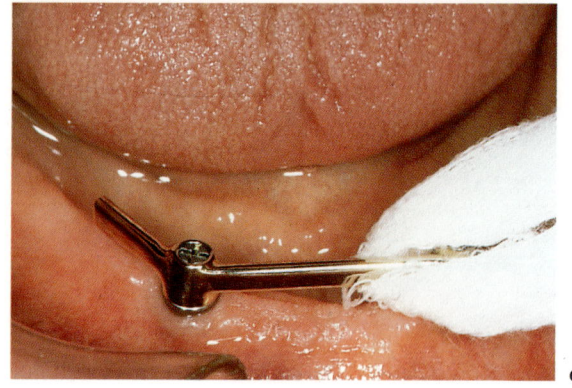

d Superfloss for cleaning the underside of the bar (difficult for patients to manipulate)
e Gauze strip for cleaning the bar

Hygiene Checklist

- Evaluate hygiene
- Identify and chart problem areas
- Place bar and screws in ultrasonic cleaner
- Remove plaque with rubber cup
- Remove calculus with special scalers of hard plastic
- Reinforce oral hygiene instructions
- Practice with the patient
- Evaluate cleanliness of the prosthesis
- Clean the denture in an ultrasonic cleaner

The bar does not have to be removed at every recall appointment, provided deposits are light and can be removed with appropriate instruments.

In many implant patients with overdentures, oral hygiene is astonishingly good, in spite of the advanced ages of most. This arises from a high level of motivation and cooperation. However, the space under the denture around the attachments can favor dead space hyperplasia, which frequently resembles stomatitis of type "Newton 3."

Plaque and calculus: Slight traces of plaque and calculus adhere to the necks of implants, but seldom extend deep into the sulcus. More pronounced accumulation of calculus is frequently found in the lingual and distal regions of the implant shoulder at the inferior margin of the gold copings. The design of the implant and attached gold coping encourages the formation of plaque in this location and hinders simple, efficient home care. This problem zone has been identified and eliminated by the Octa-system. The implant and gold coping of the Octa system have an improved design that is conducive to good oral hygiene.

Dead space hyperplasia can often be found at the junction between implant and mucosa and under the bar. It is unknown to what extent poor oral hygiene itself is responsible for this condition. (Fig. 11.**23a** and **b**). Dead space hyperplasia is also found in patients with very good oral hygiene. This leads to the assumption that there is a predisposition in certain patients. Dead space hyperplasia has no pathological effect, but renders oral hygiene more difficult and creates pseudopockets. Frequent massaging with strong saline solution is a simple, effective therapy.

Special marginal problems and implant failures are discussed in chapters 14 and 15.

Follow-Up Care of the Prosthesis

It is still quite unclear to what extent, if any, loading of the implants through the superstructure provokes unfavorable reactions of the peri-implant bone in the form of inflammation and resorption. Various studies have been

368 11 Overdentures Supported by ITI Implants

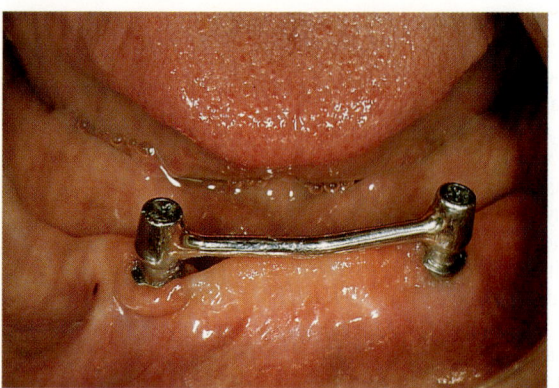

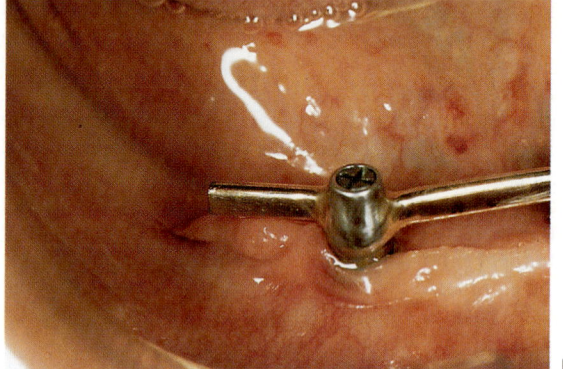

Fig. 11.**23a** Dead space hyperplasia under a bar associated with poor oral hygiene
b Mucosa covering the implant shoulder, hyperplasia under the bar extension

Maintenance Care 369

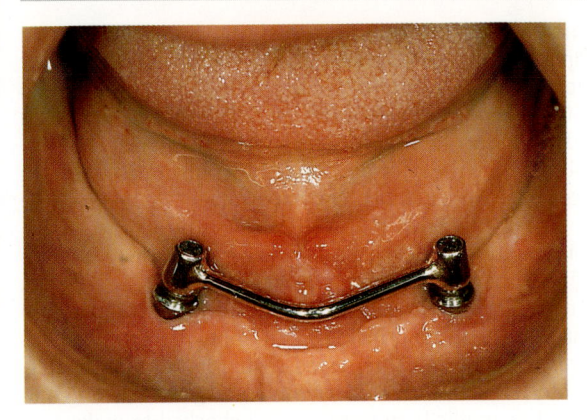

Fig. 11.**24** Pressure lesion in the lingual region. Corrections can be made easily because the denture border is made of acrylic resin

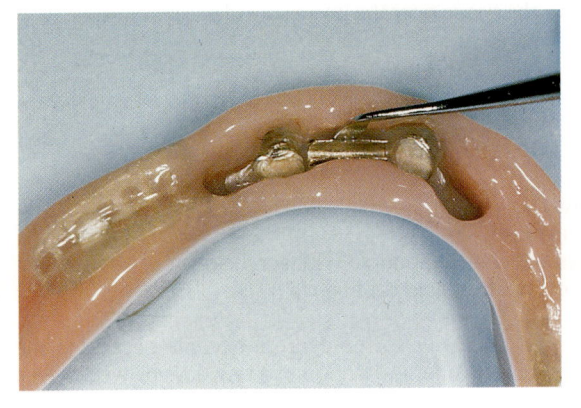

Fig. 11.**25** Checking the bar clip with a spatula

conducted on theoretical models and by measuring forces directly in patients wearing implant-borne restorations. Most of them were carried out under the assumption that forces are directed vertically, i.e., parallel to the long axis of the implant. Studies have demonstrated that vertical forces are always accompanied by horizontal force components. The highest concentration of forces is observed in the neck portion of the implant. Stresses can be induced and concentrated in the implant by imperfections in the fit of the framework that are imperceptible to the eye. Therefore an exact, passive seating of the bar is imperative. The denture itself can contribute to stability through its shape of the base and configuration of the occlusion. It is just as important that the denture-bearing tissue in the posterior portions of the ridge not be traumatized. The same principles that apply to complete dentures also apply here. The base must be tested regularly for good fit (Fig. **11.24**), and occlusal interferences corrected by remounting the dentures and occlusal equilibrating. The acrylic base must also be checked to make sure that it does not touch the implants, gold copings, or the bar. This problem is usually the result of a bar clip that is broken, loose, or lost (Fig. **11.25** and Fig. **11.26a** and **b**), but can also occur when a denture with movable attachments moves and settles into the tissue over the posterior ridge segments.

Prosthetic Follow-Up Care: Checklist

- Occlusion (remounting records)
- Base (relining)
- Pressure spots
- Bar (loose screws)
- Bar clips (broken, loose)
- Female retainers and clips remounted with acrylic resin
- Signs of wear (on implants, gold copings)

If corrections or modifications to the denture become necessary, the patient must be asked to return for evaluation in a few days or weeks. As a rule, the time period between hygiene recalls is too long.

Fig. 11.**26** Remounting the clips with self-polymerizing resin:
a The space under the bar is blocked out with wax. The screws are removed and the threaded holes are also occluded with wax. The clips are positioned on the bar. The retentive wings must not be bent out to the sides
b The inside of the denture is relieved and then tried in the mouth over the bar and clips before being loaded with resin
c The denture is removed from the mouth after the clips have been picked up with self-polymerizing resin. The bar came out with the denture, which will be refined in the laboratory

Maintenance Care **371**

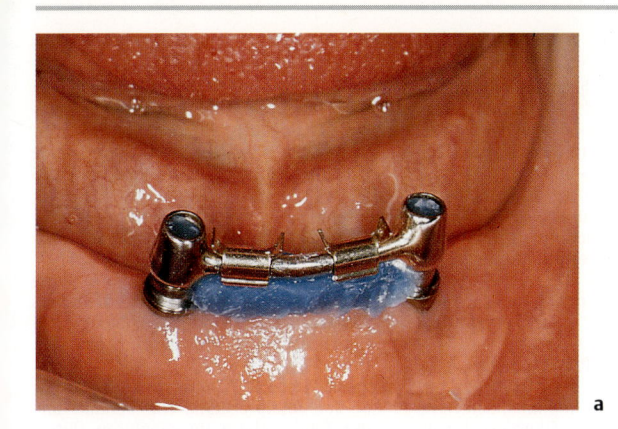

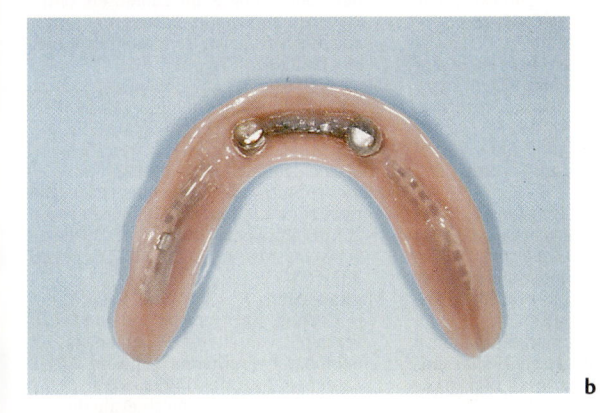

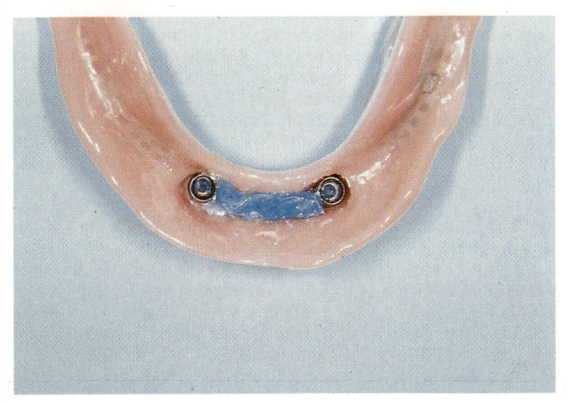

References

Ahlqvist, J., K. Borg, J. Gunne, H. Nilson, M. Olsson, P. Åstrand: Osseointegrated Implants in Edentulous Jaws: A 2-Year Longitudinal Study. Int. J. oral max.-fac. Implants 5 (1990) 155–163

Albrektsson, T., S. Blomberg, A. Brånemark, G. E. Carlsson: Edentulousness – an oral handicap. Patient reactions to treatment with jawbone-anchored prostheses. J. oral Rehab. 14 (1987) 503–511

Albrektsson, T., L. Sennerby: State of the art in oral implants. J. clin. Periodontal. (1991) 474–481

Albrektsson, T., G. Zarb, P. Worthington, A. R. Eriksson: The Long-Term Efficacy of Currently Used Dental Implants: A Review and proposed Criteria of Success. Int. J. oral mac.-fac. Impl. 1 (1986) 11–25

Apse, P., G. A. Zarb, A. Schmitt, D. W. Lewis: The longitudinal effectiveness of osseointegrated dental implants. The Toronto Study: Peri-Implant mucosal response. Int. J. Periodont. 11 (1991) 95–112

Atwood, D. A.: Reduction of residual ridges: A major oral disease entity. J. prosth. Dent. 26 (1971) 266–279

Buser, D., H. P. Weber, U. Brägger, Ch. Balsiger: Tissue Integration of One-Stage ITI Implants: 3-Year Results of a Longitudinal Study with Hollow-Cylinder and Hollow-Screw Implants. Int. J. oral max.-fac. Implants 6 (1991) 405–412

Cox, J. F., G. A. Zarb: The longitudinal clinical efficacy of osseointegrated dental implants: a 3-year report. Int. J. oral max.-fac. Implants 2 (1987) 91–100

Enquist, B., T. Bergendal, T. Kallus: A Retrospective Multicenter Evaluation of Osseointegrated Implants Supporting Overdentures. Int. J. oral max.-fac. Implants 3 (1988) 129–134

Geering, A. H., M. Kundert: Farbatlanten der Zahnmedizin, Bd. 2. Total- und Hybridprothetik. Thieme Stuttgart 1991

Jacobs, R., A. Schotte, D. van Steenberghe, M. Quirynen, I. Naert: Posterior jaw bone resorption in osseointegrated implant-supported overdentures. Clin. oral Impl. Res. 3 (1992) 63–70

Jacobs, R., D. van Steenberghe: Comparative evaluation of the oral tactile function by means of teeth or implant-supported prostheses. Clin. oral Impl. Res. 2 (1991) 75–80

Jemt, T., L. Carlsson, A. Boss, L. Jörneus: In Vivo Load Measurement on Osseointegrated Implants Supporting Fixed or Removable Prostheses: A Comparative Pilot Study. Int. J. oral max.-fac. Implants 6 (1991) 413–417

Ledermann, P.: Kompendium des TPS-Schraubenimplantates im zahnlosen Unterkiefer. Quintessenz, Berlin 1986

Lindqvist, L., B. Rocker, G. E. Carlsson: Bone resopriton around fixtures in edentulous patients treated with mandibular fixed tissue-integrated prostheses. J. prosthet. Dent. 59 (1989) 59–63

Mericske-Stern, R., A. H. Geering: Implantate in der Totalprothetik. Die Verankerung der Totalprothese im zahnlosen Unterkiefer durch zwei Implantate mit Einzelattachment. Schweiz. Mschr. Zahnmed. 98 (1988) 871–876

Mericske-Stern, R.: Die implantatgesicherte Totalprothese im zahnlosen Unterkiefer. Eine klinische Longitudinalstudie mit Ergebnissen nach vier Jahren. Schweiz. Mschr. Zahnmed. 98 (1988) 931–936

Mericske-Stern, R.: Osseointegration. Bericht zum 1. Münchner Symposium vom 20. bis 22. Januar 1989. Eine Übersicht, Schweiz. Mschr. Zahnmed. 99 (1989) 567–573

Mericske-Stern, R., J. Kowalski, K. Liszkay, A. H. Geering: Nachsorgebefund und Recallverhalten von älteren Patienten mit abnehmbaren Prothesen. Schweiz. Mschr. Zahnmed. 100 (1990) 1053–1059

Mericske-Stern, R.: Clinical evaluation of overdenture restorations supported by osseointegrated titanium implants. A retrospective study. Int. J. oral max.-fac. Implants 5 (1990) 375–383

Mericske-Stern, R., A. H. Geering, W. Bürgin, H. Graf: Three-Dimensional Force Measurements on Mandibular Implants Supporting Overdentures. Int. J. oral max.-fac. Implants 7 (1992) 185–194

Mericske-Stern, R.: Zahnärztliche Implantate – Künstliche Zahnwurzeln. Uni Press 71 (1991) 38–40

Mericske-Stern, R.: Klinische Erfahrungen bei der Verwendung von ITI Implantaten im zahnlosen Unterkiefer. Eine Retrospektive nach 8 Jahren. Schweiz. Mschr. Zahnmed. 102 (1992) 1215–1227

Mericske-Stern, R. G. A. Zarb: Overdentures supported by Implants: an alternative treatment methodology. Int. J. Prosthodont. 6 (1993) 203–208

Mericske-Stern, R.: Forces on implants supporting overdentures: morphological and cephalometric considerations. A preliminary study. Int. J. oral max.-fac. Implants 8 (1993) 254–263

Mericske-Stern, R., A. Wedig, J. Hofmann, A. H. Geering: In vivo measurements of maximal occlusal force and minimal pressure threshold on overdentures supported by implants or natural roots. A comparative study. Part I; J. oral max.-fac. Implants 1993 8: 641–649

Mericske-Stern, R.: Oral tactile sensibility in overdenture wearers with implants or natural roots. A comparative study. Part II; Int. J. oral max.-fac. Impl. 1994 8: 63–70

Mericske-Stern, R., T. Steinlin Schaffner, P. Marti, A. H. Geering: Periimplant mucosal aspects of ITI-implants supporting overdentures. A five year-longitudinal study. Clin. oral Impl. Res.: 5

Mericske-Stern, R., D. Milani, A. Olah, A. H. Geering: Periotest Measurings and Osseointegration of mandibular Implants supporting Overdentures. Clin. oral Impl. Res.

Mericske-Stern, R., E. Mericske, H. Berthold, A. H. Geering: Die zahnärztliche prothetische Versorgung von Patienten mit oralen Defekten nach Tumorresektion. Eine retrospektive Studie. Schweiz. Mschr. Zahnmed. 104 (1994) 59–68

Mobelli, A., R. Mericske-Stern, R.: Microbiological features of stable osseointegrated implants used as abutments for overdentures. Clin. oral Impl. Res. 1 (1990) 1–7

Naert, I., M. De Clercq, G. Theuniers, E. Schepers: Overdentures supported by osseointegrated fixtures for the edentulous mandible: a 2.5-year report. Int. J. oral max.-fac. Implants 3 (1988) 191–196

Olivé, J.: The Periotest Method as a Measure of Osseointegrated Oral Implant Stability. Int. J. oral max.-fac. Implants 5 (1990) 390–400

Quirynen, M., I. Naert, D. van Steenberghe, J. Teelinck, C. Dekeyser, G. Theuniers: Periodontal aspects of osseointegrated fixtures supporting an overdenture. A 4-year retrospective study. J. clin. Periodontol. 18 (1991) 719–729

Quirynen, M., D. van Steenberghe, R. Jacobs, A. Schotte, P. Darius: The reliability of poket probing around screw-type implants. Clin. oral Impl. Res. 2 (1991) 186–192

Richter, E. J., M. Meier, H. Spikermann: Implantatbelastung in vivo. Untersuchungen an implantatgeführten Coverdenture-Prothesen. Z. zahnärztl. Implantol. 8 (1992) 36–45

Sennerby, L., G. E. Carlsson, B. Bergman, J. Warfvinge: Mandibular bone resorption in patients treated with tissue-integrated prostheses and in complete-denture wearers. Acta Odontol Scand. 46 (1988) 135–140

Smith, D., G. A. Zarb: Criteria for success of osseointegrated endosseous implants. J. prosthet. Dent. 62 (1989) 567–572

Tallgren, A.: The continuing reduction of the residual alveolar ridge in complete denture wearers. A mixed-longitudinal study covering 25 years. J. prosthet. Dent. 27 (1972) 120

Teerlinck, J., M. Quirynen, P. Darius, D. van Steenberghe: Periotest: An Objective Clinical Diagnosis of Bone Apposition Toward Implants. Int. J. oral max.-fac. Implants 6 (1991) 55–61

Zarb, G. A., A. Schmitt: Osseointegration and the edentulous predicament. The 10-year-old Toronto study. Brit. dent. J. 170 (1991) 439–444

Zarb, G. A., A. Schmitt: Terminal dentition in elderly patients and implant therapy alternatives. Int. Dent. J. 40 (1990) 67–73

Zarb, G. A., A. Schmitt: The longitudinal clinical effectiveness of osseointegrated dental implants: The Toronto study. Part II: The prosthetic results. J. prosthet. Dent. 64 (1990) 53–61

Zarb, G. A., A. Schmitt: The longitudinal clinical effectiveness of osseointegrated implants. The Toronto study. Part I: Surgical results. J. prosthet. Dent. 62 (1989) 451–470

Zarb, G. A., A. Schmitt: The longitudinal clinical effectiveness of osseointegrated implants. The Toronto study. Part III: Problems and complications encountered. J. prosthet. Dent. 64 (1990) 185–194

12 Fixed Prosthetic Restorations

U. Belser, J. P. Bernard, J. P. Martinet, and D. Hess

Implant-supported prosthetic treatment of the edentulous jaw with fixed-detachable prostheses has been an integral component of the restorative-therapy spectrum for years (Brånemark et al. 1985). Excellent long-term results have been reported for this type of treatment in controlled prospective studies (Adell and co-workers, 1991). More recently, this has encouraged the focusing of increased attention on treatment of the partially edentulous jaw. A number of recent investigations have addressed the question of whether and under what conditions implants can be expected to be as successful in partially edentulous patients as in those that are totally edentulous (Jemt et al. 1989, van Steenberghe 1989, van Steenberghe et al. 1990, Buser et al. 1991, Buser et al. 1992, Naert et al. 1992, Schmitt and Zarb 1993, Zarb and Schmitt 1993a, Zarb and Schmitt 1993b). Even though the clinical observation period is definitely shorter than for implants in edentulous jaws in general and in the interforaminal region of the lower jaw in particular, the authors mentioned above basically agree that with favorable local conditions and suitable restoration design, a similarly favorable prognosis can be expected in the partially edentulous patient. Some of the pertinent local factors are the quantity and quality of bone, while the prosthetic aspects include the number and positioning of the implants and the design and configuration of the superstructure.

Principles of Superstructure Design

Careful, systematic treatment planning is an indispensable prerequisite for successful fixed prosthodontic treatment (Lang 1988). This is no less true when implants are included in the restoration. In the following, it is assumed that endosseous implants are inserted only within the context of a structured overall treatment plan and that all active pathologic processes have been eliminated during the preprosthetic treatment phase. With the exception of special situations, the generally recognized rules of fixed prosthodontics apply also to implant-borne fixed restorations. The forming of an implant-borne restoration is likewise influenced by function and form, but even greater attention must be given to achieving optimum cleansability (Brägger et al. 1990). A primary concern is to make restoration margins, proximal areas, axial contours, and pontics accessible for simple, thorough routine cleaning procedures. Specific hygiene aids such as Superfloss and fine interdental brushes have proven to be effective in facilitating this task in the visible areas of the mouth where aesthetics cannot be compromised. In this regard, the necessity of adequate follow-up care that includes regular evalutaion of the condition of the peri-implant soft tissue and intensive instruction of the patient regarding personal and professional oral hygiene is indisputable (Marinello et al. 1993).

With increasing clinical experience, there is also a continuously increasing amount of literature concerning the practical prosthetic aspects of implant-borne superstructures (Literature review: Beumer et al. 1993). The literature deals primarily with questions of biomechanics relative to the design (Babbush et al. 1988, Cibirka et al. 1992, Davis et al. 1988, Gracis et al. 1991, Gunne et al. 1992, Matheus et al. 1991, McGlumphy et al. 1992, Rangert et al. 1991, Richter 1989, Stewart et al. 1992, Sullivan et al. 1986, Sutter et al. 1988, Sutter et al. 1993, Watson et al. 1991, Weinberg 1993), as well as the clinical procedures (Assif et al. 1992, Carr 1991).

Specific Indications

In the following sections, the respective prosthetic procedures will be explained and illustrated through concrete examples that are typical for cases in which two-part ITI implants are indicated (12.**1a–b**).

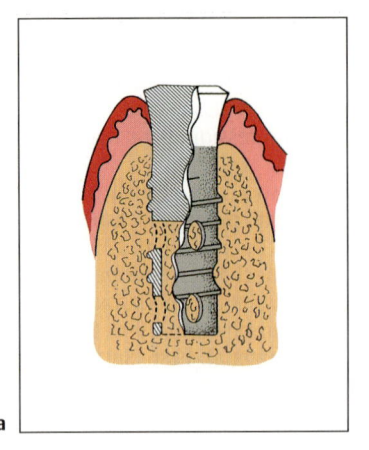

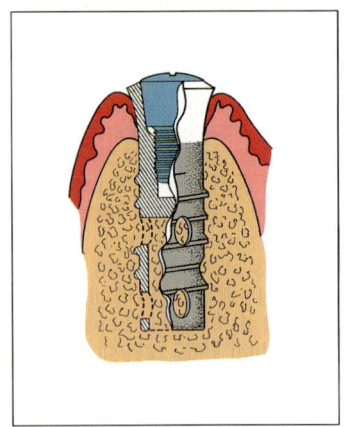

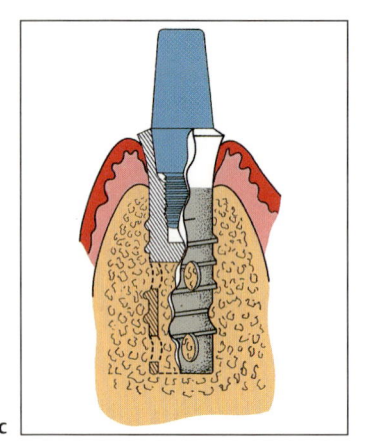

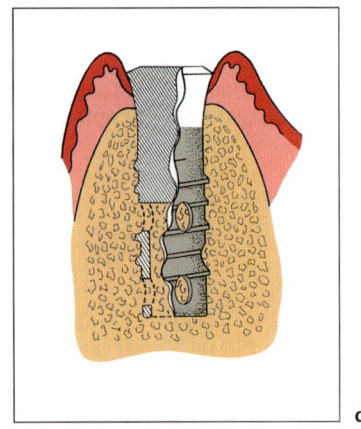

Fig. 12.**1a** Hollow screw (HS) implant with supramucosally located shoulder
b The supramucosal location of the implant shoulder permits the use of an internal occlusal closure screw during the healing phase
c HS implant after completion of tissue integration. The standard conical secondary component (abutment) allows the prosthetic superstructure to be attached with either cement or a screw
d A more deeply placed HS with the shoulder located submucosally

Specific Indications

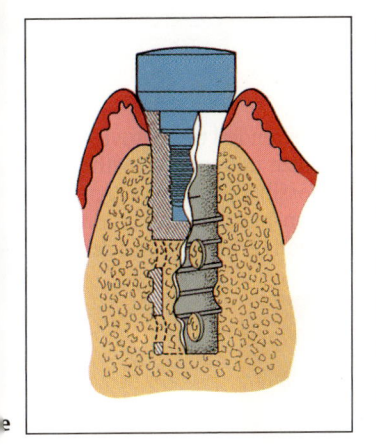

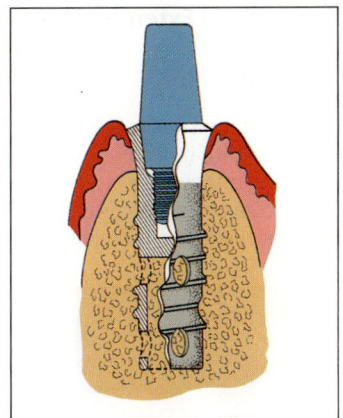

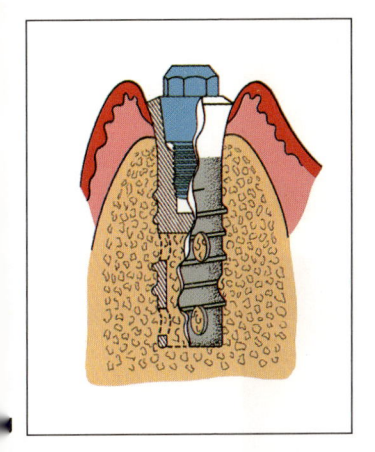

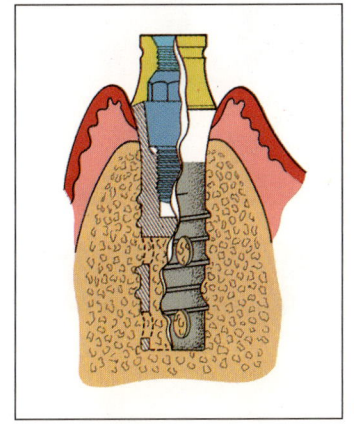

- **e** During the healing phase, a properly contoured titanium healing cap conditions the peri-implant soft tissue
- **f** HS implant after completion of tissue integration with a standard abutment screwed to place. Making an accurate impression of the submucosal implant shoulder can prove troublesome
- **g** HS with an Octa secondary component screwed to place. This allows the relationships in the mouth to be transferred to the working cast by means of integral laboratory analogs and also accommodates prefabricated elements
- **h** HS implant with submucosal shoulder, Octa secondary component, and prefabricated gold coping to which gold alloy can be cast to form the prosthetic superstructure

Mandibular Distal Extension Cases

Cemented Restorations
(Fig. 12.**2a–e**)
If a distally shortened lower dental arch is to be extended to improve masticatory function and, more importantly, to stabilize unopposed teeth (with aesthetics being relatively less important) it is possible to proceed according to the basic concept (supragmucosal restoration margins and traditional prosthetic procedures, i.e., conventional impression techniques and cement-

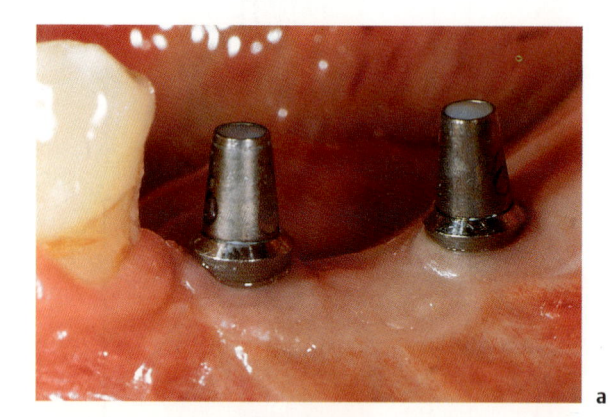

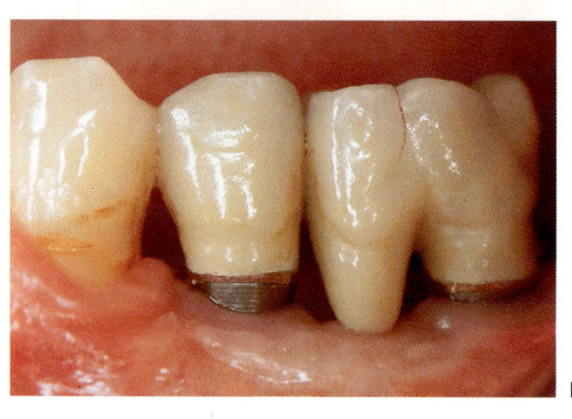

Fig. 12.**2a** Lower dental arch that is shortened posteriorly on the left side. Two ITI implants have been placed in the second premolar and first molar areas and fitted with standard 6° posts. The implant shoulders are located supramucosally

b A three-unit ceramo-metal bridge has been cemented. The ease with which the prosthetic superstructure can be cleaned is apparent

Specific Indications **379**

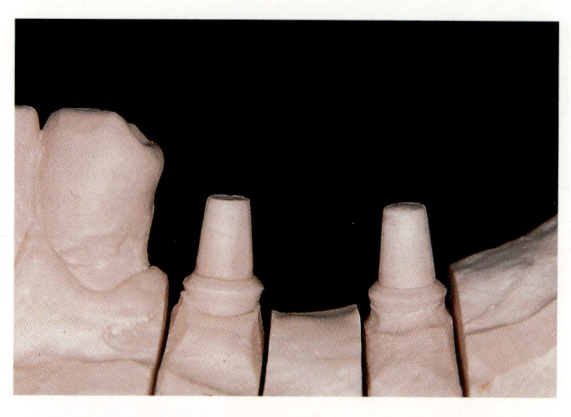

c The master cast is formed in die stone from a conventional impression

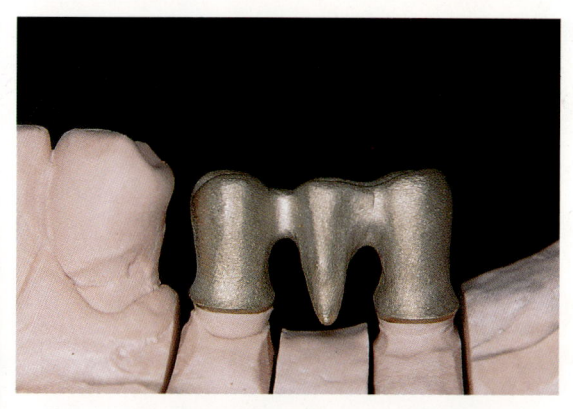

d Three-unit metal framework on the sectioned cast

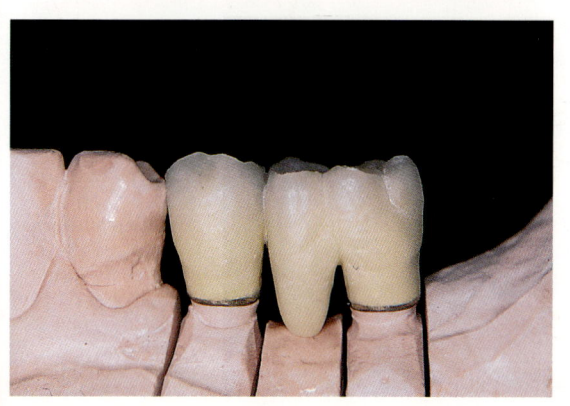

e Unglazed ceramometal bridge ready for trial insertion

380 12 Fixed Prosthetic Restorations

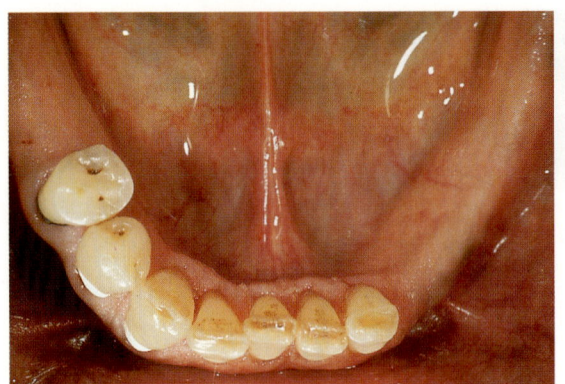

Fig. 12.**3a** Occlusal view of a bilaterally shortened lower dental arch. The prognosis for a removable partial denture is poor because of the absence of the strategically important canine on the left

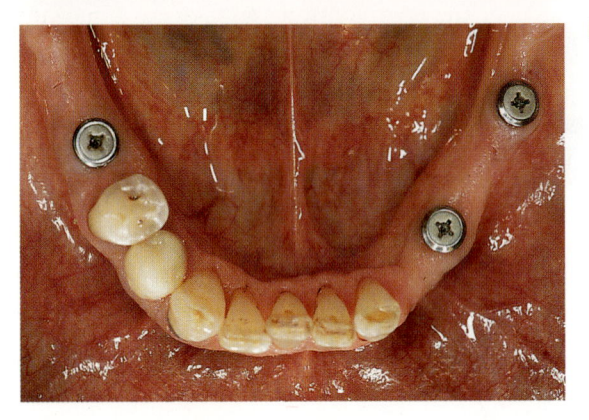

b The placement of three implants makes fixed partial dentures possible

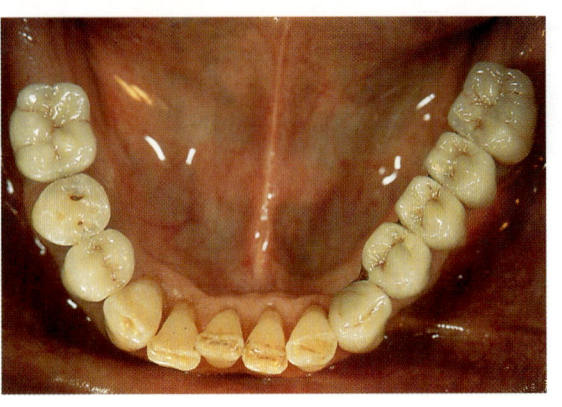

c Clinical view following cementation of a purely implant-borne five-unit ceramo-metal restoration # 18–22 (FDI numbers 34–37) with a mesial cantilever. There are also individual crowns on tooth # 28 (FDI 44) and implant # 30 (FDI 46)

ed fixed superstructures). The primary advantages of this method are that it is simple (the operator does not need to alter his or her accustomed fixed prosthodontic techniques), and the transition from restoration to implant is located in a region that presents no cleaning problems for the patient (Buser et al. 1988). In cases with severely compromised initial conditions (Fig. 12.**3a–c**), the use of implants may make it possible to avoid a prognostically poor removable partial denture.

Fixed-Detachable Restorations (Fig. 12.**4a–g**)
The primary indication for fixed-detachable implant-borne superstructures are presented in chapter 12, page 383 ff. Compared with fixed (cemented) retainers, their advantages and disadvantages are as follows:

Advantages

- They can be removed at any time, which makes it easier to monitor mobility, probing depths, etc.
- In case of a failure (e.g. loss of an implant), a new implant can eventually be placed and the existing superstructure reused or modified to fit the new situation with minimum expense
- The remaining precision attachments can be used to anchor a more conventional distal extension prosthesis

Disadvantages

- Screws can come loose or break
- Organic debris in the gaps that are always present undergo bacterial decomposition to form foul-smelling compounds
- There is a greater tendency for plaque to accumulate
- The laboratory work is technically more complex and expensive

Figures 12.**4h–m** show two examples of the construction of fixed-detachable distal extension bridges (precision sliding attachment and screws) in the mandible.

382 12 Fixed Prosthetic Restorations

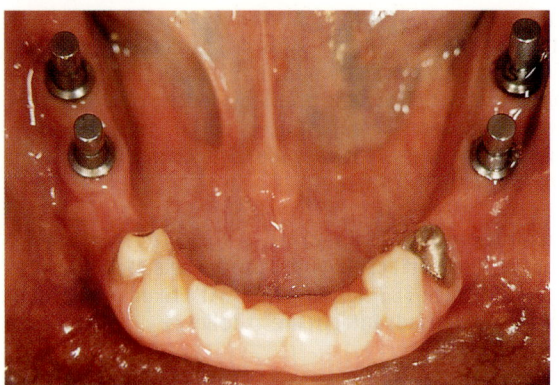

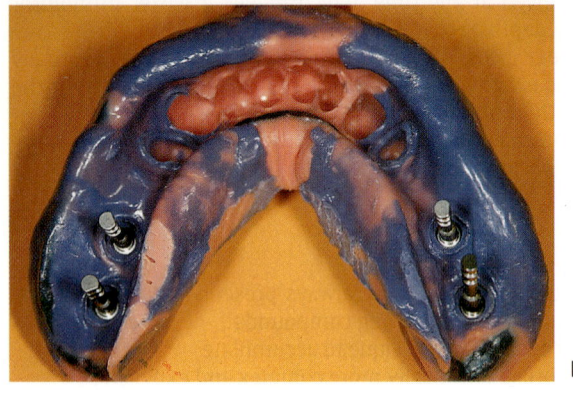

Fig. 12.**4a** Bilaterally shortened lower dental arch. Two distally located implants were placed on each side because there was an inadequate transverse bulk of bone in the areas of the missing second premolars. The impression cylinders have been screwed onto the four 15° standard abutments in order to transfer the occlusal threads to the working cast to accommodate the planned fixed-detachable superstructure
b Full-arch lower impression with impression cylinders repositioned and laboratory analogs screwed into them (manipulation implants)
c Lower master cast
d Sectioned cast with metal frameworks. Note that the implant superstructures are not connected to the copings on the natural first premolars
e Occlusal view of the ceramo-metal restorations in the unglazed state

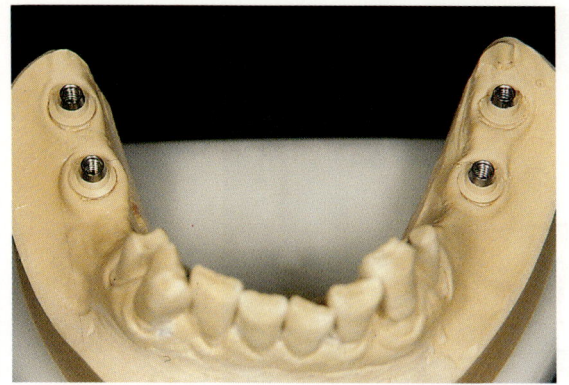

Specific Indications **383**

c

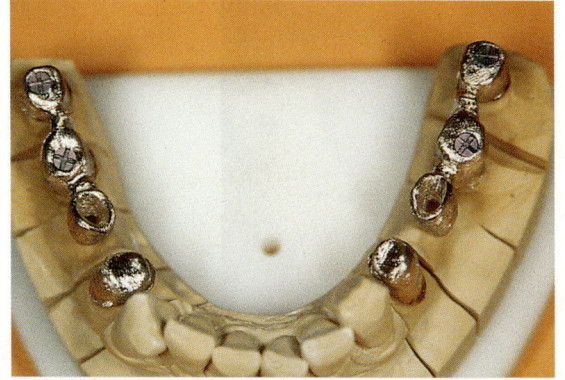

d

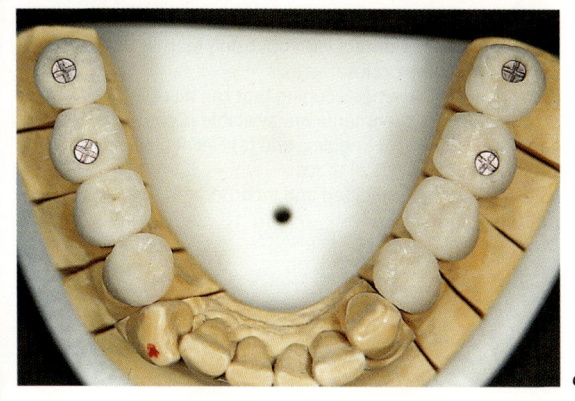

e

384 12 Fixed Prosthetic Restorations

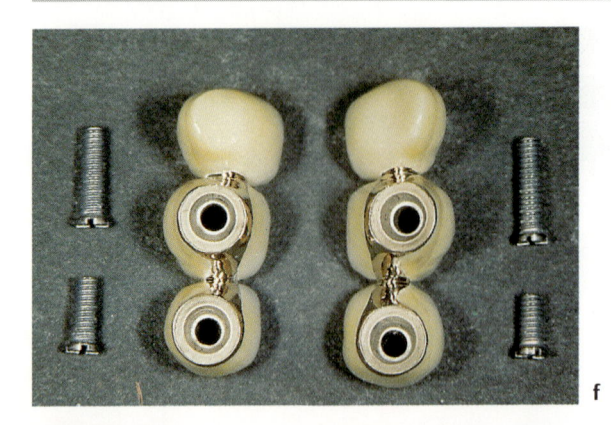

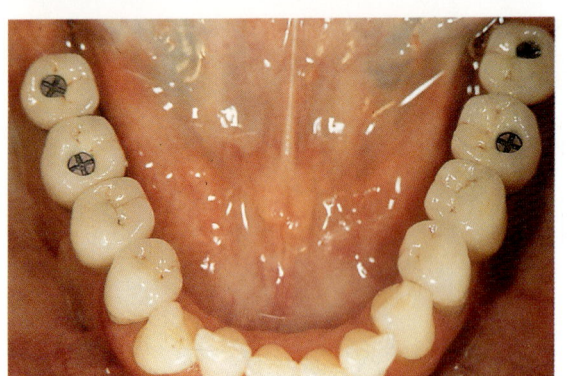

f Underside of both fixed-detachable implant-borne superstructures
g View of the restored mandibular arch. Contact with opposing teeth is to be avoided in the areas of the slightly countersunk occlusal screws
h Implant abutment fitted with a precious metal coping that can be cast to
i Various models of precision sliding attachments are available (Cendres et Métaux, CH-2501 Biel, Switzerland): (a) Conex, (b) Regulex, and (c) Flecher. Selection of the attachment depends on the available vertical space
j In this case, a Regulex attachment was selected and incorporated in the casting of the crown on the first premolar tooth

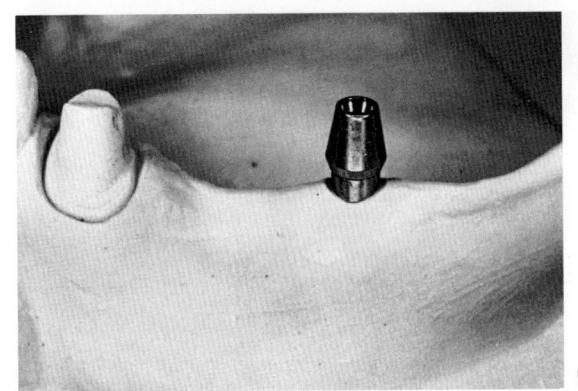

Specific Indications **385**

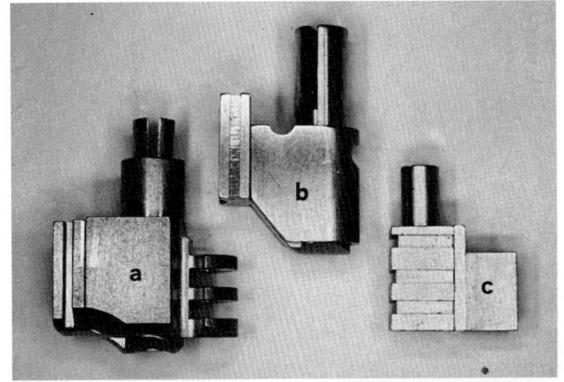

h

i

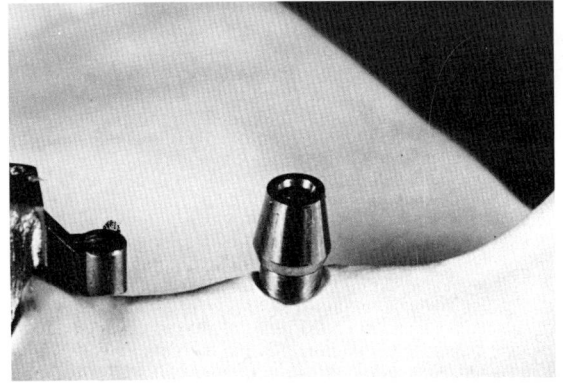

j

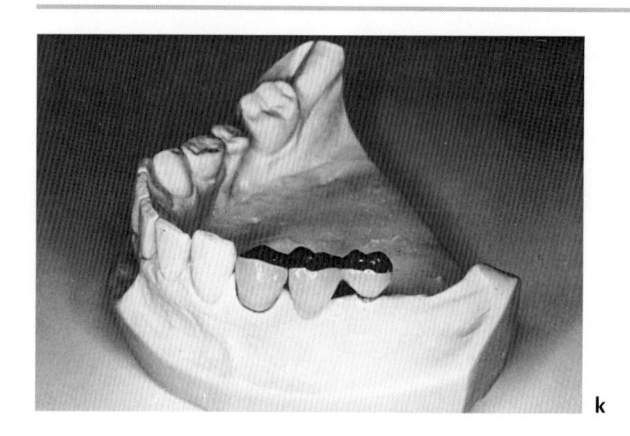

386 12 Fixed Prosthetic Restorations

k

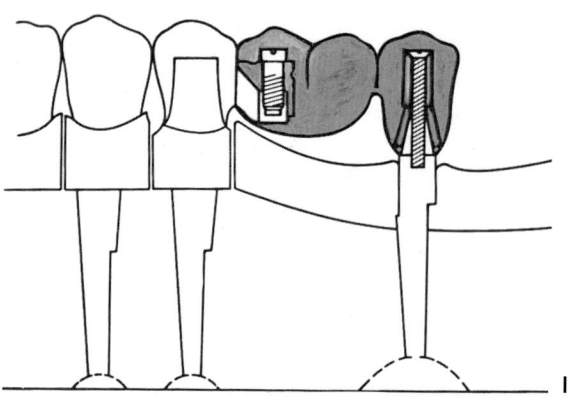

l

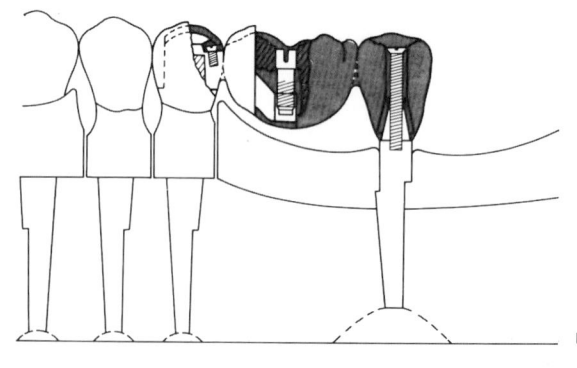

m

Fixed (Cemented) Prostheses

Advantages
- They are stable and do not loosen
- There are no gaps to retain debris
- They are simple to clean
- They are less expensive

Disadvantages
- Limited ability to monitor the implants
- Practically no possibility of adding to or modifying the prosthesis in case of a failure, such as loss of an implant

The advantages and disadvantages presented here for the two types of construction are not all of equal importance.

There is a basic difference between natural abutments and implant abutments in regard to resiliency. The mobility of a natural abutment due to the presence of a periodontal ligament is in contrast to the rigid anchorage of an osseointegrated implant abutment. According to Ericsson and co-workers (1986), this fundamental difference presents a possible risk for biomechanical complications in a fixed partial denture with mixed support. Rangert and co-workers (1991) have succinctly posed the questions associated with mixed-support restorations as follows:

- Does the mobility of the tooth prohibit it from sharing the occlusal forces with the implant, leading to implant overload and/or inadequate stimulation of the tooth?
- Is an additional implant-integrated elastic element necessary to compensate for the periodontal attachment?

Several recent clinical and theoretical studies have contributed to a better understanding of mixed-support restorations. In the first of these works, published by Erickson and co-workers (1986), good results were reported with this type of restoration, although the authors also reported some biomechanical problems. Astrand et al. (1991) and Gunne et al. (1992) came to an interesting conclusion in their long term studies. They found that

---

k Buccal view of completed bridge
l Schematic drawing of a longitudinal section through the construction
m Representation of a relatively complex, technically demanding restoration with precision attachment and screw in the pontic (laboratory technicians: Carisch, Waldenburg, and Flury, Bern)

implant abutments of mixed-support restorations exhibit less bone resorption radiographically than do corresponding abutments of purely implant-borne bridges. A possible explanation of this result was presented by Rangert and co-workers (1991) in their in vitro study: A Brånemark implant, due to the flexibility between the implant body and implant abutment, exhibits a resiliency similar to that of a natural abutment tooth. In the same article, the authors recommend that in restorations with mixed support, the span be made as long as possible to keep the load on the implant as small as possible (due to the elasticity of the bridge structure). The opposite opinion was expressed by Weinberg (1993). He refers to the law of levers and recommends that the bridge span be kept as short as possible, or that a stress breaker be incorporated into the pontic area.

Because the literature in the area of mixed restorations is sparse—especially lacking are longitudinal clinical studies over several years—and the interpretations are sometimes contradictory, it seems wise to approach mixed restorations with a certain amount of caution. Whenever possible, the problem should be circumvented by not connecting implants and natural abutments in the same prosthesis. Fig. 12.**4a** shows a mandibular case after the insertion of two posterior implants. Even though crowns were planned for the two natural first premolar abutment teeth, the implants were not connected to the natural teeth for the reasons mentioned above. The purely implant-borne restorations will consequently include a mesial cantilevered pontic with the size of a premolar. The increased risk of loosening of the superstructure in this situation, in addition to the limited intermaxillary space, make a fixed-detachable prosthesis advisable. The various components of the standard system (Sutter et al. 1988, Flury et al. 1991) are well suited for use in the technical procedures. It is especially important that the threaded occlusal opening be transferred to the master cast through an appropriate standardized impression procedure (Fig. 12.**4b** and **c**).

Maxillary Distal Extension Cases

It is frequently possible for a distally shortened dental arch in the maxilla to be expanded through the pemolar regions by means of implants. The specific characteristic of the two-part ITI implants (large surface areas for comparatively short lengths) makes them well suited for this kind of situation (limited vertical bone height, spongy bone structure) (Fig. 12.**5a** and **b**). If the initial tooth positions are favorable, even a maxilla with a minimal number of remaining teeth can be restored with a fixed prosthesis (Fig. 12.**6a–h**).

Specific Indications **389**

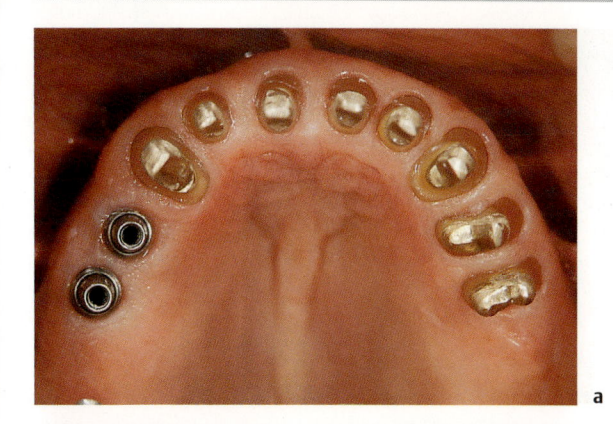

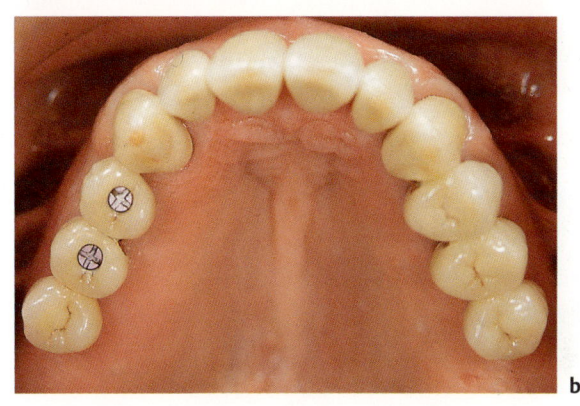

Fig. 12.**5a** Occlusal view of a bilaterally shortened maxillary dental arch. The patient preferred fixed restorations. The natural teeth from the right canine through the left second premolar are nonvital and have been fitted with gold post-and-cores. Two implants have been placed in the right first and second premolar areas

b Completed case after insertion of a ceramo-metal full arch reconstruction: Individual crowns from right canine through left lateral, four-unit cantilever bridge from left canine through left first molar, and a cantilevered pontic in the right first molar region supported solely by the two premolar implants

390 12 Fixed Prosthetic Restorations

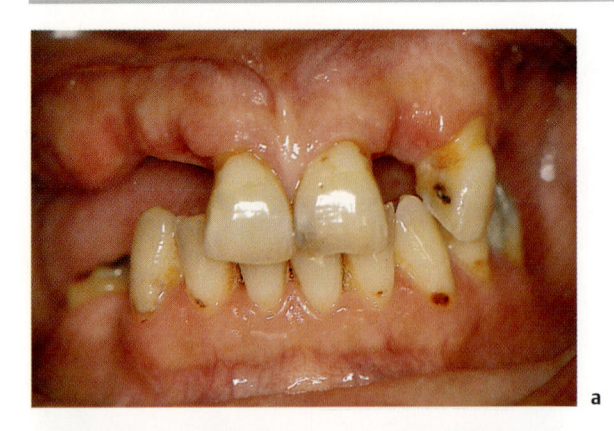

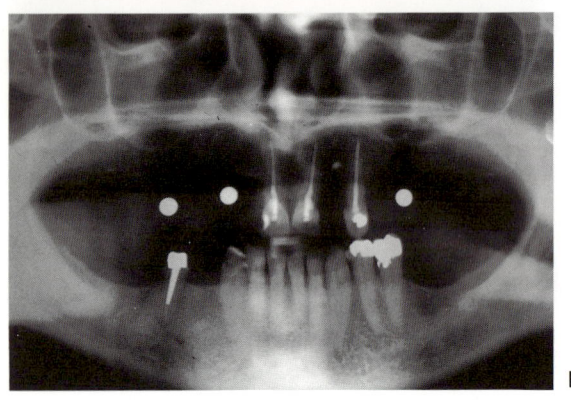

Fig. 12.**6a** Frontal view of a 42-year-old female patient who has lost multiple teeth
  b Corresponding panoramic radiograph. Steel balls of known diameter attached to a vacuum-formed template help to evaluate the vertical height of bone in the prospective implant sites
  c In order to precisely locate the ideal implant sites, a diagnostic waxup extending through the premolar regions has been made
  d The indispensable surgical template is shown in place during the surgical phase
  e Occlusal view after completion of the healing phase with implants in areas 4, 5, 7, 12, and 13 (FDI numbers 15, 14, 12, 24, and 25)

Specific Indications

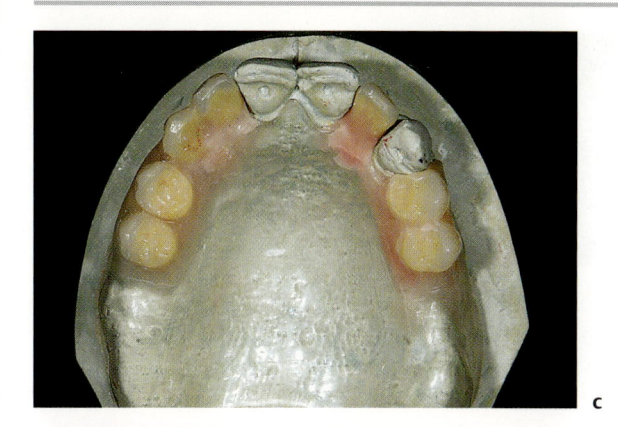

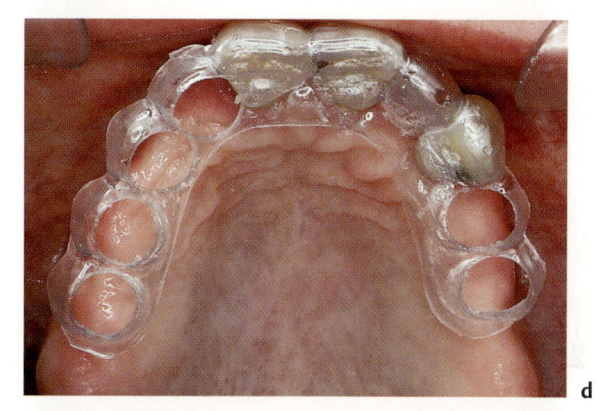

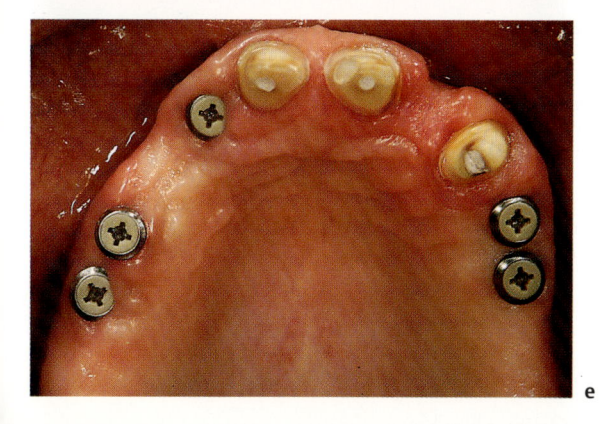

392 12 Fixed Prosthetic Restorations

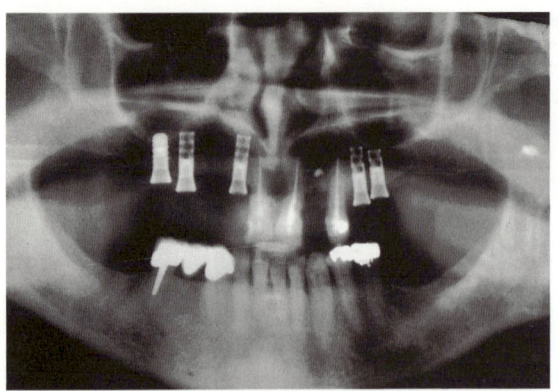

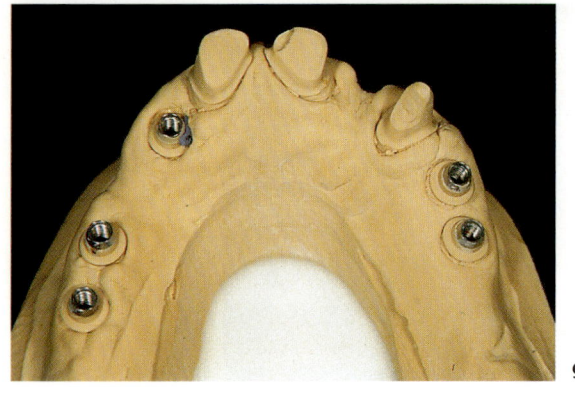

f Radiograph prior to implant loading
g Maxillary working cast. While the laboratory analogs reproduce the occlusal threads, an impression must be made of all of the preparation finish lines and implant shoulders in a conventional manner. This can prove difficult, especially when there are multiple abutments
h Sectioned cast with metal frameworks
i Completed maxillary case ready for clinical try-in
j Occlusal view of the maxillary arch after insertion of the metal-ceramic construction. Restorations are cemented on the natural teeth, but attached to the implants with screws. The slightly counter-sunk occlusal screws will be covered with acrylic resin

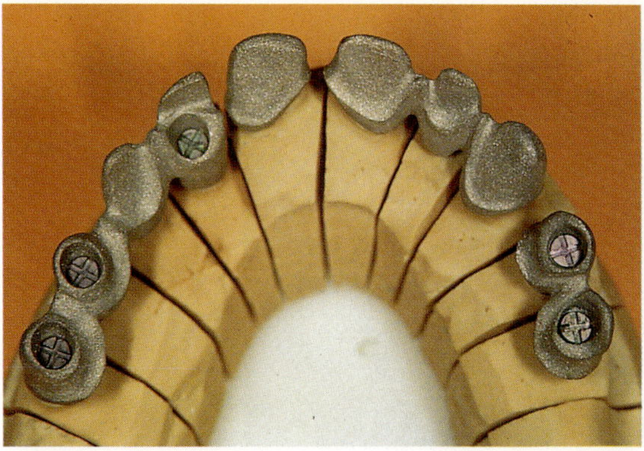

Specific Indications **393**

h

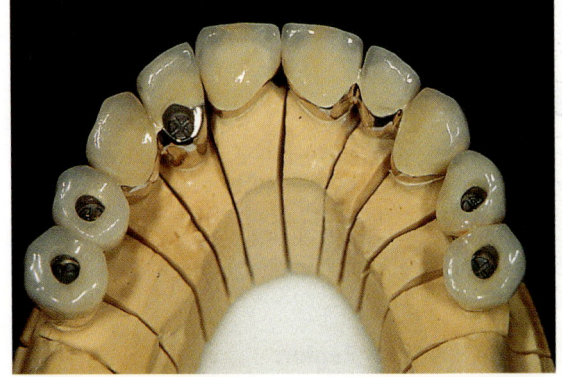

i

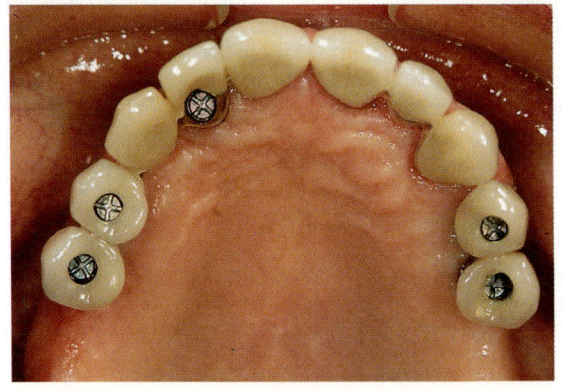

j

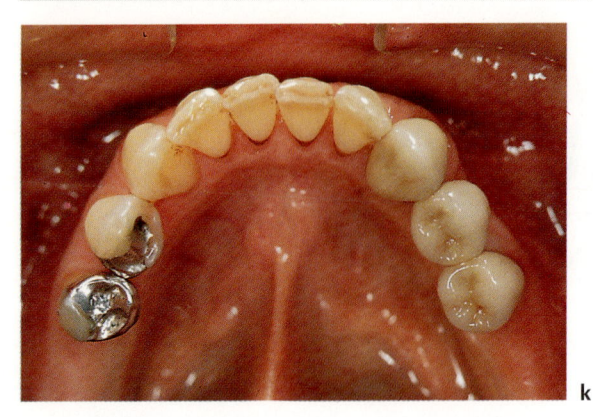

k View of the completed lower arch. Staying consistent with the premolar occlusion concept, none of the missing molars were replaced

The Edentulous Mandible

As explained in chapters 9 and 11, severely resorbed edentulous mandibles are preferably restored with removable overdentures supported by two to four anterior implants with spherical retention elements or bar attachments.

In selected cases, in which the patient express the desire for a fixed prosthesis, this can be provided by placing implants in the posterior regions as well (Fig. 12.**7a–g**).

Edentulous Spaces in the Posterior Region

Long-span fixed partial dentures on natural abutment teeth present an increased risk of failure. The most frequent causes of failure in these cases are loss of retention and fractures of abutments and frameworks. Carefully considered placement of endosseous implants in these situations often permits the fabrication of fixed restorations with a more favorable prognosis (Fig. 12.**8a** and **b**).

Fig. 12.**7a** Initial condition of a 62-year-old female patient who wished to have the lower arch treated with a fixed prosthesis if possilbe
b The diagnostic panoramic radiograph shows that even in the postforaminal region, there is adequate bone height for implants
c Radiograph taken immediately after the placement of six HS implants

Specific Indications **395**

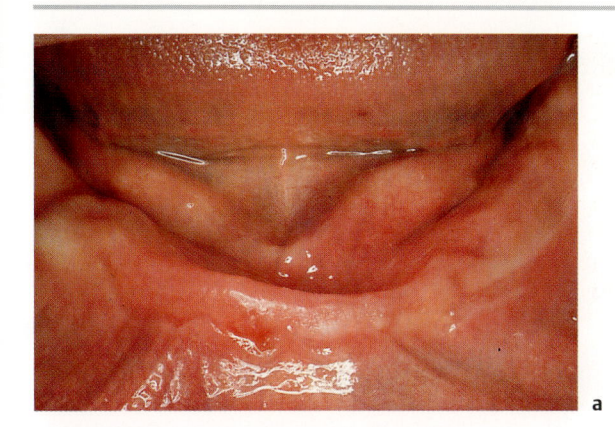

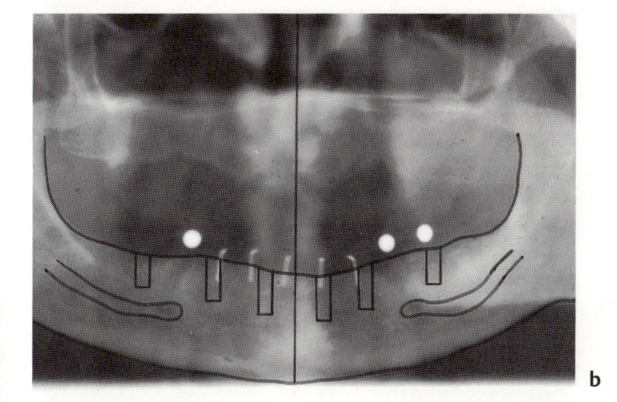

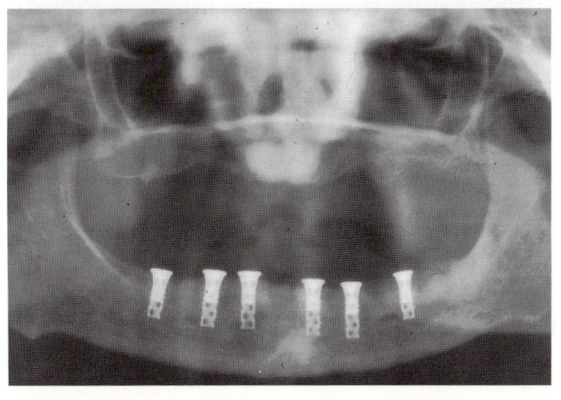

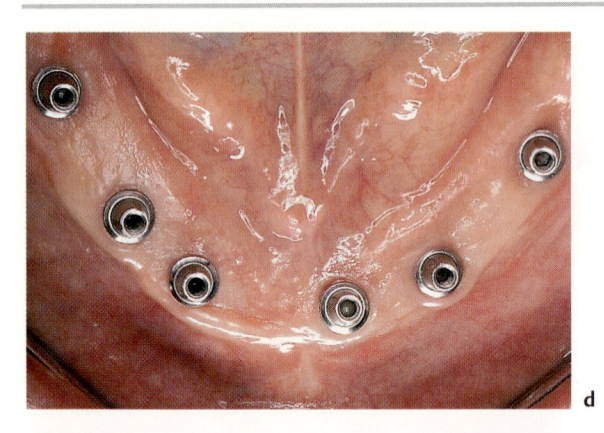

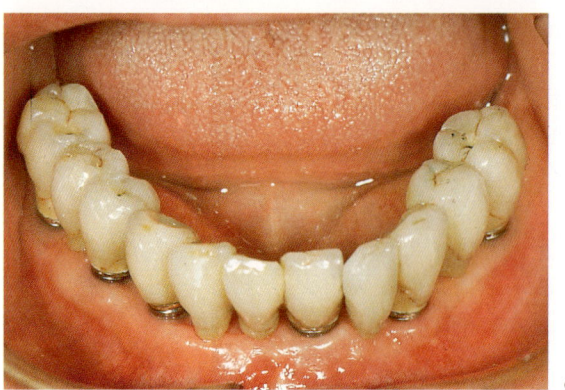

d After successful tissue integration, the appropriate standard posts are screwed to place
e The prosthetic superstructure was prepared in three segments and veneered with resin

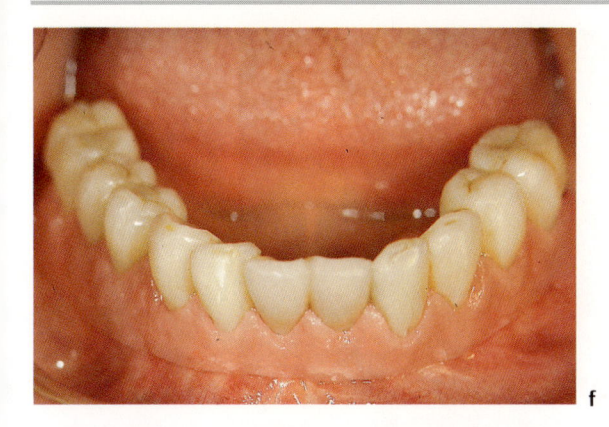

f At the patient's request, a removable silicone gingival epithesis (mask) was made to improve aesthetics and provide lip support

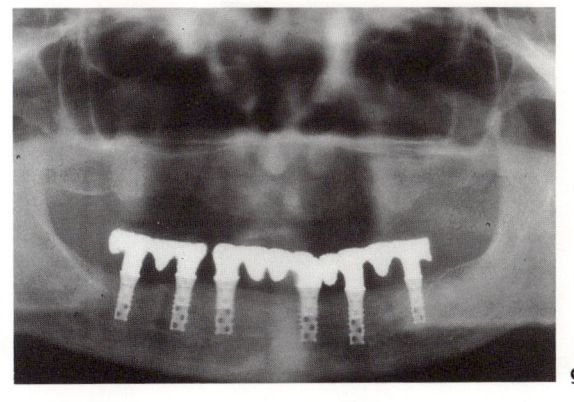

g Recall radiograph made 3 years after insertion of the prosthetic superstructure

398 12 Fixed Prosthetic Restorations

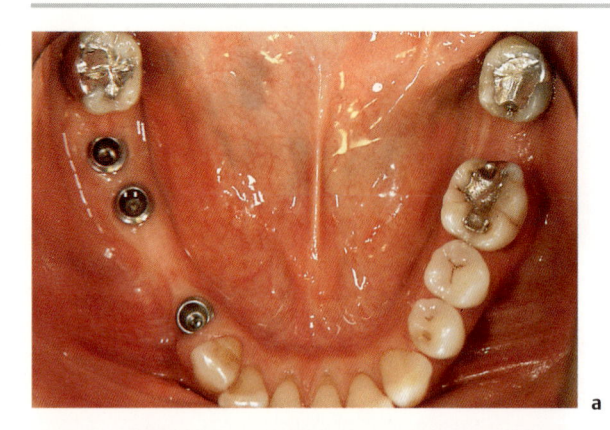

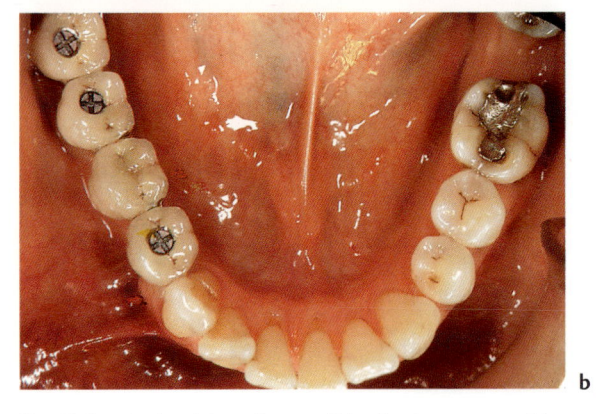

Fig. 12.**8a** Occlusal view of a mandible after integration of three HS implants within an extensive tooth-bounded space on the right side. The small space in the left second molar region was considered stable and required no restoration
b Completed case after insertion of an entirely implant-borne fixed-detachable four-unit bridge

Fig. 12.**9a** Frontal view of an edentulous space in the maxillary anterior region. Two endosseous implants were placed slightly submucosally in the areas of the right lateral and left central incisors. Before the impression was made, Octa abutments were screwed into place
b The gold copings of the Octa system are made in an alloy that can be cast to. They are available in two configurations: with (left) and without (right) the internal octagon shape. For fixed partial dentures, caps with the round internal configuration are usually employed

Edentulous Spaces in the Maxillary Anterior Region

Conventional Configuration

There are additional aesthetic considerations that must be taken into account when placing implant-supported restorations in the maxillary anterior region. These will be discussed in detail in the next section (single-tooth spaces). It has been unanimously agreed upon that the transmucosal ITI implant must be inserted more deeply to avoid visible metal in the cervical region. Consequently, a secondary component must be used in these cases that permits a simple, reproducible transfer of the spatial relationships in the mouth to the working cast (integral laboratory analogs) and allows fabrication of the superstructure by means of prefabricated elements (Sutter et al. 1993) Fig. 12.**9a–f**).

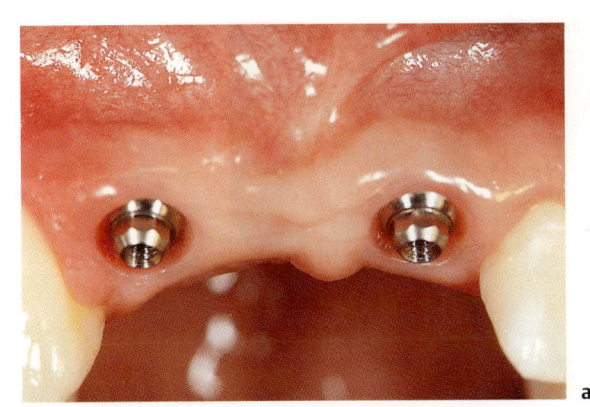

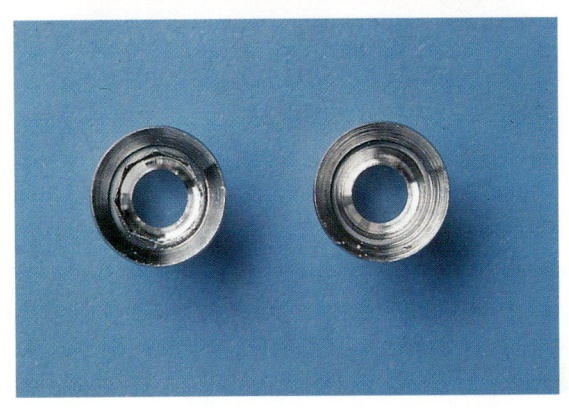

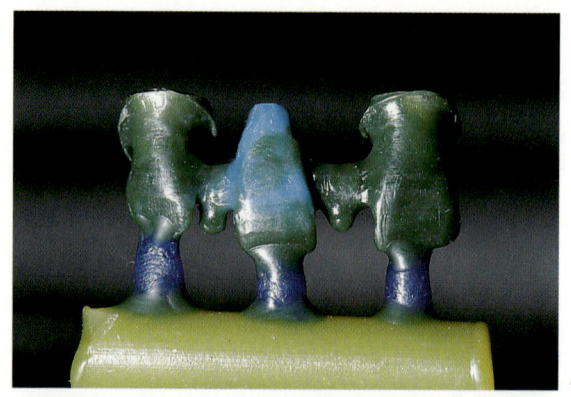

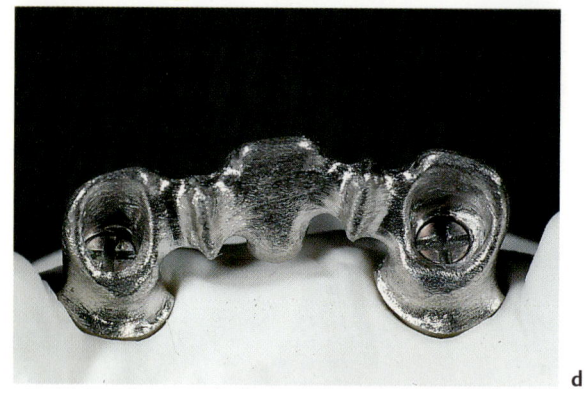

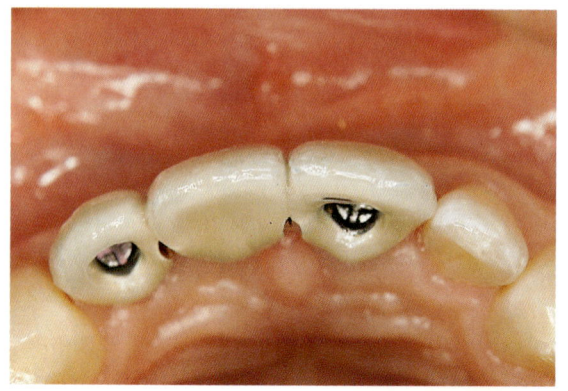

12 Fixed Prosthetic Restorations

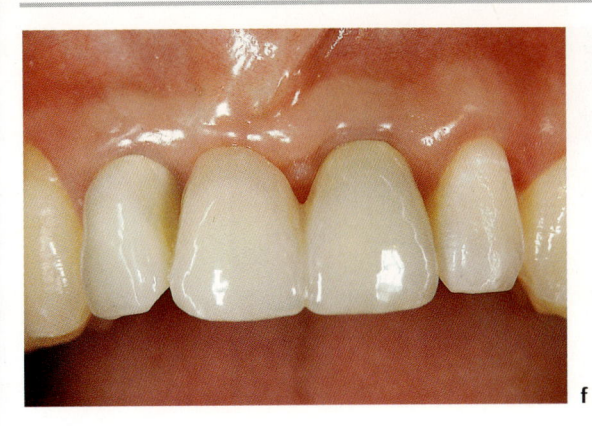

f Labial view of the same case

Compensation for Lost Tissue

In edentulous anterior jaw segments with pronounced loss of alveolar ridge and associated soft tissue, a gingival façade can be made part of the superstructure to provide an aesthetically and phonetically acceptable result (Fig. 12.**10a–g**). This, of course, must not compromise the cleansability of the prosthesis.

Single Tooth Spaces

Mandibular Posterior Region

In order to produce superstructure contours that are optimum–i.e., that are appropriate for the given dimensions of the standardized implant shoulder and that are easy for the patient to keep clean–the edentulous space should correspond to a premolar unit in the buccal segment (Sidler 1983) (Fig. 12.**11a–d**).

c Wax pattern of the three-unit fixed partial denture ready to be invested. The prefabricated elements can be recognized in the retainers
d Completed framework repositioned on the master cast
e Occlusal view of the implant-borne, metal-ceramic fixed partial denture before the screws are covered with composite resin

402 12 Fixed Prosthetic Restorations

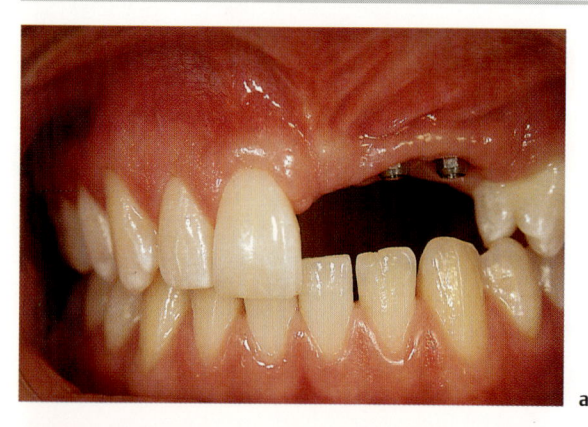

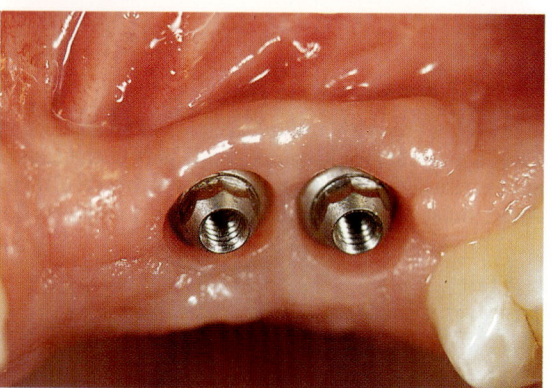

Fig. 12.**10a** The upper left central, lateral, and canine have been lost in an accident. Despite extensive damage to the alveolar bone and soft tissues, it was possible to insert two imlants following an augmentation procedure.
b Close-up view of the two implants fitted with Octa abutments after successful tissue integration
c To compensate for the loss of tissue, an artificial gingival façade was added to the fixed-detachable prosthesis, and to compensate for the excessive mesiodistal space, a proximal ceramic veneer will be bonded to the natural right central incisor
d This postoperative labial view documents the symmetrical result that was achieved
e Frontal view in maximum intercuspation

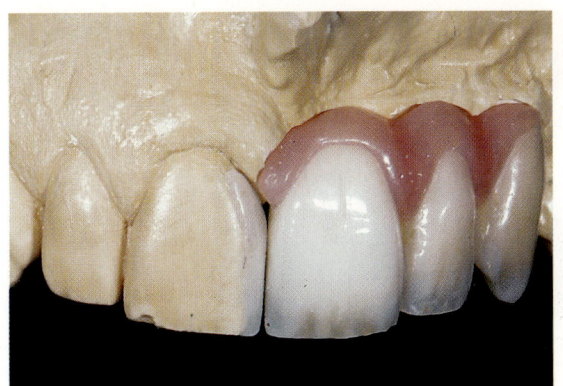

Specific Indications **403**

c

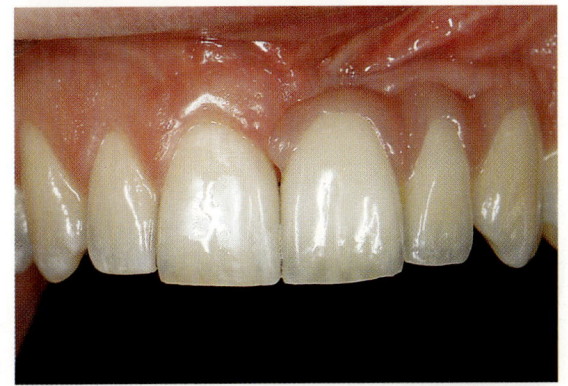

d

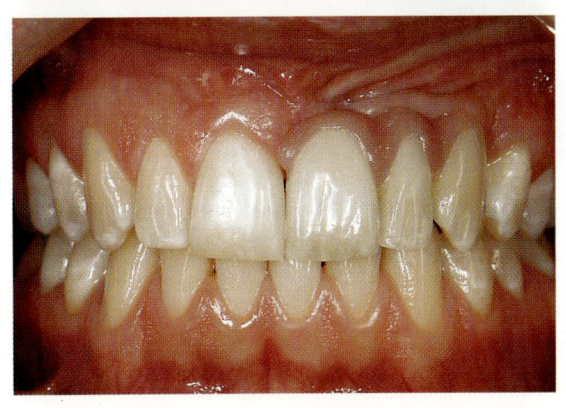

e

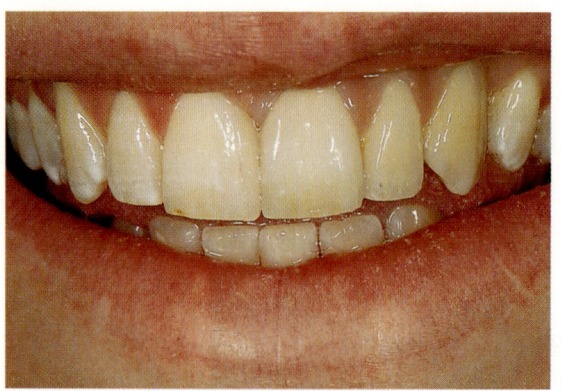

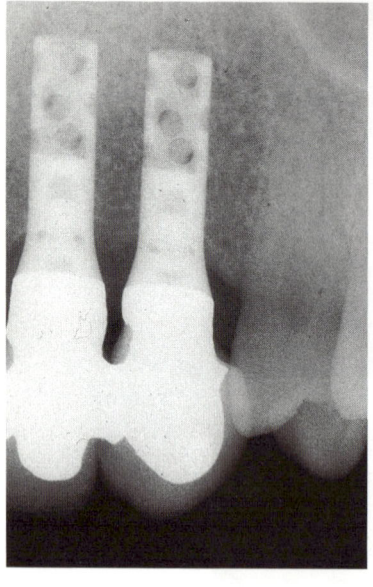

f When the patient smiles, the transition from gingival façade to alveolar mucosa is not discernible

g Follow-up radiograph 2 years after implantation

Specific Indications **405**

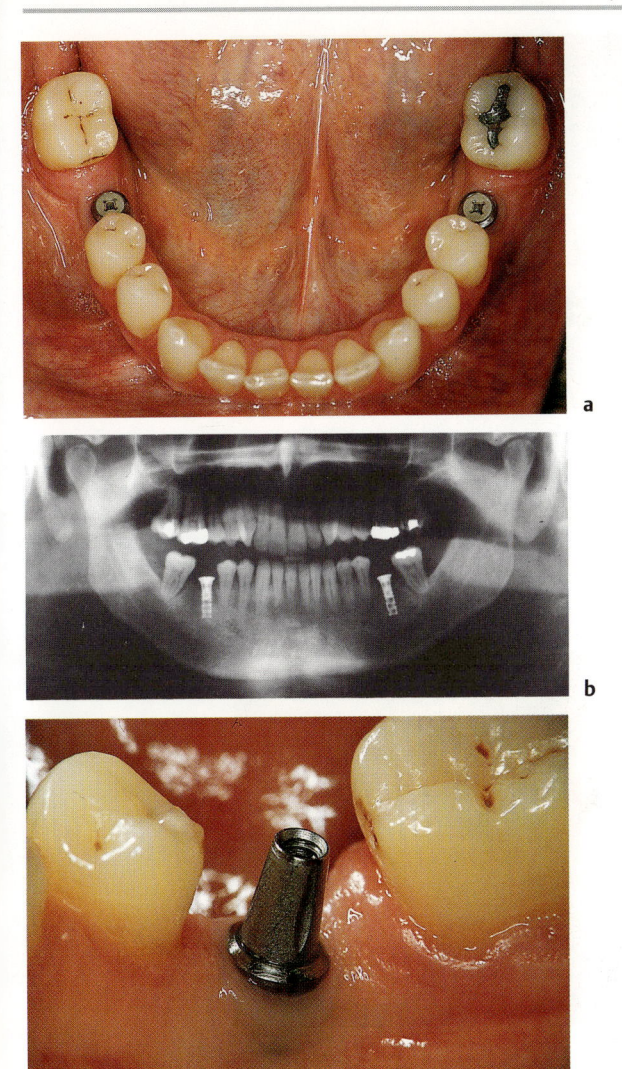

Fig. 12.**11a** Bilateral single-tooth spaces in the lower first molar regions treated with implants
b Postoperative panoramic radiograph
c Lingual view of one of the implants placed in accordance with the basic concept (supramucosal implant shoulder) with a conical post screwed in place. For cemented superstructures, the threaded occlusal opening is closed with composite before the impression is made

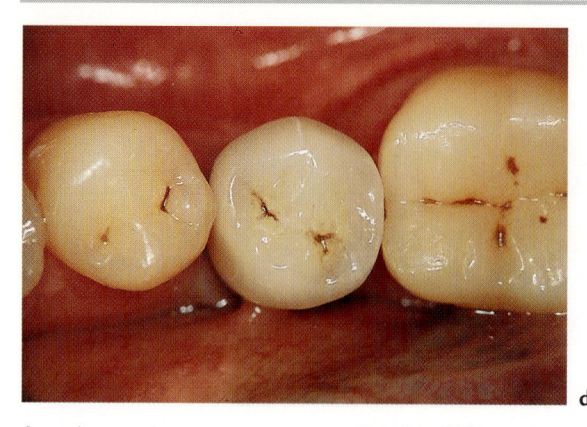

d Final view after cementation of a metal-ceramic crown with the dimension of a premolar

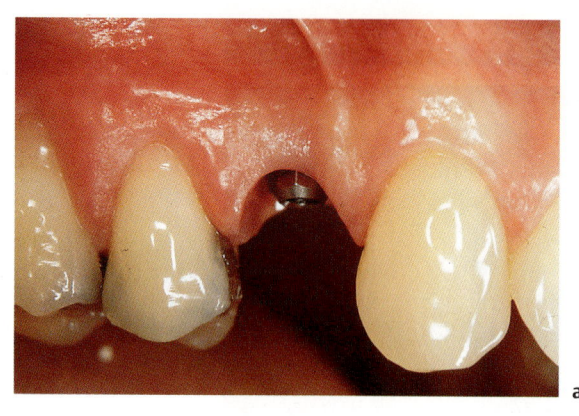

Fig. 12.**12a** Implant treatment of a single-tooth space created by loss of an upper right first premolar. Primarily for aesthetic considerations, the shoulder of the implant has been placed submucosally
b and **c** This type of restoration margin is difficult to clean using normal measures, but can be effectively reached with Superfloss, provided the axial contours of the crown are correct
d The use of prefabricated metal copings allows optimum adaptation of the margins, as this radiograph made one year after insertion of the restoration shows

Specific Indications

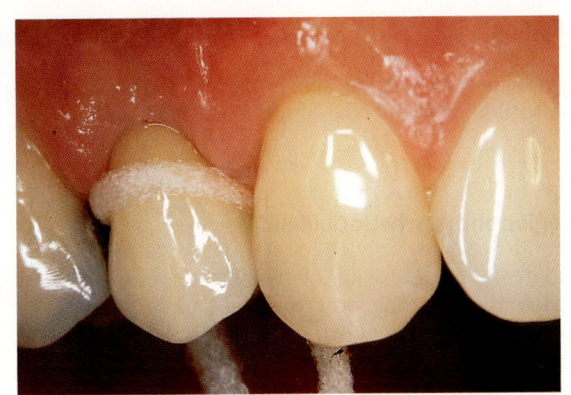

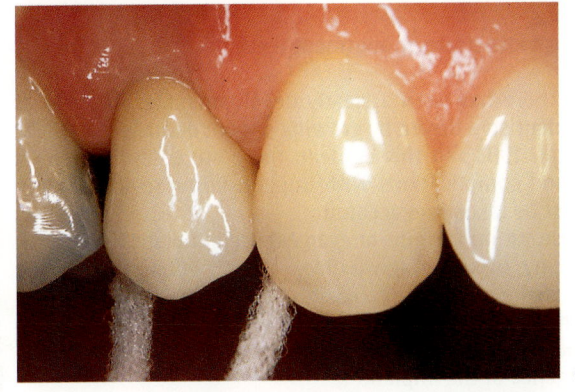

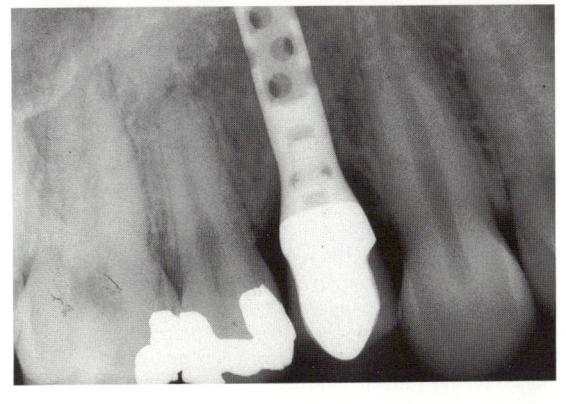

Maxillary Posterior Region

In addition to the guidelines mentioned above, there are also aesthetic requirements in the visible zone of the upper posterior region (Fig. 12.**12a–d**).

Maxillary Anterior Region and Aesthetic Guidelines

An implant-supported dental prosthesis in the maxillary anterior region is especially indicated when the following local conditions are present:
- Intact adjacent teeth
- Inadequate prospective abutment teeth (endodontic problems, unfavorable morphology, existing prosthetic restorations)
- Excessively long edentulous span
- Multiple diastemas
- Absence of one or more strategic abutment teeth

In recent years, there has been a steady development in the field of aesthetic restorative dentistry, driven by growing patient demands (Nathanson 1991, Magne et al. 1993). In this context, there are certain potential aesthetic problems and complications with implant-borne restorations in visible areas that must be taken into account:
- Visible metal (restoration margins or even exposed implant shoulders)
- Disturbed harmony of the gingival line (abrupt differences in the gingival level, loss of papillae)
- Altered axial profile (for example, in form of an excessive ridge lap because of an inadequate amount of labial bone or as the result of a too-far palatal emergence of the implant.

To avoid possible aesthetic complications, careful analysis of the prospective implant locations, complemented by a systematic treatment plan and a surgical template, is indispensible (Bernard et al. 1992, Bernard et al. 1993). To obtain an optimum aesthetic result in certain cases, a "site development" or "site conditioning" procedure is indicated, sometimes by employing the principle of guided tissue regeneration (Buser et al. 1993).

Fig. 12.**13a** Two implants have been integrated in the spaces created by the congenital absence of both maxillary lateral incisors. Placement of the Octa abutments makes the submucosal location of the implant shoulders apparent

b Impression copings are attached with guide screws to permit precise transfer of the relationships in the mouth to the casts

c Trial insertion of the impression tray with openings at the predetermined sites

Specific Indications

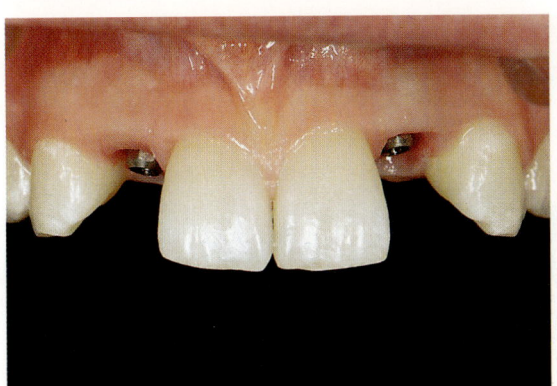

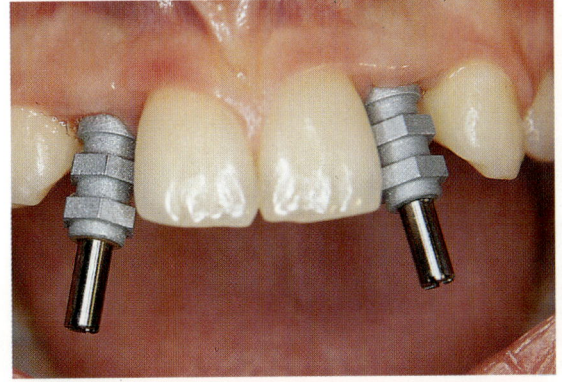

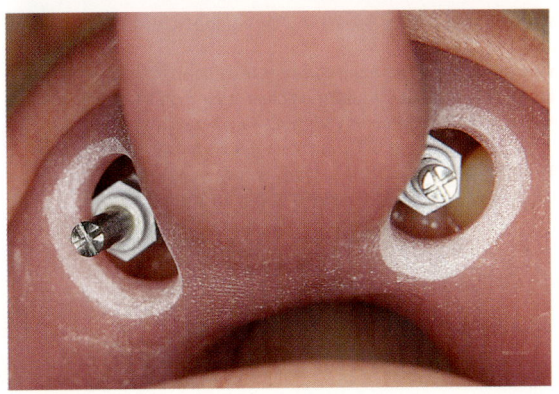

410 12 Fixed Prosthetic Restorations

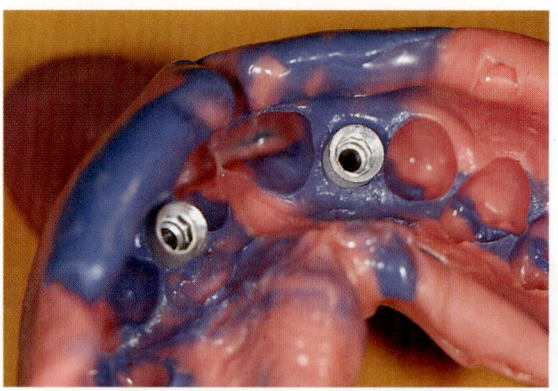

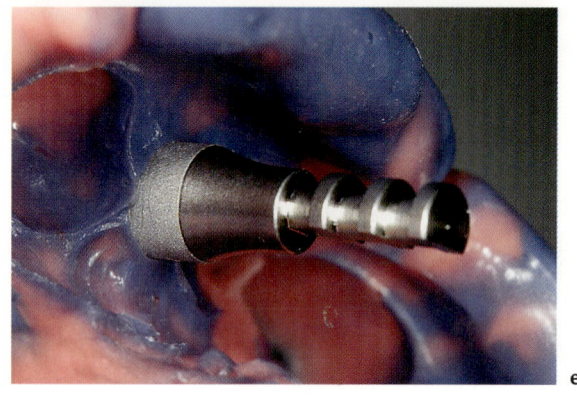

d The impression has been removed after loosening the guide screws. The copings remain in the impression
e Before the impression is poured, implant analogs are screwed into the copings
f The subgingival position of the implant shoulders is clearly seen on the working cast
g Fabrication of a removable silicone replica of the mucosa is recommended as an aid in forming the correct flat emergence profile in the superstructure and to facilitate access to the shoulders of the implants
h Occlusal view of the fixed-detachable single crowns ready for try-in

Specific Indications **411**

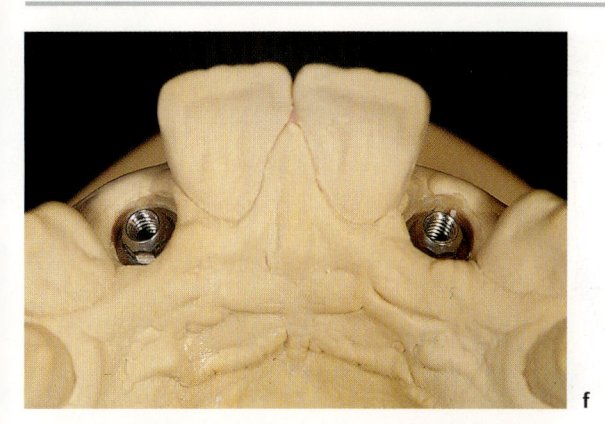

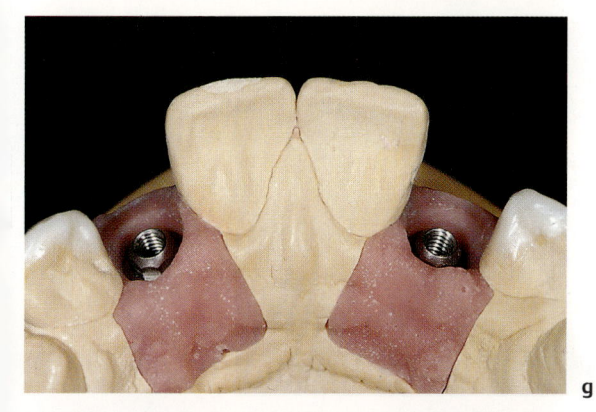

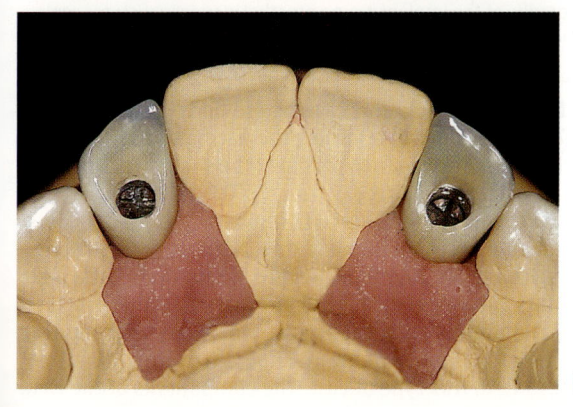

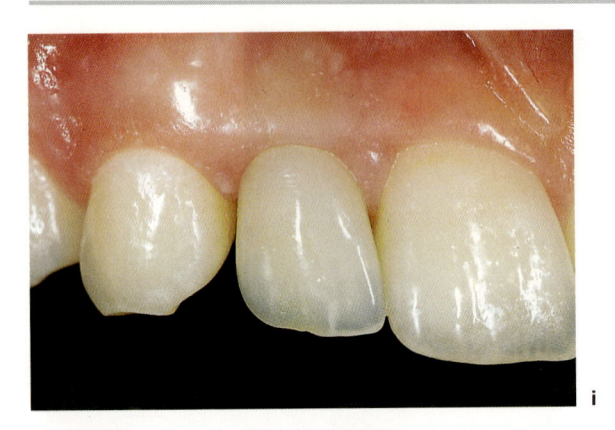

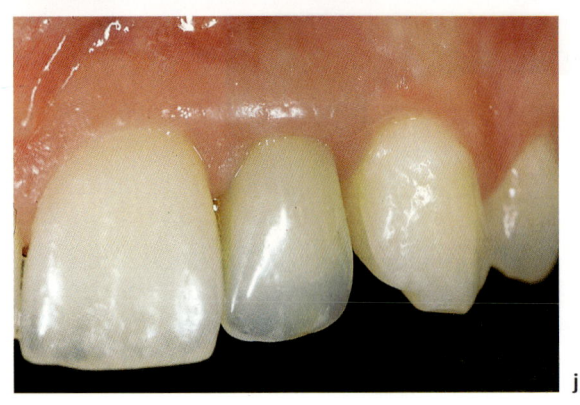

i and **j** Close-up photographs of the implant-borne prosthetic superstructures replacing the right and left lateral incisors

Figures 12.**15a–d** document a clinical case where both preimplant and preprosthetic conditions were ideal. In addition, the harmonious flow of the gingival margin and the correct emergence profile of the superstructure contribute to the excellent aesthetic result.

In accordance with their basis concept, ITI implants are placed transmucosally, with the junction between implant shoulder and superstructure usually lying supramucosally. In segments where aesthetic criteria take precedence, the implants can be set deeper to conceal unaesthetic restoration margins. Special titanium healing caps may then be used to condition the peri-implant soft tissues, allowing a future superstructure with proper axial contours (Fig. 12.**13a**). In this type of case, the components of the Octa

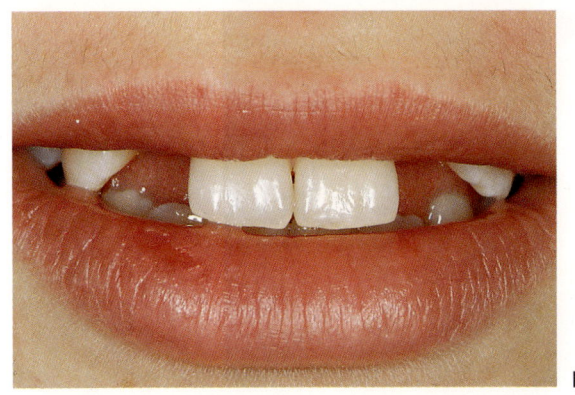

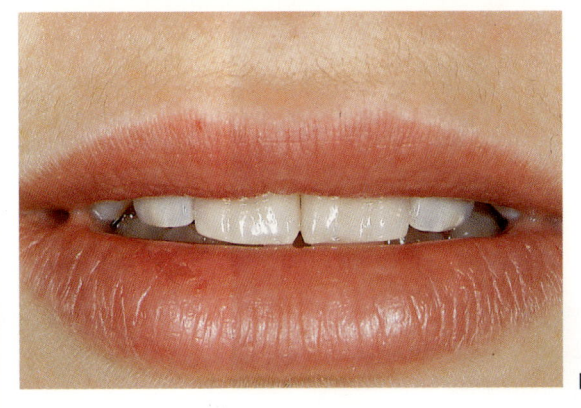

k and **l** Comparison of the patient's preoperative and postoperative smiles

system are used (Sutter et al. 1993) (Fig. 12.**13a–l**, 12.**14a–d**). To facilitate a good reproduction of the subgingival implant shoulder, prefabricated impression copings are screwed onto the Octa abutments (Fig. 12.**13b**). The actual impression is made with a custom impression tray that has openings over the implants, allowing the removal of the guide screws that hold the impression copings (Fig. 12.**13c** and **d**). In the laboratory, the one-piece implant analogs are then screwed into the impression copings and the master cast is poured in die stone (Fig. 12.**13e** and **f**). Preparing a removable reproduction of the gingivae in silicone makes it easier for the technician to develop the correct axial contours (Fig. 12.**13g–j**).

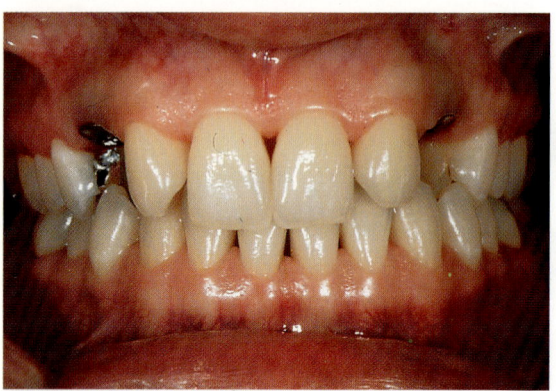

414 12 Fixed Prosthetic Restorations

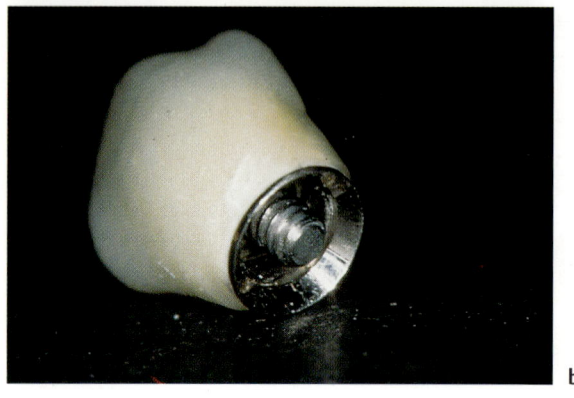

Fig. 12.**14a** Frontal view of a 25-year-old female patient with congenitally missing upper lateral incisors. The canines have been moved mesially and implants placed in their former locations
b When implant shoulders are to be placed deeper, prefabricated copings offer the important advantages of precise fit and excellent surface quality

In conclusion, it can be stated that the presence of certain preoperative conditions is essential to providing an aesthetic implant-borne restoration. If these preconditions are met, the deeper placement of ITI implants in combination with the various components of the Octa system allows the achievement of aesthetically pleasing results.

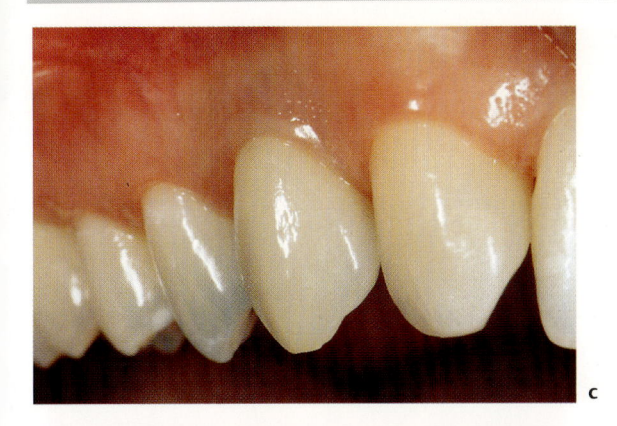

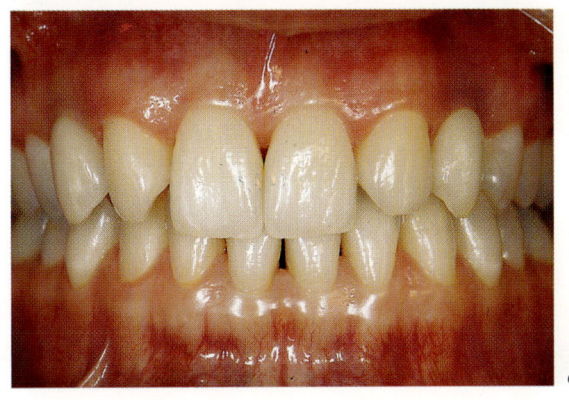

c This close-up view of the screw-attached implant-borne crown in the canine position demonstrates the quality of the esthetic result that is possible with careful planning and execution of treatment

d Completed case 2 years after insertion of the implants

416 12 Fixed Prosthetic Restorations

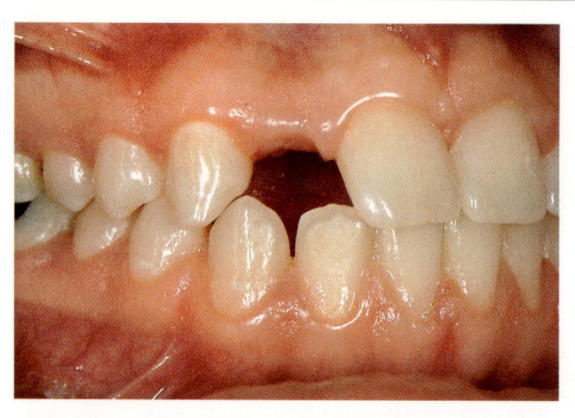

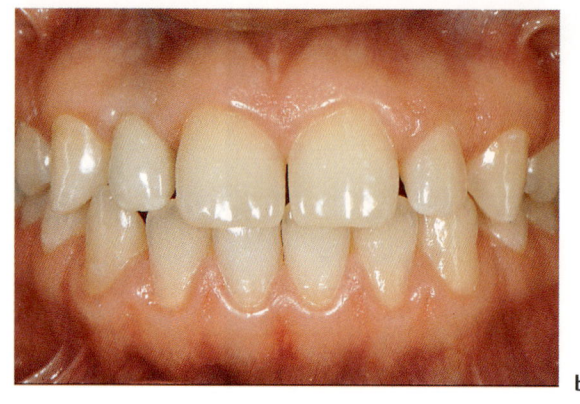

Fig. 12.**15a** The upper right lateral incisor is congenitally absent. Local conditions are optimal for an implant-supported restoration
b Frontal view 2 years postoperatively

Specific Indications 417

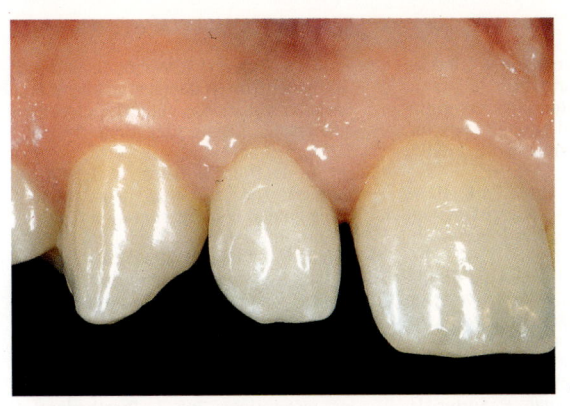

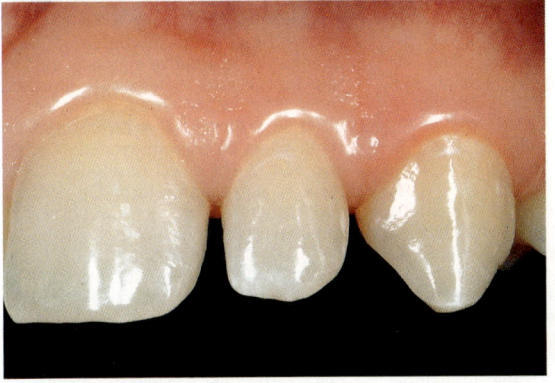

c and d Compare the ceramo-metal lateral incisor crown on the right side with the natural lateral incisor on the patient's left

References

Adell, R., B. Eriksson, U. Lekholm, P. I. Brånemark, A. Jemt: A long-term follow-up study of osseointegrated implants in the treatment of totally edentulous jaws. Int. J. oral max.-fac. Implants 5 (1991) 347–359

Assif, D., A. H. Fenton, G. A. Zarb, H. A. Schmitt: Comparative accuracy of implant impression procedures. Int. J. Periodont. Rest. Dent. 12 (1992) 113–121

Babbush, C. A., A. Kirsch, P. J. Mentag, B. Hill: Intramobile cylinder (IMZ) two-stage osseointegrated implant system with the intramobile element (IME): Part I. Its rationale and procedure for use. Int. J. Oral max.-fac. Implants 2 (1988) 203–216

Bernard, J.-P., J.-P. Martinet, F. Sutter, U. Belser: Implants endo-osseux non enfouis. Le système ITI Bonefit. Cah Proth/Impl 1 (1992) 5–15

Bernard, J.-P., J.-P. Martinet, F. Sutter, U. Belser: Réhabilitation esthétique sur implants non enfouis. Cah Proth-Impl 2 (1993) 49–58

Beumer III, J., M. O. Hamada, S. Lewis: A prosthodontic overview. Int. J. Prosthodont. 6 (1993) 126–130

Brägger, U., D. Buser, N. P. Lang: Implantatgetragene Kronen und Brücken. Schweiz. Monatsschr. Zahnmed. 100 (1990) 731–740

Brånemark, P. I., G. A. Zarb, T. Albrektsson: Tissue integrated prosthesis. Osseointegration in clinical dentistry. Quintessence Publishing, Chicago 1985

Buser, D., U. Brägger, N. P. Lang: Implantologie – die implantologische Versorgung der Freiendsituation im Unterkiefer. Schweiz. Monatsschr. Zahnmed. 98 (1988) 747–757

Buser, D., A. Schroeder, F. Sutter, N. P. Lang: The new concept of ITI hollow-cylinder and hollow-screw implants. Part II: Clinical aspects, indications, and early clinical results. Int. J. oral max.-fac. Implants 3 (1988) 173–178

Buser, D., H. P. Weber, U. Brägger, C. Balsiger: Tissue integration of onestage ITI-implants: 3-year results of a longitudinal study with hollow-cylinder and hollow-screw implants. Int. J. oral max.-fac. Implants 6 (1991) 405

Buser, D., F. Sutter, H. P. Weber, U. Belser, A. Schroeder: The ITI dental implant system: Basics, indications, clinical procedures and results. Clark's Clin. Dent. 5 (1992) 1–23

Buser, D., K. Dula, U. Belser, H. P. Hirt, H. Berthod: Localized ridge augmentation using guided bone regeneration. 1. Surgical procedure in the maxilla. Int. J. Periodont. Rest. Dent. 13 (1993) 29–45

Carr, A. B.: A comparison of impression techniques for a five-implant mandibular model. Int. J. oral max.-fac. Implants 6 (1991) 448–455

Chiche, G. J., A. Pinault: Considerations for fabrication of implant supported posterior restorations. Int. J. Prosthodont 4 (1991) 37–44

Cibirka, R. M., M. E. Razzoog, B. R. Lang, C. S. Stohler: Determining the force absorption quotient for restorative materials used in implant occlusal surfaces. J. prosthet. Dent. 67 (1992) 361–364

Davis, D. M., R. Rimrott, G. A. Zarb: Studies on frameworks for osseointegrated prostheses: Part. 2 The effect of adding acrylic resin or porcelain to form the occlusal superstructure. Int. J. oral max.-fac. Implants 3 (1988) 275–280

Flury, K., U. Brägger, F. Sutter, N. P. Lang: Implantate: Technische Aspekte. Schweiz. Monatsschr. Zahnmed. 101 (1991) 879–885

Gracis, S. E., J. I. Nicholls, J. D. Chalupnik, R. A. Youdelis: Schock absorbing behaviour of five restorative materials used on implants. Int. J. Prosthodont. 4 (1991) 282–291

Gunne, J., P. Astrand, K. Ahlen, K. Borg, M. Olsson: Implants in partially edentulous patients. A longitudinal study of bridges supported by both implants and natural teeth. Clin. oral Implan. Res. 3 (1992) 49–56

Jemt, T., U. Lekholm, R. Adell: Osseointegrated implants in the treatment of partially edentulous patients: A preliminary study on 876 consecutively placed fixtures. Int. J. oral max.-fac. Implants 4 (1989) 211–217

Lang, N. P.: Checklisten der Zahnmedizin. Checkliste: Zahnärztliche Behandlungsplanung, 2. Aufl. Thieme, Stuttgart 1988

Lewis, S., S. Arera, M. Engleman, J. Beumer III: The restoration of improperly inclined osseointegrated implants. Int. J. oral max.-fac. Implants 4 (1989) 147–152

Magne, P., M. Magne, U. Belser: Restauration des dents antérieures. Rev. mens suisse odontostomatol 103 (1993) 319–327

Marinello, C. P., E. Kundert, C. Andreoni: Die Bedeutung der periimplantären Nachsorge für Zahnarzt und Patient. Implantologie 1 (1993) 43–57

Matheus, M. F., L. C. Breeding, D. L. Dixon, S. A. Aquilino: The effect of connector design on cement retention in an implant and natural tooth-supported fixed partial denture. J. prosthet. Dent 65 (1991) 822–827

McGlumphy, E. A., D. M. Robinson, D. A. Mendl: Implant superstructures: A comparison of ultimate failure force. Int. J. oral max.-fac. Implants 7 (1992) 35–39

Naert, I., M. Quirynen, D. van Steenberghe, P. Darius: A six-year prosthodontic study of 509 consecutively inserted implants for the treatment of partial edentulism. J. prosthet. Dent. 67 (1992) 236–245

Nathanson, D.: Current developments in esthetic dentistry. Current opinion in Dentistrsy 1 (1991) 206–211

Nevins, M.: Periodontal prosthesis reconsidered. Int. J. Prosthodont 6 (1993) 209–217

Parel, S. M., D. Y. Sullivan: Esthetics and osseointegration. Osseointegration seminars (1989) 14–16

Rangert, B., J. Gunne, D. Sullivan: Mechanical aspects of an Brånemark implant connected to a natural tooth: An in vitro study. Int. J. oral max.-fac. Implants 6 (1991) 177–186

Richter, E. J.: Basic biomechanics of dental implants in prosthetic dentistry. J. prosth. Dent. 61 (1989) 602–609

Schmitt, A., G. A. Zarb: The longitudinal effectiveness of osseointegrated dental implants for single-tooth replacement. Int. J. Prosthodont 6 (1993) 197–202

Sidler, P.: Planung der implantatgetragenen Suprakonstruktion. In J. R. Strub, B. E. Gysi, P. Schärer: Schwerpunkte in der oralen Implantologie und Rekonstruktion. Quintessence, Berlin 1983

Stewart, R. B. et al.: Fatigue strength of cantilevered metal frameworks for tissue-integrated prostheses. J. prosthet. Dent 68 (1992) 83–92

Sullivan, D. Y.: Prosthetic considerations for the utilization of osseointegrated fixtures in the partially edentulous arch. Int. J. oral max.-fac. Implants 1 (1986) 39

Sutter, F., A. Schroeder, D. Buser: The new concept of ITI hollow cylinder and hollow screw implants. Part I: Engineering and design. Int. J. oral max.-fac. Implants 3 (1988) 161–172

Sutter, F., H. P. Weber, J. Sörensen, U. Belser: The new restorative concept of the ITI dental implant system: Engineering and design. Int. J. periodont Rest. Dent 13, 5 (1993) 409–413

Van Steenberghe, D.: A retrospective multicenter evaluation of the survival rate of osseointegrated fixtures supporting fixed partial prostheses in the treatment of partial edentulism. J. prosthet. Dent. 61 (1989) 217–223

Van Steenberghe, D., U. Lekholm, C. Bolender, T. Folmer, P. Henry, I. Herrmann, K. Higuchi, W. Laney, U. Linden, P. Astrand: The applicability of osseointegrated oral implants in the rehabilitation of partial edentulism. A prospective multicenter study on 558 fixtures. J. oral max.-fac. Implants 5 (1990) 272–281

Watson, R. M., D. M. Davis, G. H. Forman, T. Coward: Considerations in design and fabrication of maxillary implant-supported prostheses. Int. J. Prosthodont 4 (1991) 232–239

Weinberg, L. A.: The biomechanics of force distribution in implant-supported prostheses. Int. J. oral max.-fac. Implants 8 (1993) 19–31

Zarb, G. A., A. Schmitt: The longitudinal clinical effectiveness of osseointegrated dental implants in anterior partially edentulous patients. Int. J. Prosthodont. 6 (1993) 180–188

Zarb, G. A., A. Schmitt: The longitudinal clinical effectiveness of osseointegrated dental implants in posterior partially edentulous patients. Int. J. Prosthodont 6 (1993) 189–196

13 Follow-Up-Care and Recall

G. Krekeler

The actual implantation procedure is completed with the dressing of the wound and the postoperative radiograph. There after, the follow-up care begins. The patient is informed about the course of the surgical operation. The home-care instructions that were previously discussed are repeated. To facilitate undisturbed healing, it is advisable to give the patient an instruction sheet to take home to ensure that instructions are understood and followed.

Local prophylaxis against swelling is started as soon as the surgical procedure has been completed. The simplest preventive measure is the application of an ice pack for several hours. Internally administered prophylaxis against swelling is usually not necessary. However, when it is anticipated that an implantation procedure will be more extensive and lengthy than usual, systemic medication may be started on the evening before surgery. If severe swelling is expected because of extensive soft-tissue involvement, administration of corticosteroids (e.g., betamethasone, 1.5 mg daily to start, decreasing over 4 days) is recommended (van der Zwan et al. 1982). Additional antibiotic protection will reduce the danger of infection that is to be expected in these cases.

Antibiotic coverage is not absolutely necessary under normal circumstances–although it has been discussed whether prophylactic antibiotic administration aids healing (Gristina et al. 1989)–but when indicated because of local complications, it can be quite important. In these cases, we recommend perioperative administration of 5 million IU of penicillin over 2 days. As an alternative medication, clindamycin (Cleocin HCI, 1–1.5 gm per day) for 2–3 days can be recommended. In particularly delicate situations, the necessary antibiotic protection can be provided by high-dosage administration of an effective broad spectrum antibiotic once or twice daily.

To minimize local irritation of the wound, no tooth replacement should be worn during the first 8 days. When one-piece implants are used, we recommend that the bar not be inserted until after the soft tissue has completely healed. Meanwhile, the implants are covered with the matching plastic caps. When two-piece implants are used, care must be taken that the covering screws do not lead to plaque retention.

Local desinfection is accomplished with appropriate mouth rinses; we recommend 40-second rinses with undiluted 0.2% chlorhexidine solution (Gahlert et a. 1990).

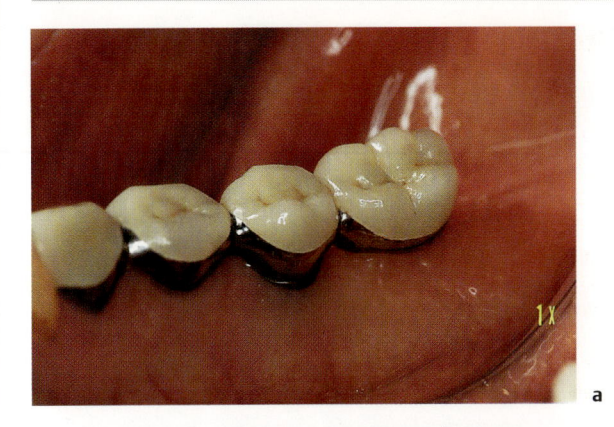

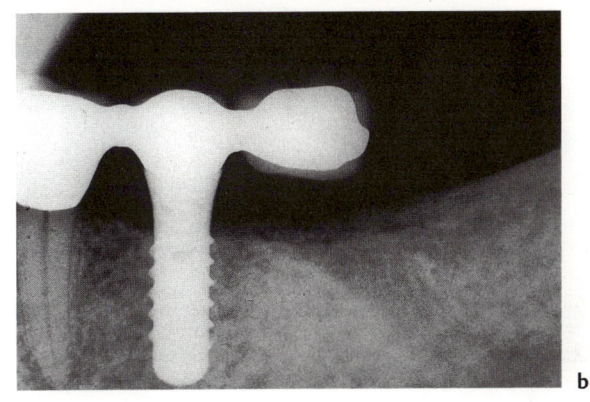

Fig. 13.**1a** Cantilever bridge in the lower right quadrant after 4 years with no evidence of peri-implant patholgoy
b Radiograph at 4-year recall

After 8 days, the sutures are removed and the wound is inspected. It is advisable to recall the patient periodically and evaluate the implants clinically and radiographically. They should be absolutely firm in the bone. An additional clinical evaluation after 4 weeks allows an updated determination of the clinical condition of the peri-implant structures. A re-evaluation should be carried out every 4 weeks until the superstructure is inserted. If there are no problems, the patient is placed in the regular recall system. Ideally, the follow-up care for these patients should include evaluations first at quarterly intervals, then semiannually, and finally once a year.

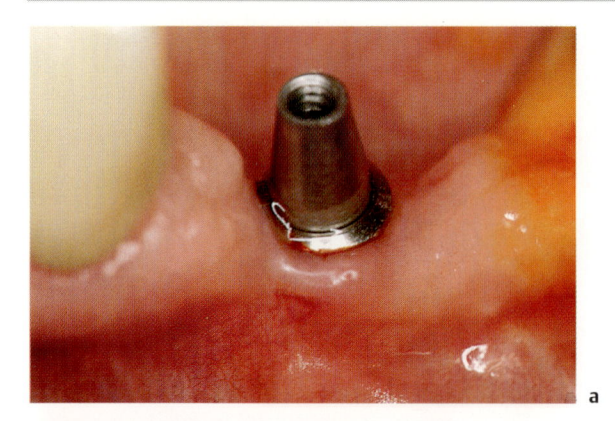

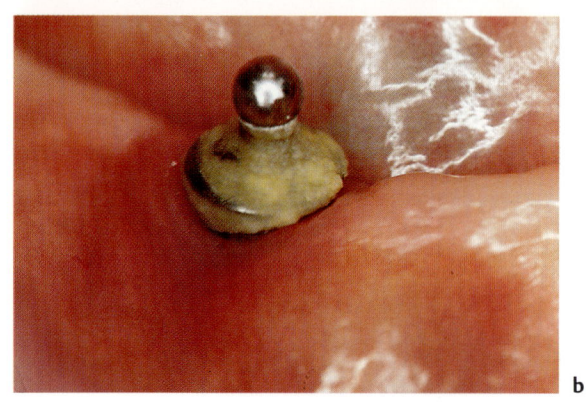

Fig. 13.**2a** Bleeding points give the first evidence of marginal inflammation
b A significant accumulation of debris on the implant has caused extensive peri-implant inflammation

This type of recall system is a condition *sine qua non* for long-term implantation success. It provides a basis for diagnostic procedures, as well as for necessary therapeutic steps involving both dentist and dental hygienist (Braugh-Muzzin et al. 1988, Stefani 1988).

An implantation can be considered successful if the patient has no complaints, the peri-implant tissue is healthy, the implant shows no mobility, and the radiograph reveals nothing abnormal (Fig. 13.**1a** and **b**). The following parameters are used to test whether these criteria of success are met:

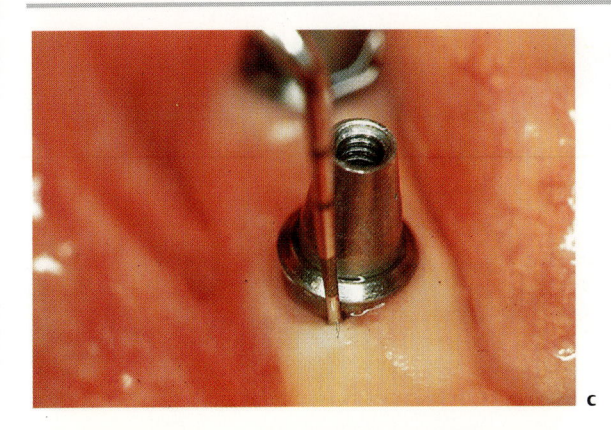

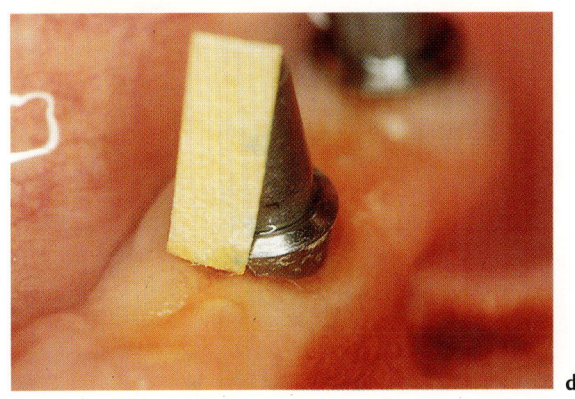

c Minimal probing depth indicates good soft tissue condition
d Sulcular fluid flow rate can be measured with a strip of filter paper

- Sulcus bleeding index to evaluate the peri-implant mucosa (Fig. 13.**2a**)
- Plaque index to determine the extent of local debris accumulation (Fig. 13.**2b**).
- Probing depth to test the adherence of the soft tissue cuff (Fig. 13.**2c**)
- Sulcular-fluid flow rate (Fig. 13.**2d**)

The amount of osseous anchorage is evaluated with the Periotest device (Schulte et al. 1986). The annual follow-up radiograph monitors the quality of the bone structure (Fig. 13.**3a** and **b**).

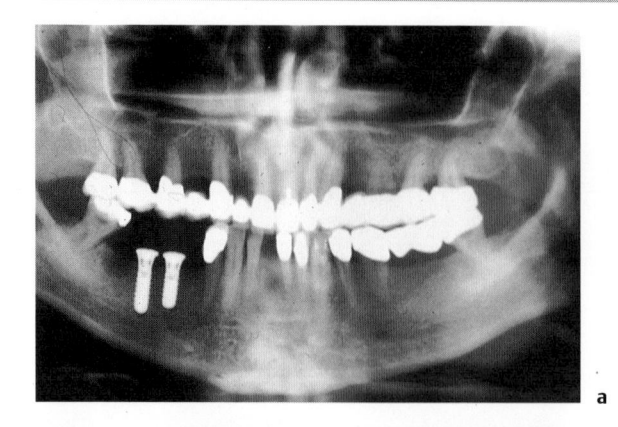

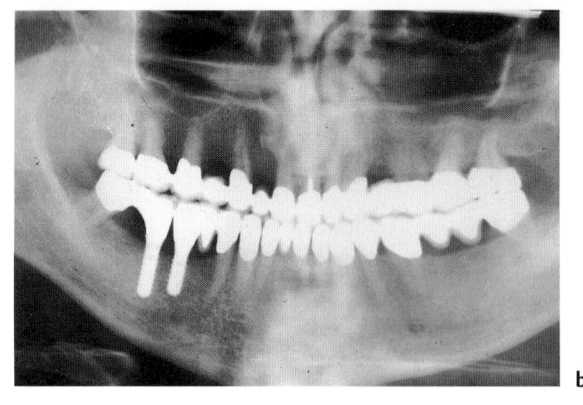

Fig. 13.**3a** Follow-up radiograph 3 months after implantation
b Annual radiograph. The bone structure around the implants is completely normal

The functional efficiency of the superstructure must also be checked. The occlusion and articulation are evaluated through occlusal analysis (Fig. 13.**4a** and **b**).

Various therapeutic measures may be necessary at recall, depending upon these diagnostic data. The implants usually require a thorough cleaning. This can be done with Superfloss or G-floss. A simple strip of gauze or an interdental brush can also be used to clean the cervical region of the implant (Fig. 13.**5a** and **b**).

Follow-Up-Care and Recall 425

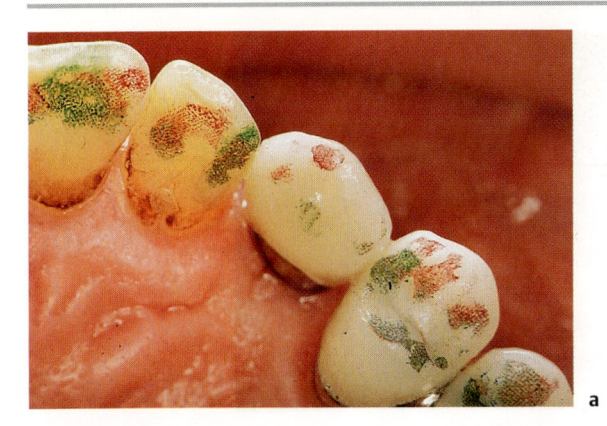

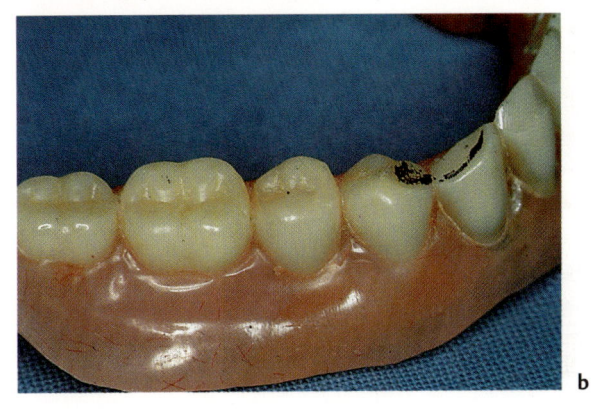

Fig. 13.**4a** A clinical functional analysis provides information about the load distribution, the superstructure, the occlusion, and articulation
b Excessive abrasion on the canine and premolar indicates parafunctional loading of the superstructure

Plastic hand scalers or ultrasonic scalers with plastic tips are recommended for the mechanical removal of calculus from the surfaces of the implants and superstructure. Titanium scalers have also been recommended for this purpose (Fox et al. 1990). Localized inflammation can be treated by rinsing the pocket with a 0.2–0.5% chlorhexidine solution twice daily for ten days. If no improvement is seen after this treatment, appropriate surgical intervention is necessary.

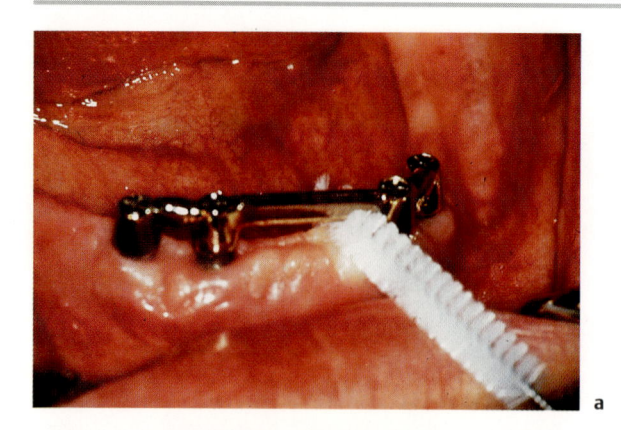

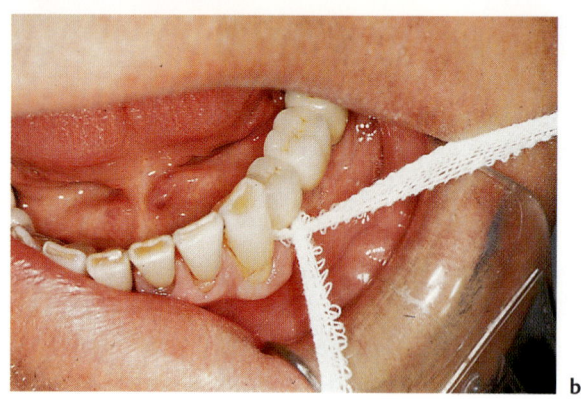

Fig. 13.**5a** Cleaning the bar with an interdental brush
b Frequently, good cleaning can be achieved with a gauze strip

The data collected during recall appointments and follow-up treatment must be accurately recorded and maintained if they are to be useful for formulating a definite statement on the long-term fate of an implant. Modern record-keeping procedures are therefore indispensable (Otten et al. 1989).

References

Brough-Muzzin, K. M., R. Johnson, P. Carr, P. Daffron: The dental hygienist's role in the maintenance of osseointegrated titanium implants. J. dent. Hyg. 62 (1988) 448

Fox, S. C., J. D. Mariaty, R. P. Kusy: The effects of scaling a titanium implant surface with metal and plastic instruments. J. Periodontol. 61 (1990) 485

Gahlert, M., K. Pelz, G. Krekeler: Die Wirksamkeit von Chlorhexidin auf das Keimspektrum parodontaler Taschen – eine in-vitro-Studie. Quintessenz (1990) 7248

Gristina, K. In L. Switalski, K. Hööh, E. Beachey: Molecularmechanisms of microbial adhesion. Springer 1989

Otten, J. E., G. Krekeler, H. Niederdellmann: Die Dokumentation in der oralen Implantologie. In M. Heners, K. Walther: Dokumentation und Planung in zahnärztlicher Praxis. Quintessenz 1983

Schulte, W.: Messung des Dämpfungsverhaltens enossaler Implantate mit dem Periotestverfahren. Z. zahnärztl. Implantol. 2 (1986) 22

Stefani, L. A.: The care and maintenance of the dental implant patient. J. dent. Hyg. 62 (1988) 464

van der Zwan, J., G. Boering, H. Wesseling, D. T. Smit-Sibinger, L. T. van der Weele: The third molar and antiphlogistics. Int. J. oral Surg. 11 (1982) 340

14 Peri-implant Problems

G. Krekeler

The 20 years of experience that we have accumulated with ITI implants show that the success rate with this titanium plasma-coated implant is extraordinarily favorable (Krekeler et al. 1990, Buser et al. 1990). Its high level of acceptance (Spiekermann et al. 1991) speaks for its dependability. To make it even more dependable, it is necessary to determine the causes of failures. These are primarily associated with the reaction of the peri-implant tissues. This affects the bone, as well as the soft tissue around the neck of the implant; implant fractures are rare.

Anchorage of the Implant Body

The root of a natural tooth is functionally anchored in the bone by the periodontal membrane, a complex attachment apparatus. With implants, we attempt to achieve a bond that transmits forces directly to bone. This rigid anchorage, called osseointegration has proven effective but its achievement is dependent upon many factors. As described in the previous chapter, osseointegration can be expected only if the vitality of the bone is preserved through careful cutting of the implant bed, if the implants fits the prepared bed closely, and if the implant has the proper shape and surface characteristics. If these prerequisites are met, one can expect a harmonious bond with the surrounding bone structure that will become well adapted to functional loading.

The durability of this force-transmitting anchorage depends upon the integrity of the surrounding bone, and this can be endangered by mistakes during preparation, improper loading of the implant, or infection of the marginal mucosa.

Thermal Trauma

Thermal trauma has a more profound effect upon healing than any other factor. If heat-induced resorption occurs, primary stability of the implant during the healing phase cannot be assured, and osseointegration is jeopardized (Fig. 14.**1a** and **b**). Avoiding thermal trauma demands a drastic reduction in the rotational speed of the drilling instruments, pressure-free osteotomy, the use of sharp drills, and copious amounts of coolant (Fig. 14.**2**).

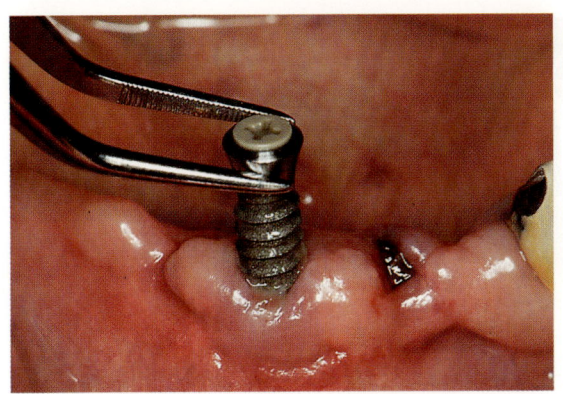

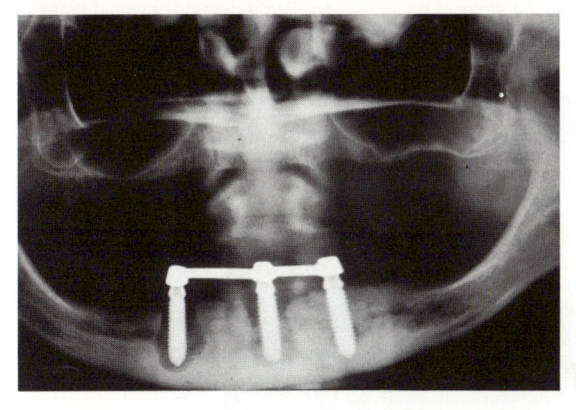

Fig. 14.**1a** Thermal injury to the implant bed is leading to premature loss of the implant due to lack of primary stability
b Typical example of bone resorption in the depth of the drill channel in the lower right canine area. Around the other two implants, osteolysis has reached the marginal regions. These implants cannot be saved

Extensive research has shown that both internal and external cooling can be effective, and that heat necrosis can be dependably avoided only if the cooling fluid reaches the cutting instrument all the way to the bottom of the drill hole. The shape of the drill has a significant effect on the effectiveness of the coolant. Internal cooling of a spiral drill is not very effective due to the inefficient removal of drill chips from the spiral grooves (Fig. 14.**3**). With this drill, we are limited to external cooling (also see page 430).

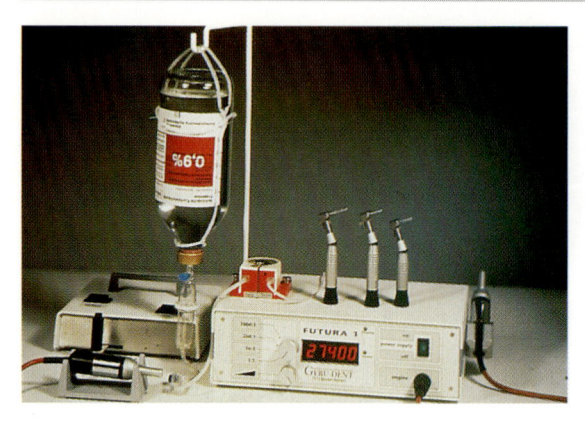

Fig. 14.**2** Modern engine handpieces provide controlled reduction of speed that can be read from the display window. Suitable pumps provide external irrigation with saline solution

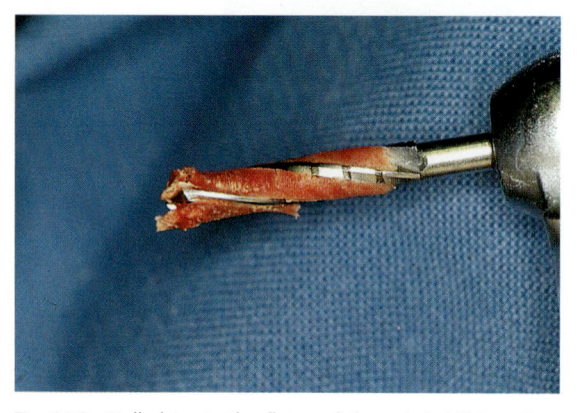

Fig. 14.**3** Drill chips in the flutes of the spiral drill interfere with adequate internal coolant flow

A certain amount of trauma to the implant bed is unavoidable even with a conservative osteotomy technique. Significant resorptive processes, which extend to a depth of approximately 500 μm (depending on the bone structure) can always be observed during the healing phase. The danger from this lively osteoclastic activity becomes apparent if the implant is loaded prematurely.

Improper Loading

An implant has no organized fiber apparatus to cushion forces that it is subjected to, whether physiologic or unphysiologic. There is no stress breaker to ensure long-term durability. This raises the question of whether osseointegration makes sense at all from the standpoint of mechanical loading.

It can currently be assumed that the force-intercepting bony attachment of an implant cannot be equated with absolutely rigid healing. Even an osseointegrated implant has a certain mobility of its own, which is analogous to that of an ankylosed tooth.

Experiments with animals (Göz, 1987) have shown that our concept of a "shock-absorbing periodontal membrane" is obviously in need of correction. Loads within the physiologic range are not intercepted first by the periodontal membrane alone, but also by the attachment of the membrane to bone, regardless of the direction of the force. Although to a reduced extent, ankylosed teeth experience a yielding movement, which is similar to that of a tooth suspended in a healthy periodontal membrane. (Fig. 14.**4**). This elasticity of the bone dispels the fear that osseointegrated implant's attachment to bone would be immediately lost through improper loading. An osseointegrated implant can withstand heavy forces, even if directed away from its long axis (Schramm-Scherer et al., 1989).

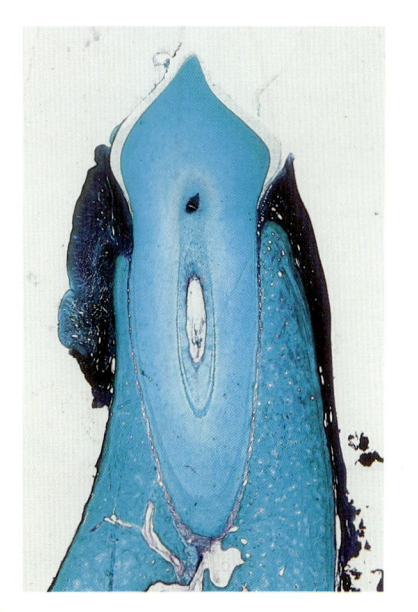

Fig. 14.**4** Periodontium of a natural lower premolar in a beagle (prepared by Göz, Tübingen Germany)

432 14 Peri-implant Problems

The shape of the implant is certainly of great importance in preserving the functionally oriented bone structure. Rounded, rotationally symmetrical implants exhibit only minimal stress-concentration points when loaded. No disruptive problems have been observed at the interface due to elasticity of the implant body itself.

As with natural teeth, a great danger to the osseous attachment is presented by infection of the marginal mucosa. With the absence of a periodontal membrane and its dense network of blood vessels, the defense against infection is reduced. A significantly more rapid osteolysis can thus be expected around an implant due to direct bacterial damage.

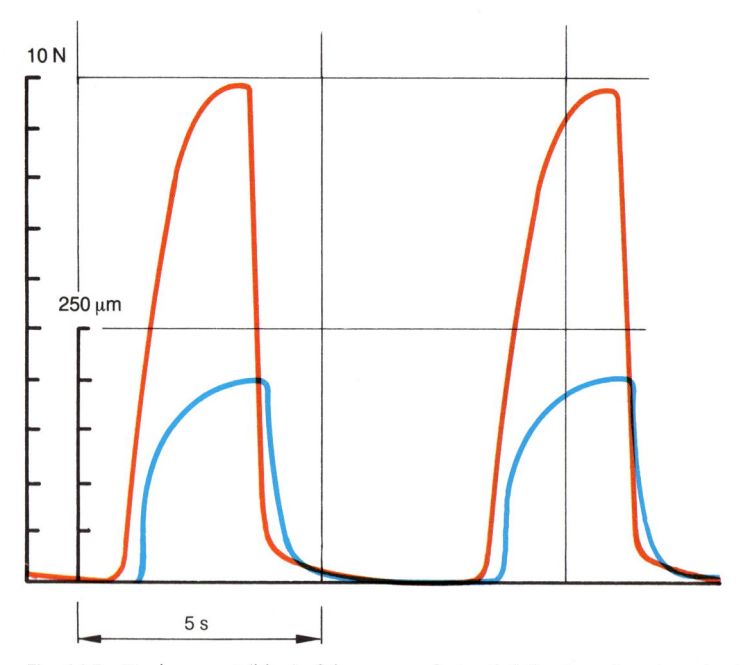

Fig. 14.**5** Displacement (blue) of the crown of a tooth following a force impulse (red). Magnitude of force: 10N, duration of force: 3 seconds (from Göz 1987)

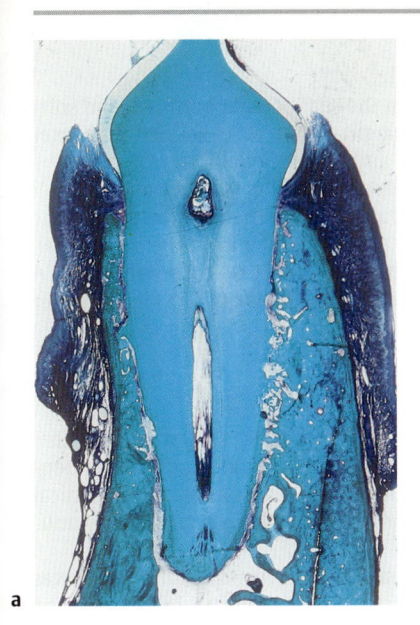

TextTextTextTest **433**

Fig. 14.**6**
a Premolar of a beagle with ankylotic changes
b Crown displacement (blue) of an ankylosed tooth following a force impulse (red).
Impulse magnitude: 10N,
impulse duration: 4 seconds.
Compare with Fig. 14.**5**. (Preparation by Göz, Tübingen Germany)

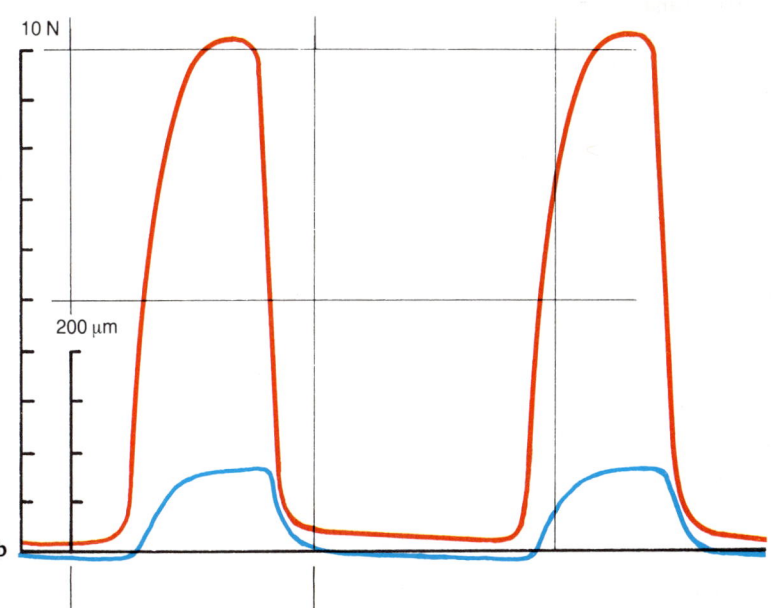

The Gingiva-Implant Seal

It is important to permanently maintain the seal between implant and soft-tissue cuff to prevent infection of the marginal bone. As described in chapter 6, both a connective-tissue attachment and an epithelial attachment can be expected within the biological width. The fine architecture of the junctional epithelium has its weak points. The parallel arrangement of the cells to the surface creates vulnerable intercellular spaces leading from the sulcus that, although patrolled by granulocytes, are still subject to bacterial attack. A high cell turnover rate seems to ameliorate this situation, however (Diemer 1984, Fig. 14.**7a–d**).

Microbial Plaque

The important peri-implant problems are, as a rule, caused by marginal infection. A significant question is whether bacterial inoculation is influenced by the implant material, its shape, or surface characteristics. The clinical impression is that ceramic materials are less susceptible to plaque accumulation than are metals (Fig. 14.**8**).

This impression was only conditionally proven in a clinical study. It was shown that when the bacterial plaque was allowed to grow undisturbed, the different materials were covered to the same extent (Fig. 14.**9**). No purely morphologic differences could be observed with the scanning electron microscope. Only microbiological analysis of the materials provided information on the different clinical conditions. While the plaque-building cocci made up approximately one-fourth of the total microbial mass of plaque growing on ceramic material, they comprised more than one-half of the flora on titanium (Krekeler et al. 1990). These data seem to indicate that the material with which the implant is made has no decisive influence on the type and quantity of bacterial growth, but possibly does effect its adherence. The phenomenon observed by Wise and Dykema (1975), that plaque could be more easily brushed from a ceramic material, might be explained by this difference in the proportion of streptococci.

Implant Surface

It is also possible that the clinically observed increase in the adherence of plaque to titanium is caused by the physical characteristics of the material's surface. The previously described bonding of organic structures to titanium (chemisorption) suggests the possibility of the adhesion of an organic matrix that then serves as a foundation for colonization of bacterial growth, consisting predominantly of gram-positive cocci and rods, the types of organisms found in the oral environment. In ceramics, this foundation slips off. These two facts form the basis for present attempts to reduce the incidence of

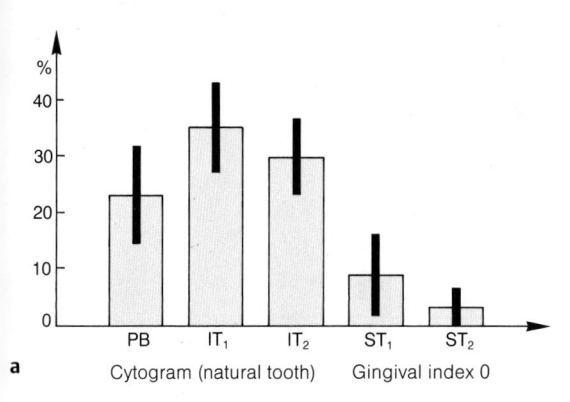

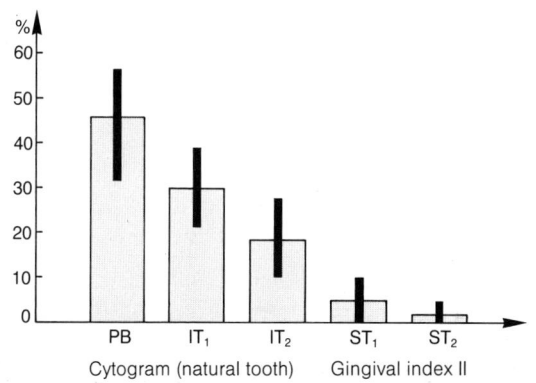

Fig. 14.**7a–d** Cytogram of the cellular content of the sulcus
a Marginal gingiva of a natural tooth free of clinical inflammation. Typical distribution of the parabasal cells (PB), the types I and II intermediate cells, and the types I and II superficial cells
b Moderate inflammation around a natural tooth. Cells from the deeper layers, such as parabasal cells and intermediate cells predominate. There is a distinct shift to the left.
c Gingiva of an implant clinically free of inflammation
d Distinct shift to the left with moderate inflammation around an implant

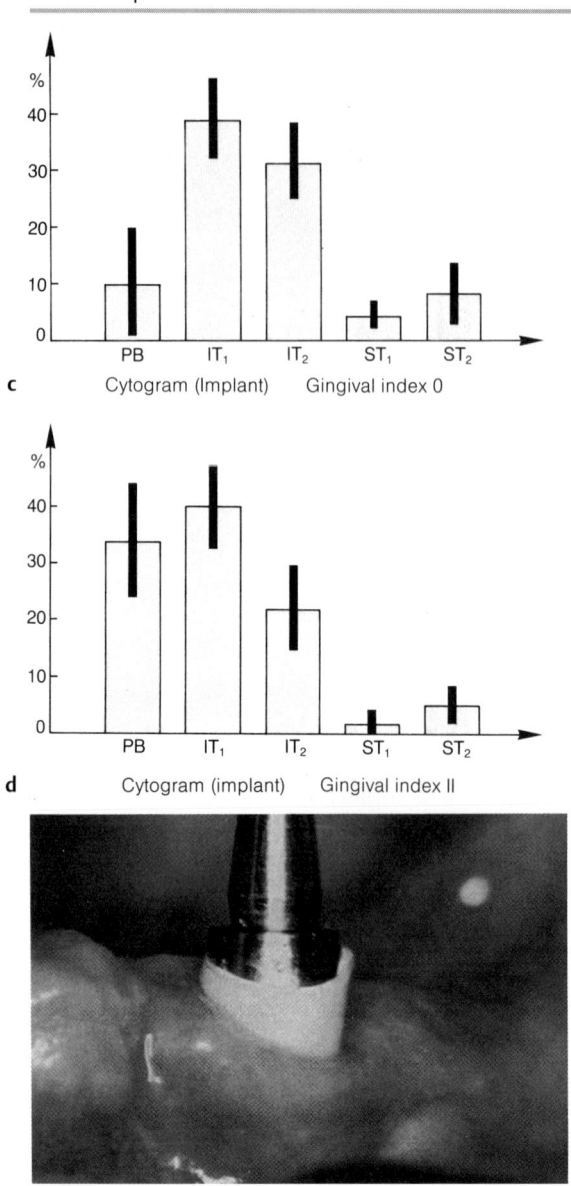

Fig. 14.**8** Tübinger implant with gingiva free of clinical inflammation. The surface of the implant is macroscopically free of plaque

Implant Surface **437**

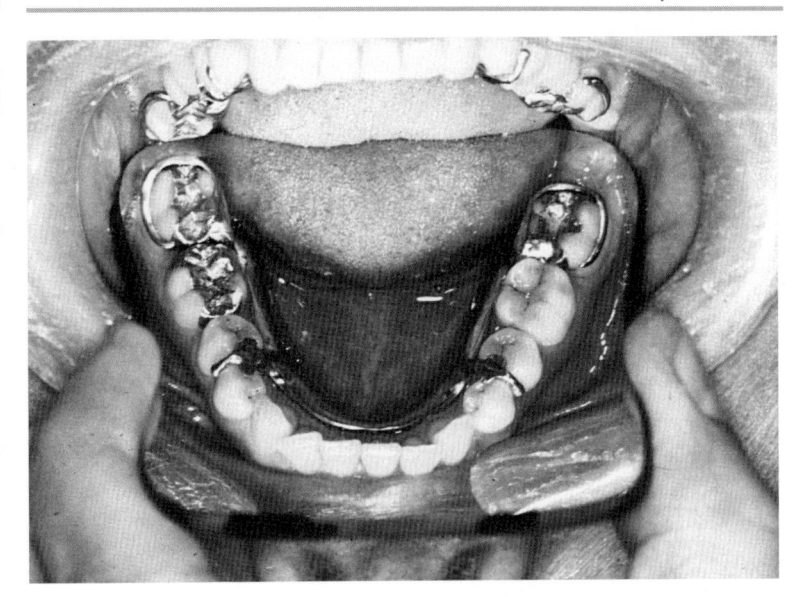

Fig. 14.**9a** Experimental arch with the various test materials in place

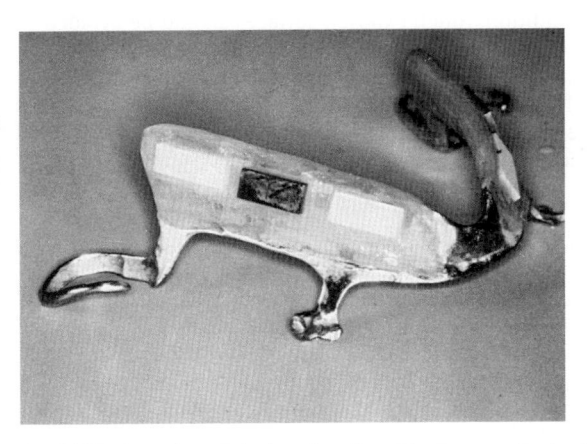

Fig. 14.**9b** Samples of hydroxylapatite, titanium, and aluminum oxide ceramic (saphire) are attached as test materials

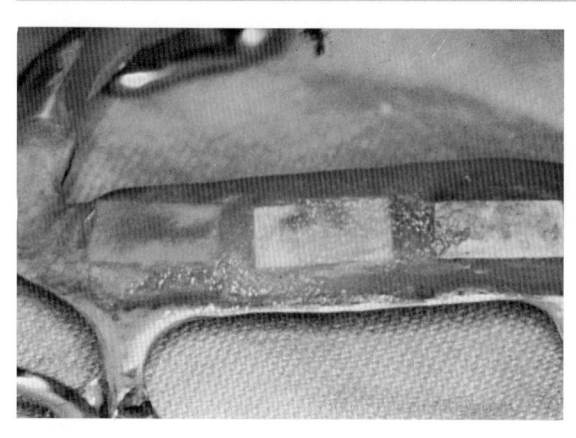

Fig. 14.**9c** The different test specimens are equally coated with plaque

plaque by modifying the surface properties of the implant where it is exposed to the bacterial flora of the oral cavity through electrochemical conditioning or by coating it with ceramic material (Krämer et al. 1989,) Petzow and Gibbesch, 1989). In addition, rough exposed surfaces should be avoided to reduce plaque adherence.

Besides these material-related properties, the shape of the implant also plays a decisive role in plaque accumulation. Retentive holes and gaps between implant elements must not interfere with cleaning. These generally lead to substantial accumulation of plaque accompanied by marginal infection (Fig. 14.**10**).

Marginal Infection

By virtue of a multitude of clinical investigations, we now know that there is a relationship between plaque accumulation and inflammation around implants, as well as around teeth (Adell et al. 1986, Günay et al. 1989). Because supragingival and subgingival plaque on implants are the same as on natural teeth (Rams and Link, 1983, Krekeler et al. 1986, Mombelli et al. 1987), a possible breakdown of an implant's epithelial attachment and formation of a pocket (depending on time and the host situation) must be taken into account. Although it is often observed clinically that these processes occur more rapidly and aggressively in the young than in the old, we are not justified in assuming that plaque plays no decisive role in elderly patients (Fig. 14.**10** and 14.**11**).

Marginal Infection **439**

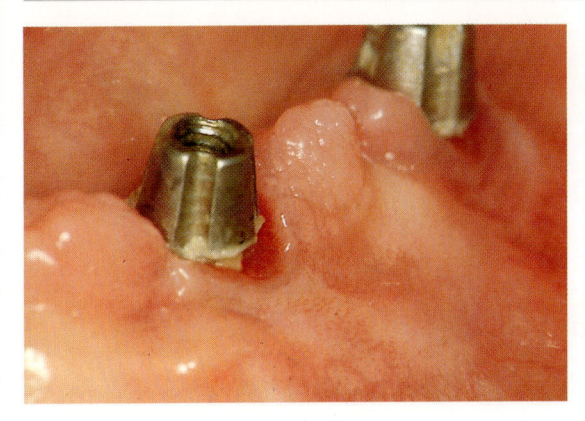

Fig. 14.**10** Constrictions around the implant neck and longitudinal grooves in the implant head are areas that favor plaque retention. The redness of the margins indicates severe localized inflammation

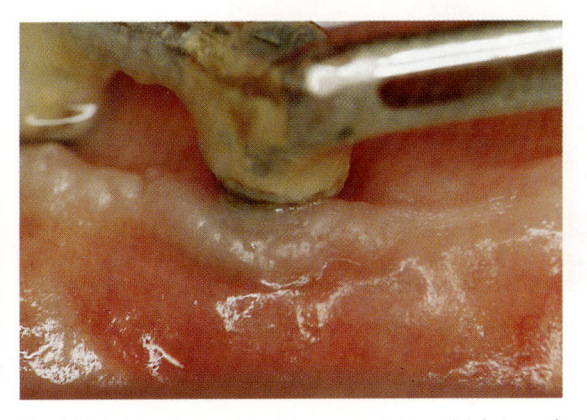

Fig. 14.**11** Despite considerable accumulation of debris on the superstructure, only a slight mucosal reaction is observed in this 86-year-old patient

14 Peri-implant Problems

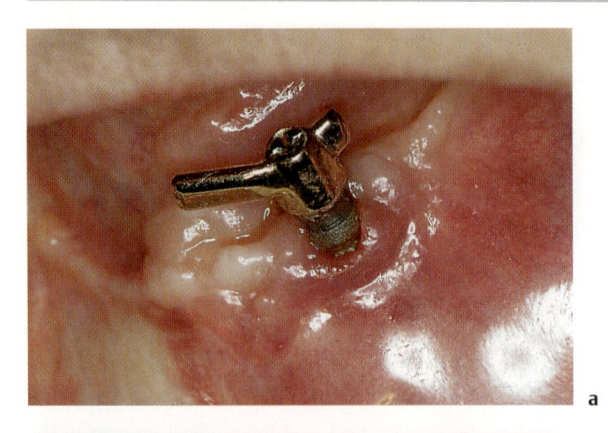

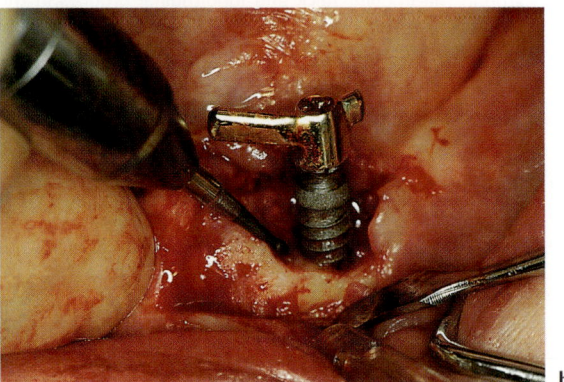

Fig. 14.**12a** Severe peri-implant inflammation. **b** The considerable bone destruction resulted in loss of the implant

Once a pocket has established itself, the local milieu is altered and with it the makeup of the bacterial population. Gram-negative anaerobes predominate among the subgingival flora. Soft tissue destruction and bone resorption accompanied by progressive enlargement of the pocket are the result. If the infection reaches the peri-implant bone, there is grave danger to the implant because of the progressive nature of these events (Lekholm et al. 1986) (Fig. 14.**12a** and **b**).

The Mucosa

Peri-implant problems can very easily appear when the mucosal conditions favor the accumulation of plaque. Pocket formation is especially observed where pronounced fibrous or hyperplastic structures are present in the posterior region, unless these are excised. For transgingivally inserted implants, it is especially important that correct soft tissue contours be present, and this frequently requires thinning and shortening the mucoperiosteal flap.

A functional gingivoimplant seal with adhesion of the soft tissue will most predictably form where the implant lies in an adequately wide zone of keratinized mucosa. If the soft tissue structures are immovably fixed around the implant, oral hygiene measures that are only average may suffice, especially in elderly patients.

Conversely, when oral hygiene is good, healthy conditions can be observed even with mobile peri-implant mucosa (Krekeler et al. 1985, van Steenberghe 1988, Mericske-Stern 1988). In these cases, there is no urgent need for a surgical correction to widen the keratinized mucosa (Fig. 14.**13** and 14.**14**).

Conclusions

Peri-implant problems that can seriously endanger the retention of an osteointegrated implant can usually be traced back to surgical trauma and/or marginal infection. In order to ensure reliable healing around an implant, the surgical fundamentals described in chapter 10 must be observed. To maintain the secondary stabilization, i.e., osteointegration and the functional implantogingival seal, prophylactic measures against infection must be pursued. These consist of:

1. proper shape of the implant;
2. attention to the soft tissue condition;
3. fixation and formation of the superstructure;
4. oral hygiene.

The shape of the implant must permit thorough plaque control as described earlier.

The condition of the soft tissues is evaluated within the context of the oral hygiene. If there is no assurance that good oral hygiene will be carried out, then an adequately wide band of keratinized mucosa must be created. This can be accomplished most reliably with a free-mucosal graft (see pages 264 ff).

Correct superstructure design is especially important for avoiding peri-implant problems. Moist spaces under complete overdentures with bar retention often cause severe marginal inflammation and pocket formation, thereby causing eventual loss of the implant. Completely implant-borne

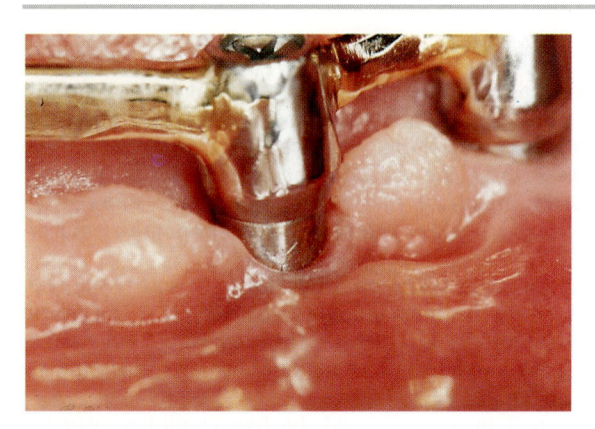

Fig. 14.**13** Good oral hygiene results here in inflammation-free peri-implant conditions despite the absence of keratinized mucosa

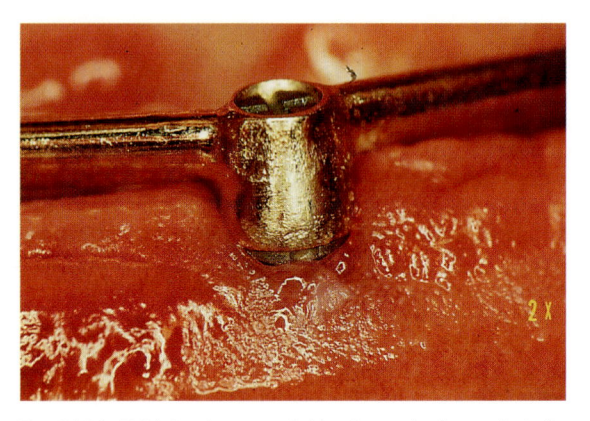

Fig. 14.**14** With inadequate oral hygiene, the hyperplasia beneath this bar-retained complete overdenture leads to considerable marginal irritation

restorations should be given preference whenever possible. If implants are to be connected with natural teeth, care must be taken to maintain a healthy periodontium around the abutment teeth to minimize the discrepancy in mobilities between the two types of abutments. Mobility of periodontally healthy teeth is 30–50 µm, and even more if periodontal disease is present, whereas the mobility of an osseointegrated implant is approximately 20 µm.

The connection between implant and superstructure can also be a source of problems because peri-implant changes can be brought about by galvanism (Hild 1986, Lukas 1987). These changes may be involved in late complications. Investigations by Hild (1986) revealed, for example, that currents with magnitudes of 0.1 to 1 µA can be measured between a titanium implant and its gold alloy superstructure.

This "battery" is created when the implant and the superstructure are in conducting contact in an electrolyte and discharge over their metallic polarization resistance. This electrochemical process makes the region around the implant neck more alkaline, producing a measurable increase in the pH of from 1 to 2 units. Long-term exposure can be assumed to injure the soft tissues.

The decisive factor in maintaining the health of the peri-implant structures is oral hygiene. In young implant patients, optimum oral hygiene is required. For older patiens, certain allowances must be made. In these cases, cleaning must be facilitated by the shape of the implant and the superstructure. Adequate oral hygiene must be established through appropriate training, and hygiene must be monitored with an effective recall system.

References

Adell, R., U. Lekholm, B. Rockler, P. I. Brånemark, J. Lindhe, B. Ericsson, L. Sbardane: Marginal tissue reactions at osseointegrated titanium fixtures. Int. J. oral. max.-fac. Surg. 15 (1986) 39

Bienick, K. W., H. Spiekermann: Zahnärztliche Implantologie – eine statistische Standortbestimmung. Dtsch. zahnärztl. Z. 46 (1991) 642

Buser, D., H. P. Weber, N. P. Lang: Tissue integration of non-submerged implants. Clin. oral Impl. Res. 1 (1990) 33

Diemer, J.: Klinische Untersuchung zum Verhalten der Gingiva am künstlichen Zahnpfeiler. Med. Diss., Freiburg 1984

Göz, G.: Die kieferorthopädische Zahnbewegung. Untersuchung zur Biologie und Mechanik. Habil. Schrift, Hanser, München 1987

Günay, H., U. Blunck, F. W. Neukam, H. Scheller: Periimplantäre Befunde bei Brånemark-Implantaten. Z. zahnärztl. Implantol. 5 (1989) 162

Hild, A.: Messung von elektrochemischen Veränderungen an enossalen Implantaten aus Metall und Aluminiumoxidkeramik. Med. Diss., Freiburg 1985

Krämer, A., H. Weber, J. Geis-Gerstorfer: Plaqueansammlung an Implantat- und prothetischen Werkstoffen, eine klinische Studie. Z. zahnärztl Implantol. 5 (1989) 283

Krekeler, G., W. Schilli, H. Geiger: Das TPS-Implantat, ein zuverlässiges Retentionselement? Z. zahnärztl. Implantol. 6 (1990) 229

Krekeler, G., W. Schilli, J. Diemer: Should the exit of the artificial abutment tooth be positioned in the region of the attached gingiva? Int. J. oral. Surg. 14 (1985) 504

Krekeler, G., K. Pelz, M. Rediker: Die Plaquehaftung an verschiedenen Werkstoffen. Z. zahnärztl. Implantol. 6 (1990) 191

Krekeler, G., K. Pelz, R. Nelissen: Mikrobielle Besiedlung der Zahnfleischtaschen am künstlichen Zahnpfeiler. Dtsch. zahnärztl. Z. 41 (1986) 569

Lekholm, U., R. Adell, J. Lindhe, P. I. Brånemark, B. Ericsson, B. Rockler, A. M. Lindval, T. Yaneyma: Marginal tissue reactions at oseointegrated titanium fixtures. II. A crossectional retrospective study. J. oral max.-fac. Surg. 15 (1986) 53

Lukas, D.: Grundsätzliche Überlegungen zu Strommessungen zwischen Titanimplantaten und deren Suprakonstruktion. Z. zahnärztl. Implantol. 3 (1987) 24

Mericske-Stern, R.: Die implantatgesicherte Totalprothese im zahnlosen Unterkiefer. Schweiz. Mschr. Zahnheilk. 98 (1988) 931

Mombelli, A., M. C. A. van Osten, E. Schusch, N. P. Lang: The microbiota associated with successful of failing osseointegrated titanium implants. Oral. Microbiol. Immunol. 2 (1987) 145

Petzow. W., B. Gibbisch: Titan-Aluminiumoxidverbunde für Implantate. Vortrag anläßlich des 2. Symposiums des SFB Implantologie der Universität Tübingen (1989)

Rams, T. E., C. C. Link jr.: Microbiology of failing dental implants in humans: electromicroscopic observations. J. oral. Implantol. 11 (1983) 93

Siegele, D., U. Soltész: Numerical investigations of the influence of implant shape on stress distribution in the jaw-bone. Int. J. oral. max.-fac. Impl. 4 (1988) 333

Schramm-Scherer, B., N. Behneke, Th. Reiber, P. Tetsch: Röntgenologische Untersuchungen zur Belastung von Implantaten im zahnlosen Unterkiefer. Z. zahnärztl. Implantol 5 (1989) 185

Van Steenberghe, M. D.: Periodental aspects of osseointegrated oral implant ad modum Brånemark. Dent. Clin. A. Amer. 32 (1988) 355

Sutter, F., G. Krekeler, A. E. Schwammberger, J. F. Sutter: Das ITI-Bonefit-Implantatsystem – Implantatbettgestaltung. Quintessenz 42 (1991) 1

Watzek, G., M. Matejka, W. Lill, G. Mailath: Efficiency of different clinical procedures regarding optimal implant integration. Saunders, Philadelphia 1988

Wise, M. D., R. W. Dykema: The plaqueretaining capacity of four dental materials. J. prothet. Dent. 2 (1975) 178

15 Complications with ITI Implants

D. Buser and B. Maeglin

Although the ITI system has distinguished itself with reliable long-term results (p. 482 ff), complications have been documented with a frequency of 5–10%. This clinical experience is caused in part by the fact that the implant is implanted as a *foreign body* into *living tissues.* These tissues must be handled as gently as possible during the surgery, and after a specified healing period, they are subjected to heavy loading forces. Consequently, there are opportunities for complications to arise if the established and clinically proven guidelines are not observed during both the surgical and prosthetic treatment. In addition, the level of oral hygiene that is necessary for maintaining the health of the peri-implant tissues places a heavy responsibility on the patient if the implant is expected to function successfully for many years. The total number of complications observed with implants will undoubtedly rise in the future because of the great increase in the number of implants placed. Therefore, the topic *complications with ITI implants* is important and presented here to give the clinician some information on the best way to proceed when complications do arise.

In this chapter, the theoretically possible complications will be presented systematically with distinctions being made between intra- and postoperative complications.

Intraoperative Complications

Hemorrhage

If the operation and incision lines have been planned properly, there is little occasion to fear severe bleeding from the soft tissues. Hemorrhage can occur from the spongiosa, however, during reduction of a sharp alveolar ridge crest. This type of diffuse bleeding usually stops spontaneously. Moderate bleeding that occurs as the endosseous implant bed is being prepared, is stopped by insertion of the implant. The occurrence of severe bleeding during preparation of an implant bed in the posterior mandibular region indicates that the mandibular canal has been entered and a blood vessel damaged. An X-ray, with the depth gauge in place, can clarify the situation.

Intraoperative Nerve Damage

As a rule, significant nerve damage occurs only in the mandible. It can involve the inferior alveolar nerve, the mental nerve, or the lingual nerve. To avoid injuring the inferior alveolar nerve, the anatomical course of the mandibular canal and the vertical dimension of the available bone must be precisely determined before surgery (p. 263). To safely protect the mental nerve, the mental foramen must be widely exposed when operating in this region. When implants are placed in the posterior molar region, the lingual nerve can also be jeopardized. To avoid injury to this nerve, a thin periosteal elevator may be inserted between the lingual surface of the bone and a mucoperiosteal flap to protect the nerve as the bone is being prepared.

Perforation of the Antrum or Nasal Cavity

During treatment planning, the relationship between the proposed implants and the maxillary sinus and nasal cavity must be determined radiographically. If the antrum or nasal cavity should become perforated during bone preparation, the available vertical bone height must be determined as precisely as possible. For this purpose, a radiograph can be made during the surgery with a depth gauge in place. The use of hollow cylinder or hollow screw implants is not recommended in such cases because the open structure of these types of implants comes into direct contact with the perforated antrum or nasal cavity, creating an unnecessary risk of retrograde infection. Therefore, the solid screw implant is preferred in these situations.

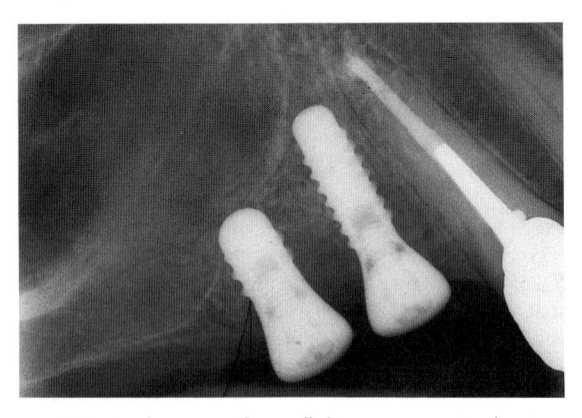

Fig. 15.**1** Implantation of a small-diameter screw implant in upper right first premolar region and a 6-mm-long standard screw implant in the second premolar region at the floor of the maxillary sinus

The screw threads maintain the vertical position of the implant, preventing it from slipping into the antrum or nasal cavity. The implant's position must be selected for maximum utilization of the available bone. The end of the implant should rest near the floor of the sinus or nasal cavity or extend only slightly into the cavity (Fig. 15.**1**).

Damage to Adjacent Teeth

The danger of damaging adjacent teeth as the implant bed is being drilled into the bone is greatest during implantation in a single-tooth space. Protection from this danger is provided by making a correct radiographic assessment of the topography, selecting an implant of appropriate dimensions, and taking the course of the long axes of the adjacent teeth into consideration. An intraoperative radiograph with a gutta-percha point inserted into the bone can also be useful by indicating the exact direction of the implant (Fig. 15.**2a–c**).

Failure to Obtain Primary Stability

Although excellent primary stability of ITI implants in the bone can usually be achieved by employing standardized drills and burs, this is sometimes prevented by improper manipulation during bone preparation. As a rule, implants with primary mobility do not integrate in the bone and therefore should be removed immediately during the surgery.

Following tooth extraction, the standard implantation procedure must be delayed until the alveolar bone has healed. Nine to 12 months are required for healing, depending on the width of the alveolus and age of the patient. A radiograph must be made before implantation to evaluate the extent of healing. An alternative is offered by the guided bone regeneration procedure with Gore-Tex membranes (p. 318 ff). This allows the healing period to be shortened to 2–3 months so that when the soft tissue cover is reestablished, implantation can be carried out earlier than with normal healing.

Fracture of Implant or Instrument

Fractures of ITI implants are not expected during surgery. Fractures of instruments usually result from incorrect manipulation, too many sterilization cycles, overheating, and sometimes material defects. Fragments of fractured implants and instruments that remain embedded in the bone must be removed with as little sacrifice of bone as possible.

448 15 Complications with ITI Implants

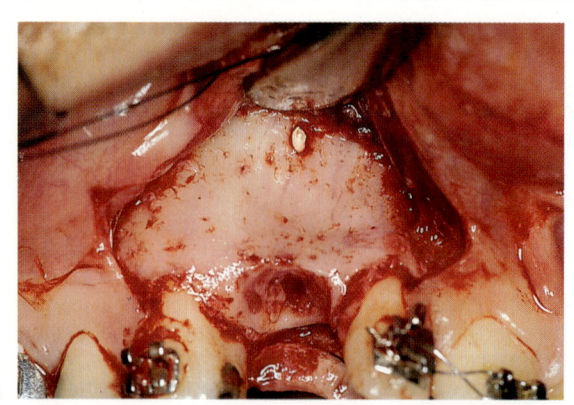

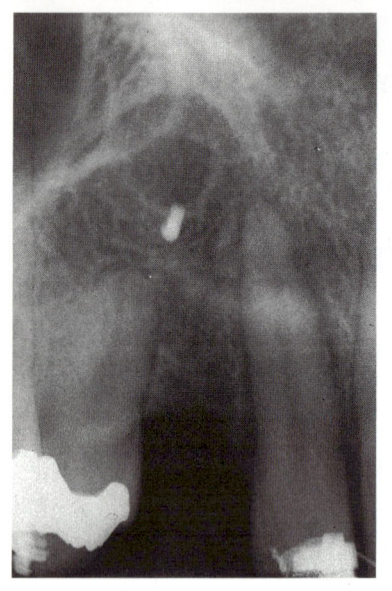

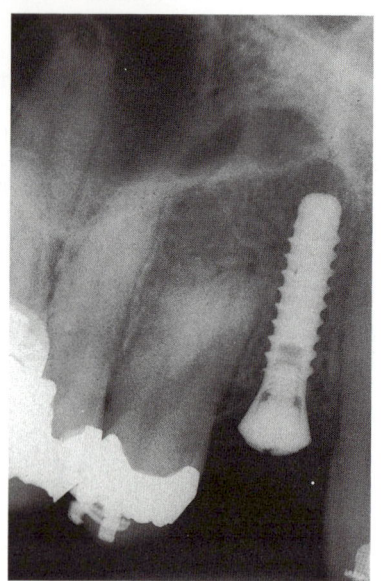

Fig. 15.2 Implantation in the space of an upper right canine with narrow spatial relationships
  a Status during the operation with a gutta-percha point as an orientation indicator for the preparation of the implant bed
  b Intra-operative radiograph to monitor the correct position of the gutta-percha point
  c Postoperative radiograph confirming that the reduced diameter implant has been placed without damaging the neighboring teeth

Foreign Bodies

Foreign bodies in immediate proximity to the implant jeopardize its success. Foreign bodies identified on radiographs, such as root fragments, root-canal filling materials, fractured endodontic instruments, etc. must be removed without exception before implant insertion. Precise localization of the object prior to the surgery (by means of radiographs made in two planes perpendicular to one another) is essential. Localization of the foreign body also influences the decision of whether the object must be removed before the implant surgery or if it can be removed at the same time without disturbing the implant bed and thereby interfering with primary stability. If exposure of the foreign body creates a large defect in the bone, this should be filled in with a material such as collagen fleece (Pentapharm AG, CH-4051 Basel) and allowed to heal before an implant is placed. Here again, an alternative would be to use the GBR (guided bone regeneration) technique with a Gore-Tex membrane.

Emphysema in the Face and Neck Region

Bone preparation with a turbine handpiece is contraindicated and can result in emphysema of the soft tissues of the face and neck. Emphysema can also be caused by sneezing, blowing the nose, or rinsing the wound with hydrogen peroxide.

The typical clinical symptom of emphysema is characterized by the sudden appearance of swelling on one side of the face with palpable crepitus in the soft tissue. The swelling can extend into the neck and sometimes into the thorax. This type of soft tissue emphysema is usually harmless. The patient who is shocked by his or her bloated appearance simply needs to be reassured. Cold compresses for the face and neck region can be prescribed, as well as prophylactic administration of an antibiotic.

Preventive measures against the occurrence of soft tissue emphysema consist of avoiding the use of turbine handpieces, which are also contraindicated for other reasons, avoidance of wound rinsing with hydrogen peroxide, close suturing of the soft tissue wound, and finally, advising the patient against raising the intraoral pressure by sneezing or nose blowing during the first few postoperative days.

Postoperative Complications

A basic distinction is made between *early complications* that are directly connected with the surgical procedure, and *late complications* that usually have only an indirect connection, if any, with the surgical procedure itself.

Early Complications

Listed among early complications are:
- wound edema;
- postoperative bleeding and hematoma;
- loosening of the implant;
- early infection;
- nerve damage.

Wound Edema

Surgical procedures on the jaws are frequently associated with edematous swelling of the soft tissues. This swelling is dependent on the duration of the operation and the extent of soft tissue trauma during surgery:

The quicker and gentler the surgery, the less swelling will occur. Soft tissue edema immediately adjacent to the surgical wound can result in dehiscence of the soft tissues. There is usually no need to resuture the wound. Healing of the dehiscence by secondary intention will occur with granulation and epithelization, and this can be accelerated by regular application of Solcoseryl Dental Adhesive Paste (Solco Basel AG, CH-4127 Birsfelden, Switzerland).

Wound necrosis is usually the result of sutures that are too tight. To counteract the tendency of necrotic tissue to become infected, the wound is carefully wiped with a small sterile swab soaked in 1% hydrogen peroxide solution. Topical application of Solcoseryl Dental Adhesive Paste can also accelerate wound healing in this situation.

Postoperative Bleeding and Hematoma

When delayed bleeding cannot be stopped with simple pressure (applied by an appropriately instructed patient) the wound must be revised under local anesthesia following conventional principles.

The more extensive the wound and surgical field is, the more likely it is that a postoperative hematoma will appear. The risk of infection also increases. Fresh hematomas between the bone surface and the mucoperiosteal flap should be opened and evacuated with suction. One can prevent the space created by the hematoma from refilling by placing an extra-oral pressure dressing over the soft tissues.

Proper hemostasis during surgery and the early local application of cold packs help to prevent the formation of hematomas. If, however, the discoloration that is characteristic of a soft tissue hematoma does occur in the skin and mucosa, external application of a heparin-containing cream is indicated. It can also be prescribed to fasten the resorption of such soft tissue hematomas.

Loosening of the Implant

Loss of primary stability of an initially firm implant is usually the result of improper technique during preparation of the implant bed. The development of heat above the critical limit of 47 °C (116.6 °F) in the adjacent bone causes coagulation of the intraosseous blood vessels and leads to necrosis of the peri-implant bone. This "heat necrosis" results in loosening of the implant after 2 to 4 weeks. This is typically seen in the radiograph as extensive bone resorption around the implant. If such an implant is splinted and stabilized by an implant bar connector, there is some chance that it will become stable again through ankylosis. Loosening of an implant that is free standing and not splinted always leads to loss of the implant. These implants can be classified as early failures and should be removed as soon as possible. This can usually be done without extensive surgery. A long delay leads to loss of more bone and exfoliation of the implant. Through early removal, the bone defect can usually be kept small so that implant insertion can be attempted again at a later time.

Early Infection

Although infections are rare with implant procedures, they do occasionally occur. Soft tissue infection manifests itself through local pain, increased swelling, tearing out of sutures, and purulent exudation from the wound, and can be treated by removing one or two sutures and rinsing with chlorhexidine-digluconate (0.12% three times a day). In addition, prescription of an antibiotic for at least 5 days is recommended. Rinsing of the wound should be continued three times daily until symptoms have ceased.

Early infection can also lead to loosening of an implant through secondary infection of the peri-implant bone tissues. When this occurs, the implant cannot be saved and should be removed as soon as possible.

Nerve Damage

In rare cases, severe edema or hematoma in the region of the mental nerve can cause sensory disturbances. A radiograph should always be made to determine if the nerve was damaged during implant placement or if there is contact between the implant and the nerve. Pain upon loading of the implant is usually an indication of direct contact of the implant with the nerve lying under it. If this is the case, the implant must be removed.

A gradual appearance of sensory disturbances in the mentalis region (Vincent's sign) in conjunction with an infection in the surgical field suggests the possibility of an osteomyelitis.

Late Complications

Late complications include:
- gingival recession;
- loosening of the implant;
- implant fracture;
- peri-implant infection.

Gingival Recession

Recession of the peri-implant mucosa can be caused by resorption of the buccal bone wall, tension from the buccal or labial frenulum, and/or incorrect brushing technique. Details of this soft tissue complication and its treatment through plastic surgery are discussed in chapter 10.

Loosening of the Implant

Very seldom does an ITI implant that has become ankylosed within healed bone loosen as the result of functional loading. This excellent clinical record is attributed primarily to the TPS layer on the ITI implant. In comparison to smooth or finely textured titanium surfaces, the TPS layer provides a clearly superior attachment to bone (p. 80 ff). At the Department of Oral Surgery University of Bern, only two cases have been observed in the past 10 years in which secondary loosening of an ITI implant occurred without accompanying peri-implant inflammation (Fig. 15.**3**). Occlusal factors were implicated in the etiology of these two failures. For this reason, utmost attention must be given to achieving optimized loading conditions in both centric occlusion and excursive jaw movements.

Peri-implant infection

Peri-implant infections do not develop overnight. They are much more likely to develop gradually (Newman and Flemmig 1988). This emphasizes the importance of regular clinical evaluations of the patient in the context of a well-organized recall system. Any inflammatory changes can thus be recognized as early as possible. If such an infection is recognized early, there is a good chance that the inflammation can be treated successfully. If, on the other hand, a peri-implant infection is not treated, it will lead (sooner or later) to loss of the implant.

Because of the low frequency of peri-implant infections, the clinical experience in treating them at the Department of Oral Surgery, University of Bern is limited, and the treatment philosophy presented here is based upon experience with only a few patients. The treatment recommendations that follow carry only limited weight, therefore, and could be revised in the future by further clinical experience.

As of this writing (February 1993), the following course of treatment is recommended when acute peri-implant inflammation with suppuration is discovered at a routine recall appointment (Table 15.**1**).

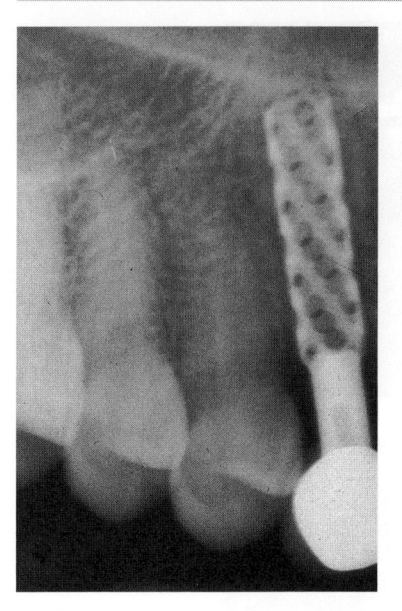

Fig. 15.**3** A secondarily loosened type F hollow cylinder implant in the upper right canine region with no clinical signs of peri-implant infection. This radiograph, made 7 $^1/_2$ years after implantation, reveals a narrow zone of bone resorption around the implant

The purpose of *antibiotic therapy* is to eliminate the acute inflammation as quickly as possible. Because acute peri-implant infection, as an opportunistic infection, exhibits an elevated component of anaerobic pathogens (Krekeler et al. 1986, Mombelli et al. 1987), a specific antibiotic must be selected that is effective against these organisms. Therefore, for antibiotic treatment of acute suppurative peri-implant infection, we prefer a mixture of antibiotics with amoxycillin (Clamoxyl; 375 mg t.i.d. orally) and metronidazole (Flagyl; 250 mg t.i.d. orally). This treatment has also been recommended for refractory periodontitis (van Winkelhoff et al. 1989). The antibiotic treatment is continued for 10 days and is combined with regular rinsing of the soft tissue pocket with chlorhexidine digluconate 0.12–0.2% three times daily for 3 weeks), which serves as an efficient local disinfectant (Mombelli and Lang 1992). The patient is instructed to flush the soft tissue pockets around the implants regularly with a fine-tipped irrigating syringe. With this therapy, the acute inflammation should rapidly subside (Fig. 15.**4c** and **d**, Fig. 15.**5c–e**). Finally, following precise reinstruction and remotivation, the patient is enrolled in a tightly controlled recall program. These patients are also given a chlorhexidine gel (Plak-Out Gel 0.2%, Hawe-Neos AG, CH-6925 Gentilino), which has been proven effective as an adjunct to mechanical plaque control. So far, impressive clinical results have been obtained in the few patients treated with this antibacterial therapy. Two

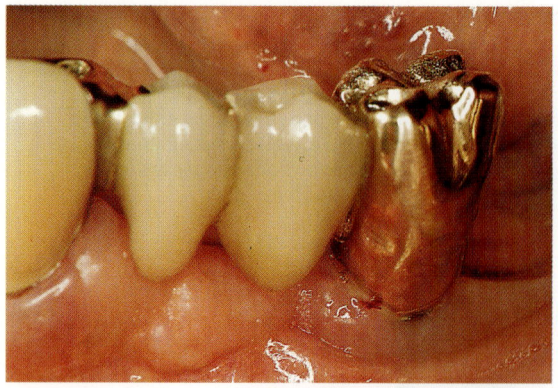

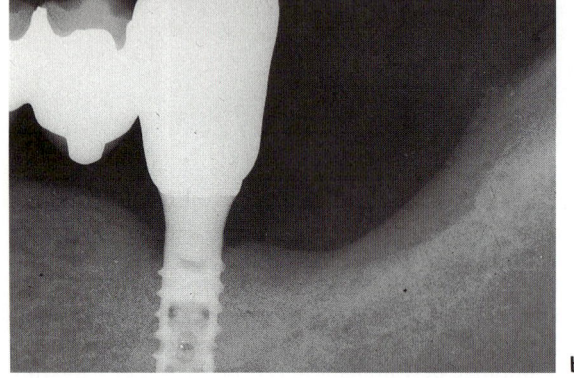

Fig. 15.4 Antibacterial treatment of an acute infection around a lower first molar implant
a Peri-implant infection with suppuration 4 years after implant insertion
b Radiograph showing a small crater-shaped area of bone resorption

Postoperative Complications **455**

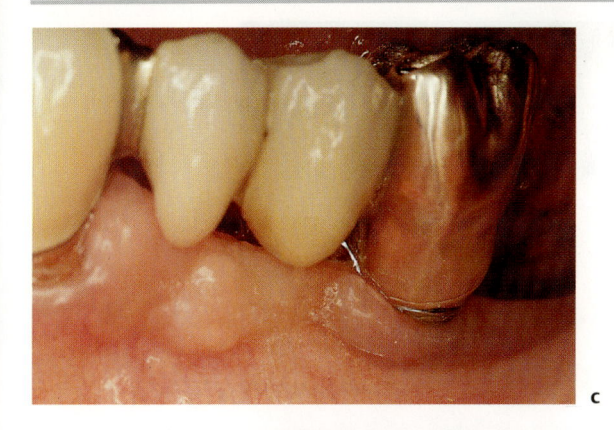

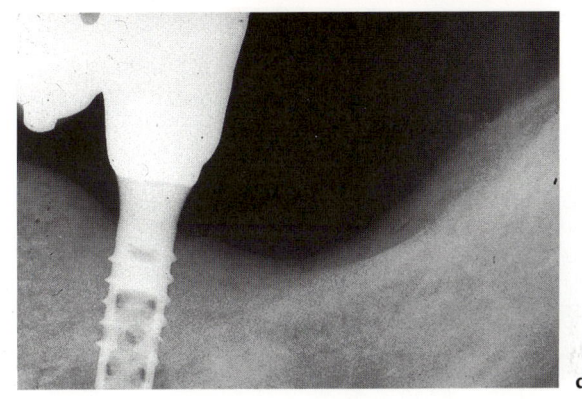

c One year after antibacterial treatment, the soft tissues are clinically free of inflammation (condition 5 years after implant insertion)

d Radiograph showing remineralization of the previously osteolytic region (condition 5 years after implant insertion)

456 15 Complications with ITI Implants

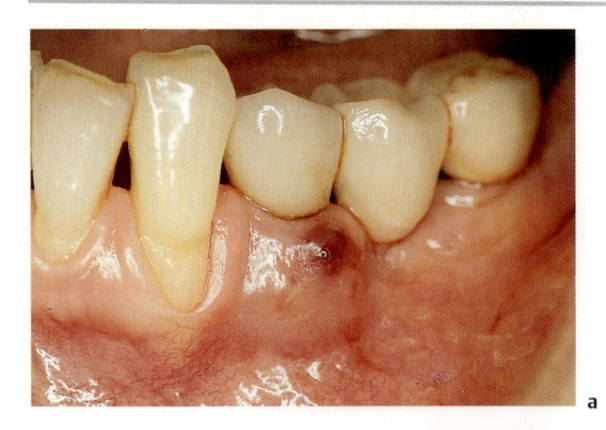

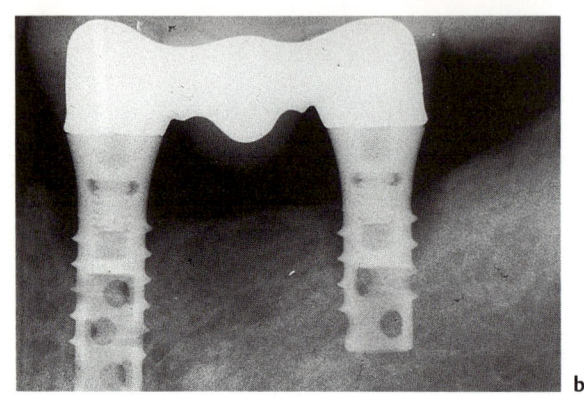

Fig. 15.**5** Antibacterial therapy of an acute infection around implants in the lower first premolar and first molar positions
a Condition at the 3-year recall. There is acute peri-implant infection around both implants. A pronounced swelling and fistula are present over the premolar implant
b The radiograph shows crater-shaped osteolytic defects around both implants (3-year recall)
c Four days after inception of antibacterial therapy with amoxycillin and Flagyl there is already an improvement in the clinical condition. A gingivectomy was performed subsequently to eliminate the fistula
d Three weeks following antibacterial therapy, there is no longer any clinical evidence of acute infection
e One year after the acute infection, there is no sign of recurrence. The peri-implant soft tissues are clinically healthy (4 year examination)

Postoperative Complications

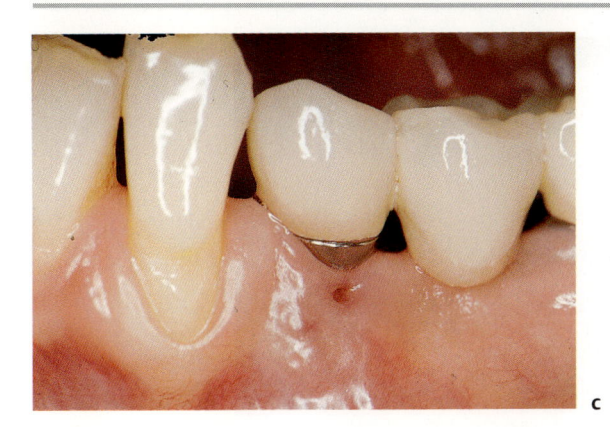

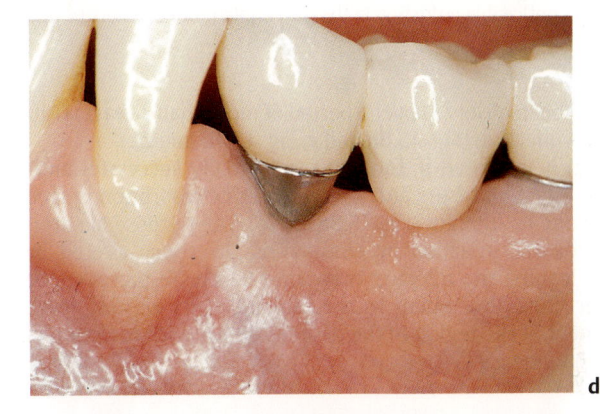

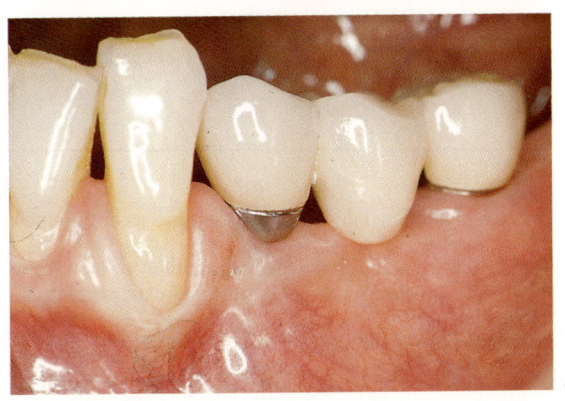

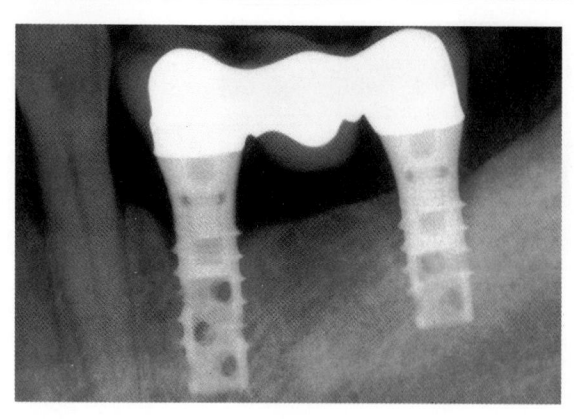

f The radiograph shows noticeable reduction in the peri-implant bone craters (4 year examination)

patients have already been observed over a period of more than 3 years without recurrence of the infection (Fig. 15.**6b** and **c**, Fig. 15.**7b** and **c**).

Surgical revision is indicated if, following an initially successful antibacterial treatment, infection recurs and advancing bone resorption is seen radiographically around an implant (Fig. 15.**8a** and **b**). The purpose of surgical revision is to stop the infection by eliminating the tissue altered by inflammation and cleaning the infected titanium surface. To preserve the remaining ankylotic bone attachment to the implant at its existing level, conservative treatment of the region of the osseous defect with resection of the bony walls is recommended.

Table 15.**1** Current treatment concept for peri-implant infections

---
1. Antibacterial treatment with systemic antibiotics (combination of Clamoxyl and Flagyl) and oral rinses with 0.2% chlorhexidine.
2. Surgical correction
3. Removal of implant

Fig. 15.**6** Antibacterial therapy of an acute infection around a lower second premolar implant
- **a** Acute peri-implant infection with suppuration and fistula formation one month after implant restoration. Treatment consisted of a gingivectomy to eliminate the fistula in conjunction with antibiotic therapy
- **b** The tissues are free of inflammation 4 years after implant insertion. During the entire observation period, no recurrence of infection was detected
- **c** Radiograph showing normal bone structure 4 years after implant placement

Postoperative Complications

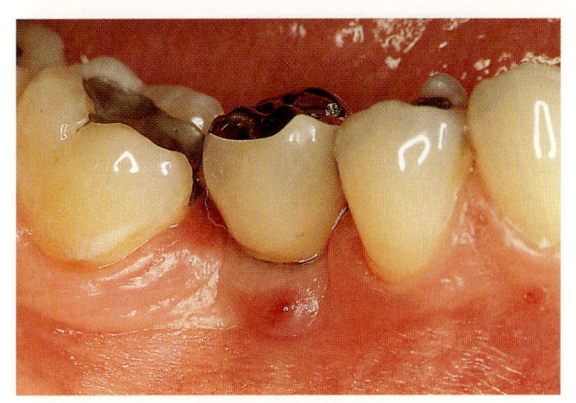

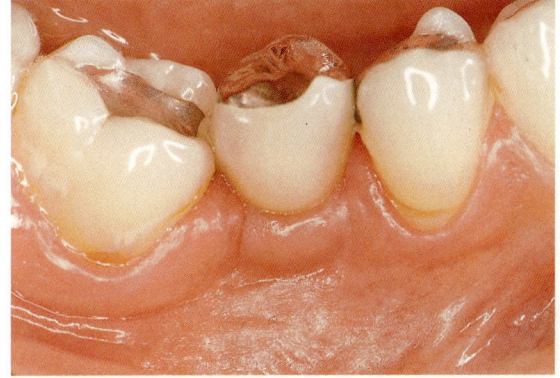

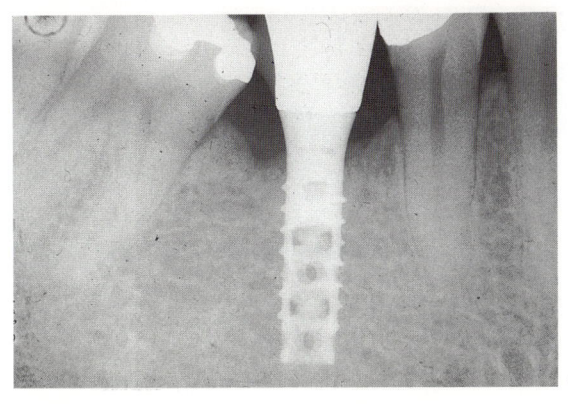

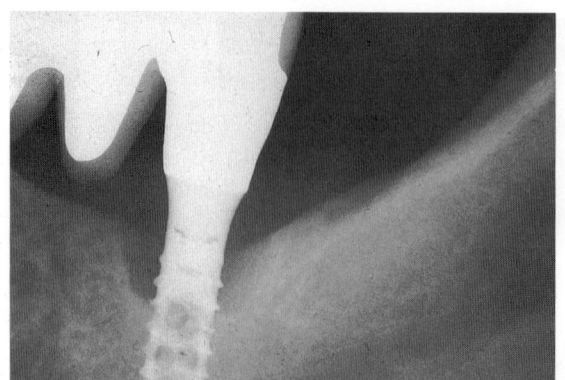

460 15 Complications with ITI Implants

a

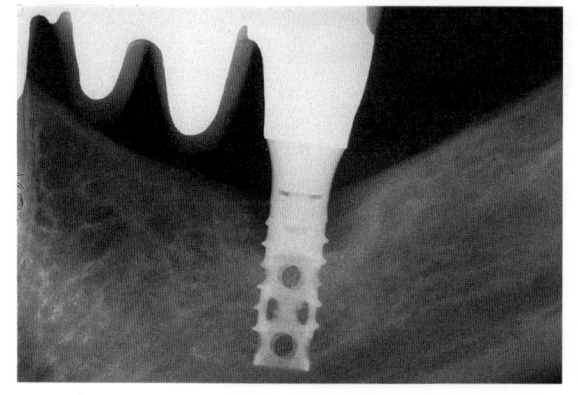

b

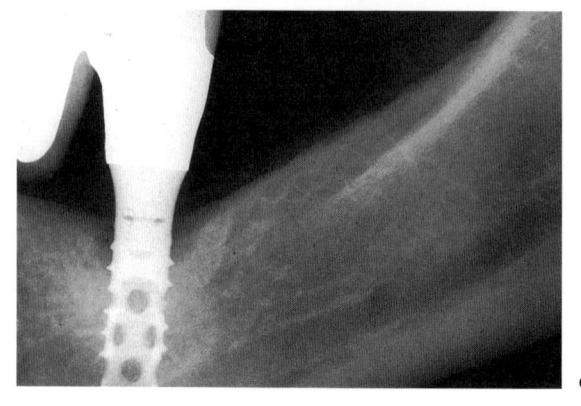

c

During the revision, a flap is reflected, the inflamed peri-implant soft tissue is excised, and the bony walls are flattened until there is good access to the surface of the implant. Following removal of all granulation tissue, the infected titanium surface is cleaned. Cleaning of the porous TPS layer presents a special problem and cannot be carried out with the usual periodontal hand instruments. Various methods for cleaning infected titanium surfaces have been presented in the recent literature (Zablotsky et al. 1992). One possibility is the use of an air powder abrasive (e.g., Prophy Jet), which cleans the contaminated titanium surface well but does not make it smooth (Fig. 15.**8c** and **d**). This device must be used with care because occurences of serious complications with air emboli have been reported in the literature. As an alternative, we currently use a flame-shaped white Arkansas stone in a low-speed handpiece to carefully remove the TPS layer with a generous stream of physiologic saline solution as a coolant. This can be done without pressure and not only decontaminates the titanium surface, but also smooths it (Fig. 15.**9a** and **b**). After the titanium surface has been cleaned mechanically, a chlorhexidine gel (Plak-Out Gel 0.2%) is applied for 5 minutes to provide topical disinfection (Fig. 15.**8e**). Next, the mucoperiosteal flap is repositioned apically, adapted closely to the implant, and fixed with interrupted sutures (Fig. 15.**8f**). Finally, a periodontal dressing is applied to hold the flap in place (Fig. 15.**8g**). The surgical revision is carried out under antibiotic coverage with the medications mentioned above. The positive result of this procedure (applied so far in four patients) has demonstrated that peri-implant infection can be arrested successfully (Fig. 15.**8h–k**).

◀ Fig. 15.**7** Antibacterial therapy of an acute infection around a lower left molar implant
  a Radiograph (May 1990) from a case of acute peri-implant infection showing a large semilunar area of bone resorption (3 $^1/_2$ years after implantation). Antibacterial therapy as described above was instituted and was repeated after 3 months
  b This radiograph made 6 months later (November 1990) already shows some reossification in the crater area
  c Radiograph 2 $^1/_2$ years after the infection (6 years after implant insertion) showing marked reduction of the peri-implant bone defect. No clinical evidence of recurrence of infection was found

462 15 Complications with ITI Implants

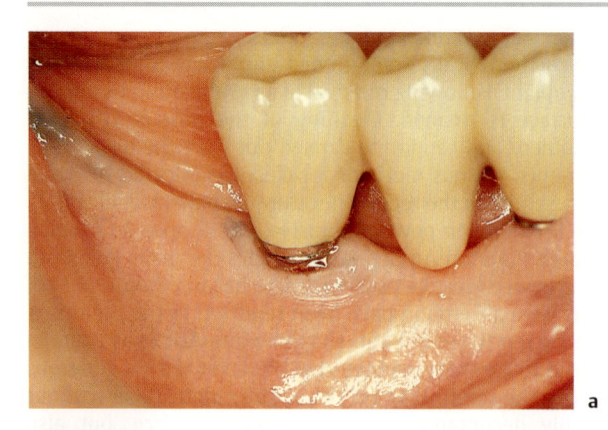

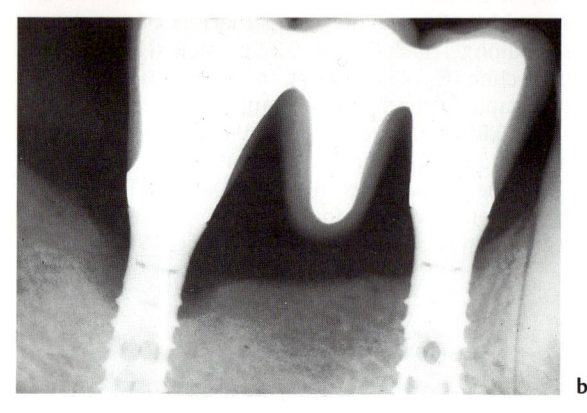

Fig. 15.**8** Surgical treatment of a chronically recurring infection around a lower right first molar implant
a Clinical view of repeatedly infected soft tissues
b The radiograph reveals an extensive semilunar crater in the bone around the distal implant
c This intraoperative view confirms the presence of an extensive crater-shaped defect
d Condition after reduction of the walls of the bony defect and cleaning of the TPS surface of the implant with a Prophy-Jet®
e Application of chlorhexidine gel (Plak-Out Gel 0.2%) for 5 minutes to provide chemical disinfection

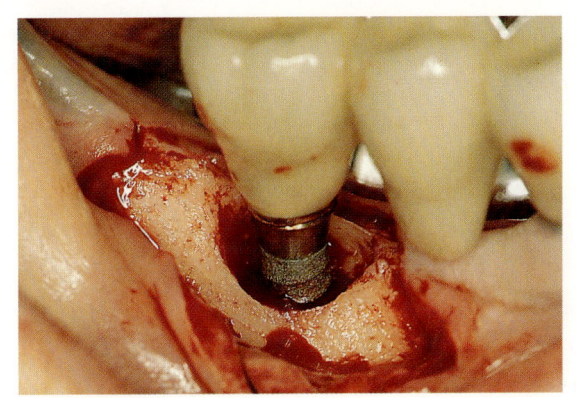

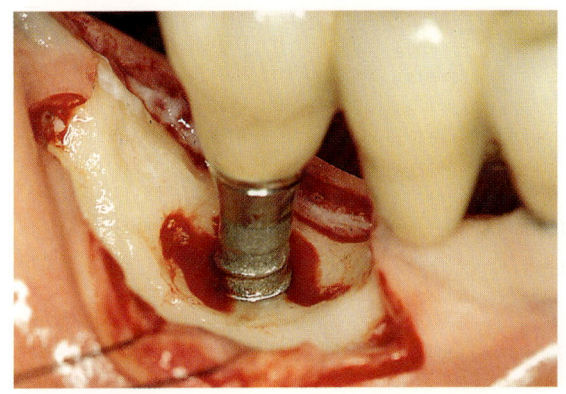

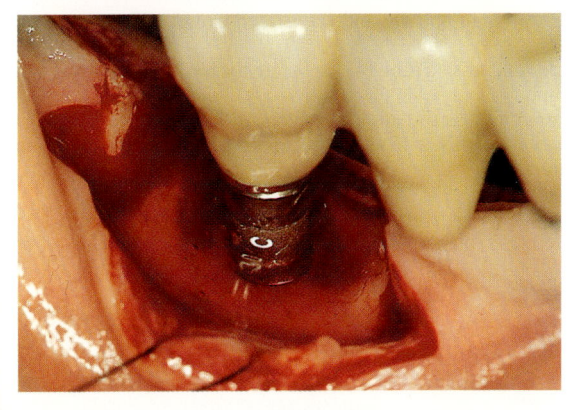

Postoperative Complications 463

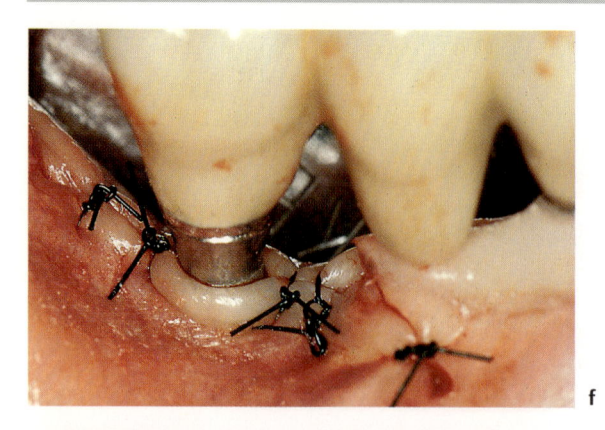

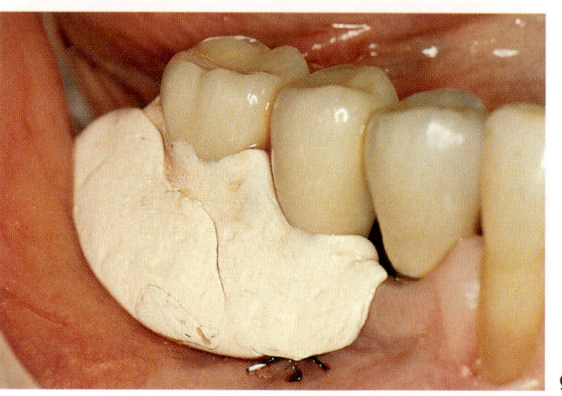

f The flap has been repositioned apically and the wound closed with interrupted sutures
g Application of a periodontal dressing (Coe Pak) to secure the position of the flap
h Postoperative radiograph
i Clinical appearance 4 months after the surgical revision
j Clinical condition 3 years after revision (6 years after implant placement). There is no sign of recurrence of infection

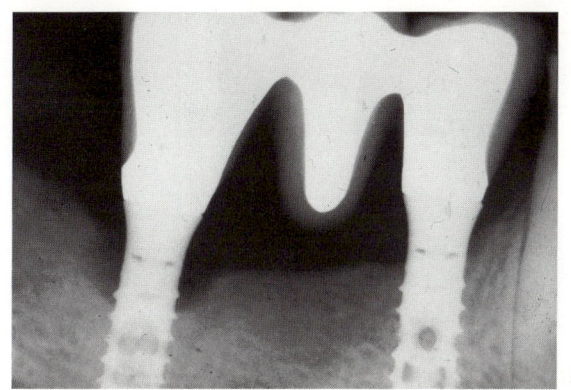

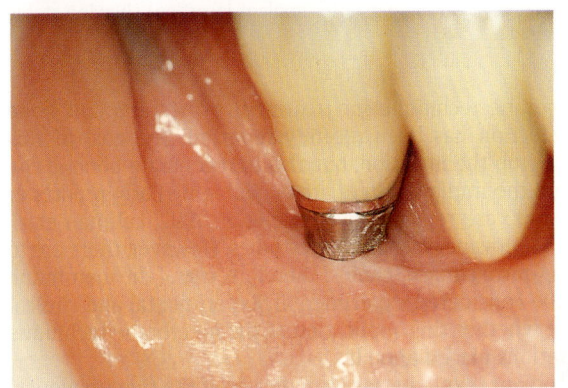

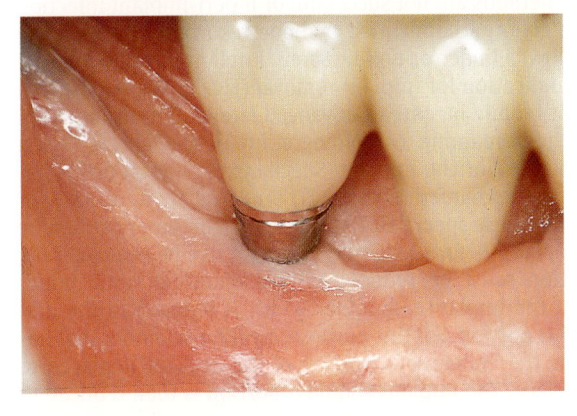

Postoperative Complications **465**

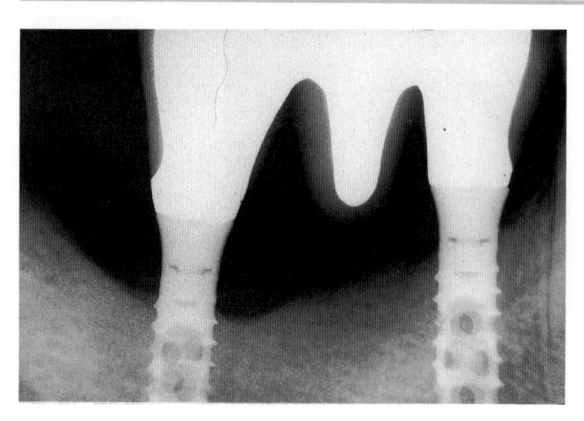

k Radiograph 3 years after revision (6 years after implant insertion) showing stable peri-implant bone levels

Use of the membrane technique for treatment of peri-implant bone defects caused by infection has been recently reported. The goal of this therapy is not only to stop the infection, but also to regenerate bone in the osseous defect around the implant. There are encouraging early reports in the literature in form of case reports (Jovanovic et al. 1992, Lehman et al. 1992) and experimental (Jovanocic et al. 1992) studies. However, there are to date no data from long-term clinical studies. Therefore, use of the membrane technique must still be considered experimental. Experimental and clinical studies must indicate whether this application of the membrane technique can fulfill the expectations placed upon it.

Removal of an implant (explantation) is indicated if the two previously described treatment methods are not successful or if peri-implant infection returns. Spread of infection accompanied by bone resorption through the perforations of a hollow cylinder or hollow screw implant into the internal space is an absolute indication for implant removal (Fig. 15.**10a** and **b**). The implant is usually not mobile in spite of advanced lateral and intraimplant osteolysis because the remaining osseointegration in the apical region provides adequate fixation for the implant. Special explantation drills that are matched exactly to the diameters of the ITI implants are necessary for implant removal. To use these special drills, the superstructure must first be removed from the implant. Before a two-part implant can be removed, the wider shoulder portion must be reduced with a diamond stone under copious coolant until the implant's shoulder width is reduced to the diameter of its endosseous portion. For this purpose, a guiding cylinder that has the same diameter as the endosseous portion of the implant is placed to serve as a guiding surface. The implant shoulder portion is then reduced to

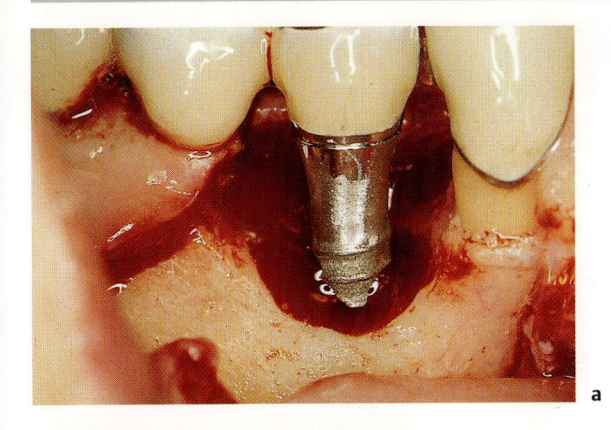

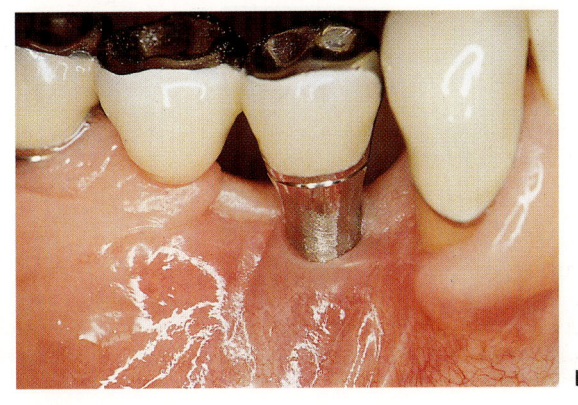

Fig. 15.**9** Surgical revision of a chronically recurring infection around the lower right first premolar implant
a The implant's TPS layer has been smoothed with a flame-shaped Arkansas stone
b Appearance 4 months after treatment. The smoothed titanium surface can be seen in the region of the marginal mucosa

the width of the guiding cylinder using a diamond or carbide drill of adequate shape (Fig. 15.**10e**). Next, a mucoperiosteal flap is reflected under local anesthesia so that the cervical part of the implant and surrounding bone can be clearly seen (Fig. 15.**10d**). The explantation drill, attached to a contra-angle handpiece, is now guided over the exposed implant with the guiding cylinder in place (Fig. 15.**10e**). The bony attachment still present around the apical portion of the implant is cut with the explantation

468 15 Complications with ITI Implants

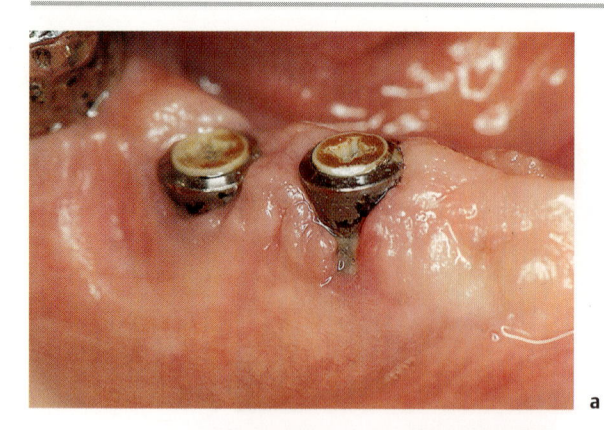

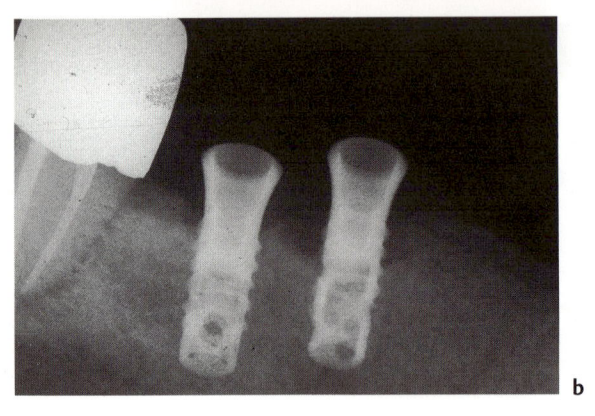

Fig. 15.**10** Removal of two HS implants that had been inserted in the lower right first and second premolar regions at a different place
a Chronic recurring infection of the first premolar implant
b Radiograph showing an extensive loss of bone around the first premolar implant
c After placement of the special guiding cylinder, the implant shoulder is eliminated with a diamond stone
d After removal of the shoulder and reflection of a flap, this intraoperative view shows an extensive bone defect around the first premolar implant with exposure of one of the perforations in the implant body
e The ankylotic bone anchorage remaining in the apical region of the implant is removed with the special explantation trephine

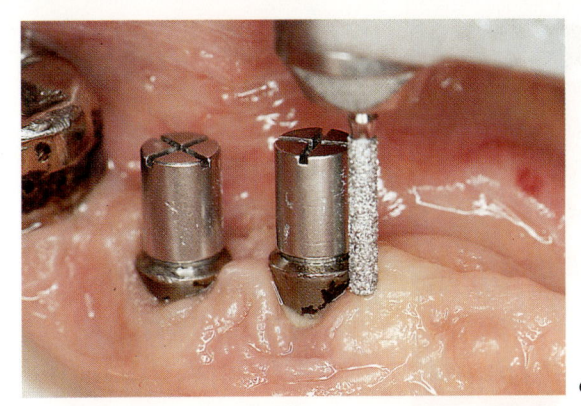

Postoperative Complications **469**

c

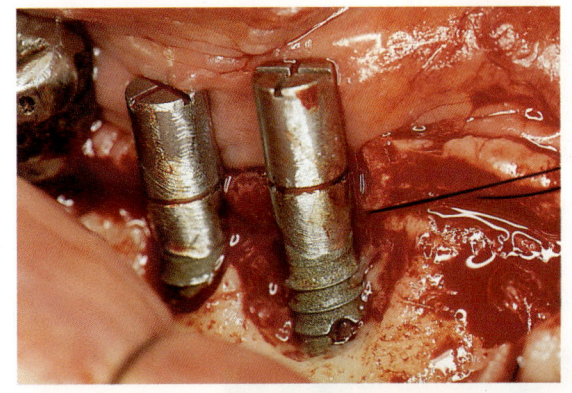

d

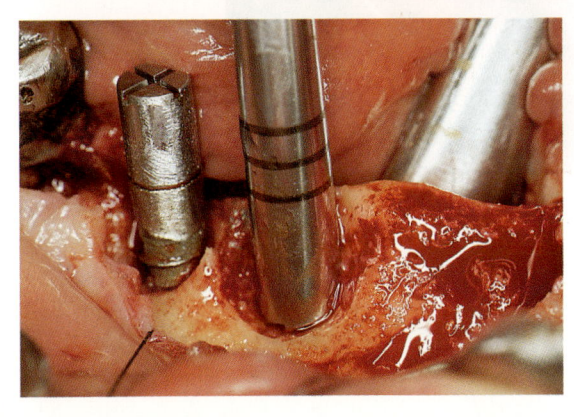

e

470 15 Complications with ITI Implants

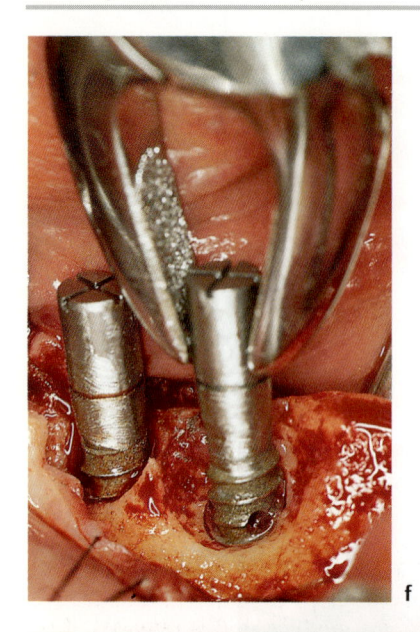

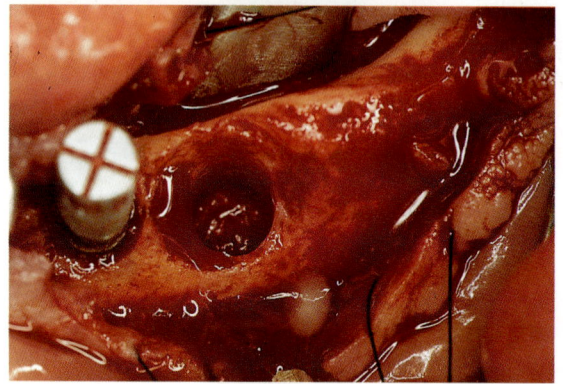

f After preparation with the explantation trephine, the implant is loosened with an extraction forceps with careful rotation
g This occlusal view shows the bone defect after removal of the implant

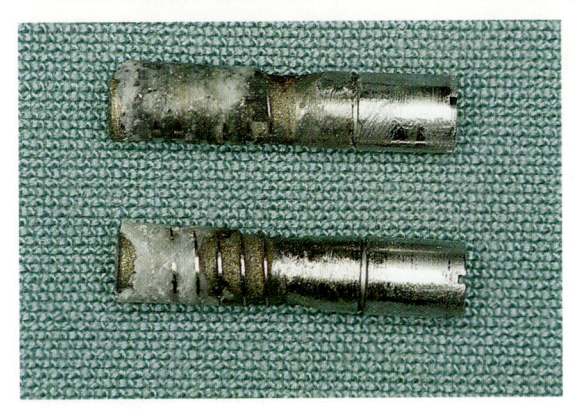

h The two implants that have been removed

trephine using a maximum rotational speed of 800 rpm and abundant cooling solution. Application of light intermittent pressure of short duration is required so that the drill does not bind and heat does not build up. The laser markings on the trephine indicate the preparation depth. After the predetermined depth has been reached, the trephine drill is removed. If the implant is still firm, it can be loosened and removed from its bed by carefully rotating it with an extraction forceps (Fig. 15.**10f**). All granulation tissue is now removed from the explantation defect (Fig. 15.**10g** and **h**). It is advisable to carefully freshen the internal bony walls of the former implant site with a medium sized round bur. The bony defect is then filled with collagen fleece (Pentapharm AG, CH-4041 Basel) to stabilize the blood clot. Finally, the periosteal flap is repositioned, and its margins are closed with interrupted sutures.

The explantation technique presented here in detail ensures that a minimum amount of bone will be sacrificed through the removal procedure. If implant removal is delayed too long, extensive osteitis, or even osteomyelitis could develop. Complications associated with infection can also arise because of anatomical relationships. Adjacent regions, such as the maxillary sinus, nasal cavity, and the contents of the mandibular canal could become involved, leading to a maxillary sinusitis, or to a neuritis of the inferior alveolar nerve.

Implant failures in edentulous mandibles in which the implants have been made to engage the cortex at both ends (bicortical stabilization, which was formerly the standard procedure) warrant special mention (Fig. 15.**11a**). When these long implants are removed with the explantation drill, the mandible (in some situations) can be extremely weakened so that–as has been experienced by one of our own patients–a fatigue fracture can occur

(Fig. 15.**11b** and **c**). In this situation, it makes sense to remove only the coronal portion of the implant and leave the apical portion in place. This unfortunate experience has reinforced our conviction that in edentulous mandibles, no more than two-thirds of the available bone height should be utilized. This will ensure that the danger of a fatigue fracture of the mandible needs no longer be a concern.

Implant Fractures

Fractures of ITI implants have rarely been reported. In cases where bone resorption is already advanced, implant fractures can occur as the result of mechanical overloading. Because of their macroscopic form, hollow cylinders and hollow screw implants are at greater risk than are solid screw implants. The thin walls of hollow implants can experience fatigue fracture in the area of the most coronal perforations. At the Department of Oral Surgery University of Bern, four implant fractures out of more than 1000 implants placed over the past 10 years has been observed (Fig. 15.**12a–c**). Based upon feedback from the implant manufacturer (Institut Straumann AG, CH-4437 Waldenburg), implant fractures have been reported only with hollow cylinder and hollow screw implants with standard diameters. A striking number of these fractured implants were fitted with ball attachments. It appears that with this type of prosthetic treatment, the loading force is increased (Jäger and Wirz 1993). Therefore, these abutments should be used only in combination with solid screw implants (4.1 mm) in order to minimize the risk of fracture.

In therapeutic terms, the question alway arises as to whether the broken endosseous implant fragment should be surgically removed or if it can be left alone. If a new implant is to be placed in the same area, then the fractured implant remnant must be removed with the appropriate drills. Otherwise, with the consent of the patient, it can be left in place.

Fig. 15.**11** Fatigue fracture of the mandible following removal of a bicortically placed ▶ Type F hollow cylinder implant
a Chronic peri-implant infection around the lower left first premolar implant with crater-shaped defect of the bone (10 years after implantation)
b Radiographic appearance of the bone defect after implant removal
c Fatigue fracture of the bone in the first premolar region

Postoperative Complications **473**

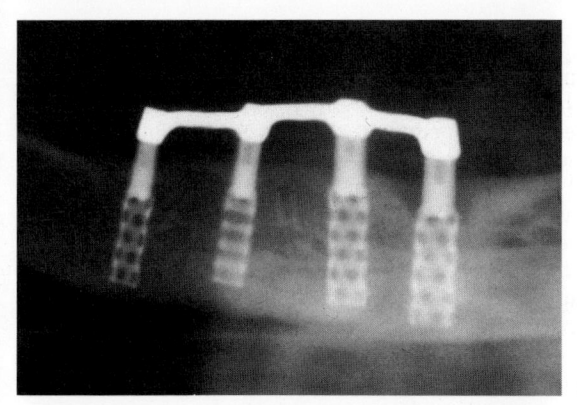

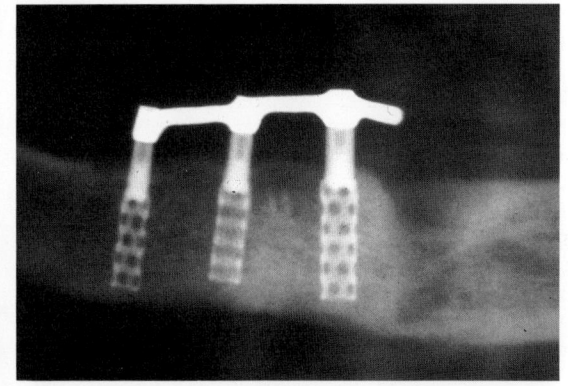

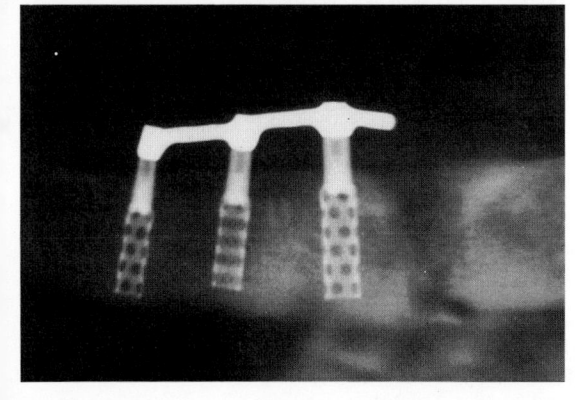

Closing Remarks

In summarizing the possible causes of complications that are encountered, it can be stated that they are of very different types. Inappropriate surgical procedures and corresponding operative techniques are certainly significant factors. There are also important anatomical conditions that, unless closely attended to, can lead to undesired consequences. Additional factors that can contribute to the development of complications are mistakes in treatment planning, loading the implants too soon, transmission of excessive forces from the prosthesis through the superstructure, and misjudging the patient's readiness to cooperate in maintaining an adequate level of oral hygiene and returning for recalls.

Fig. 15.**12** Fracture of a left first molar implant subjected to unfavorable occlusal loads ▶
- **a** Radiograph 3 years after implantation (August 1990) showing horizontal bone resorption measuring approximately 2–3 mm. There are no clinical signs of inflammation
- **b** One year later (August 1991) increasing bone destruction is observed that now has a vertical component also. During the meantime, the patient chews only on this (left) side, since he lost masticatory function on the right side through fractures of natural teeth
- **c** Three months later (November 1991) a fracture line has appeared on the radiograph through the first perforations resulting from metal fatigue. There is also an even larger area of peri-implant osteolysis apparent

Postoperative Complications **475**

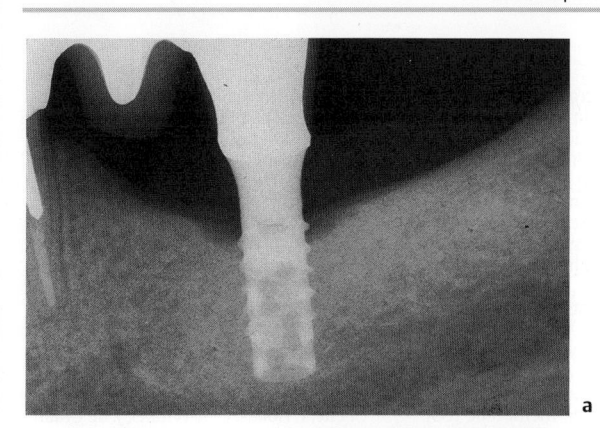

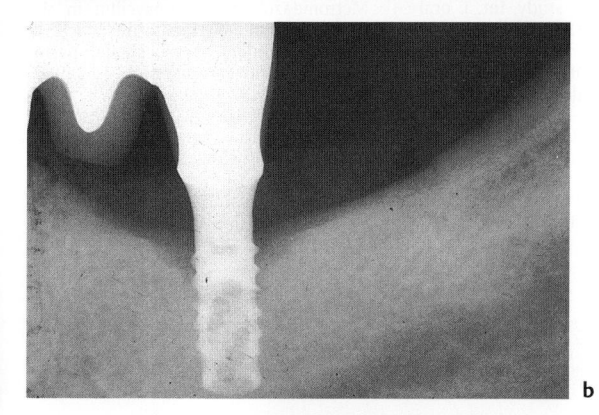

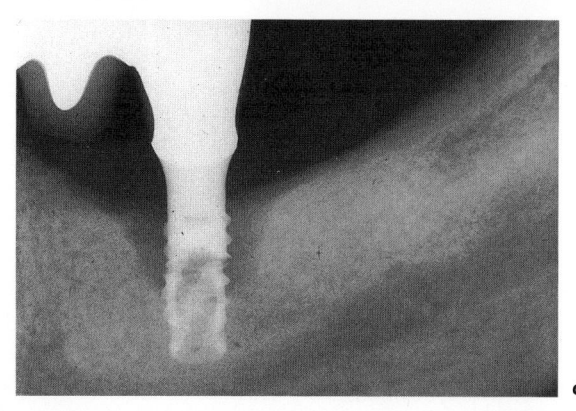

References

Jäger, K., J. Wirz: In-vitro-Spannungsanalysen an Implantaten in Abhängigkeit von den hybridprothetischen Suprakonstruktionen. Z. zahnärztl. Implantol. 9 (1993) 42–49

Jovanovic, S., H. Spiekermann, E.-J. Richter, M. Koseoglu: Guided tissue regeneration around titanium dental implants. In: Laney, W. R., D. E. Tolman (eds.): Tissue integration in Oral, Orthopedic, and Maxillofacial Reconstruction. Quintessence, Chicago (1992) 208–215

Jovanovic, S., E. B. Kenney, F. A. Carranza, K. Donath: The regenerative potential of plaque induced peri-implant bone defects treated by a submerged membrane technique. A experimental study. Int. J. oral max.-fac. Implants. 8 (1993) 13–18

Krekeler, G., K. Pelz, R. Nelissen: Mikrobielle Besiedlung der Zahnfleischtaschen am künstlichen Titanpfeiler. Dtsch., zahnärztl. Z. 41 (1986) 569–572

Lehmann, B., U. Brägger, Ch. F. Hämmerle, I. Fourmousis, N. P. Lang: Treatment of an early implant failure according to the principle of guided tissue regeneration. Clin. oral Impl. Res. 3 (1992) 43–48

Mombelli, A., M. A. C. van Oosten, E. Schürch, N. P. Lang: The microbiota associated with successful of failing osseointegrated titanium implants. Oral. Microbiol. Immunol. 2 (1987) 145–151

Mombelli, A., N. P. Lang: Antimicrobial treatment of peri-implant infection. Clin. oral Impl. Res. 3 (1992) 162–168

Newman, M. G., T. F. Flemmig: Periodontal considerations of implants and implant associated microbiota. J. dent. Educ. 52 (1988) 737–744

Tetsch, P.: Enossale Implantationen in der Zahnheilkunde. Hanser, München 1992

van Winkelhoff, A. J., J. P. Rodenburg, R. J. Goené, F. Abbas, E. G. Winkel, J. de Graaff: Metronidazole plus amoxycillin in the treatment of Actinobacillus actinomycetemcomitans associated periodontitis. J. clin. Periodontol. 16 (1989) 128–131

Zablotsky, M., D. Diedrich, R. Meffert: Detoxification of endotoxin-contaminated titanium and hydroxyapatite-coated surfaces utilizing various chemotherapeutic and mechanical modalities. Implant. Dent. 1 (1992) 154–158

16 Documentation and Statistics

A. Schroeder and G. Krekeler

"According to the classic definition, *documentation* includes the collection, understanding, organizing, and interpretation, as well as the storage and retrieval of information. Its purpose is to store (to document) the knowledge gained from experience in such a way that it can be used to gain new understanding. This means that retrieval, and not storage, is the central issue" (Dudek 1984).

It is not necessary to add to this complete explanation of the concept of documentation. Where would the acquiring of new knwledge from a growing body of experiential information be more important than in a field that is still very young, such as endosseous implantology? It is imperative that imprecise statements such as: "This technique has proved to be clinically successful for many dentists over a long period of time," or "Operators report from long experience...," be replaced by precise and verifiable data. This is not possible without reliable, complete documentation.

On the other hand, documentation is only reasonable when it is also feasible. Pages of questions that must be routinely filled out are a large burden for colleagues in private practice. The complexity of some of the questions frequently makes it difficult to delegate the documentation to office staff, as they may not be sufficiently educated for the task.

A critical point in designing a documentation system is to make it relevant to clnical practice. For this purpose, parameters must be used that are easy to comprehend and that are stated in such a way that they cannot be misinterpreted. This will enable them to be accurately recorded and clearly evaluated, even in a later analysis. At the same time, documentation must be adequate for scientific evaluation of the cases.

Parameters of Documentation

The number of parameters should be kept rather small without losing important information. Nonetheless, in addition to the obvious entries about the patient, date of operation, surgical team, etc., the documentation should include preoperative, intraoperative, and postoperative data.

Preoperative data relate to the mucosa (mobile, fixed, keratinized) and the radiographic findings from an orthopantograph, intraoral films, and, in some cases, a cephalometric projection. The latter is useful in edentulous patients to determine the actual form and height of the anterior part of the alveolar ridge.

Intraoperative and immediate postoperative conditions and procedures are recorded in detail in the progress notes. These should include premedication, anesthesia, incision location, the structure and volume of the bone, bone manipulation, the placement and removal of sutures, and any postoperative medications. The actual list of questions for data collection should cover at least the form, material, and coating of the implant, as well as complications, if any.

Postoperative documentation. The pre- and intraoperative documentation, and to some extent also the short-term postoperative documentation belong in the mandatory records of every physician and dentist. Subsequently, precise entries should also be made describing the superstructure, the time of insertion, and the type of restoration with information on, among other things, the:
– material;
– fixation (permanent or retrievable);
– type of retention (e.g., bar, crowns, telescopes, ball attachments);
– veneering material (resin, porcelain).

Important data from the *long-term postoperative* experience over many years serve to test procedures that were (in part) new at the time they were performed. Some central characteristics will fail to come to light during this process if the spectrum of parameters is too narrow.

To reiterate, the essential information to be gathered at the recall appointment concerns:
– clinical performance and patient complaints;
– status of the peri-implant soft tissue ("gingiva");
– pocket depth;
– plaque and calculus accumulation;
– radiographic findings;
– condition of the superstructure.

Collection of Data

As emphasized earlier, the foundation of every information system is data collection. The information contained in the documentation and the validity of all retrospective evaluations depends upon expert decisions as to which characteristics to consider and how much weight to give to each (Zehnder 1980). In our system, determination of the items to be recorded is not the concern of the software specialist but that of the surgeon and/or restoring dentist. A detailed documentation system has been produced by the Council on Implantology within the German Dental Society (Tetsch et al. 1985). It attempts to collect and evaluate as much experiential data as possible on a broad basis over *various* types of implants and systems, while each group that developed its own implant system concerns itself (and will continue to concern itself) primarily with a documentation system designed specifically for its own implant (e.g., blade implants, Brånemark, Tübingen, IMZ).

Likewise, a one-page, simpler questionnaire for the ITI system has been drawn up that can be filled out in hardly more than a minute by marking the boxes. The explanatory text has been reduced to a minimum (Fig. 16.**1**).

All relevant pre- and postoperative data, including that relating to the proposed superstructure, are recorded on this "implantation form." For long-term data collection, recall appointment forms are available with spaces for recording details of the completed overlying restorations, plus a checklist for the information to be gathered at the semiannual recall examinations (Fig. 16.**2**). These questionnaires (code sheets) are examined using electronic data-processing. For the colleague who has placed one or more implants in the same patient, the procedure is very simple: He or she fills out the questionnaire and sends it with the radiographs in the special envelope to the appropriate documentation center. The center's computer transfers the data from the questionnaire to a smaller format, the so-called "X-ray film card" (front side). The radiographs placed with it are copied (negative paper copies) and stuck to the back side of the card. A duplicate of the card is returned to the sender in the same envelope. It is then his responsibility to make a photocopy of the questionnaire he filled out or to obtain a carbon copy, which is usually not very satisfactory.

The patient is now "stored." Due to the uniform docmenation, the data can be retrieved from the computer at any time for scientific purposes. Present software allows any combination of selection criteria.

The system functions extremely well, but is dependent upon the documenation center. If problems should occur there, the concept would be unusable, which means other solutions would have to be sought.

Statistics

Data collection and the rapid, dependable retrieval of this data constitute the basis for statistical statements relative to the individual parameters and also provide an overall picture of success and failure. This presumes, however, that there is agreement on the definition of success and failure. While one person might categorize a slight peri-implant soft-tissue inflammation as a failure, another might not declare a failure until the implant has to be removed. A comprehensive presentation of this many sided problem can be found in Fallschüssel (1986).

16 Documentation and Statistics

ITI DOCUMENTATION	Implantation Form	No.
Clinic or Office	Operator(s)	Patient Last name First name ☐ Male ☐ Female Date of Birth: _____
Implant type HC HS S ☐ ☐ ☐ ☐ ☐	Procedure: One stage ☐ Two stage ☐	Implant region(s) FDI tooth numbers, e.g., 46 or 43/41/31/33 etc.
Date of operation	Anesthesia Nerve local infiltration ☐ La ☐	Antibiotic Yes ☐ No ☐
Mucosa Immobile ☐ Mobile ☐	Mucogingival surgery before implantation Yes ☐ No ☐ Type:	Surgical result/Prognosis Very good ☐ Satisfactory ☐ Questionable ☐
Proposed superstructure Individual crowns ☐ Bridges ☐ Fixed ☐ Detachable ☐ From To Bar ☐ Combination ☐	Opposing jaw +− Natural dentition ☐ Partial denture ☐ Complete denture ☐	☐ ☐ ☐ With implants where?

Hygiene   good ☐
            average ☐
              poor ☐
	An early
	explantation ☐
	Date:
		Reason for implant removal:

Remarks (risk factors)		
Supporting radiographs	Individual radiographs ☐ OPG ☐	Number of films: Number of films:
Place and date	Signature / Stamp	

Fig. 16.1 Implantation form

ITI DOCUMENTATION			Recall appointment sheet
Clinic or Office	Patient Last name First name		Refer to Implantation Form No.

Date of implantation:

Superstructure:
started on   Post-op.   completed on:

                Bridge from   to
                    Single crown ☐
Function   Fixed ☐
good ☐   Fixed-detachable ☐
average ☐   Bar ☐
poor ☐   Combination ☐

Remarks:

RECALL APPOINTMENT   Date:

Gingiva
  Taut ☐   Overall success ☐   No inflammation ☐
  Mobile ☐   Failure ☐   Inflamed ☐
                                                Bleeding ☐

Pocket depth   Mobility   Bone   Hygiene
2–3 mm ☐   Slight ☐   Apposition ☐   Good ☐
4–6 mm ☐   None ☐ Resorption/Invasion ☐   Avg. ☐
More ☐ Severe (vertical also) ☐   Poor ☐

Supplemental treatment on:
Antibiotics ☐   Mucogingival surgery ☐   Curettage ☐

Implant removed on Date:	Reason for removal:

Supporting radiograph(s):	Single films ☐ Panoramic ☐	Number of films: Number of films:

Place and date:	Signature or stamp:

Fig. 16.**2** Recall appointment sheet for recording long-term data

17 Long-Term Results of ITI Implants

C. M. ten Bruggenkate

The development of the implant system described in this book began in the early 1970s., before the officid foundation of the ITI team.

Numerous variations of the hollow cylinder principle (chapter 5) were conceived by A. Schroeder and F. Sutter, and starting in 1974, these were tested clinically within a small group of colleagues. At about the same time, the titanium plasma-sprayed (TPS) screw implant was designed for treating edentulous mandibles and was clinically tested. These clinical tests showed that the rotationally symmetrical ITI implants (Type F hollow cylinder implant and TPS screw implant) gave the best results. Subsequently, these two implants served as the foundation for the integrated and fully standardized ITI System that was developed in 1985 and 1986.

The quality of an implant system must scientifically be judged on the basis of long-term results. Since 1978, there have been many proposals on the definition of implant success rates. None of these proposals have led to a clear consensus because all suggested success criteria have met some variety of objection. Buser and co-workers (1990) have drawn up a list of useful, rigid criteria for success, and these have been used for evaluating the long-term results of the clinical trials presented below (Table 17.1).

The data used to evaluate the results of a system can be differentiated in quantitative or qualitative data. The concern how purely quantitative results many implants were inserted and how many were available for inspection at recall, compared with how many were either lost or had to be removed. To gather qualitative data, the implants available for inspection were evaluated both clinically and radiographically (Table 17.1).

The evaluation of an individual implant can change over time. An implant might appear on a checklist as a failure when it temporarily causes a problem, but later if the problem has been successfully resolved, the same implant can be listed as a success.

Table 17.1 Success criteria for ITI implants (Buser and co-workers 1990)

1. Absence of persisting subjective complaints such as pain, foreign body sensation, and/or dysesthesia
2. Absence of recurring peri-implant infection with suppuration
3. Absence of any detectable implant mobility
4. Absence of a continuous radiolucency around the implant

Table 17.2 Numbers of various types of implants inserted

	Bern	Boston	Darmstadt	Freiburg	Geneva	Leiden	Total
Implantation period				1977–1988		1984–1988	
TPS screws				872 (only for bars)			872
Type F						102	102
Implantation period	8/1985–2/1989	3/1990–12/1992	10/1985–5/1993	1988–5/1993	4/1989–5/1993	5/1988–5/1993	
ITI implants:							
HC-I	78	–	24	28	–	344	474
HS-I	23	–	27	–	–	6	56
SS-I	–	–	134	423	–	15	572
HC-II	28	60	65	14	129	806	1102
HC-A	15	15	59	50	51	146	336
HS-II	105	130	210	24	331	220	1020
SS-II	–	24	613	1739	9	121	2506
SS-3.3	–	12	312	991	4	101	1420
Total inserted	249	241	1444	329	524	1759	7486

HC Hollow cylinder
HS Hollow screw
SS Solid screw
I One-piece implant
II Two-piece implant
A Angled abutment implant

Table 17.3 Superstructure (number of implants at the time of prosthetic treatment)

	Bern Super-structure	Bern Impl.	Boston Super-structure	Boston Impl.	Darmstadt Super-structure	Darmstadt Impl.	Freiburg Super-structure	Freiburg Impl.	Geneva Super-structure	Geneva Impl.	Leiden (F-type) Super-structure	Leiden (F-type) Impl.	Leiden Super-structure	Leiden Impl.
Bar attachments	26	99	4	11	56	185	532	2092	11	29	9	68	327	1222
Ball attachments	1	2	2	4	13	26	64	128	45	90			30	70
Crowns	42	42	100	100	474	474	99	99	75	75	7	7	163	163
Bridges	49	105	51	124	345	759	283	950	145	330	13	26	141	304
Total		248		239		1444		3269		524		101		1759

Participating Clinics

The following clinics have generously made the results of their long-term studies available for compiling the information in Tables 17.**2**–17.**4**:

Bern	Clinic for Oral Surgery, University of Bern, Switzerland (PD Dr. Daniel Buser and co-workers)
Boston	Division of Implantology, Harvard University, Boston, Massachusetts (Dr. Hans-Peter Weber, Dr. Joe P. Fiorellini)
Darmstadt	Clinic for Oral and Maxillofacial Surgery Darmstadt, Germany (Dr. Dr. Dr. Christian Foitzik)
Freiburg	Clinic for Oral and Maxillofacial Surgery, Section for Periodontal Surgery University of Freiburg im Breisgau, Germany (Prof. Dr. Gisbert Krekeler)
Geneva	Dental Institute of the University of Geneva, Switzerland (Prof. Dr. Urs Belser, Dr. Jean Pierre Bernard)
Leiden	Clinic for Oral and Maxillofacial Surgery, St. Elisabeth Hospital, Leiden, The Netherlands (Dr. Christiaan M. ten Bruggenkate)

Note regarding Tables 17.**2**–17.**4**: The calculated rates of success are based upon the principle that the drop-out rate is not added to the failure rate. This appears to be legitimate, because not all unmonitored implants can be recorded as lost. This category also includes, for example, implants of deceased patients that were in successful function until the time of death. However, we have included all inserted implants in the statistics so that these clinical data may also be interpreted in correlation with the drop-outs.

Our calculation of success is based upon the implants that were actually evaluated; i.e., failures were only registered if early or late loss had occurred, if patient complaints arose, or if implant mobility or radiographic changes were registered.

Table 17.**4** Length of time the ITI implants had been in place

Year	Bern	Boston	Darmstadt	Freiburg	Geneva	Leiden
$1/3$–1	–	134	146	687	234	273
1–2	–	79	181	991	169	431
2–3	–	26	298	525	95	451
3–4	–	–	312	507	26	344
4–5	68	–	261	352	–	220
> 5	158	–	246	207	–	40

Table 17.5 Number of implants lost, qualitative data, and success rate

	Bern	Boston	Darmstadt	Freiburg		Geneva	Leiden	
Number placed	249	241	1444	872 TPS	3269 Bonefit	524	102 Type F	1759 Bonefit
Implantation period	8/1985–2/1989	3/1990–12/1992	10/1985–5/1993	2/1977–6/1988	5/1988–1993	4/1989–5/1993	1984–5/1988	5/1988–5/1993
Implants lost during healing phase	1	2	2	46	109	2	1	6
Number of loaded implants	248	239	1442	826	3160	522	101	1753
Implants lost after loading	5	1	22	19	65	1	–	21
Unable to monitor	17	7	491	204	359	7	5	202
Monitored implants still present	226	231	929	603	2736	514	96	1530
Patient complaints	–	–	10	5	6	6	1	16
Acute infection	2	–	18	2	4	6	–	22
Implant mobility	–	–	8	–	–	–	–	–
Radiolucency	–	–	23	9	–	3	4	42
Success rate (%)	96,5	98,5	93,5	88	94	98	94,7	94,5

Discussion and Conclusions

In this multicentered study, the results of implantation in six clinics were reported. Detailed data are abundantly available in the literature.

It should be pointed out that among the qualitative evaluations recorded in Table 17.**5**, the same implant is sometimes counted in more than one of the categories (patient complaints, acute infection, implant mobility, and radiolucency). For example, if there is acute inflammation associated with one implant, the same implant could also be associated with pain and radiolucency. These cases have been taken into account in calculating the success rate.

When the results are evaluated according to Buser's criteria for success, the success rates are found to be about the same in most of the participating clinics. The earlier types of ITI implants, such as the F hollow cylinder implant or the TPS screw implant, still show good results over relatively long observation periods. It can be concluded that based upon the literature and the results compiled in this chapter, the ITI system represents a simple, modern, and dependable method of oral implantology.

References

Albrektsson, T., G. Zarb, P. Worthington, A. R. Eriksson: The long-term efficacy of currently used dental implants: a review and proposed criteria of success. Int. J. oral max.-fac. Implants 1 (1986) 11–25

Babbusch, C. A., J. N. Kent, D. J. Misch: Titanium Plasma-sprayed (TPS) Screw Implants for the Reconstruction of the Edentulous Mandible. Int. J. oral max.-fac. Surg. 44 (1986) 274–282

ten Bruggenkate, C. M., W. A. M. van der Kwast, H. S. Oosterbeek: Success criteria in oral implantology (a review of the literature). Int. J. oral Implant. 7 (1990) 45–51

ten Bruggenkate, C. M., K. Müller, H. S. Oosterbeek: Clinical Evaluation of the ITI (F-Type) Hollow Cylinder Implant. Oral Surg. Oral Med. Oral Path. 70 (1990) 693–697

Buser, D., A. Schroeder, F. Sutter, N. P. Lang: Das neue ITI-Implantatkonzept – Indikationen und klinische Aspekte. Quintessenz 40 (1989) 17–34

Buser, D., H. P. Weber, N. P. Lang: Tissue integration of non-submerged implants. 1-year results of a prospective study with 100 ITI hollow-screw and hollow-cylinder implants. Clin. oral. Impl. Res. 1 (1990) 33–40

Buser, D., H. P. Weber, U. Brägger, Ch. Balsiger: Gewebeintegration von einphasigen ITI-Implantaten: 3-Jahresergebnisse einer prospektiven Langzeitstudie mit Hohlzylinder- und Hohlschraubenimplantaten. Parodontol. 3 (1992) 189–199

Buser, D., F. Sutter, H. P. Weber, U. Belser, A. Schroeder: The ITI Dental Implant System. Basics, Clinical Indications and Procedures, Results. In Hardin, J. (ed.): Clark's Clinical Dentistry. Lippincott, Philadelphia. Vol. 5, 52 (1992) 1–23

Fallschüsssel, G.K.H. Zahnärztliche Implantologie. Quintessenz, Berlin (1986).

Krekeler, G., W. Schilli, H. Geiger: Das TPS-Implantat, ein zuverlässiges Retentionselement. Z. zahnärztl. Implantol. 6 (1990) 229

Ledermann, P. D.: Das TPS-Schraubenimplantat nach siebenjähriger Anwendung. Quintessenz. 35 (1984) 1–11

Mericske Stern R., T. Steinlin Schaffner, R. Marti, A. H. Geering: Periimplant mucosed aspects of ITI implants supporting overdentures Clin. Oral Impl. Res. 5 (1994) 9–18

Schnitman, P. A., L. B. Shulman: Recommendations of the consensus devel-opment conference on dental implants. J. Amer. dent. Ass. 98 (1979) 373–377

Schroeder, A., O. Pohler, F. Sutter. Gewebsreaktion auf ein Titan-Hohlzylinderimplantat mit Titan-Spritzschichtoberfläche. Schweiz. Mschr. Zahnheilk. 86 (1976) 713–727

Schroeder, A., B. Maeglin, F. Sutter: Das ITI-Hohlzylinderimplantat Typ F zur Prothesenretention beim zahnlosen Kiefer. Schweiz. Mschr. Zahnheilk. 93 (1983) 720–733

Smith. D. E., G. A. Zarb: Criteria for success of osseointegrated endosseous implants. J. prosth. Dent. 62 (1989) 567–572

Sutter, F., A. Schroeder, F. Straumann: Technische und konstruktive Aspekte der ITI-Hohlzylinderimplantate. Zahnärztl. Welt/Ref. 90 (1981) 50–59

Sutter, F., A. Schroeder, D. Buser: Das neue ITI-Implantatkonzept – Technische Aspekte und Methodik. Quintessenz 39 (1988) Teil I: 1875–1890. Teil II: 2057–2061

Vermeeren, J. i. J. F., G. J. van Beck, c. m. ten. Bruggenkate, A. V. Gool: ITI-Implantate in den Niederlanden. Z-Zahnärztl. Implantol. 11 (1995) 145–148.

Weber, H. P., D. Buser, J. P. Fiorellini, R. C. Williams: Radiographic evaluation of crestal bone levels adjacent to nonsubmerged titanium implants. Clin. oral Impl. Res. 3 (1992) 181–188

18   Legal Considerations

A. Schroeder

Since this book is intended for readers from *various countries*, who are interested in implantology, the actual legal questions cannot be treated, in view *of differing judicial systems*. We must hence restrict ourselves to some fundamental observations which are primarily related to the *behavior of the implanting physician* as a doctor. The following important and generally valid points can be singled out from various publications in recent years:

According to Günther (1984), the following parameters are crucial in the appraisal of whether the implantological standard was maintained (in the case of a claim for compensation):
- postgraduate training;
- undertaking of the treatment;
- establishing the indication;
- performance of the therapy;
- assurance of the continuity of total care of the patient (postoperative care and follow-up).

"The various forms of *medical information* provided to the patient without which legally binding consent (informed consent) and thus a treatment in conformity with the legal position is not possible "apply at various points in this chain.

"In order ... to safeguard an implant operation in legal terms, the dentist must inform the patient of the diagnosis in the individual case, the probable further course of the disease, offering his/her dental assistance according to the present state of knowledge of implantologic treatment, and advising the patient of the advantages and disadvantages of the method" (Fibelkorn 1980).

Postgraduate Training

"In the case of new methods of treatment, the ... amount of postgraduate training required must ... be increased to include all means of obtaining medical knowledge of the new treatment in order to be able to assume responsibility for recommending and applying it in an individual case." (Fibelkorn). Expressed in less legalistic terms, the dentist or the maxillofacial surgeon who is practically concerned with implantology or is intending to take up this discipline must secure adequate training. Since, at least for the time being, implantology is not a component of undergraduate training, he/she must acquire the necessary knowledge and technical surgical skills in *postgraduate training courses*. Serious training and extensive experience in oral surgery will appreciably facilitate his/her moving into this new field.

Practical exercises, e.g., on plastic jaws, are quite suitable in order to familiarize the novice with the procedures for creating the implant bed. However, they do not of course simulate the actual clinical situation.

For this reason, whenever possible, instruction by one or several experienced colleagues must precede the first implantation operation of one's own. It is not always easy to arrange this; however it is worthwhile and avoids the typical "pioneer period" with its unnecessary failures.

Undertaking of the Treatment

The clear statements of Günther can be quoted literally here: "Assuming responsibility for the treatment generally includes reviewing one's own personal competence. Negligence has been demonstrated by the physician when he has not foreseen that the treatment of a not completely improbable complication will overtax his/her abilities or the technical and staff conditions of his/her practice, or when he/she has undertaken the treatment for commercial reasons or for reasons of prestige despite this foresight. In the latter case, one of the rare examples of *premeditated bodily harm* is involved when damage for the patient results from this behavior. This form of negligence is often completed by nonobservance of the *duty of referral*."

Establishing the Indication

The indications for the ITI implants are stated in Chapter 10, "Indications and Contraindications" (see pp. 262ff.).

In general, however, alternatives – whether in the form of other types of implants or implant-free solutions – must be considered in each case and discussed with the patient. This is part of the duty of informed consent, without making it into a "sacred cow," as feared by Feigel (1985). On the contrary, what Günther writes on this point appears to us to be completely true: "Whoever chooses the less safe method because he/she does not have mastery of the method affording more safety is acting negligently". Let us select a given case from daily practice for illustration: a patient with an otherwise complete dentition is lacking the two premolars in the right mandible. The teeth 43 and 46 are intact in periodontal terms. In order to construct a bridge from 43 to 46, however, the molar would first of all havel to be treated endodontically. This treatment should be given priority, because experience shows that this is by and large a safe method. It would be ethically questionable and a contravention of the objective duty of information not to inform the patient who has heard about implants and imagines that the problem of closing the gap might be solved in this way. This despite the fact that it appears to be simpler (and possibly more lucrative) to extract the tooth and to insert an implant in its place. In the present case, lack of endodontic experience is no excuse.

The principle "no art only for the sake of art" thus applies also to implantology.

The best basis for establishing the indication is the relation of trust between the dentist and patient. If such a relationship is optimal, then the declarations of consent signed by the patient (see, for example, Fallschüssel 1986), which might prevent court actions in case of failures, are actually superfluous.

Performance of the Therapy

Even the excellently trained, most experienced and careful physician or dentist can make mistakes. It is always to be borne in mind that he/she is working in a "biological medium." He/she cannot give a guarantee in the sense that everything will turn out as he/she and the patient wish. "Medicus curat, natura sanat!" For this reason, failure may occur even in the best circumstances, whether this is the physician's own fault or not. Insurance companies and judges must rely on appraisals of neutral and highly competent experts if matters come to that stage; i.e., the matter cannot be settled reasonably between the dentist and patient by mutual concessions.

Postoperative Follow-Up

The lifetime of any dental prostethic reconstruction will be shorter, if one leaves the patient to himself without further care after completion of treatment.

Only careful postoperative follow-up and continuous monitoring ultimately justify the effort and expense of an oral reconstruction that has been conscientioulsy planned and performed in accordance with all the rules of the art.

This applies even more so when implants are involved. Postoperative treatment immediately following the operation has already been discussed on pages 344ff. What we are concerned with here are the measures of follow-up and management over many years; these measures are indispensable to avoid the risk of a perfect primary result of implantation suddenly turning into a failure. The continuity of medical treatment is difficult to ensure, especially when the patient must be referred or when a team consisting of oral surgeon and prosthodontist is responsible for the treatment from the beginning. One of the two (usually the person responsible for prosthetic reconstruction) must assume the responsibility of the postoperative follow-up and keep the entire documentation. When he/she passes on the treatment to a third party, he/she must provide this party with all treatment documents.

Günther notes on this: "Holding back treatment documents can be rated as severe negligence in legal terms. As a rule, it is a behavior not consistent with professional ethics."

To summarize, the person engaged in implantology takes on additional responsibility of which he/she must be aware from the beginning. He accepts this responsibility by fully taking into account the specified five points (see p. 348) in his duty of care. He has thus done all that is humanly possible to reduce the danger of being involved with legal problems to a minimum.

References

Fallschüssel, G. K. H. Zahnärztliche Implantologie. Quintessenz, Berlin: 1986 (p. 434)

Feigel, A. Die Implantologie im "deutschsprachigen Raum". Eine kritische Betrachtung. Swiss. Dent. 6 (1986) Nr. 5

Fibelkorn, W. Forensische Probleme der Implantologie. Hanser, Munich 1980 (p. 183ff.)

Günther, G. Schwerpunkte des Arzthaftrechts – bezogen auf die Implantologie. Fortschr. Zahnärztl. Implant. 1 (1984) 5

Maeglin, B. Kritische Stellungnahme zur Problematik der zahnärztlichen Implantate. In J. F. Strub, B. E. Gysi, P. Schärer. Schwerpunkte in der oralen Implantologie und Rekonstruktion. Quintessenz, Berlin: 1983 (p. 15ff)

19 Final Remarks

A. Schroeder

In the foreword to this book, it was stated that it was the intention of the authors not only to present one implantation system in detail, but also to discuss general problems of oral – endosteal – implantology. Related to this intention was the idea of making the reader aware that implantology is subject to more problems than one might assume at first glance. This is not surprising if we reflect on the venture in quite fundamental terms: We countersink a foreign body into the bone in order to obtain one or several posts on which we can then attach a prosthesis in some form or other; the foreign body must be accepted and integrated by the bone and soft tissues covering it in such a way that it can take over the function of a natural tooth over years and decades.

In view of the evident audacity of this idea, the question of sceptics as to whether it is indeed a "figment of the imagination" is entirely justified. Even an enthusiastic implantologist does by no means need to be ashamed of such heretical reflections, especially when he/she is confronted by an unexplained failure.

In the course of time, he/she will observe that failures can be largely avoided when one is prepared to learn from the errors which everyone makes in his/her first years of implantological work.

A "residual risk" always remains because our partner is the human body; we cannot expect that it will tolerate our intervention under all circumstances.

The insertion of implants must be carried out in each individual case against this almost philosophical mental outlook if one wants to avoid disappointments.

What one should avoid:
- implantation without unequivocal indication, without records which are adequate in all respects, without meticulous overall planning and thus without the ability to appraise the prognosis beforehand;
- operating without sufficient training and experience in oral surgery and without observation of asepsis to the extent possible in the oral milieu;
- overheating of the bone because of excessive drill speed or inadequate cooling;
- imprecise depth measurement;
- tilting and force in insertion of the implant;

- lack of care in the wound closure;
- lack of postoperative control and patient care;
- putting weight onto the implant during the 3-month healing phase (exception: implants splinted with a bar in the front of the mandible);
- inadequate instruction and check-ups for oral hygiene.

This list of possible errors of omission is incomplete and does not apply to the superstructure; it does, however, record the most frequent mistakes which lead to failures. If one looks for the causes of a failure, it will be observed in most cases that one or several contraventions of rules were committed and that the implantation system as such cannot be considered responsible for it.

Index

Note: page numbers in *italics* refer to figures and tables

A

abutments
  alveolar mucosa against 310
  bridge 231
  connecting to natural teeth 246
  ITI bonefit implant 140, *142*, 186, 187
  overdentures supported by ITI implants 349, *351*
  periodontium 93, *94*
  prosthetic 179
  see also conical abutment system; Octa abutments
acid etching 91, 92
aesthetic guidelines
  fixed-detachable restorations 408, *409-12*, 413, *414-17*
  implant locations 408
  implant-borne crown *415*
  restoration margin concealment 408
aesthetics
  of anterior teeth 236
  Octa system 205, 212
age
  bone availability 248
  limitations for ITI implants 227
air powder abrasive 461, *462*
alloplastic membranes 318
aluminium oxide 6, *7*
alveolar artery
  anterior superior 30, *31*
  inferior 30-1, *32*
  middle superior 30, *31*
  posterior superior 30, *31*
alveolar bone
  healing 447
  reduced 193
alveolar nerve
  anterior inferior 20, *21*, 27, *28*, 29, 30
  anterior superior 25
  inferior 26, 27, *28*, 30
  middle *29*
    superior 25
  posterior superior 24, *29*
alveolar process
  atrophy of mandibular 20
  maxillary 11-12, *13*

alveolar ridge 11
  atrophy avoidance by tooth root retention 336
  augmentation 178
  bone
    deficiency correction 318
    grafts 178
    layer thickness 318
  curvature 241
  elderly patients 333
  GBR technique 298
  implant selection 263
  inclination 241
  ITI implant 79
  posterior edentulous mandible preparation 281
  small diameter screw implant 298
alveolar vein, inferior/superior 33
alveolar wall
  cancellous bone 22, *23*
  compact bone alterations 22, *23*
  structure 18
amino acids 56
anaesthesia 261
anchor
  and arrowhead pin 62
  ball 262, *352*, *353*, 354
  bar 262
  Dalla Bona 349, 354
anchoring
  ankylotic *see* osseointegration
  bone 80, 423
  element 114, *133*
  implant body 428
  overdentures 240-1, *330*, 331
    supported by ITI implants 349, 351
ankylosis, functional 80
ankylotic bond 9, *81*, *82*, 169
antibiotic therapy
  follow-up care 420
  infection 452, *454-7*, 458, *459-60*
  perioperative coverage for edentulous mandible 279
antrum perforation 446-7
articular relationships, complex 227
atropine 260
axial loading, stress distribution 170-2

B

bacterial osteolytic damage 432
ball anchor 262, *352, 353*, 354
ball attachments, implant-borne 231
bar
  anchor 262
  attachments 354-8
    fabrication 354
    movable 355
    rigid 355
  clips 348, *369*, 370
  connection 241
  interconnections 129
  overdentures *346, 347, 351*, 370
  rigid sliding attachment 355, *356, 357*
  round 355-6, *357*
  splinting 351
basal lamina 93, 96
bioceramics *8*
bioglass 54
biting force *336*, 337
bleeding
  index of sulcus *422*, 423
  postoperative 450
bone
  adequate available 248
  anchorage 80, 423
  apposition acceleration 90, *91*
  availability 227
  defect regeneration 318
  elasticity 431
  filling 449
  grafts
    alveolar ridge 178
    implant insertion depth 178-9
  growth with titanium implant 80
  height in edentulous mandible 262, 472
  infection 440
  mapping 233, 234, 236, *237*-8, *249*, 251
    single-tooth space in maxilla *249*, 251
  mechanical strength 137
  regeneration 80
    ITI bonefit system *135*, 136
    membrane-supported procedure 447
  resorption *429, 430*
    implant fractures *472*
    prevention 178
  response to implants 80-1, *82*, 83-4, *85-8*, 89-92
  structure in healing period 280
  tension rupture 83, *85-6*
  thermal damage 162-3, 428-30
    prevention 159
  transplants
    ITI screw implant augmentation 180, *181-4*
    with reconstruction plate system (THORP) 180, *185*
  vitality maintenance 162
  volume scanning with computed tomography *254*
bone-implant contact 91
bone-screw surface bonding 178
bone/implant interface
  acid etching 91
  histological reactions *5*
  proteoglycan layer 84
  sand blasting 91
  surface increase 91
  ultrastructure 83-4, *87*
Brånemark implants 62-3
bridge abutments, implant-borne 231
buccal frenum 310
buccal nerve *29*, 30
bur
  round 153, *155, 156*, 157
  trephine *302*, 307

C

calcium phosphates 9
calculus
  overdentures supported by ITI implants 367
  removal *425*
canine fossa 25
canine plexus 25, *26, 29*, 30
cantilever bridge *421*
cantilever pontic
  distal 245
  mesial 245
cardiovascular disease, surgical risk 334
cavernous sinus 33-4
cementoalveolar fiber bundles 21, *22, 23*
cephalometric radiograph 235, *236*
ceramics 3
  glass 6, *8*
  plaque accumulation 434, *436, 438*
cervical lymph nodes, deep 34
chlorhexidine 103
  digluconate 451, 453
  gel 292, 453, *454*, 461
  oral rinse 458
  solution 260, 279
    follow-up care 420
    localized inflammation treatment 425
closed mucosal system 129, *130*, 132
cobalt-chromium-molybdenum alloys 5
  sequestration tissue reaction 46
collagen fiber
  bundles 21, *22*
  fibril contact with titanium implant 84, *88*

collagen fleece 449, 471
complications 445
  early infection 451
  emphysema 449
  foreign bodies 449
  gingival recession 452
  haematoma 450
  implant fractures 472, *475*
  implant loosening 451-3, *454-7*, 458, *459-60*, 461, *462-5*, 466-7, *468-70*, 471-2
  intraoperative 445-7, 448, 449
    antrum perforation 446-7
    damage to adjacent teeth 447, *448*
    fracture of implant/instrument 447
    hemorrhage 445
    nasal cavity perforation 446-7
    nerve damage 446
    primary stability failure 447
  nerve damage 446, 451
  postoperative 449
    early 450-1
    late 452-73, *475*
  postoperative bleeding 450
  surgical revision 461, *462-5*, 466, *467*
  wound edema 450
conical abutment 187, *351*
conical abutment system 195-6, *197*, 198-9, *200-2*, 203, *204*, 205
  abutments *195*, *203*, *204*
  cemented restorations 195-6
  conicity 196, *197*, *201*
  conus guauge 199, *201*
  die stone model 203, *204*
  impression 199
  impression model cylinder 199, *200*, *202*
  master model 203, *204*
  screw-retained restorations 196, *197-8*
  sequence of operation 198-9, *200-2*, 203, *204*
  transfer pins 196, *198*, 199
  working model 203, *204*
consultation 231-2
contraindications to ITI implants 226
coolant 163-4, 262, 263, 428
cooling
  burrs *156*, 157
  external/internal 429
  trephine mill 157, *160-1*
  see also ITI internal cooling system
corrosion reactions 39, 40
  chemical compatibility 43
  metallic biomaterials 41-3
  polarization resistance 41, *42*, 43
  practically noble 41, *42*
  rate 41, 43
  thermodynamically noble 41
  tissue reaction 45

corticosteroids 420
crown displacement *432*, *433*

D

Dalla Bona anchor 349, 452
data
  collection 478-9
  intraoperative 478
  postoperative 478
  preoperative 477
  statistics 479
dead space hyperplasia 367, *368*
dental alveoli 19
dental arch, superior external 30
dental floss 364, 366, 374, 424
dental plexus *24*, 25, *29*, 30
  inferior 27
dentogingival nerves *28*, 29, 30
dentogingival rami 27
dentogingival seal 93
denture
  base with vitallium reinforcement *76*
  dead space hyperplasia 367, *368*
  evaluation 233, 236
  fixed partial 244, *245*
  provisional for healing phase 238-9
  provisional set-up in wax 239, *240*
  screw-attached fixed-detachable 361, *362-3*
  stability increase 232
depth guage 146, *147*, 150
  diameter-reduced screw implants *190*, 191
  edentulous mandible 264, *268-9*
  single-tooth space in maxilla 303
design 2
diagnostic set-up 233
diagnostic wax-up
  shortened mandibular dental arch *251*, 252
  single-tooth space in maxilla 249
Dilder bar 355
disinfection 260
  local 420
documentation
  intraoperative data 478
  parameters 477-9
  postoperative data 478
  postoperative follow-up 491-2
  preoperative data 477
  recall appointment 478
double-blade implant 63
drill
  diameter-reduced screw implants 189, *190*
  edentulous mandible 263, 264
  explantation 467, 471
  fluted *155*

drill
  fluted
    cooling system 157, *159*
    service life 164, *166*
  implant bed preparation 153, *154*
  ITI implants with 6mm anchorage 194
  rotational speed 153, 428
  solid screw implant site preparation 153
  spherical headed 145
  twist 151, 153
duty of referral 490

E

edentulous jaw
  atrophic *234*
  fixed prosthetic restorations 374
  implant-borne overdentures 232-36, *237*, 238-41, *242*
  saw-cut cast *237*
edentulous mandible 228, *237*, *242*
  antibiotic perioperative coverage 279
  bone height 262
  complications 279
  denture wearing after implants 279
  depth of bone used 472
  fabrication of final prosthesis 280
  fatigue fracture of mandible 471-2, *473*
  fixed-detachable restorations 388, 394, *395-8*, 401
  four implants 274, *275*, 276, *277-8*
    bar insertion *277*
    bone available 274, 276
    implant channel 276
    mucoperiosteal flap 274, *275*
    wound closure 276, *277*
  GBR technique 263
  implant
    evaluation 280
    healing period for osseointegration 279-80
    length 262
  inadequate soft tissue foundation *311*
  ITI implants *340*
  one-piece implant 261, 262
  oral hygiene 279
  patient behavior 279
  posterior 280-2, *283-8*, 289, *290-1*, 292-3, *294-6*
    alveolar ridge preparation 281
    bone height availability *283*
    closure screw *287*, 289, 292, 293
    follow up 292
    gingivectomy 289, 292, *294-5*
    healing *290-1*, 293
    implant insertion *286-7*, 289
    implant location preparation 281-2, *284-5*
    implants 388, *395-7*
    mucoperiosteal flap 281, *284*
    orthopantomogram 292
    preliminary drill 282
    screw thread precutting 282, *285*
    soft tissue incision 281, *283*
    transgingival healing cap 289, *290*, 292-3
    wound closure 289, *290*
  postoperative treatment 279
  primary soft tissue correction *311*
  secondary part attachment 280
  six implants 261, *278*, 279
  sugical procedure 261-296
  thread cutting *278*
  two implants 262-4, *265-73*, 274
    alveolar ridge preparation *265*
    bone cutting 263
    closure screw *272*, 274
    coolant 262, 263
    depth guage 264, *268-9*
    guide key *271*, 274
    heat necrosis avoidance 263
    implant channel *267-8*
    implant location 264, *265-73*, 274
    implant site 262-3
    instruments 263-4
    procedure *265-73*
    ratchet 264, *271*
    screwing down *271*, 274
    thread cutter 264, *269*, *270*
    wound closure *272-3*, 274
  two-piece implant 261-2
elastic properties
  bone 431
  ITI bonefit system 132, *134*
electrochemical series 39-40
emphysema 449
endosseous implant
  ankylotic anchorage 37, 102, *103*
  GBR technique 318, *322*, *323*
  optimum tissue integration 102
  oral hygiene 103
  tissue reactions 103
endosteal implant 37, 62-3
  blade 62
  cage-like 62
  healing 153
ethmoid nerve, anterior 25

F

facial index *345*
facial vein 34
fixed partial denture, implant-borne *400*

Index **499**

fixed prostheses 387-8
  biomechanical complications 387
  bridge span 388
  maxillary distal extension cases 388, *389-92*
  shortened mandibular dental arch 387
fixed prosthetic restorations 374
  cleaning ability 374
  hygiene aids 374-5
  indications 375, *376-7*
  mandibular distal extension cases 378, *379-80*, 381, *382-6*, 387-8
  stress breaker 388
  superstructure design 374-5
fixed reconstructions, implant-borne 193, *194*
fixed-detachable restorations 381, *382-6*
  advantages 381
  aesthetic guidelines 408, *409-12*, 413, *414-17*
  disadvantages 381
  edentulous mandible 388, 394, 401, *494-7*
  edentulous spaces
    in maxillary anterior region 394, *399-400*, 401
    in posterior region 38, *398*
  implant-borne superstructures 246, *384*
  maxillary anterior region 408, *409-12*, 412, *414-17*
  maxillary distal extension cases 388, *389-92*
  noble metal coping *384*
  precision attachment *386*
  single tooth spaces 401, *405-7*, 408, *409-12*, 413
  sliding attachments 381, *385-6*
follow-up care 420-6
  antibiotic coverage 420
  data collection 426
  disinfection 420
  superstructure functional efficiency 424, *425*
  swelling prophylaxis 420
  two-piece implants 420
force impulse *432*, 433
foreign bodies 449
  localization 449
fracture
  fatigue 471-2, *473*
  implant 447, 472, *475*
  instrument 447
  remnant removal 472
free-gingival graft *314*
free-mucosal grafts 310, *311*
friction lock 187
functional analysis, clinical 424, *425*

G

galvanic series 40
galvanism 443
gingiva
  inflammation 434, *436*
  lymphatic drainage 34, *35*
  sensory innervation of mandibular *29*, 30
gingival collar 93
gingival cuff
  connective tissue organization 102
  response 92-4, *95*, 96-98, *99-101*
gingival recession 452
gingival sulcus 93
gingivectomy 457
  avoidance 310
gingivo-implant seal 79, 434, 441
glass ceramics 6, *8*
gold
  bar for overdenture retention 280
  coping for Octa system 211-12, *214*, 218-19
  corrosion rate 42-3
  sequestration tissue reaction 46
Gram-negative anaerobes 440
guide key 151
  edentulous mandible *271*, 274
guided bone regeneration (GBR) technique 256, 397-8, 318-28
  bone filling 449
  edentulous mandible 263
  hollow cylinder insertion *327*
  with ITI implants 318, *319-28*
  membrane fixation 318, *320*, *325*
  one-stage procedure *319-22*
  single-tooth space 318, *319-22*, *324-8*
  surgical requirements for success *323*
  two-stage procedure *323*, *324-8*
guided tissue regeneration 318, 408

H

haematoma, postoperative 450
handpiece systems 257
hard palate, free-mucosal grafts 310
healing
  alveolar bone 447
  maintenance 441
  membrane-supported bone regeneration procedure 447
  period for bone structure 280
  period for osseointegration 279-80
  phase for provisional denture 238
  thermal trauma 428
  transgingival 238
heat necrosis
  avoidance 263

heat necrosis
  implant loosening 451
  see also thermal trauma
hemidesmosomes 93, 96
hemorrhage, intraoperative 445
histologic specimens 104-5, *106*, 107, *108*, 109-10
  chemicals 111
  counter staining 109
  cutting 105, *106*
  embedding in acrylic 104, *106*
  embedding mixture 104-5
  light microscopy 104
  polishing 107, 109
  preparation for scanning electron microscopy 109-10
  specimen hardening 105
  thin grinding 107, *108*, 109
hollow body implants, perforated 132, *133-6*, 136-7, *138-9*, 140
hollow cylinder (HC) implant 63, 64, 115-17, *118-19*, 120, *129*
  axis angulation 297
  bevelled buccal crown 120
  characteristics 132, *133-5*, 136-7, *138-9*, 140
  constructional features *136*, 137
  development 66
  fracture 472
  functional loading 115
  GBR technique *327*, *328*
  gold coping 116, *117*
  instruments 145-6, *147*, *150*
  long-term success 482, 487
  one part 115-16, *117*
  perforations *135*
  titanium 174, *175*
  two part 116-17, *118-19*, 120
    angulated 120, *121*
    beveled *118*, 120
    single-tooth space 248
    straight *118*, *121*
  wound closure *312*
hollow implant concept 66
hollow screw (HS) implant 66, 120-4, *125*, *129*
  autologous bone graft *319*
  axial pull-out tests 122
  characteristics 132, *133-5*, 136-7, *138-9*, 140
  edentulous mandible 262
  fixed prosthetic restorations *376-7*
  fracture 472
  healing period stability 178
  implant-borne restoration 229
  indications 229
  inserting device *149*, 151
  instruments 146, *148*, 149, *150*, 151
  mucosa recontouring *313*
  Octa secondary component *377*
  one part 122-3
  perforations *135*
  posteriorly edentulous mandible 281-2, *283-8*, 289
  primary stability 121
  subgingival shoulder *376*, *377*
  supragingival shoulder *376*
  thread tapping 121-2
  titanium healing cap *377*
  two-part 123-4, *125*
hydrogen peroxide
  mouth rinse 449
  wound cleaning 450
hydroxyapatite 9
  point-of-zero charge 57
hydroxyl ions 40

I

iliac crest transplants 256
implant
  abutment
    alveolar mucosa against 310
    periodontium 93, *94*
  arrangement 241
  bed
    thermal injury *429*
    trauma 430
  bed preparation 153, *154-5*, 156-7, *158*, 159, *160-1*, 162-4, *165-7*
    for diameter-reduced screw implants 189
    drills 153, *154*
    hemorrhage 445
    internally cooled solid mill *167*
    rotation speed of drills 153
    rotation-symmetrical implants 153
    temperature measurement 153, *155*, 156
    trephine mill *167*
  body anchorage 428
  cleaning 424, *426*
  connected to natural teeth 441-2
  course of bar between *242*
  distance between 241
  explantation technique 466-7, *468-70*, 471
  fractures 447, 472, *475*
    remnant removal 472
  loading 52
    conditions 452
  loosening 451
    explantation 466-7, *468-70*, 471
    fatigue fracture 471-2, *473*
    infection 452-3, *454-7*, 458, *459-60*
    membrane technique 466
    surgical revision 458, 461, *462-5*, 467

materials 174-5, *176*, 177
mobility 442
  primary 447
number 240-1
overloading 337
point of emergence 241
removal 466-7, *468-70*, 471
seal with soft-tissue cuff 434
self-threading 264
splinted 245, 242, 451
stability 451
submucosal 60
subperiosteal 61, *62*, 63
superstructure connection 443
surface 434, 438
titanium 174-5, *176*, 177
see also endosseous implant; endosteal implant
implant-bone interface
  loading 52
  shear strength 53
implant-bone structural unit
  ankylotic bond 9, 169
  biomechanics 169-73, *174*
  load spread *168*, 169
  peak pressure *168*, 169
  photoelastic stress analysis 169-72
  three-dimensional geometry 176
implant-borne restoration 374
  prosthetic aspects 375
  prosthetic superstructures *412*
implantation
  follow-up care 420-7
  form 479, *480*
  potential sites 35-6
  success 422-3
implantology 60, 493
  endosteal implants 62-3
  methods 60
  situations to avoid 493-4
  submucosal implants 60
  transfixation 60
IMZ implant 62
incisive canal 19, *21*, 34
incisor
  ceramo-metal crown *417*
  congenital absence *416*
  missing *248-50*, *252*, *253*
  nerve *see* alveolar nerve, anterior inferior
indications 490-1
inertness, corrosion 45
infection
  antibiotic therapy 452, *454-7*, 458, *459-60*
  bone resorption *458*, *460*
  chronic *467*, *468*
  development 452
  early postoperative 451

marginal 434, 438, *439*, 440, 441
membrane technique 466
monitoring 452
osseous defect treatment 458
prophylactic measures 441
recurrence *458*
surgical revision 458, 461, *462-5*, *467*
titanium surface cleaning 461, 463
treatment 453, *454-7*, 458, *459-60*, 461, *462-5*, 466-7, *468-70*
inflammation, marginal 441, *442*
infraorbital artery 30, *31*
infraorbital nerve 24, 25, 26, *29*, 30
infrazygomatic ridge 11-12
instruments
  edentulous mandible 263-4
  fracture 447
  internal cooling system 153, 156, 157, *158*, 159, *160-1*, 162-4
  kit 258-9
  life 164, *165-6*
interdental brush 375, 424, *426*
interincisor rami 31, *32*
intraoral inspection, clinical 233, 234, 236
intraoral pressure 449
ITI bonefit implant 63-4, 114
  6mm anchorage 192-4
    instruments 194
  abutments 140, *142*
  accessories 140, *142*
  age limitations 227
  alveolar ridge 79
  ampoules 219, 220
  anaesthesia 261
  anchorage element volume 114, *133*
  animal experiments 64, 66
  ankylotic bonding *82*
  bar interconnections 129
  basic design *129*
  bed preparation 132, *133*, 153-64, *165-7*
  blood vascularization 136
  bone
    anchorage 79
    regeneration *135*, 136
  choice 140, *143*
  combination with bone grafts 178-80, 179-80, *181-2*, 183, *184-5*, 186-7
    abutments 186
    basal screw 180, *184*, 186
    bone graft covering 187
    conical abutment 187
    friction lock 187
    mucosa cylinder 180, *184*, 186
    prosthetic parts 186
    transgingival abutment design 187
  contraindications 226
  design 66, *67*, 68-70, *71*, 114

ITI bonefit implant
  design
    force transmission 169
  development stages 66, 67, 68-70, 71-8, 79
  disinfection 260
  elastic deformation of jaw 132
  elastic properties 132, *134*
  endosseous diameters 263
  equipment 257-9
  extension types 66, 68
  GBR technique 318, *319-28*
  gingival seal 79
  gold coping 129
  healing period for osseointegration 279-80
  hollow 66
  indications 140, *144*, 227, *228*, 229
  information 219
  inserting device 220
  instruments 140, *142*, 145-6, *147-8*, 149, *150*, 151, *152*
    service life 164, *165-6*
  integrated 140, *141-4*
  length of time in place *485*
  loadability 114
  loading
    axial *141*
    characteristics 137, *138-9*, 140, *141*
    lateral *141*
    physiological 132, *134*
    time for 70, *71*, 178
  long-term results 482, *483-4*, 485, *486*, 487
  loosening by physical loading 452
  medical history 226
  mucosal seal 120
  number lost *486*
  numbers placed *483-4*
  one-part design 129
  oral hygiene 79
  osteoingration *83*
  participating clinics 485
  perforated hollow body implants 132, *133-5*, 136-7, *138-9*, 140
  plaque deposition 127
  plasma spray technique 89-90
  premedication 260
  prosthesis retention 129
  prosthetic abutments 179
  qualitative data *486*
  quality 482
  questionnaire 479, *480*
  ratchet 220, *221*
  removal 68
    from ampoule 259
  residual tension 141
  site preparation 114
  soft tissue surgery 310, *311-17*
  solid screw implants (S) 125, *126*, *127*, 128, *129*, 137
  splinting 70, *71*
  sterile packaging 219-20
  sterilizing indicator 219-20
  stiffness *134*
  success 428
    criteria *482*
    rate *486*
  superstructure design 79
  supracrestal portions 94
  supracrestal region 102, 103
  surgical augmentation for screw 180, *181-4*
  surgical procedure 256-7
  surgical team preparation 260
  tensile stress 132, *134*
  thread
    configuration 140
    profile 137, *138-9*, 140, *141*
    tap 140, *142*
  titanium 177
    plasma coating 114
  transgingival *131*, 132, 408
    extension sleeve 179-80, 183
    healing 256-7
  two-part
    conical abutment system 195-205
    design 129-30, *131*, 132
    Octa system 205-19
    reconstruction 195
  types 114-17, *118-19*, 120-5, *126-7*, 128, *129*
    Type C 66, *67*
    Type F 70, *71*
    Type H extension 69, *70*
    Type K extension 68, *69*
  see also complications; hollow cylinder (HC) implant; hollow screw (HS) implant; surgical procedure for primary indications
ITI internal cooling system 153, 156, 157, *158*, 159, *160-1*, 162-4
  coolant 262, 263, 428
  supply *162*
  cooling medium 163-4

J

jaw defects 227
junctional epithelium 93, 98, *99*, *101*, 102
  weak points 434

L

labial frenum 310
  insertion *316-7*
legal considerations 489-92

lingual artery, deep 31, *32*
lingual nerve *29*, 30
load
  plasma spray coating 52
  spread in implant-bone structural unit *168*, 169
  transmission in rough porous surface of implant 172, *174*
loading 52, 54
  axial *141*, 170-2
  characteristics of ITI implants 137, *138-9*, 140, *141*
  conditions 452
  implant/bone interface 52
  improper 431-2, *433*
  lateral of ITI implants *141*
  loosening implant 452
  Octa system 217-18
  osseointegration 89
  physiological 132, *134*
  tension lines for horizontal *173*
  time for ITI implants 70, *71*, 178
  titanium implant 52, 53, 54, 89

M

macroglossia 227
mandible
  age-related changes 16-20, *21*
  atrophy *333*
  bone structure 16-20, *21*
  configuration *14*, 16-17
  fatigue fracture 471-2, *473*
  form changes 19-20
  gingival sensory innervation *29*, 30
  implant number 241
  intraforaminal region extent 241
  ITI implant indications *228*, 229
  poorly fitting prosthesis 19-20
  posterior region single tooth spaces 401, *405-6*
  single-tooth replacement *228*
  tooth axes *14*, 17-18
  see also edentulous mandible
mandibular alveolar process atrophy 20
mandibular angle 20
mandibular arch 17
mandibular canal 20
  course *17*, 18-19
mandibular dental arch
  shortened *228*, 251-3
    diagnostic wax-up *251*, 252
    extension 378
    first appointment 251-2
    fixed partial dentures *378-80*
    fixed prostheses 387
    implants 253
    second appointment 252-3
    template fabrication 253
mandibular distal extension cases
  cemented restorations 378, *379-80*, 381
  five-unit ceramo-metal restoration 380
  fixed prosthetic restorations 378, *379-80*, 381, *382-6*, 387-8
  fixed-detachable restorations 381, *382-6*
  mixed restorations 388
  three-unit ceramo-metal bridge *378-9*
mandibular teeth
  arteries 30-1, *32*
  innervation 26-7, *28*, 29
  lymphatic drainage 34, *35*
  venous drainage 33-4
marginal infection 434, 438, *439*, 440, 441
materials *2*, 3
  biocompatibility 3, 5
  bone compatibility 5
  elongation values *4*
  groups 5-6, 9
  mechanical properties 3
  tensile strength values *4*
maxilla
  alveolar wall 12, 14-15
  bone structure 11-12, *13*, 14-16
  gingival sensory innervation *29*, 30
  implant number 241
  ITI implant indications *228*, 229
  posterior region single tooth spaces 401, *406-7*
  single-tooth replacement *228*
  single-tooth space 247-8, *249-50*, 251, 297-8, *299-306*, 307-8, *309*
  sinus extent 241
  tooth axes 12, *13*
maxillary alveolar process 11-12, *13*
maxillary anterior region
  axial contours 408, *409*, 413
  edentulous spaces 394, *399-400*, 401
  fixed-detachable restorations 408, *409-12*, 413, *414-17*
  gingival facade 401, *402-4*
  implant analogs *410*, 413
  implant prefabricated copings *414*
  implant-borne prosthetic superstructures *412*
  implant-supported dental prosthesis 408
  impression tray 408, *409*
  lost tissue compensation 401, *402-4*
  Octa system 408, *409*
    abutments *399*, *402*
  prefabricated elements 394, *399-400*
  subgingival position of implant shoulder *411*

maxillary arch 17
maxillary artery 30, *31*
maxillary cast 240
maxillary dental arch, shortened 253, *254*
maxillary distal extension cases
  fixed prostheses 388, *389-92*
  fixed-detachable restorations 388, *389-92*
maxillary molars, cancellous bone 14, *15*
maxillary sinus, maxillary teeth relationship 15-16
maxillary teeth
  arteries 30, *31*, *32*
  innervation 24-6
  lymphatic drainage 34, *35*
  relationship to maxillary sinus/nasal cavity 15-16
  venous drainage 33-4
maxillary veins 33
medical history 226
medical information 489
membrane-supported bone regeneration procedure 447
mental artery 31
mental canal 19
mental foramen 19
mental nerve *28*, 29
  damage 451
  protection 446
metal ions 40
metal oxide
  solubility in electrolytes 43-4
  surface reaction 56
metallic biomaterials, corrosion 41-3
metalloprotein complex formation *46*
mill, internally cooled solid *167*
missing teeth, fixed replacement 232
mobility
  of implant 442
    osseointegration 431
    primary 447
  teeth 442
molar, infection around implant *454*
morphological conditions, unfavourable 227
mucoperiosteal flap
  posterior edentulous mandible 281, *284*
  single-tooth space in maxilla 298, *300*
  surgical revision 461
  suturing over 129, *130*
mucoplasty *313*
  indications 310
mucosa
  condition 102-3
    for plaque accumulation 441
  infections 432
  keratinized 441, *442*
  oral hygiene 441
  peri-implant 179

pocket formation 441
mucosal seal 120
mucosal thickness determination *250*
  intraoral measurement *250*, 251
mylohyoid nerve 27, 29

N

nasal artery, lateral 30
nasal cavity
  maxillary teeth relationsip 15-16
  perforation 446-7
nasal nerve, lateral *21*, 25
nasal septal artery, posterior 30, *31*
nasal wall, lateral *21*, 25
nasociliary nerve 25
nasopalatine nerve *29*, 30
negligence 490
nerve damage 451
  intraoperative 446
niobium 6
noble metal alloys 5
nose blowing 449

O

occlusal relationships, complex 227
Octa abutments *206*
  edentulous mandible *273*
  maxillary anterior region *398*, *401*
  overdentures supported by ITI implants *342*, *358*
  prefabricated impression copings 408, *409*
  screw-retained restoration *296*
Octa system 205-19
  aesthetics 205, 212
  axial contours 408, *409*
  base 211-12
  connection 205
  conus-screw combination 214, *215*, *216*, 217
  fit of prefabricated gold/plastic copings 212, 214, *215-16*, 217-18
  gold coping 211-12, *214*, 218-19
  guide screw *208*, *209*
  impression 207, *209*
    coping *208*, *210*
    technique modelling 205
  loading 217-18
  maxillary anterior region 408, *409*
  microcrevice 205
  operation procedure 207, *208-10*, 211-12, *213*
  oral hygiene 367
  overdentures supported by ITI implants 337, 356

Index **505**

secondary component *206*
  hollow screw implant *377*
single-tooth space in maxilla 297
stone model 207, *210*
titanium base copings 212, *213*
transfer pin 207, *210*
transmucosal healing caps 212, *213*
open transmucosal system 129, 130, *131*, 132
operating light 257-8
ophthalmic nerve 25
opthalmic vein, superior 34
oral hygiene
  aids 374-5
  care 333
  edentulous mandible implants 279
  endosseous implant 103
  importance 443
  ITI implant 79
  monitoring 443
  mucosa 441, *442*
  Octa system 367
  overdentures supported by ITI implants 364, *365*, 366-7
  patient motivation 227
  patient responsibility 445
  soft tissue condition 441
orthopantomogram 234, *235*
  posterior edentulous mandible 292
osseointegration 37, 79, 80, 102, 103
  acetabulum 89, *90*
  bone vitality 162
  during transgingival healing 238
  force transmission 92
  healing period 279-80
  implant loading 89
  mobility of implant 431
  problems 428
  submicroscopic structure/bodies *55*
  thermal trauma 428
  titanium 37, 51-4
  titanium plasma spray coating 169
osseous anchorage 79, 423
osseous attachment, damage 432
osteoblasts
  activity with titanium implant 80
  implant surface 81
osteoclastic activity 430
osteoclastic resorption with titanium implant 80
osteocytes, implant surface 81
osteogenesis
  bond 6, 9
  contact 6, *7*
  distant 5-6
  implant surface 90, *91*
osteointegration *see* osseointegration
osteolysis *429*

bacterial damage 432
remineralization *455*
osteolytic defects *456*
osteomyelitis, incipient 451
osteosynthesis development 5
osteotomy
  conservative 430
  pressure-free 428
overdentures 231
  gold bar for retention 280
  implant number for anchoring 240-1
  implant-anchored *330*, 331
  implant-borne 232-36, *237*, 238-41, *242*
  planning 239
overdentures supported by ITI implants
  abutments 349, *351*
  anchorage 349, 351
  attachment
    device 349
    of overdenture to implants 348
  ball anchors *352*, *353*, 354
  bar *346*, *347*, *351*, 370
    attachments 354-8
    clips 348, *369*, 370
  base 370
  calculus 367
  cast metal framework 348
  cleaning 364, *365*
    aids 364, 366
  clip remounting 370, *371*
  contraindications 334-5
  custom tray *340*, *341*, *343*
  Dalla Bona anchor 349, 354
  dead space hyperplasia 367, *368*
  denture wax-up *344*
  design 337
  edentulous mandible *340*
  elderly patients 332
  exlusion criteria for patients 334-5
  expectations of patients 330
  extensions 357-8
  fabrication 337-8
  facial index *345*
  facial morphology 337
  follow-up care 367, 370
  force perception 337
  forces 370
  function 336-7
  hygiene 364, *365*, 366-7
    checklist 367
  impressions *340*, *341*
  indications 331-4
  individual attachments 354
  life expectancy 330-1
  lingual morphology 337
  load on implants 351
  maintenance care 364, *365*, 366-7

Index

overdentures supported by ITI implants
  mandibular implant 337
  master cast *344, 348*
  medical conditions in patients *335*
  movement 333
  occlusion 370
  Octa abutments *342, 359*
  Octa system 337, 356
  orthopantomogram *358, 362*
  overdenture insertion 348-9
  patient finances 331, 332
  patient selection 330-4, *335*
  plaque 367
    accumulation 364
  pressure
    lesion *369*
    spots 370
  prognosis 334
  prosthesis
    delivery 349, *350*
    in place *359-60*
  prosthetic procedures 336-63, *339*
  retention 349, 351
  retentive attachments 354-8
  retentive device 349, 351, 354
  selection criteria 331
  sensory feedback 336
  splinting bars 351
  stability 336-7
  supporting tissue replacement 337
  terminal abutments 358
oxidizing strength of solution 41

P

palatal lymphatic tracts 34
palatal region, bone thickness 234
palatine artery, descending 30, *32*
palatine nerve 30
  greater *29*
parotid lymph nodes 34
partial dentures
  fixed bridge replacement 232
  implant-borne 231
partially edentulous jaw, fixed prosthetic restorations 374
patient, ascertainment of desires 231-2
periodontal ligament 12, 21-2, *23*
periodontal membrane
  healthy *431*
  shock absorbing 431
periodontitis, marginal 22
periodontium
  force exertion control 337
  sensory feedback 336
periosteal elevator 446

periosteal sheath, mandibular 26, 27
Periotest device 423
pH effects of galvanism 443
pharyngeal lymph nodes, lateral 34
phosphates 54
photoelastic stress analysis 137, *139*, 140, *141*, 169-72
pilot drill *see* twist drill
plaque
  accumulation of different materials 434, *436, 438*
  deposition in ITI bonefit system 129
  index *422*, 423
  microbial 434, *436*
  mucosal conditions 441
  overdentures supported by ITI implants 367
plasma coating *see* titanium, plasma spray coating
pocket formation 438, 440-1, 453
polarization resistance 41, *42*, 43
polymethylmethacrylate (PMMA) 5
postgraduate training 489-90
postoperative follow-up 491-2
pre-drill 145, 153, *155*
  cooling system 157, *158*
premedication 260
premeditated bodily harm 490
premolar
  ankylotic changes *433*
  units 242, *244*
premolar/molar region, implant-borne fixed reconstructions 193, *194*
preoperative diagnosis 231
Prophy-Jet 461, *462*
prosthesis
  bar supported 193
  provisional 238-9
    planning 233
  retention in ITI bonefit system 128, 129
pterygoid plexus 33
pterygopalatine canal 34
PTFE membrane 318

R

radiograph
  intraoperative 446, 447
  panoramic 251, 252
radiographic survey 233, 234-6
ratchet 149
  edentulous mandible 264, *271*
reactive metal 43
recall 421-6
  appointment
    checklist 479, *481*
    documentation 478

data collection 426
  implant cleaning 424, *426*
  therapeutic measures 424
record keeping 426
rehabilitation of the mouth 2
reossification *460*
retention elements 241
retention mechanism 241
retromandibular vein 33
retromolar trigonum 16-17, 20
retromolar tuberculum 12, *13*
rigid sliding attachment bar 355, 356, *357*
rotation-symmetrical implants 153
round bar 355-6, *357*
round burr 153, *155*
  cooling system *156*, 157

S

sand blasting 91, *92*
scar ring 102
screw implants (S type) 124-5, *126-7*, 128, *129*
  diameter-reduced 187, *188*, 189, *190*, 191
    depth guage *190*, 191
    drilling 189, *190*
    insertion 189, *190*, 191
    preparation 189, *190*
    thread cutting 191
  edentulous mandible 262, 264, *265-73*, 274
  head design 125
  length 125, *126-7*, 128
  one-part 125, *126*
  posteriorly edentulous mandible 281, 289, *290-2*, 292-3, *294-6*
  prosthesis retention 128
  reduced diameter *294-6*, 298
  thread profile *127*
  two-part *127*, 128, *129*
screw retained restoration *see* Octa system
sedatives 260
sensory disturbance 451
sequestration tissue reaction, corrosion 45-6
Sharpey's fibers 21-2
shear force resistance, gingival collar 93
silver, sequestration tissue reaction 46
single-tooth implant
  immediately adjacent 244, *245*
  labial frenum insertion *316-17*
single-tooth space
  GBR technique 318, *319-22*
  mandibular posterior region 401, *405-6*
  maxillary posterior region 401, *406-7*
single-tooth space in maxilla 247-8, *249-50*, 251

bone support 297
channel preparation 298, *301-2*, 307
conditions 297
depth guage *303*
diagnostic wax-up *249*
first appointment 248, 250
GBR technique 297-8
hollow cylinder implant 248
implant channel beveling *304*, 307
implant position 298, *301*
mucoperiosteal flaps 298, *300*
Octa system 297
  secondary piece placement *309*
plaque control 297
postoperative treatment 307-8
preliminary drill *302*, 307
procedure 298, *299-306*, 307-8, *309*
second appointment *249-50*, 251
sectioned cast *249, 250*, 251
surgical procedure 297-309
transgingival healing cap *305*, 307, 308
trephine burr preparation *302*, 307
wound closure *305*, 307, 308
sneezing 449
soft tissue
  contours for transgingival implants 441
  cuff 102, *103*
    depth probing 423
    seal with implant 434
  emphysema 449
  hematoma 450
  infection 451, *462*
  maintenance of soft tissue 92
  peri-implant 310
  pockets 453
  recontouring 310
  response 92-4, *95*, 96-8, *99-101*
  surgery 310-18
    ITI implants 310, *311-17*
  swelling 450
Solcoseryl Dental Adhesive Paste 450
solid screw implants 137
  anchorage depth 151, *152*
  antrum/nasal cavity perforation 446-7
  instruments 151, *152*
  site preparation 153
  two-part diameter-reduced 187
  see also screw implants (S type)
sphenopalatine artery 30, *31*
splinting of implants to natural teeth 245, 246, 453
  ITI implants 70, *71*
stability, primary 447
stabilization, secondary 441
stainless steel 5, *6*
  corrosion rate 42
  sequestration tissue reaction 46

standard electrode potential electrochemical series 39, 40
stress breaker 246
  fixed prostheses 388
stress distribution with axial loading 170-2
subepithelial connective tissue 93, 95
  build-up 103
subgingival flora 440
sublingual artery 31, 32
submandibular lymph nodes 34, 35
submental artery 31
submental lymph nodes 34
submucosal implants 60
subperiosteal implants 61, 62, 63
success 428
  criteria 482
  long-term 2-3
    for screw implant 482, 487
  rate 487
  titanium plasma spray coating 428
sulcus
  bleeding index 422, 423
  cell turnover 434, 435
  epithelium 98, 99
  fluid flow rate 423
  gingival 93
  peri-implant 97-8, 99, 101
superfloss 374, 424
superstructure 441, 443
  design for ITI implant 79
  implant connection 443
supracrestal connective tissue 93, 101
  formation 103
supragenoid ramus 31, 32
surface morphology 2
surgical instruments *see* instruments
surgical procedure for primary indications
  edentulous mandible 261-96
  GBR techniques 328-38
  single-tooth space in maxilla 297-309
  soft tissue surgery 310-18
surgical team preparation 260
surgical trauma 441
sutures 450

T

tantalum 6
teeth
  fixed replacement for missing 232
  intraoperative damage 447, 448
  mobility 442
  see also tooth root retention
tensile stress, ITI bonefit system 132, 134
tension lines, horizontal loading 173
thermal trauma 159, 162-3, 428-30

see also heat necrosis
THORP reconstruction bridging system 178, 180, 185
thread cutter, color-coded 148, 149
thread cutting 191, 278, 282, 285
  edentulous mandible 264, 269, 270
thread profile 127
  depth 137
  flank inclination 137, 138, 140
  holding flank 137, 138
  load bearing surfaces 137
  photoelastic stress anlaysis 137, 139, 140, 141
  pitch 137
thread tap 140, 142, 149
tissue response 80
  bone 80-1, 82, 83-4, 85-8, 89-92
  histologic specimens 104-5, 106, 107, 108, 109-10
  reactions to endosseous implant 103
  soft tissue 92-4, 95, 96-8, 99-101
titanium 6, 37
  behaviour in electrolyte 43-4
  biologic compatibility 45-6
  body load 47
  bond
    with bone 51
    model 55-7
  characteristics 37
  chemical behaviour 47
  chemical compatibility 39-43
  corrosion 39-43
  elastic module 174, 175
  hollow cylinder design 174, 175
  hydride 48-9
  as implant material 47-8, 174-5, 176, 177
  ingestion 47
  ions in solution 44
  ITI-system 63-4
  maximum loads 38
  mechanical properties 37, 38, 137
  microstructure 177
  neutral species in solution 44
  osseointegration 37, 51-4
  physico-chemical bond 55
  plasma spray coating 48-9, 50, 89-90, 175, 176, 177
    ankylotic bond 169
    bond strength 49
    compatibility 49
    electrochemical behavior 49
    gun 176, 177
    implant success 428
    loads 52
    pull-off resistance 52-3
    pull-off strength 177
    screw implant long-term success 482, 487

shear/torsion resistance 52, 173, *174*
surface of implant 49, *50*
technique 89-90
practical scale 41
reactive *43*
shear/torsion resistance of smooth surface 173, *174*
strength 37, 38
surface morphology of anchorage element 175, *176*, 177
surface oxide 47
tensile strength *174*, 175
tissue gluing *55*, 56
tissue levels 47-8
unalloyed 38
titanium implant
abutment surface characteristics 102
acid etching 91, 92
anchoring ability 52, *53*
ankylotic union 81, *82*
apatite crystal contact 83-4, *88*
blood vessel ingrowth 80
bone
contact *85*
growth 80
permeation of surface 83
remodelling 54
collagen fibril contact 84, *88*
connective tissue
fibers 94, 96, *97*, *98*
membrane absence 92
endosseous portion surface *87*
epithelial attachment 96-8, *99-101*
force transmission 92
functional force support 53-4
loads 52, 53, 54, 89
osteoblastic activity 80
osteoclastic resorption 80
plasma layer 83
production technique 177
rough porous surface load transmission 172, *174*
sand blasting 91, 92
shape 81, *82*, 83
stress flow 54
tension rupture in bone 83, *85-6*
time of loading 54
tissue integration 102
torque for unscrewing 92
transgingival 97-8, *99-100*
titanium oxide
amphoteric hydroxylated 56
solubility in electrolytes 43-4
surface reaction 56
titanium-blade implants 62
tooth root retention 336
force perception 337

retentive attachments 336
toothbrush 364, *365*, 366
toxic reactions, corrosion 45
toxicity of elements 46
training 489-90
transfixation 60
transgingival extension sleeve 179-80, 183, 187
transgingival healing 238, 256-7
transgingival healing cap 289, *290*, 292-3
GBR technique *321*, *327*
single-tooth space in maxilla *305*, 307, 308
transmucosal system, open 129, 130, *131*, 132
treatment
continuity 491
failures 491, 494
performance 491
postoperative 491
undertaking 490
treatment planning 232-6, *237*, 238-41, *242*
biomechanical guidelines 244-5
evaluation criteria 241, *242*
partially edentulous jaw 242-8, *249-50*, 251-3, *254*
practical procedure 246-7
premolar units 242-3, *244*
primary indications 246
secondary indications 247
trephine
edentulous mandible 263
explantation 467, 471
service life 164, *165*
trephine mill 145-6, *147*, 153, *155*
cooling system 157, *160-1*
implant bed preparation *167*
trigonal distance 17
Tübingen immediate implant 62
turbine handpiece 449
twist drill 151, 153

U

undercut palpation 236

V

vestibuloplasty 310
anterior *311*
Vincent's sign 451
viscoelastic elements 246
vitallium subperiosteal implants 60, *61*, 62

W

Wolff's law 54
wound
　closure 289, *290*, *464*
　edema 450
　healing acceleration 450
　necrosis 450

Z

zygomatic process 11